## PRAISE FOR *SACRED WOMAN*

"Queen Afua is an extraordinary healer, teacher, mother, and keeper of our legacy. Through *Sacred Woman*, she has given us the sacred tools we need to live our lives in this new century."

—HAZELLE GOODMAN, actress

"Just when I thought I was all alone, I found myself walking with a group of conscious women who were taking sacred steps and speaking sacred words. We were on our way to Queen Afua's Global Sacred Woman Village. Come with us, there's Maat—balance and order—there."

—ERYKAH BADU

"*Sacred Woman* offers profound wisdom to all who seek healing and transformation. . . . Queen Afua is a national treasure."

—BOB LAW, author, radio personality, and vice president of WWRL

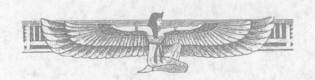

BY QUEEN AFUA

*Sacred Woman:*
*84 Day Healing Journal*

*Man Heal Thyself:*
*Journey to Optimal Wellness*

*Planet Healing:*
*What Would You Do to Heal Planet Earth?*

*Circles of Wellness:*
*A Guide to Planting, Cultivating and*
*Harvesting Wellness*

*Overcoming an Angry Vagina:*
*Journey to Womb Wellness*

*The City of Wellness:*
*Restoring Your Health Through the Seven*
*Kitchens of Consciousness*

*Sacred Woman:*
*A Guide to Healing the Feminine Body,*
*Mind, and Spirit*

*Heal Thyself for Health and Longevity*

# SACRED WOMAN

# SACRED WOMAN

A GUIDE TO HEALING THE FEMININE BODY, MIND, AND SPIRIT

## QUEEN AFUA

ONE WORLD
NEW YORK

2021 One World Trade Paperback Edition

Published in the United States by One World, an imprint of Random House,
a division of Penguin Random House LLC, New York.

ONE WORLD and colophon are registered trademarks of Penguin Random House LLC.

Originally published in hardcover and in different form in the United States by Ballantine Books,
an imprint of Random House, a division of Penguin Random House LLC, in 2000.

Grateful acknowledgment is made to Alfred A. Knopf, an imprint of the
Knopf Doubleday Publishing Group, a division of Penguin Random House LLC,
and Harold Ober Associates Incorporated for permission to reprint an excerpt from
"Harlem" from *Collected Poems* by Langston Hughes. Copyright © 1994
by the Estate of Langston Hughes. Used by permission.

ISBN 978-0-345-43486-9
Ebook ISBN 978-0-307-55951-7

Printed in the United States of America on acid-free paper

oneworldlit.com
randomhousebooks.com

41st Printing

I dedicate
*Sacred Woman*
to the first mothers
and healers of the planet,
the Afrakan woman,
and women globally
who are in need of
wellness

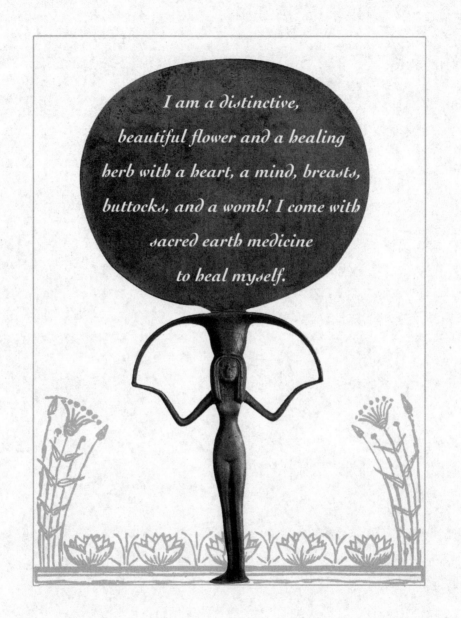

# AUTHOR'S NOTE

Over the past two decades I have seen hundreds of women, and through my holistic work with women's wombs I became known as the Mother of Womb Wellness. As the Mother, I observed through consultations, workshops, and seminars. In *Sacred Woman* I use the stories from sacred women and the wisdom I have gained from years of experience to offer programs for the body, mind, and spirit for the divinely sacred woman. These recommendations are not a prescription, and you should not implement any of these strategies without first consulting your healthcare practitioner. I have included them because I believe healthcare is self-care—the more informed you are, the better you will be able to collaborate with your doctor to come up with a treatment plan that suits your individual needs. If at any point you feel any of your symptoms are a sign of any serious issues, immediately go see a doctor.

# CONTENTS

# INTRODUCTION TO THE TWENTIETH
# ANNIVERSARY EDITION

The arms of *Sacred Woman* are far reaching. *Sacred Woman* embraces the least of us, to the best of us, to the most blessed of us who are seeking wellness. *Sacred Woman* arms are wrapped around the brokenhearted, the most disappointed, the Hood Girls, the Vixen Daughters, the Angry Mad Daughters, the Strippers, and the Fallen Angels. The Wise Woman, Medicine Woman, Sacred Sisters, Sanctified Woman, Goddess Woman, Holistic Devotee Mothers and Daughters: They are all embraced within this book. They are flexitarians, pescatarians, lacto-ovo vegetarians, vegans, non-hybrid vegans, sun-fired raw foodists, chlorophyllians, juicetarians, and fruitarians. Baby Boomers (born 1941 through 1964), Generation X (born 1965 through 1979), Xennials (born 1975 through 1985), Millennials (born 1985 through 1994), and Generation Z (born 1995 through 2015) are in the *Sacred Woman* family. From the corporate woman who hit the glass ceiling to the entrepreneur fighting for her freedom; from the creative artist, among those who influence social media, to the liberation advocates, the home care providers, and the Velvet Sword Clan: There are multitudes of tribes, clans, and circles united by *Sacred Woman*. There are Christian, Rastafarian, Hebrew Israelite, Muslim, Buddhist, Yoruba, Akan, Nuwaubian, Universalist, and Khamite Sacred Women, all on a path to healing the collective body, mind, and spirit of Woman.

*Sacred Woman* heart wraps its love around you as you take your holistic transformation journey. You are being called to take your Sacred Seat of Power, that we women—a unified mighty force of nature—may uplift ourselves, our families, and all of humanity.

## SACRED WOMEN, WE ARE CALLED!

**"We are the Women who lighten the darkness. We have come to lighten the darkness. It is lightened. We have overcome the destroyers. We are there for those who weep, who hide their faces, who sunk down. They looked upon us then. We are the Women. We are the Healers."**
—PAPYRUS OF ANU

*Sacred Woman* has touched womenfolk everywhere. The Ancient Mothers answered our call to heal us: to overcome our "pained body"; to overcome Willie Lynch's command of divide and conquer; to overcome the legacy of those stolen from ancient Afraka, the Motherland; to overcome Jim Crow, colonization, domination, social injustices, broken homes, and broken hearts. We called and shouted, and she answered. The year 2000 was a major shift for women. My friend and comrade Lloyd Strayhorn, a world-renowned astro-numerologist and author of *Numbers and You,* forecast that the year 2000 was the opening, the era, the Rise of the Woman. He was spot-on. Together we cheered the arrival of Sacred Woman as she traveled through the birth canal of our Celestial Sky Mother Nut. She appears here, in this text.

*Sacred Woman: A Guide to Healing the Feminine Body, Mind, and Spirit* was born April 4, 2000, on a warm Spring Solstice day, when the flowers in Brooklyn's neighborhood parks and community gardens began to blossom. After seven years of writing longhand, channeling, fasting, editing and re-editing, Fire Breathing, weeping, and truth telling, the *Sacred Woman* book with all her charm, her peace, her love, her knowledge, her hope for us to heal, to unify, and to empower ourselves was born. After four hundred years, eight generations of chattel slavery, this book arrived to help us become whole, particularly those women who survived the Middle Passage and the Door of No Return. The book's purpose was to overcome our sorrow, our great loss, our woundedness, our separation from our homeland. *Sacred Woman* would reawaken us from unconsciousness to wakefulness. Through the text itself, and *Sacred Woman* book circles and Sacred Woman Rites of Passage workshops, we would be born again. We have, for over twenty years, become more radiant with each page read, more vibrant with each level of detoxification, more hopeful through each Gateway lesson, more prayerful and confident with each step. As we live the Sacred Woman observances, we become healers once again. We remember ancient times, when the air, water, and food were pure and our hearts were balanced, as light as feathers on the Scale of Maat. Courageously, we return to our original selves when we are revered by our men and respected as Mothers of our Nation. We were not always hurt and angry, vengeful despondent Women. We were the "Woman who lightened the darkness . . ." As we have turned the pages of *Sacred Woman* over the years, from 2000 to now, following the calling, we are remembering, we are returning, we are overcoming.

Over the twenty years from 2000 to 2020, over three generations we began to rise forward. We heard the call, came alive, and shared our newfound self with our mothers, daughters, and sister-friends. Many of the women call *Sacred Woman* the Woman's Bible, a guiding light for us all. As we turned these pages, thousands of us began to receive our treasures and were given a second chance, another pathway paved in blue wombs, yellow radiance, green hearts, lavender self-trust, pink harmony—a pathway paved with moonstone, topaz, crystals, malachite, emeralds, and rose quartz. A pathway to the home inside ourselves, where we stand transformed. Some of us tiptoed through the gateways of Sacred Word, Sacred Food, Sacred Relationships, nervously facing our own awesomeness. Some of us ran with bated breath into the Sacred Woman Rites of Passage circles. Some of us fell into the Gateways. Some of us went at it alone with a cup of herbal tea, a candle, and a prayer. Some of us fell away and then rose again from Sacred Women of Antiquity to rejoin as Sacred Women of the Renaissance. We vowed to never fall asleep again; with newfound wisdom we would live the lifestyle of a Sacred Woman to be saved, spared, rejuvenated.

We heard the call and we reached out to one another and were taken into the Global Sacred Woman Village, our safe haven where the healers come and get charged. Into the Global Village where we laugh, cry, dance, sing, and share to celebrate our womanness, our sisterhood. Our sacredness is a place where we get strong for our families and for ourselves. Our communities connect through us and they heal because of us, and together we learn how to live as healers. From all spiritual houses we fiercely gather. We become Sacred Sisters (Ast and Nebt-Het), dwelling on common ground, united in this Sacred Sister Circle. With love, respect, and honor, we women gather to receive healing from our sister tribes and clans. From the four directions—East, North, South, and West—we come to be restored within the Sacred Woman Mothership. From 2000 to 2020, *Sacred Woman* expanded from Sacred Woman Rites of Passage to Sacred Woman Muts (Mothers) to Sacred Woman Elders to Sacred Woman Master Teachers. From 2000 to 2020, three generations of women took their journey from daughters to mothers to grandmothers, bonding as healers of themselves and their families and to one another. In the spirit of "each one, teach one," we gathered, and we healed.

## SACRED WOMAN WAS PRESENT

Over the last twenty years, women witnessed movements from Black Girls Rock, to the Million Woman March on Philadelphia and Washington, to the shouts of the Me Too Movement. *Sacred Woman* was there as President Obama and First Lady Michelle Obama were sworn into office to take the seat of Ast, the Great Mother, and Asar, the Great Father of Turtle Island (miscalled the United States). *Sacred Woman* witnessed the Rise of the Goddess and the Fall of Wall Street. She was there when the mainstream embraced holistic living, making huge profits as natural fruit and vegetable stands became the norm. *Sacred Woman* was there when mother's sons were horrifically shot across "the land of the free." There she was as the people took to the streets from city to city chanting "No Justice, No Peace!" *Sacred Woman* was there at the birth of my granddaughters, Atnnt, Maati, and Satraya, each from their mother's holistic womb. Big Mama *Sacred Woman* was there at the helm to welcome her brother and sister books, from *City of Wellness* to *Overcoming an Angry Vagina: Journey to Womb Wellness* (now called *Sacred Womb Awaken*), *Man Heal Thyself: Journey to Optimal Wellness*, *Circle of Wellness*, and *Planet Heal*. Thereby *Sacred Woman* will continue to restore the women, and so restore all our relations now and throughout all time.

## SACRED WOMAN THE MOVEMENT

*Sacred Woman* became a social justice movement, a holistic wellness movement, a peace movement, a Healer's movement, and a sisterhood. It is an Ast and Nebt-Het movement, an entrepreneur movement, a womb wellness movement, and a Womb Yoga Dance movement. Through her trials, tests, and tribulations as a lotus out of the mud, *Sacred Woman* has withstood because sacred sisters, sacred mothers and daughters, Nubian woman, soul sisters, and homegirls have cried out for healing, waiting on our prayers to be answered. This is our time to heal, the movement we've been waiting for to live, to rise! *Sacred Woman* cannot be stopped! From Baby Boomers to Generation X to Millennials: Sacred Women are and will always fulfill our needs as women, mothers, and daughters. We are relevant and cannot be played out.

*Sacred Woman*, from its birth in the 1990s to the book's release, was presented to a Global Sacred Woman Village. In the summer of 2019, myself and Queen Esther, the dean of the Goddess Sacred Woman Village, my sister, Ast and Nebt-Het, came to the understanding that Sacred Woman is indeed a movement.

I started my personal healing journey, my inner movement, in 1969 in the wake and birth of a multitude of movements: Holistic Health Movement, Vegetarian Movement, Transcendental Meditation Movement, Quantum Physics Movement, Black Power and Panther Movement, African Liberation and Cultural Movement, and, through Dr. Martin Luther King, a nonviolent Civil Rights Movement. Students were doing sit-ins at colleges and riding the Freedom Bus, while people marched in cities set on fire protesting racism and hatred. We protested to Sweet Honey in the Rock, an a cappella woman's civil rights group singing "We Who Believe in Freedom Cannot Rest"; to James Brown's "Say It Loud, I'm Black and I'm Proud"; and to Richie Havens's hip, soul-out "Freedom." At the iconic Woodstock, Pharoah Sanders sang "The Creator Has a Master Plan." I later came to realize that each one of us carries the freedom song within. We can overcome, we can heal our personal, family, community, and global conditions. As it was in the 1960s, and is still true now: "All Power to the People."

These songs of inspiration, like the movements, shaped me and others. When the time came to birth the Sacred Woman Movement Spirit, we had the strength to bring forth a movement of profound magnitude that transformed the masses of ready women. We, the Women, continue to rise up to make the shift from mass dis-ease to massive wellness. We the healers lock arms as we quilt together to become trailblazers for Global Wellness.

## SACRED WOMAN EVOLVED TO A WOMB WELLNESS REVOLUTION

Over several decades of working with women's wombs holistically, I became known as the Mother of Womb Wellness. As the Mother, I observed through consultations, workshops, and seminars that 98 percent of all women are challenged with one to three womb issues in their lifetimes. Gateway 0 Nut represents the Universal Sky Mother who rebirths women on our pathway to holistically gain control of our wombs.

With devotion we heal our wombs to wellness, boldly taking responsibility to free our wombs of disease and toxicity and generate womb wellness awareness.

In the 1980s, the New York City Health Department honored myself, along with the eldest black woman obgyn of New York City—Dr. Josephine English, who delivered Malcolm X's children as well as my own babies in Brooklyn—and Dr. KaKayi, a longtime comrade in wellness. Since then, Dr. English has transitioned into an honorable Ancestor, continuing to guide us.

The acknowledgment strengthened our work in women's reproductive health. Sacred Womb Wellness work has revolutionized the field of women's reproductive health and uterine care. From the guidance in "The Spirit of the Womb" and "The Care of the Womb" (chapters 3 and 4) in *Sacred Woman*, women have courageously rejuvenated and detoxified their wombs from fibroid tumors (of crystallized mucus), vaginal cysts, heavy menstrual bleeding, chronic PMS, vaginal discharge of yellow and white vaginal slime, vaginal burning, and itching. Change has come to women challenged with stressed-out infectious wombs, various forms of STDs, acidic vaginas, infertility, toxic living, mood swings, and depression. It has come to women from young to middle-aged to elderly and menopausal. It has come to women suffering from day and night sweats, vaginal or uterine wall thinning, and prolapsed uterus, which can lead to a hysterectomy or the chronic pain of endometriosis—all of which are related to a toxic physical, mental, emotional, and dietary lifestyle.

Over the last decade, I've observed women across the board and around the world who live a lifestyle of womb wellness through the *Sacred Woman* way of life. These Sacred Women are empowered because they have the knowledge to protect, nurture, and nourish their wombs with nature's elements. From 2000 through 2020, I've witnessed Sacred Woman Womb Wellness Works attract and connect doulas, nurse-midwives, conscious obgyns, yoga teachers, energy workers, and nutritionists to the Nut Womb Wellness Gateway. Womb Wellness Teachings save, carry, and deliver returning ancestors (babies) to the world. With the rise of black women dying from childbirth and infants dying in various ways, even with advancements in technology and medicine, expectant mothers of color are in a crisis and are falling through the cracks with little to no help in sight. Through *Sacred Woman*, we women are banding together, expanding our knowledge, and learning to live our lives holistically to help end the health disparity of our wombs.

## SACRED WOMAN AS A HOLISTIC THERAPY BY WOMEN FOR WOMEN

Over the past twenty years, Sacred Woman has grown as a holistic therapeutic treatment in and of itself, much like polarity therapy, acupuncture, massage, reflexology, colonic irrigation therapy, and zone therapy. Sacred Woman as a therapy has proven an effective holistic treatment gifted to us from the Mothers of Antiquity to uplift their daughters; women are transforming from death to resurrection. With the renewal of the ancient concept of Healer as Woman, there is bound to be a change in the landscape and the approach to women's healing, giving us choices that broaden our scope and our awareness as Healers of ourselves. Women are awakening in a mighty way and beginning to take responsibility for their well-being, particularly women of color, and remembering the way of the Grandmother Spirit. We walk in her footprints, and form sister circles, wellness meetings, and *Sacred Woman* book clubs. We are setting up our homes as wellness centers for our families, based on Sacred Space charged from Sekhmet the Healer's Gateway and through the teachings in this text.

From 2000 through 2020, I've witnessed women using alternative medicine to heal themselves. These women radiate with illuminating possibilities. I've observed numbers of women overcoming disease. Many of the graduates of Sacred Woman Rites of Passage go on to higher holistic education by training to become Sacred Woman Practitioners and form Sacred Woman Sister Circles as a way to reach out to women in need of wellness throughout our world community. Women are growing with the Sacred Woman Movement and studying within our holistic university, and thereby are gaining confidence as the bedrock of the family, restoring all those from mates to children, parents to friends, elders to neighbors and coworkers to a newfound wellness.

I have found over the last twenty years that "Healer" and "Woman" are synonymous. With the activation of women's innate nurturing spirit and realignment with nature's elements—air, fire, water, and earth—women are able to heal themselves and aid other women to do the same. Sacred Woman is now carrying the movement to issues of Free Choice—of a woman having the right to choose her approach to healing herself and so choose her caretakers, be it allopathic care or holistic care.

Women, let's lobby this together. I'm inspired to bring this to the halls of Congress thanks to my birth daughter, Sherease Rasheida Maat, an advocate who opened my mind to stand for change and justice. For Woman, for Free Choice, to heal ourselves now: All Power to the Woman.

## SACRED WOMAN STILL ON TOP

The power of *Sacred Woman* never ceases to astound me. In its very early years, *Sacred Woman* appeared as an *Essence* magazine bestseller for six months. It was recognized by *The New York Times* and the BlackBoard bestsellers list. Even now, twenty years later, *Sacred Woman* has appeared on the Amazon Best Sellers list. Twenty years later women and men who love us are buying into wellness in great numbers. We are "healing thyself."

## THE GREAT SHIFT: SACRED WOMAN FROM OLD SCHOOL TO NEW SCHOOL

From 1989 through 2014, Sacred Woman Rites of Passage was taught only face-to-face. Women came to train for twelve weeks from the Bronx, Manhattan, Long Island, New Jersey, and as far as Philadelphia and Washington, DC. Women came to heal, rebuild, recover, and overcome in the Sacred Woman Circle. We looked at one another heart-to-heart, eye-to-eye. We cried, hugged, and lifted one another up every spring and summer, fall and winter during our Rites.

In the early years, the Rites attracted ten or fifteen students each semester and was taught once a year. This was old school. After the *Sacred Woman* guide was released in April 2000, the Rites of Passage attracted forty to fifty students each semester—all, again, old school.

The spring/summer 2015 new-school Sacred Woman Rites marked a change, a shift, a transition, an expansion. Through Instagram, Facebook, Twitter, Zoom, and conference calls, we opened the door for online Rites of Passage trainings. Every season a hundred students enroll, from the United States, Canada, Brazil, United Kingdom, the US Virgin Islands, and Africa.

Before social media, I called the graduates of Sacred Woman, Sacred Women of Antiquity; after 2015, we changed the name to Sacred Women of the Renaissance. During the Renaissance period, I trained Sacred Woman practitioners to take the teachings within this text to the masses to uplift humanity. We were becoming a powerful women's movement. With the support of Queen Esther, the Dean of the Global Sacred Woman Village Movement; Dr. Jewel Pookrum, our surgeon general and master teacher of brain balancing; Sacred Woman Priestess Sappora; and many other devoted Sacred Women, we were able to touch women globally. Together we survived the storms, hurricanes, and mudslides of Sacred Woman, with the many trials and tribulations of growing up as a holistic woman's movement and a Sacred Woman university within the Queen Afua school of holistic learning.

## SACRED WOMAN IS ON THE MOVE

Social media comes with its challenges, but for Sacred Woman it has championed our unity and oneness, and has strengthened the fact that Sacred Woman is still, after twenty years, on the move. Because of Sacred Woman's steady growth, we launched the book *Man Heal Thyself: Journey to Optimal Wellness*, written nine years ago. The counterpart to *Sacred Woman*, *Man Heal Thyself* used twelve-week Rites of Passage training to create Wellness Warriors, complementing the rebirth of the amazing Sacred Woman mothers, daughters, and wives. Family-to-family we heal ourselves.

Sacred Woman has officially opened the way to planetary healing and humanity. It's 2020 and we are right on time. Sacred Woman was in the Beginning. Sacred Woman is now, and Sacred Woman will always be. It will help set us free.

From 2000 to date I observed the following transformations:

### Sacred Woman as Holistic Medicine / Woman as Healer / The Gateways as Holistic Medicine

I Am a Woman of Womb Enlightenment
I Am a Woman of Divine Intelligence
I Am a Nature Woman
I Am a Woman of Sacred Spirit Dance
I Am a Woman of Grace and Beauty
I Am a Woman of Intuitive Skill
I Am a Woman of Natural Medicine
I Am a Woman of Harmony and Balance
I Am a Woman of Supreme Love
I Am a Woman of Vision
I Am a Woman on Cosmic Time
I Am a Woman on Purpose

### Nut: Womb Wellness as Personal Medicine, Gateway 0 Ruled by the Womb

Personally: Over a twenty-year span, I observed women begin to live the Gateways in numerous fashions. I witnessed women heal themselves from a multitude of womb issues. Living a womb wellness lifestyle allowed them to overcome fibroids, infertility, cyst, chronic PMS, and emotional womb trauma. Professionally: Nine years after the birth of *Sacred Woman,* I wrote, directed, and performed a one-woman play called *Overcoming: If Your Vagina Could Speak, What Would She Say,* originally inspired by *Sacred Woman* chapters on Womb Wellness.

My aim with the play was to help rebirth women's wombs from pain to peace; from brokenness to wholeness. The play traveled from New York to Philadelphia, Atlanta, and London, offering awareness to women that we could use art to inspire healing of our wombs. Together in celebration throughout the play, myself and the audience laughed, cried, sang, danced, and leaped as we embraced the holistic healing of our wombs.

### Tehuti: Word as Medicine, Gateway 1 Ruled by the Throat

Personally: Women within Tehuti used their voices to speak out for family and community justice. Women began to speak themselves into their renewed life of wholeness with every word, healing physically and metaphysically. Professionally: I observed women begin to birth their inner scribe and birth the books that were lying dormant inside of them.

### Ta-Urt: Food as Medicine, Gateway 2 Ruled by the Digestive System

Personally: In Ta-Urt, Food as Medicine, we learn how to use foods from the garden to heal ourselves and our families. Professionally: Some women are making careers as vegan chefs and others adapting a plant-based garden lifestyle to live optimally.

### Bes: Sacred Movement as Medicine, Gateway 3 Ruled by the Circulatory System

Personally: Women perform the Womb Yoga Dance to become ageless beauties by maintaining their youth and vitality with each movement and breath, while reversing the aging process by releasing past pain. Professionally: Over the last two decades, women have become Womb Yoga Dance practitioners through my certification.

### Het-Hru: Sacred Beauty as Medicine, Gateway 4 Ruled by the Young Heart

Personally: To tap into your authentic beauty is to connect to your inner child, find out where your pain began, and connect with, accept, and take your inner child on the Sacred Woman healing journey; over time, beauty will shine through. Professionally: Some women take on beauty as a career and design and tailor and present fashion shows, offering consultations on how to bring forth your beauty.

## Nebt-Het: Sacred Space as Medicine, Gateway 5 Ruled by the Pineal Gland / Ujah

Personally: Through Nebt-Het, women discover that the power to heal all things is within as they connect with and learn to trust their inner voice. Professionally: Some women become very intuitively powered and offer counseling as Sacred Woman practitioners.

## Sekhmet: Sacred Healing as Medicine, Gateway 6 Ruled by the Bloodstream

Personally: Through Sekhmet women may lower their blood pressure, relieve their anger, and fortify the Healer within. Professionally: Women became herbalists, energy workers, Sacred Woman practitioners, Reiki healers, massage therapists, and naturopaths to transform their communities to wellness. Inspired by Sekhmet, women, in general, become fully empowered as awakened Healers of themselves and their families.

## Maat: Sacred Relationships as Medicine, Gateway 7 Ruled by the Mature Heart

Personally: We've learned to balance our hearts on the scales of Maat. We've learned to forgive and overcome together. We create and attract relationships now that support our wholeness as women, mothers, and daughters. Professionally: Some Sacred Women may be inspired to become psychotherapists or relationship counselors.

## Ast: Sacred Union as Medicine, Gateway 8 Ruled by the Crown

Personally: We balanced our left brain of intelligence and materialism, and the right brain of creativity and spirituality. It took a decade after the *Sacred Woman* text was written before I realized that Gateway Ast was also a Gateway of Wealth and Prosperity. Once a woman has fully accessed her brain, she is able to materialize all things.

## Nefer Atum: Enlightenment as Medicine, Gateway 9 Ruled by the Pituitary

Personally: Those who have trained as Sacred Women have a particularly magical spirit that is recognizable by others. The way a Sacred Woman expresses herself, interacts, connects, and shares all she does is uplifting. She has a radiant, natural glow from rising out of the mud of suffering through the healing waters to reach the sunlight of a vibrant life.

## Seshat: Cosmic Time as Medicine, Gateway 10 Ruled by the Skeleton/Muscles/Joints

Personally: Sacred Time of Seshat measures our life by what we accomplish and how we use time in order to receive the best of life—from awakening in morning meditation at Nebt-Het hour to receive our treasure chest from 4 to 6 A.M.; to receiving our vision of full creation at midday; to the closing of the day in Het-Hru as we nurture ourselves with baths and massages and vegan dinner; and finally to Nut time, evening, when we rest so that we may knit and heal to awaken again at 4, in Nebt-Het's hour, and go higher and higher with each day.

## Meshkenet: Sacred Work as Medicine, Gateway 11 Ruled by the Birthing Womb

Professionally: Woman discovers her purpose, her life mission, her life's work, her healing balm, her joy, peace, and prosperity. Her work may come in the form of service or of a product; of working as a writer, a motivational speaker, a CEO, or a partner in a joint vision supported by the worldwide web of Sacred Women and loved by her family and her community.

*Sacred Woman* has seasoned me for over three decades from day to day and moment to moment. With each breath *Sacred Woman* continues to propel me, nurture me, cleanse me, hold me, comfort me, direct me, love me. *Sacred Woman* has a healing balm from the beginning of time (NTRT Hmt) and will always be a healing tool in these days to help us attain our wholeness. From Gateway to Gateway, we rise. All Power to the People.

**All hail to Maat
*(the Indwelling Guardian of Heart Harmony)*,**

**HOTEP QUEEN AFUA**

# . . . NEVER BE THE SAME!

Sacred Women make lemons into lemonade. Throughout the Global Pandemic, we, Sacred Women, did not just accept the fear from the death toll due to the virus; we rose up and bonded with nature's healing balm.

We energetically transformed the lockdown and isolation of quarantine into the Spirit of a Healing Home Retreat. Our homes became Wellness Spaces. Our families throughout the land became holistically renewed from the teachings offered throughout this *Sacred Woman* text.

Sacred Women and their families left behind dietary toxicities that create an inner environment contributing to the breakdown of the immune and respiratory systems. Sacred Women fully embraced a vegetarian and vegan, mindful, Natural Living, plant-based way of life to strengthen our bodies against the Virus. We, Sacred Women, live a lifestyle that allows us and our families to be bold in the midst of the Global Pandemic.

Sacred Women in Wellness Leadership have become shape shifters, game changers, and holistic liberators, protecting ourselves, our families, and our communities.

Sacred Women is a fierce movement, a force of nature for social justice We have reached over 100,000 families through social media. We did not lay down our lives due to the Virus. We fought back and stood up, with "food as medicine" as our motto. We are becoming more and more empowered in our Holistic Wellness Lifestyle.

Due to the times we find ourselves in, I was further compelled to train Sacred Women to become certified Emerald Green Holistic Practitioners to aid the masses to Holistic Recovery.

During this time, we had home births, homeschooled our children, and detoxed our families.

We became entrepreneurs and used social media to expand our Sacred Work, our Meskhenet.

To further empower the people holistically, Queen Esther Hunter-Sarr and I hosted our first Heal Thyself Rally in July 2020 at The Legacy Center in Atlanta, Georgia. We partnered with the CEOs of The Legacy Center in the plight to make Atlanta the Mecca of Wellness, the first City of Wellness, through this event.

Little did we know while planning for the Heal Thyself Rally that family man George Floyd of Minneapolis would be murdered at the hands of a group of racist police officers. His lynching, lasting a long 8 minutes and 46 seconds from a knee on his neck, would become an outcry and the catalyst for numerous Freedom Rallies that rose up throughout the world. Like a Great Awakening, people from all ages and all races banded and bonded together in unity throughout America, Europe, and Africa against violence toward Brown and Black people. We, the people, as one mighty force, marched the streets, shouting "No justice! No peace!" The people rose up for freedom, for justice, and now for our healing.

We, the people, are shouting, "No more Jim Crow! No more free labor!" The prison system has filled its cells with millions of Brown and Black people enslaved in a modern day plantation.

We know that our voices as women, mothers, daughters, and wives globally will be heard, respected, and honored if we unify.

We, Sacred Women, follow in the redeeming footprints of our African Ancestors as we shout, "We are the women who lighten the darkness. We have come to lighten the darkness. It is lightened. We have overcome the destroyers. We are there for those who weep. Who hide their faces. Who sink down. They looked upon us then. We are the women. We are the healers."

# I AM THE WOMAN, I AM THE HEALER

**I am the Woman who lightens the darkness.
I have come to lighten the darkness, it is
lightened. I have overthrown the destroyers.
I have adored those who are in the darkness. I
have been made to stand for those who weep,
who hide their faces, who sunk down. They
looked upon me then.
I AM A WOMAN
I AM A HEALER**

**— PAPYRUS OF ANI**

## PREPARING TO ENTER THE GATES— SACRED WOMAN TRAINING

*Ring . . . ring . . .* "344-HEAL. This is Queen Afua. May I help you?"

The sister on the other end of the phone began to weep. "I'm so frightened. My doctor told me that my ovaries are dead . . . I'm only twenty-nine years old, and I feel like I'm going through menopause. What am I to do?" she pleaded.

*Ring . . . ring . . .* "344-HEAL. This is Queen Afua. May I help you?"

A sad, quiet voice said, "The gynecologist I just saw tells me that I have to have a hysterectomy. I'm only thirty years old, with one daughter. I was hoping to get married again and have more children. In 1982 I was diagnosed with pelvic inflammatory disease and regenerating fibroid tumors. The tumors didn't cause me any major problems for six or seven years, but now they've grown. What can I do? Do you think you might be able to help me—in a natural way? I don't want to lose my womb."

*Ring . . . ring . . .* "221-HEAL. This is Queen Afua. May I help you?"

There was a deep sigh from the caller. "Hello, Queen. I guess I'm finally ready to try the natural way—nothing else has worked. I'm getting heavy bleeding, with only about ten days between my periods. In between I'm in constant PMS, and a screaming lunatic with my family and coworkers. I just can't go on this way."

As the Founder and Director of the Heal Thyself Center, and a Holistic Health Consultant, Colon Therapist, Polarity Practitioner, and Lay Midwife, I have experienced a Natural Living lifestyle for more than forty-five years, and I have guided thousands along the Path of Purification for more than forty years. But nothing in my experience as a Minister of Purification and a Nubian Khamitic Priestess of the Temple Nebt-Het, initiated through the Shrine of Ptah, could have prepared me for the epidemic of womb disasters that began to appear at the Heal Thyself Center.

The issue of African American women's health has always been one of my primary concerns. I know how chilling the statistics are. There are more than 550,000 hysterectomies performed each year in the United States. Yet, as Dr. Michael E. Toaff, creator of the Alternative to Hysterectomy website, comments, "In the vast majority of these cases, the indications for surgery are benign, non life threatening conditions. Only 10% of hysterectomies are performed for cancer."

Due to this widespread practice, the National Black Woman's Health Project's Public Education and Policy Program has highlighted the following issues among its top priorities for African American women's health: "Reproductive health and rights issues such as high rates of breast and cervical cancer and STD's; and excessive hysterectomies."

Their efforts are critical when we consider the fact that by the age of sixty more than one-third of the women in the United States have had a hysterectomy. An article on indications for hysterectomy found that African American women and women with male gynecologists are more likely to undergo hysterectomies.[1]

Research has also shown that "African American women are more likely than white women to have a hysterectomy, are hospitalized longer, and are at a higher risk for complications and death. Based on 1986 to 1991 hospital data from the State of Maryland, researchers found that African American women are 25 percent more likely to have a hysterectomy than are white women the same age. The study also indicated that African American women undergoing the same procedure are more likely to experience complications, remain hospitalized longer, and have a higher risk of death than white women."[2]

## Judgment Day Is Every Day—as Our Ancestors Have Told Us

Many of the health books on the market today convey a sense that we need only to treat health as an accessory, one that we can buy at a department store, just as we'd buy a pair of earrings. Well, it's simply not true. We get confused by our consumerist way of thinking, which says that if only we have this car, or that brand-name clothing, or this stereo system, or that house—all things outside of the self—then everything will be fine.

But you can't buy good health, no matter how much money you have, what kind of possessions you have, how many degrees you've earned, what job title you hold, or what neighborhood you live in. You have to plan and cultivate good health. You have to commit to good health. You have to live good health because it comes from the inside out. It comes from what you bring to your life: positive, empowering thoughts, prayers and affirmations, uplifting company, and high-quality, life-giving foods.

To have excellent health you must invest time and energy into the transformation of your Sacred Body Temple. And once you've acquired excellent health, you must maintain it vigilantly. That's the true divine challenge—one that you can and must meet.

## THE STATE OF YOUR WOMB REFLECTS THE STATE OF YOUR LIFE

The womb is the gateway of all human life. When the womb is honored and respected, she becomes a channel of power, creativity, and beauty—and joy reigns on earth. When her voice goes unheard, unanswered, denied, the womb becomes a vessel of disease.

The collective state of women's wombs reflects the condition of the world. When so many women's wombs suffer from tumors, cysts, frigidity, and heavy menstrual bleeding, when so many women experience sexually aggressive acts and unnecessary hysterectomies, then disharmony covers the earth.

The condition of women's wombs also directly reflects the condition of women's minds, spirits, and actions. The womb is a storehouse of all our emotions. It collects every feeling—good and bad. Today we have collectively reached a state of "negative womb power."

Unnatural living and unhealthy lifestyles perpetuate negative womb power, and this in turn supports the conflicts of humans against the planet, humans against humans, and woman against the womb. The condition of a woman's womb also reflects the condition of all her relationships. When a woman's womb is in a healthy state, her life is a reflection of this balance.

The love and care that a woman gives to her womb reflects her true level of emotional, spiritual, physical, and mental health. Unfortunately, too many women in today's world experience some form of womb degeneration that results in disease. As we women heal and transform our wombs, we will change our destiny and the destiny of our planet.

Women, it is time to take back control. We must defend our wombs with our lives, for the womb is the birthplace of all our creative abilities.

Nonkululeko Tyehemba, a blessed nurse-midwife, spoke very eloquently about the power of the fully revitalized womb:

*As a midwife and a keeper of the shrine of Meshkenet, as one who has helped to birth countless babies of light onto this earth, I know that Sacred Woman speaks to the power of the womb. So often we women do not realize the power we possess, what ways this power can be manifested, and what factors can alter the patterning of the womb for better or for worse.*

*A female is born with all the sacred ova she will ever use in her lifetime. Each ovum is a sacred entity unto itself. Hence, it's important not only to use these words of wisdom for our woman selves, but also to use this text to assist our daughters as they move into womanhood.*

*For example, we must initiate our daughters and our own girl selves into the many practices that enhance the strength of the womb. In turn, wombs that are strong and powerful will become a sanctuary for the fertilized ovum. In this way we "break the chains" of generational womb problems, i.e., menstrual cramps, fibroids, infertility, and so on.*

In *Sacred Woman* we learn techniques from herbology to hydrotherapy to protect our wombs from inner and outer oppressions. We learn how we perpetuate harmful self-behaviors, and then we turn gratefully to the Queen Afua Method of Transformation. We learn how to spiritualize ourselves for the upliftment of the sacred womb, for when we learn to affirm ourselves, we automatically empower our womb.

## THE SACRED WOMAN MISSION

Many women's voices speak through these pages, and I believe yours will, too. My prayer is that the message of this book will ignite your transformational journey. When you open yourself up to the Sacred Woman you truly are, you will receive a higher vision of self, and the hope, help, and courage you need to go forward.

This book will be truly successful if it encourages you to help not only yourself but also another woman, sister, or friend in need of wellness. This book is your reminder from the universe that you possess the innate power to create transformation and change—personally, communally, and globally. Bring forth your Het-Hru warrior queen skills and you will be victorious in remaking yourself into a divine vision. Now is your time—the time to reclaim your self and unleash your power as a Sacred Woman.

*Sacred Woman* is a path and journey for inner freedom, a road map to Divinity. It is the road of emancipation, led by the First Mothers of the earth, Afrakan women. Sacred Woman consciousness is the ultimate answer to planetary healing. We are embarking upon a journey of liberation and our destination is freedom. The price for freedom may be high, but the price that we pay for being imprisoned and cut off from the very root of our being is even higher.

When you choose life, you must have the courage to sacrifice your old, worn-out, ineffective self. As you transform from a wounded woman to a Sacred Woman, you will evolve from a frightened, withdrawn state to a courageous one. You will move from confusion to serenity; from mistrust to trust; from spite to compassion and love; from weakness to empowerment; from

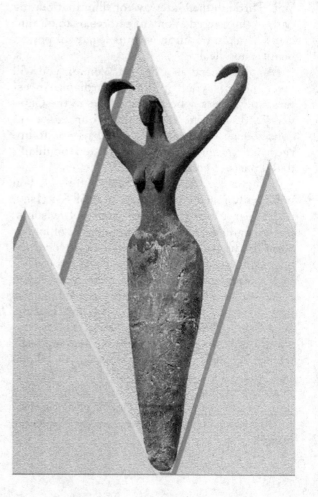

being an unconscious woman to being a wise woman. You will move from a disturbed mind to a divine mind; from restlessness to contentment; from boredom to creativity; from a suppressed woman to an expressive one. You will rise from a deflated woman to an inspired woman; from a depressed woman to a joyful one; from a disease-infested person to a disease-free one; from a dishonest woman to an honest woman; from a follower to a leader and freethinker; from a pessimist to an optimist. Like a lotus in the sun, you will blossom into a radiant Sacred Woman.

As you grow and ascend into a Sacred Woman, you will heal in countless dimensions by way of prayer, healing affirmations, visualizations, sacred dance, purification rites, fasting, eating live foods, altar work, storytelling, holistic nutrition, and nature cures filled with Mother Wit. Through the Gateways of Illumination, the path of the Sacred Woman restores us to our ancient Afrakan tradition with its legacy of power, beauty, and healing.

As you ascend as a Sacred Woman, you will meet and greet your Spiritual Guardians, Ancestors, and Elders, who hold the keys to the Gateways to heaven on earth. Your state of consciousness will soar as you journey on to uproot and purge out the deteriorated or dilapidated parts of yourself.

As you travel through each Gateway, you will finally reach your Sacred Seat of Ast (Isis), the Great Mother Afrakan Spirit of wisdom, power, and healing. In your divine seat of higher mind, body, and spirit, you will be fully charged and ready to be crowned by Nefer Atum, the Divine Lotus, who will aid and guide you as you reach out to others who are also in need. This is how, together, we will create planetary healing. As a Sacred Woman in the making, who is constantly unfolding and reinventing herself as she travels through the many Gateways to wholeness, you will weave your *seneb* shawl of beauty, health, and purity. Freedom will erupt within you, for after all, Sacred Woman, your destination is *freedom* and your quest *liberation*! Welcome home!

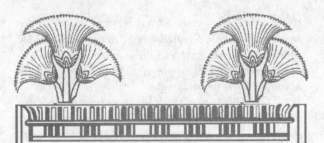

Most Divine Sacred One,
I, your daughter born Helen Robinson ascended to Queen Afua, illuminated to Mut Nebt-Het, stand in the lineage of Nebt-Het, who as the Lady of the House and the Lady of Heaven brings enlightenment and resurrection to the Sacred Body Temple.
As a Purification Priestess of Nebt-Het, I am a Guardian of the Breath, a Holder of the Ankh Key. I am a Custodian of the Seat of Ast, Founder of the Heal Thyself Natural Living Center, Spiritual Midwife to the many, holder of the Ancient Afrakan Medicine Bag, Daughter of the East Wind, Daughter of Oshun, Holder of the Sacred Feather of the Native People of Turtle Island.
As a Daughter from the loins of Ephraim Robinson and the womb of Ida Ford Robinson, I ask you, Almighty One, the Owner of the Day and of the Night, to open the way of Healing and Wholeness for all your Daughters. I pour a libation in honor of our ancestors to assist us, and guide us to our Divinity as womenfolk. I ask for blessings as we step into our Sacred Womb Circle and begin our transformation and enlightenment that will allow us to pave our way to an enlightening transformation that will bring a healing message from the hearts of all Sacred Women to the heart of the world.

# SACRED WOMAN TRAINING: HOW TO USE THIS BOOK

*Sacred Woman* is a spiritual and cultural journey. In order to begin this adventure of discovery and transformation, we must turn our compass south to the sources of the Nile River in the womb of Mother Afraka. Just as the Nile flows from south to north, which goes against our preconceived notions of how rivers flow, so too do the origins of the culture that we think of today as Egypt. Few understand or fully appreciate that the origins of ancient Egypt also flowed from the south—beginning in the black Afrakan source of Khamitic Nubia, giving rise to the celebrated culture of the north.

Today, contemporary seekers of various traditions are invoking the spiritual wisdom of their ancestors in order to revitalize such traditions in modern life. Whether it's Native Americans reconnecting with the Great Spirit, or the Chinese drinking freely from the well of Taoist tradition, or Jews debating their Talmudic roots, we have discovered that we cannot become whole unless we understand the wisdom of those upon whose shoulders we stand.

Afrakan Americans' exploration of their ancestral wisdom teachings has been painfully restricted by the absence of written records. But thanks to the unconquerable and profound legacy of our rich oral tradition, and the extraordinary efforts of Afrakan and Afrakan American historians and scholars, such as Dr. John Henrik Clarke, Dr. Yosef Ben Jochannan, Dr. Shava Ali, and Jacob Carruthers—and spiritual leaders who apply ancient Maatian principles to live by today, such as my husband Hru Sen-Ur Semahj—we have at last been able to document the true origins of Nubian-Afrakan culture and its defining and indisputable influence on Khamitic (Egyptian) culture. Armed with this knowledge, we have been able to tap into the roots of this legacy and bring its fruits to vibrant life.

*Sacred Woman* has given me the opportunity to share the spiritual traditions of ancient Khamit—the mother of Northern Egyptian culture revered in books and museums worldwide. To enter fully into Khamit and the Afrakan-Nubian tradition, one must set aside many of the preconceptions taught about "classical Egypt," its origins, history, and spiritual traditions. This may be difficult for those who question the legitimacy of the Afrakan-Nubian heritage. I can only suggest that the passport to the realm of the Sacred Woman is an open mind and heart willing to honor and experience this wisdom firsthand.

Part 1: The Ancient Ways will introduce you to the spiritual and ethical legacy left to us by our ancient Nubian-Khamitic ancestors, who have gifted us with our understanding of sacred unity. These teachings have shown us that ancient Khamit was never a polytheistic or animistic culture. This tradition viewed NTR as the undifferentiated One/All-Divine from whom all life emanates. It gave the Mother-Father aspects of the Creator/Creatress equal respect.

The Ancient Ways will also introduce you to the spiritual guidance embodied in the NTRU, such as Ast (Isis), the Great Mother Afrakan Spirit, culture bringer, and healer; Maat, who represents truth, balance, harmony, law, and cosmic order; Het-Hru (Hathor), the aspect of Divine love, beauty, and nurturing; Heru (Horus), the Sacred Warrior of Light, the aspect of will; Bes, the aspect of expansion, NTRU of dance; Sekhmet, the lion-headed patroness of healers; and finally the sacred lotus, Nefer Atum, the aspect of highest ascension and unlimited potential.

Thus the NTRU, who have been mislabeled the Gods and Goddesses, are actually manifestations of the wondrous divine attributes of NTR, the Mother-Father Source. This is especially significant to Western women, who are more accustomed to receiving their empowerment through worship of a male Godhead and the intercession of a male priesthood.

The spiritual teachings of ancient Khamit are made relevant today through Sacred Woman Training. By necessity, Sacred Woman Training provides only a brief introduction to ancient Khamit, for indeed the serious study of this civilization could take a lifetime. I offer it to you in hopes that you will be so fascinated by the truth of its teachings that you will be inspired to explore much more deeply into our rich cultural treasures.

## First-Degree Sacred Woman Training

*Gateway 0: The Sacred Womb.* The purpose of First-Degree Sacred Woman Training is to awaken us to the power of the womb as our physical and psychospiritual center. As we enter Gateway 0 we learn how to identify, cleanse, purify, heal, and honor one of the primary Gateways of our spiritual power.

Through Sacred Altar Work and Daily Spiritual Observances, and through Journaling and Dialoguing with the Spirit of the Womb, we learn how to deprogram ourselves from harmful thoughts, attitudes, habits, and relationships. Through Gateway 0 we learn the art of caring for our wombs by offering them the gift of Wellness Philosophy. This includes the Natural Living approach to food, Womb Rejuvenation Techniques, womb affirmations, womb meditations, and learning to use the Sacred Woman's Womb Scroll. Most important, we learn how to honor ourselves through an Afrakan spiritual and cultural tradition whose sole aim is to bring us into full flower.

You may experience your Womb Work by entering Gateway 0 individually or as a member of a Sacred Womb Circle of four to eight women who gather their forces together for a minimum of twenty-one days or a maximum of four months to purify and heal the womb on a physical, mental, and spiritual level. This process can be extremely rewarding and supportive, so call your girlfriends, coworkers, relatives, and/or women's group to pack their spirit bags and join you as you inaugurate this powerful ascent into your sacredness. Together you will physically purify, pray, meditate, do journal work, make music, and love and support one another as you transform your wombs from a state of disease and disharmony to one of wellness and perfection.

First-Degree Sacred Woman Training lays the foundation of womb wellness that is integral to your experience of the Gateways of Initiation. Once you have completed Gateway 0, your womb health will be better than ever before and you will be ready to begin the second stage of your Sacred Woman Training.

## Second-Degree Sacred Woman Training

*Exploring the Gateways Individually.* Each Gateway represents a spiritual rite of passage that will liberate you from your old life and usher you into a new way of being. This work requires a commitment to transform your consciousness from ignorance, denial, or grandiosity to harmonious alignment with your true divine nature as a Sacred Woman.

We do not travel the Gateways alone. At each Gateway we are accompanied by the inspiration, grace, protection, and guidance of the Spiritual Guardians, Ancestors, Elders, and Contemporaries associated with the teachings of each particular Gateway. And if we are blessed, the collective energy and transformative power of the sisters also accompany us in our Sacred Womb Circle.

Each Gateway will introduce you to a specific spiritual legacy that will serve as the next step in the cultivation of your Sacred Woman Consciousness. The Gateways and their Guardians are: Gateway 1: Sacred Word—Tehuti; Gateway 2: Sacred Food—Ta-Urt; Gateway 3: Sacred Movement—Bes; Gateway 4: Sacred Beauty—Het-Hru; Gateway 5: Sacred Space—Nebt-Het; Gateway 6: Sacred Healing—Sekhmet; Gateway 7: Sacred Relationship—Maat; Gateway 8: Sacred Union—Ast; Gateway 9: Nefer Atum—Sacred Lotus Initiation—Meshkenet and Nefer Atum / Ast and Nefer Atum; Gateway 10: Sacred Time—Seshat; and Gateway 11: Sacred Work—Meshkenet.

Exploring each Gateway requires a seven-day commitment, and conscious immersion in this profound curriculum.

*In Second-Degree Sacred Woman Training you have the option of exploring any of the Gateways as a separate course of study. The most important requirement is that the chosen Gateway serve as an answer to your prayer.*

For example, Sarah found herself in a state of constant agitation. She could only utter the harshest criticisms and complaints to her family, coworkers, and friends. When her four-year-old daughter said, "Mommy, you say too many bad words," Sarah burst into tears, for she knew that her words had indeed become lethal weapons. In the safety of her Sacred Circle she knew there was an answer to her dilemma, and she was able to seek refuge in Gateway 1: Sacred Word, where she found herself in the sheltering arms of Tehuti. As Sarah began her journey through Gateway 1 and dedicated herself to its Daily Spiritual Observances, Guided Meditations, and Journaling and Transformative Work, day by day her life began to change before her eyes.

In Second-Degree Training, the most important steps are to:

1. Read the entire text of the Gateway before you begin your work.
2. Commit to a seven-day period in which you have a lighter or more flexible schedule and can prioritize your spiritual work.
3. Make the hours of 4 A.M. to 6 A.M. sacred, no matter how challenging your daily schedule. Remember, if you put your commitment to Spirit first, all the energy you need will be gifted to you.

### Third-Degree Sacred Woman Training

*The Gateways of Sacred Initiation.* In Third-Degree Sacred Woman Training, you make a profound commitment to putting Spirit first in your life. Like the initiation of the ancient Mystery Schools, Third-Degree Training brings you to the crossroads between unconsciousness and consciousness in your life's journey. When you enter this level you are no longer protected by the safety nets of ignorance offered to beginners—this is a conscious path.

Some members of our Sacred Womb Circle described the process of embracing Third-Degree Training this way.

*First-Degree Training is like getting your BA degree. Gateway 0 contains all of the fundamentals about how to locate and maintain your Sacred Seat, and Womb Wisdom is a rigorous course of study. By the time you have completed four months you actually do become wise in the ways of your womb and you begin to understand the absolute necessity of embracing a Natural Living lifestyle.*

*Second-Degree Training is like getting your master's degree. You choose a specific Gateway of the Sacred Woman Training to concentrate on, and you delve deep. Once you begin to explore the body-mind-spirit dimensions of a particular Gateway, every part of your life begins to change. I concentrated my first experience of Second-Degree Training on Gateway 5: Sacred Space, and I watched everything in my life transform. Clutter disappeared, old, wornout possessions that I no longer had use for were joyfully released, and I found new, almost magical ways of creating Sacred Space in my life. I never realized how much I'd been holding on to until Nebt-Het revealed to me that I was hanging on to old fears like the old shoes in the back of my closet that no longer fit. When I got rid of those old shoes, I got rid of my old consciousness too.*

*I can't tell you how rewarding it was for me to spend three months in Gateway 5. Now, my sister-friend Anne had no issues in that Gateway, and she had a positive, and satisfying experience in seven days, but I needed three months! Second-Degree Training allows us to take and make our own Sacred Time. Anne reminded me that she spent six months studying and processing the teachings of Gateway 8: Sacred Union, and she didn't even have a mate at the time! We decided that the most important thing for us in Second-Degree Training was to trust that our Spiritual Guardians and Ancestors would guarantee that we ended up in the right gate at the right time.*

*Third-Degree Sacred Woman Training truly prepares you to receive your PhD. It requires a commitment of fifty-six days devoted to putting Spirit first and foremost in your life. Since the majority of the women in my circle are employed full time and care for their families as well, Third-Degree Training is a major commitment. But with the help of our Sacred Circle—commit we did!*

In Third-Degree Sacred Woman Training, aspirants meet together in the Sacred Womb Circle to journey together through each of the Gateways of Initiation in sequential order. They perform their Daily Spiritual Observances, share experience stories, discuss their encounters with the healing presence, discuss the challenges they've faced as they incorporate the Dietary Guidelines and other elements of the Natural Living lifestyle, and rate their progress with their Seven-Day Transformative Work.

They come face-to-face with suppressed emotions and share the joy of their triumph that comes from releasing old fears and healing the feminine spirit. Aspirants experience the cumulative power of making their words Sacred, making their food Sacred, making their movement Sacred, making their beauty Sacred, making their space Sacred, making their healing Sacred, making their relationships Sacred, making their union Sacred, making their time Sacred, and making their work Sacred in order to experience the culmination of the training in Nefer Atum—Sacred Lotus Initiation, which enthrones you in your Sacred Seat of Afrakan womanhood and glory—from which they journey on to making Sacred their time and their work.

Divine Queen, with your lotus status reinstated, you will walk the earth as a fully realized Sacred Woman in contact with your inner heavenly realms. Once again it will be as it was in the beginning, when you were fully empowered. Invigorated with the memory of who you were then and who you are now, you have even greater dynamic potential because of the purity of your strong cultural and spiritual lineage.

Even with all the twists and turns of our lives, always remember that Sacred Woman was our beginning. Sacred Womanness is our home. Living as a Sacred Woman is our destiny. Everything in life works in a circle. All things come from the womb. The Sacred Spirit dwells in a Sacred Woman and she will forever rise.

Let's begin.

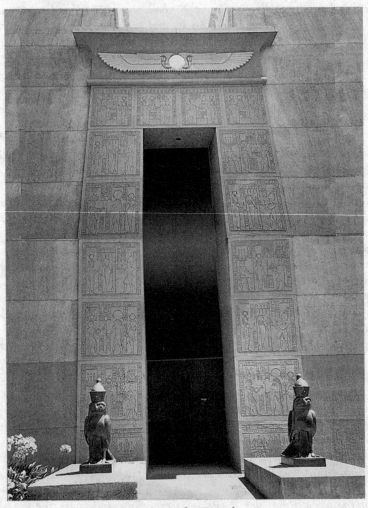

Entering the Temple

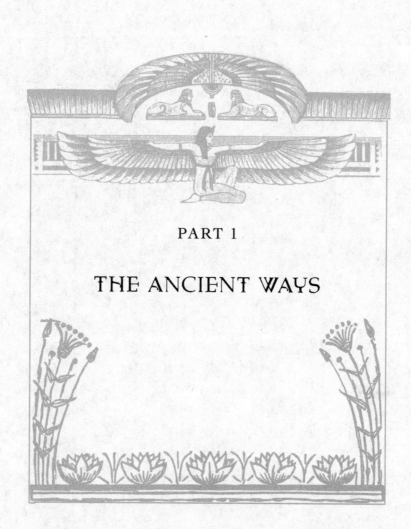

PART 1

# THE ANCIENT WAYS

# CHAPTER 1
# KHAMITIC NUBIAN PHILOSOPHY

**THEY SAY OUR WAY IS DEAD.
THEY SAY OUR WAY IS NO MORE.
THAT THE NILE VALLEY LEGACY
ALL ENDED THOUSANDS
OF YEARS AGO.
BUT WE ARE HERE,
AND WE REMEMBER!**

My people are the Elders of the earth. They are the originators of what is commonly known as "Greek philosophy," which is actually the ancient Khamitic (Egyptian) way of life. "Khamit" refers to the original Nubian Maatian culture of the Hapi (Nile) Valley Afrakans. The spelling of "Af-ra-ka" literally means "flesh [af] and soul [ka] of the hidden Sun [ra]." The more common spelling, "Africa," comes from the Arabic word *firk* or *frik*, which means separate, divide, or conquer. Like "Africa," "Egypt" is a name imposed on ancient Khamit by foreigners. The Khamitic people are the spiritual heads, teachers, motivators, and guides of the planet ordained by NTR, the One Most High Creator/Creatress.

The people of ancient Khamit had much to share thousands of years ago. We descendants and perpetuators of that sacred tradition have much to share today. The *hotep* (peaceful) ways and original holistic nature of the Khamitic people is a model that, if properly adapted, has the ability to save Planet Earth from mass destruction. It is this path, this way of life, that has so deeply inspired me and become the root of my life's work.

The ancient ways of the Khamitic people can teach all people how to become truly humane again. The Khamitic Masters came to this realization by purifying their lives. Today, as we purify our own lives, we grow closer to our divine selves, and this transformation can bring us to a state of constant bliss, peace, and wellness.

*Sacred Woman* is the entranceway I offer into that state of enlightenment. Following the path of body/mind/spirit purification can bring us to the place where we will be touched by and united with the great-great-great-grandparents of the earth—the Ancestors.

My Ancestors learned how to combine and unite the elements of earth, air, fire, water, and spirit, and they continue to teach us their methods through the carvings and inscriptions on their temple walls. They bring us the gift of the laying on of hands through the efforts of Ast (Isis) and her sister Nebt-Het (Nephthys) to restore life to the broken body of Asar (Osiris), who became a symbol of resurrection for all humanity.

Contrary to popular belief and ignorance, my Ancestors, the Black people of the Black land of the Nile Valley, did not worship many gods and goddesses. My Afrakan Ancestors viewed NTR, the Creator/Creatress, as the undifferentiated One/All-Divine from which all life emanates. However, NTR has many wondrous divine attributes, and all of these manifestations—the NTRU—are aspects of Its wholeness. Consider, for a moment, such divine emanations as Maat, the aspect of balance, harmony, truth, law, righteousness, and reciprocity; Het-Hru (Hathor), the aspect of divine love and beauty; and Nefer Atum, the Sacred Lotus, representing the highest ascension and unlimited potential. Heru (Horus) the falcon represents victory, the aspect that we can call upon to fly above all obstacles; Tehuti (Thoth) embodies the aspect of divine intelligence, and so on.

The Khamites, my ancestors, believed that within the heavenly realm the presence of the Divine is reflected in the balanced worship of NTR—the Mother/Father Creator/Creatress, where both aspects in One are given equal respect. By contrast, most present-day Western

*I will not do wrong.*
*I will not steal.*
*I will not act with violence.*
*I will not kill.*
*I will not act unjustly.*
*I will not cause pain.*
*I will not waste food.*
*I will not lie.*
*I will not desecrate holy places.*
*I will not speak evil.*
*I will not abuse my sexuality.*
*I will not cause the shedding of tears.*
*I will not sow seeds of regret.*
*I will not be an aggressor.*
*I will not act guilefully.*
*I will not lay waste the plowed land.*
*I will not bear false witness.*
*I will not set my mouth in motion*
*against any person.*
*I will not be wrathful and angry*
*except for a just cause.*
*I will not copulate with a man's wife.*
*I will not copulate with a woman's husband.*

*I will not pollute myself.*
*I will not cause terror.*
*I will not pollute the earth.*
*I will not speak in anger.*
*I will not turn from words of right and truth.*
*I will not utter curses.*
*I will not initiate a quarrel.*
*I will not be excitable or contentious.*
*I will not prejudge.*
*I will not be an eavesdropper.*
*I will not speak overmuch.*
*I will not commit treason against my Ancestors.*
*I will not waste water.*
*I will not do evil.*
*I will not be arrogant.*
*I will not blaspheme NTR, the One Most High.*
*I will not commit fraud.*
*I will not mistreat children.*
*I will not mistreat animals.*
*I will not defraud temple offerings.*
*I will not plunder the dead.*

religions recognize only the male priest and worship only a male God in a heaven of male angels. In the ancient Afrakan spiritual tradition, there is deep respect for the Mother Creatress and the female priestess as well as for the Father Creator and the male priest.

The Khamites lived the philosophy of Maat (harmony) and had respect, reverence, and honor for NTR and Its divine manifestation in man and woman and all Nature. They saw Nature and their environment as an expression of NTR, and an inspiration for self-healing—from which my "Heal Thyself" philosophy comes.

The Khamites used the element of *water* for purification rites through baptisms, fasting, and enemas. They used the element of *earth* in the form of healing foods, herbology, and aromatherapy to purify and rejuvenate the Body Temple.

My Ancestors used the element of *air*—breath—through what was called Ari Ankh Ka, now known as Hatha Yoga. The various sacred movements and poses that have been depicted on the walls of temples and pyramids were carved by my people thousands of years ago. Their records have outlasted man-made misinterpretations and outlived the libraries burned by foreigners who could not comprehend or appreciate the spiritual heights and advancement of my people.

To be recharged and purified, my people used the element of *fire* in rituals based on the powerful rays of Atn-Ra (the Sun), which blazed over the vast desert of Khamit. They used fire foods to cleanse, such as radishes, leeks, onions, and cayenne. They burned frankincense and myrrh, cinnamon and other spices, herbs, and essential oils and used them to smudge their bodies to destroy negative spiritual entities attracted to the Body Temple.

Today, we only need to look to the source of this knowledge as presented in the Forty-Two Laws of Maat.

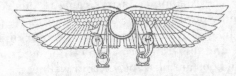

# THE FORTY-TWO LAWS OF MAAT

This moral and ethical guide is the legacy left to us by our ancient Nubian Khamitic Ancestors. Egyptologists refer to them as the "Negative Confessions" or the "Declarations of Innocence." The interpretations below came through Hru Ankh Ra Semahj, Chief Priest of the Shrine of Ptah in New York City.

Unlike the Ten Commandments, which came from an exterior power, the Forty-Two Laws of Maat inspire personal responsibility and accountability to one's own indwelling Divinity. We recite them at sunrise and sunset. In the morning we say, "I will not . . ." In the evening we say, "I have not . . ." In this way we conduct a daily moral inventory, for as Khamites, every day is Judgment Day.

*Hetepu* (Peace and Blessings).

## The Basis of Khamitic Society

Every day of my life, I maintain a healthy Body Temple as my Ancestors did before me, by blessing and consuming the four elements to protect body, mind, and spirit from disease. I activate the *element of spirit* through meditation and *hesi* (chanting). This element of spirit permeates all the elements, for NTR and Nature are One.

My earliest Ancestors were mostly vegetarians, particularly the priestesses and the priests. They understood the necessity for purity in performing spiritual work—unlike many spiritual teachers of today. The basic Khamitic diet consisted of beans, lentils, peas, barley, millet, nuts, fruits (such as dates, melons, and pomegranates), vegetables (such as onions, cabbage, and peppers), and healing herbs such as gotu kola, nettle, aloe, garlic, and parsley. And when they were invaded by Asian nomadic shepherds, the Heq Shaasu (Hyksos), more flesh foods entered the diet, thus sowing the seeds of our ultimate deterioration.

My Ancestors founded their entire society upon the Divine Spirit NTR, which kept them in a state of continual purification, meditation, wellness, and harmony of the soul, body, and mind. Everything they did was sacred and NTR-driven—from their work to their clothing, from

their relationships to their homes, temples, and government. The entire society was directed by the Forty-Two Laws of Maat, the moral code of ethics that later inspired the Ten Commandments. This belief in the sacredness of life and of all things helped them maintain a thriving nation. Like the Hunzas in the Himalayas today, my people were for thousands of years an unpoliced, peaceful people. Today, their example of a divine civilization offers us a model that could, if put into practice, create Global Healing.

## Khamitic Spiritual Practices

I rise at the hour of Nebt-Het (dawn) to call out in prayer the Forty-Two Laws of Maat to spiritually secure my day. Then I place a Maat feather in my hair to encourage me to live in right and truth throughout my day, for I am responsible for what I create.

My ancient Afrakan ancestors taught us how to love ourselves through the Divination of the Body Members, showing us that every part of us is a divine aspect of the Creator/Creatress—from our eyes of Het-Hru (beauty) to our two feet of Ptah (stability and strength). This healing ritual, which appears in our Afrakan Holy Book, the *Prt M Hru N Gher, The Book of Coming Forth by Day from Night* (misnamed *The Egyptian Book of the Dead* by Egyptologists), teaches us how to love ourselves more each day so that we can be of greater service in uplifting humanity.[1]

My Khamitic Ancestors had a powerful way of bringing our spiritual bodies into balance and healing. It was done by giving us sacred words to speak in our meditations to evoke the resurrection of our *ka* (soul). My favorite is "*Nuk pu nuk khu ami khu qemam kheperu M NTR hau*—I am that I am; a Shining Being dwelling in light, and I come from the limbs of the Most High NTR." I speak these words daily, for they make me feel spiritually confident that I am divine by nature because I am the essence of the Creator/Creatress. This fills my soul and makes me complete as a NTRT Hmt—a Sacred Woman.

My people used beauty, art, music, and dance to elevate the spirit. We were the originators of the guitar, the harp, the tambourine, and the drum. Art was seen as a beautiful, holy expression of the Divine, for my people believed that beauty and goodness are an expression of NTR, the Divine Creator/Creatress dwelling within us. So today we celebrate many ceremonies, rituals, and services artistically for the glory of NTR. To this day, our music, our voices, and our songs often tame the violent, beastly nature of all who would destroy or oppress life.

## Coming Home to Our True Selves

We are the original Lotus People, sweet, beautiful, illuminating, spiritual, and compassionate. The consciousness of one who lives in the lotus state was/is Nefer Atum, a being of pure light who evolves out of the mud of challenge, where the lotus seed is fertilized, and grows upward to blossom into a wondrously beautiful soul of light. Asar (Osiris), the first Lotus Master, is depicted on temple walls and papyrus scrolls with a lotus growing out of his feet. The priestesses were Lotus Women who wore lotus blossoms in their headbands.

Tragically, we lost our way thousands of years ago. But some of us seek to remember, to spiritually and physically grow and blossom by returning to our ancient ways. My mate is one who was touched by the ancients early in life. His first mentor was his father, James Georges (a Garveyite like my father), in Tortola, British Virgin Islands. Although he was a Christian minister, he taught and guided his son in secrecy from the age of five in our ancient Khamitic legacy, and the seed his father planted in him at such a young age has grown into a sturdy tree. Many years later, after much study and application and meditation, my husband, Sen-Ur Hru Ankh Ra Semahj, has been passing on this legacy by initiating many newly awakened Khamites into their Hapi (Nile) Valley tradition.

I myself am one of Sen-Ur's most devoted students of our ancient path. For years I kept seeking my spiritual home in many beautiful cultural and spiritual paths from other races of people. In my search I learned to love and appreciate all forms of spiritual life. Yet I was always a visitor. All those years I was on the outside looking in while I danced their dance of the spirit, chanted their words of praise, draped myself in

their garments, and spoke in a foreign tongue. But now I have been blessed to find my way back home to Self. My unique cultural expression of Divinity now lives and has its breath and being within me. I'm no longer a stranger to our ancient ways. I am soul-fulfilled because I am one with my beginnings.

After twenty years on the Path of Purification, diligently cleansing my *shai* (karma), I was blessed with a living teacher who would be my chosen mate and my guide on the pathway home. I received my Ankh, my key of life, and was initiated into my legacy by Sen-Ur Hru Ankh Ra Semahj Se Ptah, Elder, priest, and healer in Afrakan High Culture and Spiritual Life, who has initiated thousands into the ancient way of the Maatian Khamitic Nubian legacy.

I am a returning ancestor, shaking off the dust and restoring my dry bones. For my legacy says that Ankh (life) is eternal—we never die. And since I'm part of that eternity, I have been blessed to pick up where I left off thousands of years ago, because knowledge of self is in my DNA, in my melanin.

I am blessed because my people were the ones who taught the world about NTR, the One/All Creator/Creatress, about true holistic living and natural healing, and about respect for elders, nature, and community. We even taught humanity astronomy and astrology—how to read the planets and the stars. We were very spiritually attuned—before foreigners began to plague our land and our green fields, and destroy our spiritual wealth.

It is my people, the earth's Elders, who gave the world science, math, the laying on of hands, reflexology, art, music, and dance—a legacy of magnificent beauty. So it is with tremendous gratitude that we now realign ourselves with the ancient Maatian way. It brought glory to our past, and it can help us today.

## A BRIEF OVERVIEW OF PREDYNASTIC KHAMIT (EARLY EGYPT): "OUR STORY" BY HRU ANKH RA SEMAHJ

We Khamites coming into consciousness today hold in our ancestral memory a vision of the origins of Khamitic (ancient Nubian Egyptian) high culture very different from that of modern Egyptology.

One favorite Egyptological spin is the notion that Stone Age hunters fleeing a Nordic ice age wound up in the then fertile Sahara. When it dried up they migrated to the lush Nile Delta to become the founders of science, government, philosophy, religion, astronomy, architecture, and medicine.

Another favorite Egyptological belief is that the "Egyptian" people picked up the art of agriculture from the early neolithic farmers of Mesopotamia. Another error is Egyptologists' irritating tendency to speak of Afrakan and Egyptian culture as if they are two separate entities.

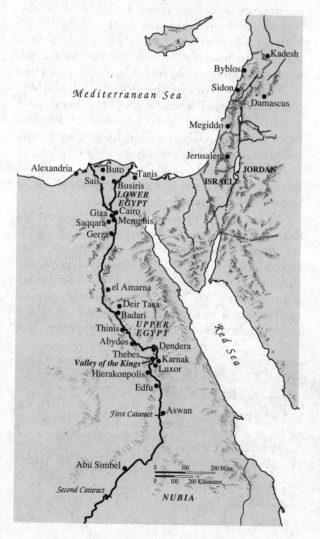

Sadly, this way of thinking seems endemic in the citadels of modern Egyptology. These scholars remain uncomfortable with anything that reveals genius coming from a central equatorial Afrakan source. Hence, terms such as "Ice Age hunters" and "Mesopotamian farmers" brainstain humanity into accepting the "gyp"tological lie of a primordial northern origin to account for the flowering of the Hapi (Nile) Valley civilization. But the Black Bones at Olduvai Gorge in Kenya (that George Leakey leaked out); the primordial bones of "Lucy" in the Afar regions of Kush (Ethiopia) and those in Monomotapa (South Africa) do not lie. Neither do the richly melanated skins of the Sahu (so-called mummies) found in the Valley of the Kings and the Valley of the Queens.

Our Annu/Twa ancestors (now insultingly labeled "pygmies") were the originators of predynastic Khamitic civilization and built the holy city of Annu (biblical On, Greek Heliopolis). These same Annu later migrated to become the Ainu of Japan and the Ta-Annu (Taino) of the West Indies.

Our exalted Afrakanubian civilization existed for untold millennia before the inhabitants of the northern zone were ever heard of. And when the northerners finally succeeded in conquering the Afrakanubian "Blameless ones"—whether Chambysis the Persian (525 BCE), the Greek Alexander (330 BCE), or the Romans Antony and Caesar (30 BCE)—they lacked the cultural and spiritual astuteness to sustain the Maatian (righteous) principles that made Khamitic civilization so lasting and great.

If one honestly seeks to learn the originators of Khamitic culture and civilization, it is to the oral history and oldest writing of Khamites themselves that one must go. In sections of *The Book of Coming Forth by Day from Night* (the so-called *Egyptian Book of the Dead*), in the Pyramid Text and in the Coffin Texts, my ancestors continuously refer to a star-born origin. The kings and queens who sat on the Lion's Throne of Heru (Horus) in the Hapi (Nile) Valley called themselves Sa-Ra (Son of the Sun) and Sat-Ra (Daughter of the Sun), respectively. Our first earth mother, Ast (Isis), was born from the Star SPDT (called Sirius); our first earth father, Asar

7

(Osiris), was born in the constellation of Sah (Orion). We Afrakans were star trekkers for untold thousands of years before Captain Kirk's *Star Trek*. Listen to Mut Hetep (Mother Peace), a Queen of the Fifth Dynasty, in a quote from her own papyrus (British Museum #10,010, Sheet 3):

> I have come forth from between the thighs of divinity (NTRU) I have been conceived by Sekhmet and I have been brought forth at the door of the STAR SPDT (Sirius) the foremost who is Long of Strides along the celestial path of Ra day after day.[2]

Listen to another Khamite (from a *sesh* [papyrus] at Paris):

> I rise like a mighty star in the Star World. Let me journey through it like the Son of Ra. . . . I am Hru—heir of Asar. I have received his Nemes crown in the Star World.[3]

To this very day the Dogon people of Mali—who trace their beginnings to the Hapi (Nile) Valley—still celebrate the orbital cycles of Sirius "B" around Sirius "A." They call Sirius "B" Potolo, the Seed Star.

Modern Egyptologists, such as Martin Bernal, the author of *Black Athena: The Afroasiatic Roots of Classical Civilization,* now admit that the people who created the early Egyptian civilization flowed from the sources of the River Hapi in Kush (Ethiopia) and Khenset (Nubian Sudan). Because southern origins are unmistakably black and Afrakan, some European Egyptologists have held that Egypt is in the Middle East.

That Egypt is part of the entire Afrakan continent is evident to all except the most voluntarily blind.

Any researcher who attempts to present a brief outline of Khamitic history is confronted by a mass of Egyptologian gobbledygook of foreign names and conflicting time lines, dynasties, and data. However, they all seem to toe the line of a first dynasty beginning at 3100 BCE.

One who graduates out of Egyptology to embrace Khamitology soon discovers, though, that the Khamitic mind deals with past, present, and future simultaneously. The story of Khamit is a cyclical one. As the Western world enters its third millennium, anyone of Khamitic consciousness who needs to celebrate dates has countless beginnings to choose from. In 10,500 BCE the Spdtian Nubian Khamites of the Hapi (Nile) Valley unified to build HRU-M-AKHET (the Sphinx) to honor Sekhmet, the lioness cosmic mother healer who had rid the land of the enemies of Maat, the Isfitians (historically called Heq-Shaasu [Hyksos], nomadic shepherd worshipers of Seth, NTR of the desert and storms). In 4240 BCE, the Hru (King) Nrmr known to Egyptologists as the "Pharaoh Narmer" or "Menes," reinstituted a lost unity and declared the Smai (unification) of Tawi (the two regions)—Khamit and Khenset (Egypt and Nubia/Kush).

In the year 2000, if we choose the provable date of an Age of Leo beginning (10,500 BCE), we would be at the halfway mark of our thirteenth millennium, 12,500 PH (Post HU—the Sphinx). If we choose Nrmr's 4240 BCE, the beginning of the Age of Taurus, we are at the one-quarter mark of our seventh millennium—since the reunification (Smai Tawi) by Nrmr, this

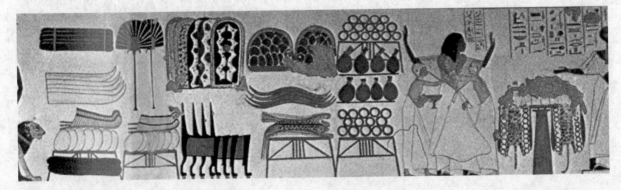

would be 6240 ST (Smai Tawi). If we choose to date from King Tutankhamen, it would be 3373 SA (since Atn-Ra).

How long have Khamites been on Planet Earth? Our traditions say, "From the first times." So we are not confused by conjectured Egyptological dates.

We look at our story to gather the lessons of our past errors so that we may correct them. But most important, we gather the enduring values of Maat (righteous healing with truth, light, and order), that we may live them and practice them.

The evidence of Khamitic glory and downfall has been captured on temple walls and *sesh* (papyrus). Khamit rose and fell because no civilization can escape the law of cycles. (What goes around comes around. What goes up comes down to rise again.) People ask, "If the ancient Egyptians were so great, how or why did they fall?" Just let them reflect and meditate on the law of cycles.

Some of the signs of the pending fall from glory are mirrored on the walls in the killing of animals for food and sacrifice, and in the killing of humans in war. The walls are replete with the story of a gloriously peaceful civilization forced to make chariots (which they did not invent) to defend themselves from the northern Asiatics and the southern Isfitians, who worked against the principles of Maat (order, righteousness, and reciprocity).

We focus on times of Smai Tawi (Unity) as our model because where there is unity, there is healing taking place. Today, humanity is disunified, therefore sick with violence, pestilence, and war. It must be healed! The rebirth of the Smai Tawi Nubian Khamitic Maat paradigm is

upon us. Once we overcome the Egyptological preoccupation with dates and dynasties, then all humanity can have access to the Smai Tawi: Heal Thyself—Know Thyself—Mer (love) Thyself—Be Thyself Maatian way of ascension and renaissance.

Oh, Khamit, what historical lies have been told of you through your present-day distorted name—Egypt! Oh, Nubian Kushite Khamitic Ancestors, Western man is claiming that he came from the north to build the pyramids (with "bricks and straw," thanks to Hollywood). Ann Baxter is Nefertiti, and Yul Brynner is Ramses. Hollywood's *Star Gate* has desecrated Ra as an epicene demon, and the "Mummy's Curse" has been unleashed, in a sorry effort to sow doubt and fear among people, all of whom need Maat (truth, righteousness, and fairness) in their lives. But they will fail to know it, because Maat is a principle hidden behind the gates of a cosmic divine high culture whose door was supposed to remain sealed by the invention of the word sound "Egypt." The biblical curses against "Egypt" would scare most people away from discovering the glittering heritage that awaits their claim.

For an even older version of our creation story, one can examine the Shabaka Stone (now preserved in the British Museum in London, England). It tells us that Ptah/Sekhmet, great Mother/Father Creator/Creatress, became the first ruler/guide of the Khamitians. Ptah and Sekhmet established the Hesepu (Nomes, the "states" or administrative divisions of the country) and constructed the temples and shrines. They fashioned the statues and figurines of the NTRU and put them in their places (Egyptologists refer to this time as the "Rule of the Gods").

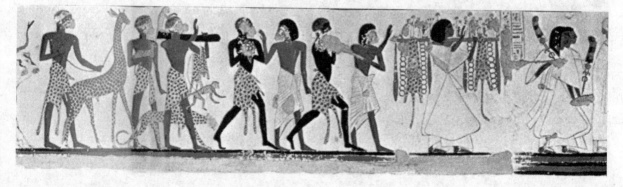

The Shabaka Stone also refers to the drowning of Asar (Osiris) and his resuscitation by his wife Ast (Isis) and her sister Nebt-Het (Nephthys).

The lives of the citizens of Khamit were centered around the temple, much like the state capitol or city hall of modern times. Reverence for the Divine permeated all aspects of life in Khamit. The culture was spiritual, not religious. Religion is modern, whereas spirituality is primordial. The very word "religion" is drawn from the Latin word *religare* or *religio,* which means to tie back or to tie again. Since the Khamites saw their lives as intrinsically connected to Divinity, there was no reason to be tied. It was those who saw themselves as alienated from the Divine who invented religion and its attendant competitive dogmas to tie them fast to their spiritual vision.

Khamitic consciousness perceives itself as surrounded, enveloped, saturated, nurtured, and immersed in divinity, like the fish in the ocean. Khamites had no need to invent religion. Spiritual immersion was the mode of existence. This view empowered our Khamitic ancestors.

They entertained no doctrine of salvation by proxy. Maat demands personal responsibility and accountability. There is no vicarious atonement. When you live in Maat, every day is judgment day.

Another fatal error of Egyptology is the use of the terms "gods" and "goddesses" to describe the attributes, aspects, and differentiations of NTR (Divinity). Western concepts of divinity give us an objective male God up in heaven somewhere ruling over a hierarchy of all male angels and little boy cherubs. This will never do for the Khamite.

From the beginning, Khamitic cosmology was Maatical (balanced). It taught of NTR, a Mother/Father Creator/Creatress. The NTRU (Divine Attributes) were likewise feminine and masculine, for example, Ptah/Sekhmet, Amen-Ra/Mut, Tehuti/Maat, Ast/Asar. This way of viewing the Divine that filtered down into everyday life was *Maat*riarchal, and women enjoyed a measure of equality unduplicated in these so-called modern times. The Greeks and Romans were appalled at the level of freedom of Khamitic women, who could own property and function as queens, high priestesses, and living oracles.

The lineage of kings was transmitted through the mother, as was inheritance. The Maatocracy (righteous government) of the ancient Khamites eclipsed the democracy of modern times, whose hallmark has been the suppression and oppression of women, coupled with a pervasive undercurrent of racism.

In order to begin to understand the spirituality of the ancient Khamites, it is important to open your consciousness and familiarize yourself with the Khamitic cosmological legacy that created the Maatocracy. If you pray for guidance as you experience the Gateways of Initiation, you will discover what your Khamitic ancestors always knew: that your so-called spiritual life and your "normal" life are truly one.

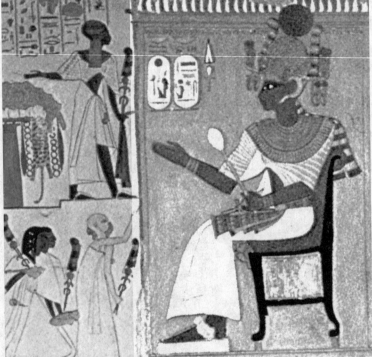

Every day is Judgment Day.

# THE NTRU: ANCIENT KHAMITIC NUBIAN SPIRITUAL ENERGIES

**Asar** (Osiris): Husband of Ast; resurrection, re-constitution, renewal of life.

**Ast** (Isis): Mother of Hru; Great Mother Afrakan Spirit; culture bringer, healer.

**Atn-Ra** (Aten/Ra/Sun): Element of Fire; Revealed Light of the Hidden Sun (Ra).

**Bast** (Bastet): Cat; masked sistrum bearer who disperses adverse energy.

**Bes:** Principle of expansion; guardian of dance.

**Geb:** Element of Earth; consort of Nut; father of Asar (Osiris).

**Hapi:** River Nile; Guardian of Lungs; Khamite name of Aquarius.

**Heru** (Horus): Sacred Warrior of Light and Victory; the faculty of Will.

**Het-Hru** (Hathor): Divine love, beauty, protection, and nurturing.

**Imhotep:** Sacred architect, physician-healer, and philosopher.

**Maat:** Truth, harmony, balance, law, righteousness, sobriety, propriety, cosmic order.

**Meshkenet** (Meshkent): Birth/rebirth; Guardian of the Womb and the birthing bricks.

**Mut:** "Eye of Ra"; consort of Amen-Ra; the personal mother principle.

**Nebt-Het** (Nephthys): Sister of Isis; protectress; midwife; Guardian of Breath.

**Nefer Atum:** Highest Ascension; unlimited potential; the Khamite Adam.

**Neith:** Weaver, warrior, defender.

**Nu:** Element of Water.

**Nun:** Primordial Waters.

**Nut** (Sky): Consort of Geb; Great Cosmic Sky Mother; Grandmother of all Gateways and re-births.

**Ptah:** Creativity; guardian of craftspeople.

**Renenet:** Name Giver; guardian of good fortune.

**Renenutet:** Sacred Cobra; nourishment, harvest.

**Sekhmet:** Consort of Ptah; lioness patron of healers.

**Selket:** Protector of organs of regeneration; guardian of small intestines.

**Sesheta** (Seshat): Consort of Tehuti; patroness of writing, architecture.

**Seth** (Osiris's Brother): Consort of Nebt-Het; strength, lord of desert, darkness, storms, usurper.

**Shu:** Element of Air; guardian of the winds; consort of Tefnut.

**Ta-Urt** (Taweret): Great Earth Mother.

**Tefnut:** Guardian of water and moisture.

**Tehuti** (Thoth): Moon, Divine Intelligence, Lord of Time; inventor of writing; patron of scribes.

# GLOSSARY OF ANCIENT KHAMITIC TERMS

**Ankh.** Symbol of Life; key of eternity and unity.

**Ari Ankh Ka.** Egyptian poses of power; predates yoga.

**Arit, Aritu.** Chakra, chakras; subtle Body Temple energy centers.

**Hesi.** Praise chants (mantras); Nubi-sonics.

**Hetepu.** "Peace unto you"; also, altar offerings, gifts.

**Hotep.** Peace, calm, tranquility; offerings.

**Ka.** Soul.

**Khamit, Kham, Khm.** Ancient Egypt.

**Khepera.** Transformation, evolution, metamorphosis.

**Mtu NTR.** Hieroglyphic language; words divine, literally, the Words of God.

**Mut.** Mother.

**NTR.** The All One, Divine Mother/Father Creator/Creatress.

**NTRT Hmt.** Sacred Woman.

**NTRU.** Sacred Aspects of NTR, the Creator/Creatress, such as Ast, Maat, Sekhmet.

**Prt M Hru M Gher.** *The Book of Coming Forth by Day from Night* (*Egyptian Book of the Dead*).

**Seneb.** Health, soundness, wellness.

**Sesh.** Papyrus.

**Shai.** Karma, destiny.

**Smai Tawi.** Union of the Double Regions.

**Sunnutu.** Physicians.

**Tua-k, Tua-Tu.** "Thank you."

**Tua NTR.** "Praise Divine."

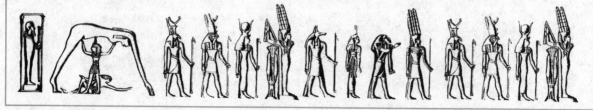

### Prayer for the "Wombniverse"

I call upon the Divine Creator/Creatress to protect
my womb and the wombs of our daughters.
Heal our wombs from all wickedness. From this
day forward we must speak up for and guard our
wombs with all our inner power as we call on the
ancient Afrakan spirit of Meshkenet, Afrakan
Guardian Angel of the Sacred Womb.
I call upon the Afrakan spirit of Maat, for
womb balance and wellness.
I call upon the spirit Het-Hru within me, to demonstrate
divine love of my womb and absolute harmony.
I call upon the spirit Tehuti within me, so that I may make wise
decisions on behalf of my womb's restoration.
I call upon Ast, the Great Afrakan Mother Spirit within me,
to inspire the continuous nurturing of my sacred womb. I affirm
that all abuse and desecration of the womb are to be no more.
My womb speaks and commands peace upon the earth and
throughout the "wombniverse."
Through the healing of my womb all wars shall cease. Through the
healing of my womb all men and wombmen shall be at peace. Earth
Mother, because of the peace within my womb, tidal waves,
hurricanes, tornadoes, volcanic eruptions, floods, and earthquakes
shall cease. According to my womb there will be peace, for it is my
womb that is the spiritual coordinator of all activity on this
sacred earth and all the worlds within the
wombniverse. Women, guard your womb and
guard it well, so wickedness will no
longer exist.

According to my womb, Peace.

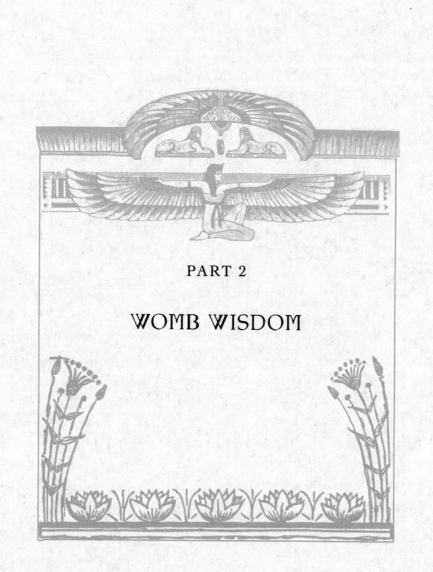

# PART 2

# WOMB WISDOM

## CHAPTER 2

# GATEWAY O: THE SACRED WOMB

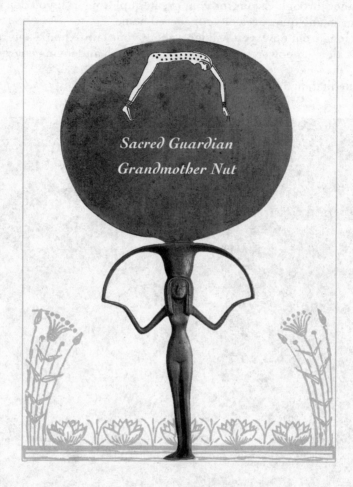

Sacred Guardian
Grandmother Nut

**Ancestors**

Biddy Mason

Queen Mother
Moore

**Elders**

Aunt Iris O'Neal

Dr. Josephine
English

**Contemporaries**

Dr. Jewel Pookrum

Nonkululeko
Tyehemba

## CREATING YOUR SACRED ALTAR

Your altar should be placed in a room undisturbed by the public. A private prayer area is best—a place where you, your family, and attuned friends can go to pray. This is the designated area where you will commune with the Creator/Creatress, receive spiritual, mental, and emotional comfort, and gain inner guidance through visions for your greater upliftment. If you don't have such a room, then set up your altar in any quiet area of your sacred home.

One day not too long from now, you will look about your entire home and realize with joy that every room is like an altar, empowered with your sacred touch and loving energy from the indwelling Sacred Spirit.

In your chosen meditation area, place the table for your altar.

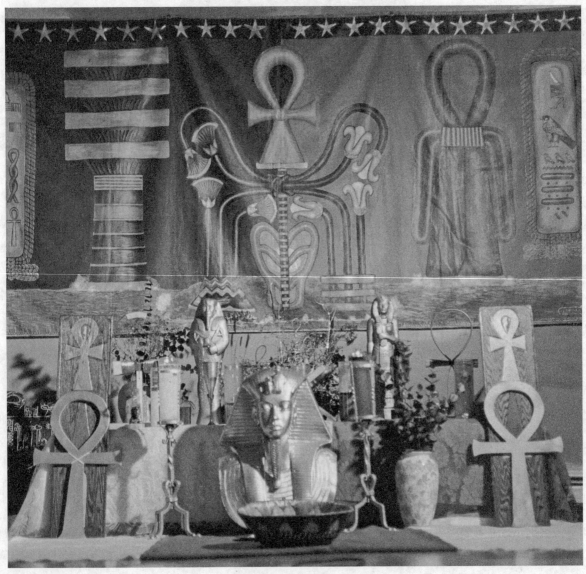

Altar Offerings

# SACRED WOMB ALTAR WORK
## Face Your Heart to the East—to the Rising Sun
### (Layout from top view)

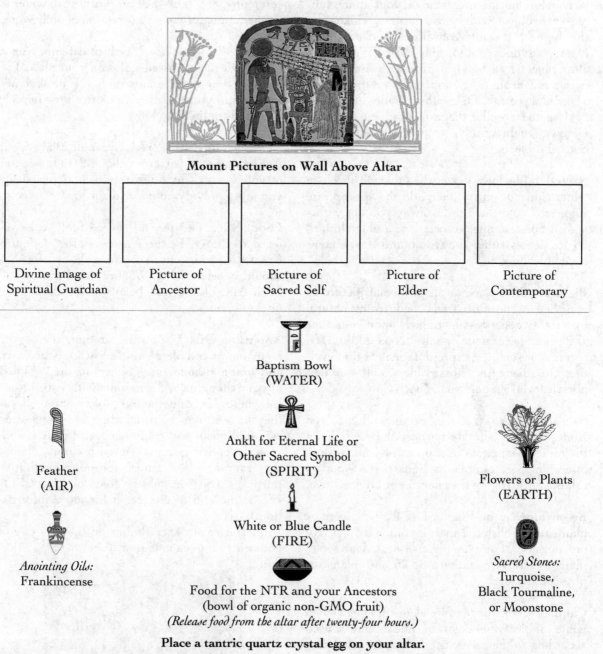

**Mount Pictures on Wall Above Altar**

| Divine Image of Spiritual Guardian | Picture of Ancestor | Picture of Sacred Self | Picture of Elder | Picture of Contemporary |

Baptism Bowl
(WATER)

Feather
(AIR)

Ankh for Eternal Life or
Other Sacred Symbol
(SPIRIT)

Flowers or Plants
(EARTH)

White or Blue Candle
(FIRE)

*Anointing Oils:*
Frankincense

*Sacred Stones:*
Turquoise,
Black Tourmaline,
or Moonstone

Food for the NTR and your Ancestors
(bowl of organic non-GMO fruit)
*(Release food from the altar after twenty-four hours.)*

**Place a tantric quartz crystal egg on your altar.**

Sacred tablecloth (white or blue) and scarf or prayer shawl to wear during altar work.
Sacred color cloth to lay before altar with your sacred instruments to be
played as you pray, i.e., harp (zither), drum, bell, rattle, etc.

# SACRED ALTAR PREPARATION

Remember to purify all of your Sacred Altar objects before positioning them on your altar. Handle each object with consciousness, emanating the highest possible vibrations and intention from your body, mind, and spirit. Wash each altar object in a bowl of purified water mixed with a few drops of frankincense and myrrh and a pinch of sea salt. Dry with a clean white cloth.

Use the specific diagram outlined for each Gateway to direct the placement of each of your Sacred Objects.

**Sacred Tablecloth.** Cover the table with a clean white cloth for purity, then add the appropriate suggested color for the Gateway you are working in. For example, you can use a blue cloth to create peace within the womb and lessen menstrual bleeding.

**Pictures.** First place an inspirational picture of your Self in a beautiful frame made from a natural material (wood, crystal, or glass) upon your altar as a reminder of your divinity. Next add framed pictures or symbolic representations of the Spiritual Guardian, Ancestors, Elders, and Contemporaries who support you at each Gateway.

**Sacred Stones.** Place the recommended sacred stones on your altar to harness the energies of the mineral kingdom in support of your healing intention. For example, rose quartz is a wonderful tool for invoking the energies of Divine Love.

**Fresh Flowers or Plants.** Use fresh flowers or plants to establish the energies of the living earth on your altar. For example, use an African violet plant to banish negativity or an aloe plant for physical healing.

**Candles.** To honor the Fire element, light a small white candle. Other colors of candles may be used according to the recommendations for the Gateway. For safety, if you are using a large seven-day candle, place it in a bowl of water in a safe place on your altar. Never leave a candle burning when you're away from home. Blow it out upon completion of your spiritual observances.

**Baptism Bowl.** Fill a crystal or wooden bowl with purified water to absorb negativity in the environment. Pour out the water after each altar ceremony, and refill the bowl with fresh water at the beginning of your next session of altar work.

**Feather.** Gently place a beautiful feather on a small pedestal or raised stand on your altar. The feather represents maintaining your balance throughout your journey no matter how fiercely the winds of life may blow.

**Ankh or Other Sacred Symbol.** Place your Ankh on a small velvet or silk cloth in the center of your altar. The Ankh represents eternal life and unity in body, mind, and spirit.

**Food.** Rinse and dry all sacred food to be offered to the NTR, the Mother/Father Creator/Creatress, and your Ancestors. Your offerings should consist of high-quality dried grains and fresh fruit placed in a beautiful wooden, glass, or clay bowl.

**Anointing Oils.** Use a small amount of essential oil to anoint and bless your forehead, your heart, and your abdomen, thus connecting the "wombs" of your thoughts and emotions with your physical womb. Use only the finest of essential oils, as they have a high spiritual vibration. Suggested essential oils: rose, frankincense, myrrh, cinnamon, lavender, jasmine. As with colors, choose the fragrance best suited for your meditative purposes. (See the master chart on pages 130–135 at the end of chapter 5 for more information.)

Refresh your sacred altar on the first day of your entry into each Gateway.

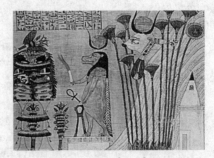

Preparing the Altar

# AND I CALL MYSELF
# A WOMBMAN

*Nekhena Evans, Sacred Woman Initiate*

How can I become a "Wombman"
when I don't know my womb?
I have never had a conversation with my womb
so how can I consider myself a Wombman?
I have been with you . . . grown with you,
been through Rites of Passage with you
from childhood, to adolescence, to adulthood, and yet . . .
I have never had a conversation with you.
You have been a victim. A consequence to an action.
A symptom of a disease.
An effect of my action.
I have never spoken to you. Consulted with you.
Inquired of you. Cared for you.
Or understood you.
And I call myself a grown Wombman.
Where have I grown? How could I have grown without talking with you?
Without acknowledging your presence and your works?
And I call myself a Wombman.
I have put you through dozens of men . . .
alien spirits/beings/entities . . . of all dimensions,
from all places and stations.
I have created and destroyed babies through you.
I have fed you all kinds of poisons, thereby creating diseases—
fibroids, tumors, cysts, and the like.
I have sexually abused you, thereby creating sexually transmitted diseases . . .
infections of all types, itching . . . burning . . . hurting . . . PAIN!
I have used you for my own purposes . . .
money, favors, alleged self-esteem, beauty, clothing, food.
I have allowed men to probe you,
doctors to drug you, while I held you down.
If I had known someone who had done all these things
I would call them the names I despise the most—
MURDERER, THIEF, LIAR, BETRAYER, DEMON.
Yes, I would . . .
And I call myself a Wombman.
Time to release. RELEASE, RELEASE.
FORGIVE ME. FORGIVE ME. FORGIVE ME.
I am complete.
I will be responsible for you, for myself . . . for my womb.
We are in relationship together.
We have been from the very, very beginning.
I will commune and communicate with you.
I will listen to you.
I will wash, cleanse, and purify you.
I will pay attention to your patterns, your moods, your signs and wonders.
I will . . . I will . . . I will . . . become the Wombman
that you made me from the beginning.

**Gateway Element: Water**

The Sacred Womb is the Gateway to all Gateways.

Each Gateway represents a spiritual exercise of ascension. The practices offered for Gateway 0: The Sacred Womb are to be performed daily for a minimum of twenty-one days to a maximum of four months. Disciplining yourself to honor this path will awaken your inner Gateways of Divinity so that you may blossom and establish your full sacred center.

The Sacred Womb lays a foundation of womb wellness that will serve as your preparation for the Gateways of Initiation. Through the twenty-one-day training, you will learn how to cleanse toxic thoughts, foods, and attitudes out of your divine Body Temple. You will present to your womb the gift of Wellness Philosophy. This includes the Natural Living approach to food, Womb Rejuvenation Techniques, womb affirmations, and womb meditations for total attunement.

### 1. The Spiritual Bath

Begin your journey into Gateway 0 by entering the depths of the ocean. One way to honor this intention is to create a dawn ritual of taking a spiritual bath with Epsom salts or Dead Sea salts when you rise between the hours of 4 A.M. and 6 A.M.

Make a ceremony out of your bath—light candles and incense, have soft, inspiring music playing. Bless your bathwater. Use the bath to release all negativity, everything that blocks the free movement of light, love, healing, and peace through your Sacred Womb and Body Temple.

Add the essential oil of frankincense to the bathwater to open your crown *arit* (chakra). Frankincense attunes you to the Divine Oneness of NTR inspiration and divine wisdom, and brings forth the Divinity and the sacredness of the womb. It eliminates confusion and depression. Place seven drops of frankincense oil in your bathwater. Also add seven drops of frankincense to a bowl of purified water on your altar

and sprinkle a few drops around your prayer space.

### 2. Your Altar

Set up your altar according to the altar preparation guidelines on page 18 and sit before it quietly and meditatively on the floor on a pillow, or in a comfortable chair.

*Anoint with frankincense.* Select only pure essential oils. Use essential oil of frankincense to anoint your crown and your third eye (in the center of your forehead between the brows), the Body Temple Gateway of supreme spirituality. Next, anoint the heart (the Body Temple Gateway of compassion and divine love). Also anoint your womb area, the palms of your hands (to make everything you touch become more sacred), and the bottoms of your feet (to spiritually align yourself for stepping out in power, promise, and faith).

*Sacred musical instrument.* Softly play a sacred instrument (drum, sistrum, shekere) to awaken the indwelling angelic host. Or you might want to use a small, clear-toned bell at that early hour, out of respect for the others sleeping in your household.

### 3. Opening the Gateway

In your prayers to each of the Gateway Guardians you may use whatever words pour from your heart. For example, here's a prayer that might be used to "Open the Way" to Gateway 0:

*Sacred and Divine Nut, Spiritual Guardian of the Gateway of the Sacred Womb, please accept my deepest gratitude for your healing presence on my altar and in my life. Thank you for your guidance and inspiration, and for your love and blessings, and please accept my love and blessings in return.* Hetepu.

### 4. Libation

A libation is the act of pouring a liquid such as water or spirits (alcohol) as a holy offering to the One Creator/Creatress. In Sacred Woman practices we use purified water that we have blessed and offered ceremonially to the Most High. For the libation in Gateway 0, pour a small amount of water from a cup, or sprinkle a few drops with your fingers from a bowl or calabash onto the earth (if you're outside), or onto a potted plant on your altar. As you pour your libation, call out this prayer of adoration (the details will change with each Gateway, but not the intent):

*I pour this libation in praise and adoration of the Sacred Mother Guardian of Gateway 0,* Nut, the Great Cosmic Mother.

*I pour this libation in praise and adoration of the Ancestors of Gateway 0,* Biddy Mason and Queen Mother Moore.

*I pour this libation in praise and adoration of the Elders of Gateway 0,* Aunt Iris O'Neal and Dr. Josephine English.

*I pour this libation in praise and adoration of my Divine Self and my Divine Contemporaries* Dr. Jewel Pookrum and Nonkululeko Tyehemba.

## 5. Sacred Woman Spirit Prayer

Gently ring your bell, or softly play another sacred instrument at the beginning and end of the prayer.

*Sacred Spirit, NTR, hold me near, close to your bosom. Protect me from all harm and fear, from the blows of life. Direct my steps in the right way as I journey through this vision. Sacred Spirit, surround me in your absolutely perfect light. Anoint me in your sacred purity, peace, and divine insight. Bless me, truly bless me, as I share this sacred life. Teach me, Sacred Spirit, to be in tune with the Universe. Teach me how to heal with the inner and outer elements of air, fire, water, and earth.*

## 6. Sacred Womb Prayer

Again, gently ring your bell, or softly play another sacred instrument at the beginning and end of the prayer.

*Divine Mother, give me the power to heal my womb. Bless the wombs of all your daughters, and assist us in the healing of our wombs. Restore our faith that we may grow in strength, power, and knowledge as we recapture the purity and sacredness of our womb. May the wombs in all women be born again to the eternal heights as womb healing and wellness spread over each and every land.*

## 7. Chanting Hesi

Chant this *hesi* from the first language, Mtu NTR, four times:

Nuk Pu Ntrt Hmt—*I am a Sacred Woman.*

## 8. Fire Breaths

Prepare for your Fire Breathing (rapid breathing) by slowly inhaling four times and slowly exhaling four times. Then, when you are totally at ease, begin your Fire Breaths. Allow each deep Fire Breath to represent the opening of the thousand-petaled lotus of illumination and radiance that will ultimately allow you to reach Nefer Atum—the ultimate Afrakan Lotus Gateway of Divinity. In Gateway 0, you will begin with fifty to one hundred Fire Breaths. And with each new Gateway, you will add a hundred more Fire Breaths until you are performing one thousand breaths of power and light.

**How to Do Fire Breaths**
- With your mouth closed, inhale deeply like a pump through your nostrils as you expand the breath down into the abdomen, then back up to expand the chest.
- Then, exhale fully as your abdomen contracts and the lungs release your breath completely.
- Practice the Fire Breath a few times slowly, and then do it fifty times as rapidly as you can fully inhale and exhale.

*Note:* If you should become light-headed or slightly breathless, which is called hyperventilating, simply breathe into a small paper bag—*not* plastic—held over your nose and mouth for a few minutes, to restore your carbon dioxide balance.

The more you practice the Fire Breath, the more you will build your capacity to do it, and so receive its amazing energizing and restorative benefits.

## 9. Gateway 0: Sacred Womb Meditation

Each day of the twenty-one days you spend working through Gateway 0, increase the length of time you spend in meditation. The longer you are in meditation, the deeper your inner peace will be, and the more vibrant your *ka* (spirit) will become. The cleaner your Body Temple, the sooner it will be able to live permanently in the peace and inner balance of the meditative state.

**The Sacred Womb Meditation**
- Visualize yourself sitting on a lotus bed rooted in the very core of your sacred center.
- Begin your attunement with Womb Wisdom right now by breathing in Nut, the Cosmic Sky Mother and the Sacred Guardian of the Womb.
- Inhale and allow Nut to breathe a blue light of serenity into your womb. Then exhale as you release and purge out emotional and spiritual blockages and toxic substances from your womb, your seat of creation and creativity. Repeat seven times.
- Now breathe in four counts, and exhale eight counts. Witness the power of womb healing, stability, and radiance flourishing as your womb grows into and learns to maintain a sense of well-being.
- Now, bless the womb of your mind, the womb of your heart, and the womb of your Sacred Seat.

**Sacred Healing Color and Stone Work**
*Color Visualization.* Visualize the color of the Gateway you're in. In Gateway 0, which honors the element of water, visualize white or blue for purification and serenity. As you perform your meditation, wear white or blue and place a white or blue cloth on your altar.

*Sacred Stone Meditation.* Hold in your palm over your womb one or all of the sacred healing stones of Gateway 0: *moonstone, turquoise,* and *black tourmaline.*

- *Moonstone* opens us up to our true femininity so that we can become one with our divine selves. Moonstone also aids in relief from tumors. It is connected to the moon and the female aspect of a woman's emotional nature.
- *Turquoise* is a symbol of the blue sky. It raises the spirit and brings us to spiritual heights on earth and in the heavenly realms. It is a blue-green semiprecious stone that gives us wisdom and brings good fortune. It can absorb negative feelings and vibrations and sends healing to the wearer. This gem represents the fifth *arit* (chakra), or energy center, which regulates the throat, which aids in divine communication, particularly when performing morning meditation between 4 A.M. and 6 A.M.
- *Black tourmaline* contains protective energy against negativity, and helps to ground you and attune you to the earth.

### 10. *Herbal Tonics*
Drink herbal tea while you're doing your altar, prayer work, and journal work in Gateway 0. Use the Heal Thyself Woman's Herbal Formula (see the product list in the appendix) for General Womb Wellness.

Dandelion tea, made from the plant's roots and leaves (*Taraxacum officinale*), is another useful tonic for Gateway 0, as it strengthens the womb. It also purifies and destroys acids in the blood, and is good for anemia.

Drink your tea for twenty-one days to receive the full benefits of attuning to Gateway 0. Enjoy your herb tea in your favorite mug during or after spiritual writing. Be sure to finish the tea before 1 P.M.

*Preparation.* Use one teabag or 1 teaspoon loose tea to 8 ounces of water boiled in a nonmetallic pot. Boil water, turn off flame, then add tea and steep. Strain herbs from water. Drink before or after your morning bath or sacred shower. Drink with joy and peace as you breathe quietly between sips, and settle into easy contemplation.

### 11. *Flower Essences*
To center, deepen, and stabilize your experience in each Gateway, work with the recommended flower essences. Flower essences are vibrational remedies that heal when a few drops of the potentized essence of aromatic flowers are placed on or under the tongue or in a small glass of water that is sipped at regular intervals. Flower essences are primarily recommended to restore balance to mental and emotional states and can offer wonderful support as we work on remov-

ing the obstacles that stand in the way of our self-healing.

*How to choose an essence.* Select among the recommended essences by reviewing the definition of the essence and matching it to the mental or emotional state you want to address. You can also use your intuition, muscle testing, or a pendulum to select from a group of essences.

*Dosage.* Place 4 drops of the recommended essence on or under the tongue or add the same amount to a small glass of purified water. Also review the characteristic qualities of the essence(s) you are working with and reflect on the impact of the essence on your state of mind and emotions. Record your observations in your Sacred Womb Journal.

*Flower essences for Gateway 0.* As presented in *Flower Essence Repertory: A Comprehensive Guide to North American and English Flower Essences for Emotional and Spiritual Well Being,* by Patricia Kaminski and Richard Katz (for this and all subsequent Gateways):

- *Alpine lily:* Promotes the ability to contact true femininity through grounding in the female organs; the integration of the feminine with the female sexual and biological self.
- *Pomegranate:* Creative expression of the feminine aspect of the Self both in procreation and in worldly creativity.
- *Star tulip:* Spiritual receptivity, opening the feminine aspect of the self to higher worlds.
- *Black-Eyed Susan:* Clearer insight into hidden or buried emotions.
- *Angelica:* To feel protected and guided, to feel spiritual guardianship during times of stress.

## 12. Diet and Movement

Daily, follow the Sacred Woman Natural Living Dietary Laws given in the Womb Wellness Cleansing Food Plan (see page 72) and do the Dance of the Womb movements presented in Gateway 3.

## 13. Sacred Journal Writing

Journal writing is best done after your sacred bath, and/or internal cleansing (with an enema), and/or meditation. When you are cleansed and centered, you can receive spiritual messages from the One Most High with grace. When in the spirit, messages travel down through your spirit mind, to your heart, into your hand, and onto the paper. (This is how I do all my writing.)

The best time to receive your spiritually written work is after you have completed your altar work, between the hours of 4 A.M. and 6 A.M. Keep a very special pen and journal by or on your altar to work with the power, force, and stillness at the coming of dawn.

At this time, write in your journal the thoughts, activities, experiences, and interactions that occurred previously in your daily life. You might also want to write down your self-inspired hopes, visions, desires, and affirmations so that you can draw on them for help and support when needed. You'll be surprised at how healing and sustaining your journal wisdom can be.

## 14. Senab Freedom Shawl or Quilt

As you enter Gateway 0, choose the Sacred Cloth that will serve as the canvas for your spiritual garment. This cloth will serve as the backdrop on which you create your Senab Freedom Shawl or Quilt (see pages 122–125). You will begin preparing the sewing materials you will need to continue your Senab quilt or shawl work throughout the Gateways of Initiation.

## 15. Sacred Tools

Wooden table or raised platform to establish the foundation for your Sacred Altar. Materials needed to set up your Gateway 0: The Sacred Womb Altar (see page 18).

## 16. Sacred Reminder

Throughout the next twenty-one days, you are to observe closely the wisdom presented in Gateway 0. For maximum results, live freely in tune with the various systems of body, mind, and spirit wellness presented.

### Closing Sacred Words

*Divine Creator/Creatress, help me to honor and treat my womb in a most sacred way. Thank you for all the blessings you have granted me on this sacred journey.*

## TO THE KEEPERS
## OF THE SACRED WOMB

Womb Wisdom is women's work, so say the ancients. As Earth Mothers from the original heavenly realms of Nut, we have the ability and responsibility to heal ourselves with natural ways using the elements of air, fire, water, and earth. Men do not have this power, nor is it their destiny to heal our wombs. Men need only to love, respect, support, come through, and give reverence to our wombs. Men can only support what women first establish through the renewal of their sacred wombs—the natural foundation of our self-discovery and recovery.

When our wombs are restored through the steady, unrelenting transformation of our thoughts and our hearts and our blood, then and only then will the destiny of the earth rise again. Due to our present degenerated state as women, we are often impotent healers of self. Lost women are women who are disconnected from their sacred center.

We must move out and harness all of our power, which has been dormant, locked away in our wombs, for we are at the crossroads of life on this planet. Whether men and women are to live or die is up to us. As women, we have the power to stop the destruction of the earth. Sacred Women, move out quickly and with absolute certainty and tenacity.

Look at the condition of our wombs; statistically, they tell the story. They hold the answer to whether or not we are to be. Most women have womb problems. Too many wombs are dead asleep. Others are filled with bacteria, imploded with stress and disease. Still others are bleeding to death. We are collectively in trouble, so say the voices of our wombs.

We women have squatted on our power for centuries. It's time for us to stand up, for full resurrection is our birthright. When we as women activate our full strength, then it will be as it was in the beginning. When women were whole, we were supreme, for we too were given the power to rule the earth. We women, Gatekeepers of Life, are the key to creating a glorious healing upon the earth, through the realignment of the ancient ways of healing, taught to us by the first mothers of antiquity.

Sacred Women, I implore you to take your life in your own hands, and take hold of your daughters' hands as best you can, and seek out your sisters, your mothers, your grandmothers, your aunts. Create a womb circle, speak womb talk, and pass it on—wombs are healing everywhere. Go heal a wounded womb, and charge a healed womb with light so that it may bear a bright future. Envision a planet of healthy minds and hearts. It is all up to us, the Peacemakers, the Keepers of the Womb. For when we as women go forth and sit on the sacred seat of Ast (Isis), the Great Mother within, then men, with all their warring over land, people, and resources, can do nothing but submit. Come sit with us in the Sacred Womb Circle, Sacred Women, and invoke your true divinity.

## WELCOME TO
## THE SACRED WOMB CIRCLE

The Sacred Womb Circle was created to re-awaken the knowledge within women's consciousness that we have an innate, natural ability to heal ourselves. It was born out of a need to reach out to women like you and me who want to take a more active and responsible role in creating and maintaining the personal wellness of our wombs.

To begin the process of womb wellness, we must first establish and become rooted in the concept and philosophy of Gateway 0: The Sacred Womb and its natural, holistic approach to creating womb wellness. It is not designed to diagnose or prescribe; it is offered to women as a loving introduction to holistic education. It is not intended to serve as a substitute for medical treatment. If you are being attended to by a physician, please continue to do so as you simultaneously begin to educate yourself about the process offered here.

Today, when so many women are faced with the threat of hysterectomy due to uterine fibroids, endometriosis, and an increase in the number of cancerous wombs, the Sacred Womb Circle is an answer to Afrakan women's collective prayers. It says, "Come to me for the prevention of chronic excessive monthly bleeding. Come to me for the elimination of womb infections. Come to me to stanch the growth of tumors, cysts, or fibroids. Come to me to summon the courage to end sexual womb abuse. Come to me to mend the painful emotional scars of unhealed abortions. Come to me to end the premature loss of your monthly cycle or the stress of menopause. Come to me to embrace and rejoice in your Sacred Wombs."

Women who take on this sacred work are striving to create wombs that work brilliantly—wombs that don't hurt, or bleed profusely, or drop, or scream. Women who take on this sacred work will end the inner "womb wars" and save their sacred seats from the dread of disease, so they can begin to heal naturally. We need powerful, tumor-free, energized, pain-free, cleansed, and spiritually charged wombs. We need wombs that don't lock in negative experiences and peo-

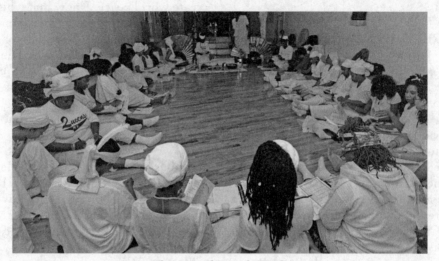

The Sacred Womb Circle

Gateway 0 empowers women by encouraging the formation of Sacred Womb Circles in order to collectively heal ourselves through womb wellness work. It urges mothers to bond with their daughters, and daughters to honor their mothers' experience and wisdom. It asks grandmothers and elder women to gather all the womenfolk of their communities to their bosoms for rebirthing by sharing ancient, "wise woman" healing traditions. These traditions allowed Afrakan women of the Americas, the Caribbean, the Motherland, and throughout the world to heed the call to heal ourselves, through Womb Wisdom, using traditional herbs, roots, leaves, berries, mud, water, air, sun, and prayer.

Gateway 0 teaches us how to establish a Natural Living Lifestyle that will strengthen and purify the "wombniversal mind"—the womb of the heart and the throne of the womb, the sacred seat of Ast.

ple, only to become diseased when all of these toxins are not safely released.

Although this Gateway does not contain all the answers to restoring the full beauty and magnificence of the womb, it does offer the first sparks of light that can ignite our sleeping spirits and take us across the bridge of womb enlightenment.

Gateway 0 speaks to all women—from the young woman who has recently been initiated into her menstrual cycle to the woman whose womb has been surgically removed. To all women, we say: "Bless the spirit of your womb, for that spirit is eternal and never dies. Charge your spiritual womb daily throughout each cycle of your womb-life with much love and peace, for if your spirit is whole, so too is the spirit of your womb."

Whatever your spiritual affiliation, philosophy, educational background, or cultural expression, the Sacred Womb Circle can work for you. It is a safe haven in which every woman may rejoice in the power of her newfound womb awareness. This is the foundation you need as you set out on the evolutionary path of the Sacred Woman.

May this book open you up to the possibilities of taking greater responsibility for the restoration and preservation of your womb. May each lesson fill you with a greater sense of wholeness.

Let's begin!

## SACRED WOMB CIRCLE

We sit in a Womb Circle to do our Work, to heal our minds, hearts, and wombs—our sacred seat. We gather from all walks of life to heal ourselves and one another, to form circles of love, trust, support, and nonjudgment that allow us to share our "womb story."

Our Sacred Womb Circle offers us the sacred space and time to affirm that we have the power to heal not only ourselves but one another as well. As we reveal our innermost secrets in the safety of the Circle, we begin the work needed to purge the past and the disharmonies that we have attracted over time to and through our wombs.

In the Sacred Womb Circle we share with one another the ways we've found that help us love, pamper, heal, and support ourselves through Womb Work. We teach one another how to forgive and let go of our past hurts; how to raise children constructively; how to love our present mates. We inspire one another to restore our divine womb life.

We meditate, pray, and do journal work together. We make music together, and sing songs full of spirit to free our souls. We dance. We read our own and other women's healing poems. We study the principles of Sacred Womb Work together, and learn which foods and herbs nurture our wombs and our nerves. We learn that a woman's Body Temple must be kept pure and clean, for as she transforms her womb, she elevates herself to enter a special sacred state of wholeness.

As we close our Womb Circle in prayer, we hold everyone's stories in our hearts as tools to help us grow. We pray for health, love, abundance, blessings, and good vibes for each of us until we meet again. We are everything and all things in this Circle of healing, sister-to-sister.

At present there are Women's Healing Circles and Sister-to-Sister Circles all over the world. The Mother/Father Spirit deep within us all is calling out for planetary wellness. Know that your Sacred Womb Circle is an indelible part of the many sacred gatherings helping to create world peace. Know that wherever there is a woman who is healing her womb, there is a household with the potential for healing and wellness. One household at a time, prayerfully, this healing will spread like a cleansing fire throughout the communities of the world.

### Setting Up a Sacred Womb Circle

- *First meeting:* At the first exploratory meeting to establish the energy of the Circle, you need to discuss what each sister feels is her individual womb wellness project, and how she feels she might benefit from joining together in a circle with other sisters. Leave plenty of time for meditation and sharing.
- *Purpose of Circle and Commitment Statement:* By the end of the evening, the Circle should have discovered its common purpose and made a commitment to work together once a week for a minimum of twenty-one days and a maximum of four months. Each sister should then write out, date, and sign her personal commitment statement:

*I commit myself to the Sisters of my Sacred Circle, and to the Divine Guardians, Ancestors, and Elders, to heal myself by taking responsibility for my womb wellness. I commit to weekly participation in this Sacred Circle and to stay focused on my mission to heal myself. I will be mindful of the distractions and challenges around me and the denial and rationalizations arising within me that will inevitably attempt to detour me from my course. I will stay strong and steadfast in the company of my Sisters because I know there is unity, power, and divinity in a holy and healthy womb.*

Name: _____

Date: _____

- *Number of women in group:* Four to eight women make an ideal number for a Womb Circle. That way everyone will have time and space to share and to speak their hearts.
- *Suggested length of meeting:* Two to three hours.
- *Where to meet:* To create a shared experience within the group, take turns meeting in one another's sacred homes.
- *Food and drink:* To support the Womb Circle, the sisters will bring potluck sharings of fresh salads and fruit, herbal teas, fresh juices, and water.
- *What you will need:* Dress comfortably so you can do the Dance of the Womb sacred movements together as a group. Bring your own musical instruments—bells, chimes, Tibetan bowl, kalimba, shekere, rattle, or drums (play lightly)—so that you may be inspired to create divine sound healing.
- *Journaling:* Bring your Sacred Womb Journal and pen for any journal work that arises out of the Circle's discussions or meditations.

## Womb Circle Activities

- *Sacred altar:* If the Womb Circle is in your home, you have the privilege of setting up the womb altar. Each sister will want to add an offering, such as flowers, incense, or essential oils, or something sacred of her own to enhance the energy of the Circle.
- *Music:* Open the Womb Circle by playing your musical instruments or singing, or both, to help establish a harmonious atmosphere for womb wellness.
- Purify the Sacred Space and yourselves by choosing one of these methods:
  - Smudging the space and one another with sage.
  - Smudging one another with frankincense and myrrh in a little fireproof pot of charcoal.
  - Anointing one another's crown (mind), heart (spirit), and womb (sacred seat) with essential oils: lotus, lavender, sage, or frankincense and myrrh.
  - Anointing one another with blessed water for sacred cleansing.
- Repeat the Womb Circle Prayer together:

*May our wombs rest on the petals of the sacred lotus. Divine Mother, help me to open up within the Sacred Womb Circle all that is buried within the womb of my mind, the womb of my heart, and the womb of my sacred seat.*

*May the stories that we share within our Womb Circle renew our wombs, lighten our hearts, and heal our minds. May we treat our Womb Circle in a sacred way and keep our shared stories within our collective, making them sacred. May we commit to traveling this road of womb recovery without wavering, that we may restore our womb balance.*

*Divine One, who is indwelling, I open myself up today for absolute womb wellness. May our Womb Circle reveal to us our Sacred Medicine, that we may heal ourselves.*

*I give thanks in advance for the wellness that surrounds my womb and the healing and the peace that surrounds and protects our Womb Circle.*

Hetepu.

Just being a part of a Sacred Womb Circle means that we are ready for healing—in our bodies, our lives, and our environment. Perhaps you'll want to offer fruit or flowers or applause as you receive or give support to the sisters in the Circle who are able to stand up against womb abuse by self and others, and to those who do their best to follow the Womb Wellness diet plan, and to those who cleanse their colons so their wombs can be as light as a feather.

Divine Wisdom dwells in the Sacred Womb Circle.

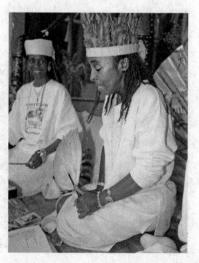

Musical Womb Circle with Queen Afua and Lady Prema

# NUT: OUR CELESTIAL SKY MOTHER

This knowledge of our divinity brings us into the celestial arms of Mother Nut, the Grandmother and Guardian of all the Gateways. You cannot complete the Gateways of sacredness that she encloses until you first go before her, the Celestial Womb.

In the original first written language—Mtu NTR, spoken by our ancient Nile Valley Ancestors—the womb was called the *khat,* which also means "to hold," or "to keep," or "to catch." According to natural law, the Sacred Woman's wellness begins in the womb and spreads out from her center like branches of a tree. She ascends to strength or descends to weakness according to the condition of her roots. In order to grow properly as a whole woman, we must spiritually return our awareness to our beginnings and draw our supply from the oldest Spirit Woman known to humankind and spiritkind—Great-Grandmother Nut.

Here is a prayer to her from the *Prt M Hru N Gher, The Egyptian Book of the Dead:*

*Grandmother Nut, grant that I may reach the heaven of everlastingness and the mountain of thy favoredness. May I be joined with the shining beings, holy and perfect. May I come forth with them to see thy beauties. Thou shinest at eventide and thou goest to thy Mother Nut.*[1]

Speaking from the Celestial Realm, Nut tells us:

*I represent the highest aspect in woman. I am Nut, Womb of the Universe. I was discovered by the first people of the Nile Valley, the Khamites. I am the Celestial Mother who stretches over the entire sky. I contain within my womb all the trillions of stars and planets. I am the Wombniversal Mother whose arms spread across galaxies upon galaxies. I cover the entire universe.*

*My arms spread far enough and wide enough to protect all my children. I am your guide and protectress. Those who come to me in their meditation experience are reborn into divine consciousness. Look for me. My body is deep blue in color and spangled with stars.*

*I can shower you with pure inner peace. Within me reside all the answers of the universe—and the answers you need in your world. I am the principle of the Creator/Creatress in womblike form. Look upon me and I will give you absolute inner serenity. Spend time with me daily in your meditation, and I will heal your body and ignite your inner star so that you may glitter gold and silver bright, just as I do, your Mother.*

All of us womenfolk have taken our turn on the birthing wheel. We are the granddaughters of Nut, the Universal Womb. Each one of us is a star of light. All the women that welcome you at the Sacred Womb Gate—the Ancestors, Elders, and Contemporaries—are representations of the countless manifestations of Nut star beings. These women, the spiritual midwives you will discover as you move through the Womb Wisdom of *Sacred Woman,* will help you through your rebirth.

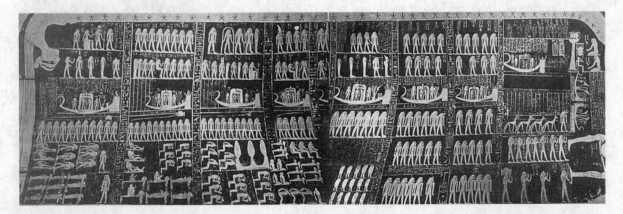

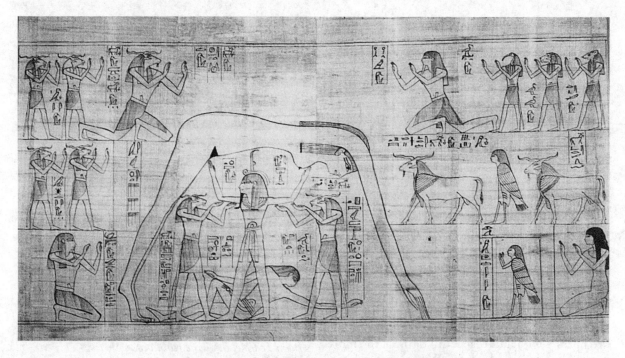

### In the Arms of the Sky Mother: A Visualization

*Daughters of Nut, with each ray of light issued to your womb, may you experience liberation as women. May you shine brighter and brighter as you meet the spiritual midwives standing at the gateway of our rebirth with their full skirts and cast-iron pots and big-bosom smiles.*

Nut, the highest principle and reflection of woman, holds the light to rebirth you into Sacred Womanhood. To start your Womb Healing, Nut speaks:

*Whatever state you are in, come to me. I, Mother Nut, will comfort you. Come fly with me. I will set you free, for I am the divinity that dwells within you. Look up to me at night or at dawn for a few moments, or as long as it takes for you to quietly seal a vision of me into your mind's eye. And when peace, stillness, and light have spread throughout your entire body, know that you have been fed from my sky bosom.*

*Gently close your eyes, sit very still, and enter into me on a higher plane. See your stars shine brightly as the light inside wells up in you and you become one with your celestial womb.*

*Sitting still and easy, breathe deep and deeper still. See your inner stars renew themselves and shine brighter and brighter until all the dark spaces in you melt into one ball of light.*

*Feel this heavenly, womblike, safe, and peaceful state of light vibrating and emanating from within you, circling your body in a womb-shaped temple of light.*

*Meditate daily with me, your Sky Mother, so that all the dark spaces in you become one light, one love.*

To energize your womb healing, hold a piece of lapis lazuli or a moonstone in your palm and over your womb as you perform your Nut Meditation. These stones are known to increase the infinite inner space of the Heavenly Spirit where Nut resides within you.

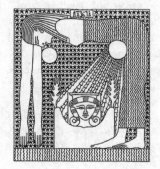

# SACRED TIME

To begin the work of Gateway 0, we must first align our body, mind, and spirit with a new sense of time. When you honor your sacredness, you begin to understand that all time is spiritual. When you live life in a more cosmic, timely, organized fashion, you are more in tune with self, humanity, and the Moon, Sun, and stars. Time moves in a circle. It is ongoing and it never ends. Even at the end of life, when we think it's all over, it begins all over again. Our Ancestors have said that life is eternal: "I am yesterday, seer of millions of years is my name, traveling along the way of Heru (the Light, the Truth)."[2]

The Sacred Clock keeps on ticking, so use your time with complete awareness and as much grace and mindfulness as possible to gain the power, clarity, wealth, and oneness in the spirit that comes in the fullness of time. The more you are in tune with and respectful of time, the more you will be blessed by time. We use every bit of time all the time, so use your moments with as much wisdom as you are able. What we do with our time will ultimately determine all our successes and all our temptations. Time is filled with all kinds of choices. Please think first, to make your choices wisely, for you will live with all your choices, good and bad, for all time. My soul has guided me to dance in the space of time to release the remains of a day gone wrong, or to dance in the space of time in praise because my inner soul was jumping for joy in my midday, or to dance gentle and easy because I survived yet another day with grace and ease.

## Prayers for the Sacred Times of Day: Sunrise, Midday, Sunset, and Nighttime

Within the course of twenty-four hours, Ast (Isis) and her sister Nebt-Het (Nephthys), our ancient Afrakan guardians, come forth to greet us at their designated time of the day, help us to maintain our spiritual, physical, emotional, and mental equilibrium, and remind us to use our time in the spirit of Maat.

*All praise to you, Mother/Father Creator/Creatress, the keeper and bestower of all time, the aspect and reflection of the Most High.*

*Divine Creator/Creatress, you have helped me to be in harmony with the seasons of time, with the time of day, the time of the Moon, the time to eat, the time to fast, the time to rest and the time to rise, the time of my womb cycle, and the time to be intimate and nurtured. May I be in tune with the lesson of time and use it well and with divine intelligence. May I keep time with the ebb and flow of my emotions so that I am able to maintain inner harmony.*

## Nebt-Het: Sunrise

*Adoration to you, Nebt-Het—you who appear between 4 a.m. and 6 a.m.—the female guardian of the darkest hour before dawn, the balance between night and day. You appear at the earliest morning light, standing as the gatekeeper of this twilight time. Honor to you, Nebt-Het, the Lady of the House and sister of Ast, the Lady of Heaven, for living within us as we tune into a new day coming that we as women may carry our house, our Body Temple, in divine right order.*

## Nebt-Het Ritual

The time of Nebt-Het is the time that our melanin, symbolic of our spiritual force of enlightenment, flows strongest. During Nebt-Het's sacred appearance at dawn, sit in quiet meditation. You may place a purple or white prayer shawl upon your head as you meditate on the cosmic Sacred Lady of the House coming through you in a state of cleanliness and Maat. Upon the roof of her house she is crowned with a bowl representing purification, completion (wholeness). And at the gate of her house is the Maat feather of peace and harmony, which will touch and anoint you upon entry into your divine self.

Ring a bell to summon the heavenly host, that they may come around you and within you. Burn incense of frankincense and myrrh to prepare for a purified day.

## Ast: Midday

*All praise to you, Ast, the Great Mother. Time reflects through you as the brightest light of midday, when the Sun is highest and strongest in the heavens, on earth, and within us, giving us great vitality and vigor. Ast, I thank you for this potent charge of light from you at the* time of day you have set aside for my complete blossoming. Beloved Creator/Creatress, help me to stay in tune with time, to be on time with life, and with the commitments I make to be shared with the world of time.

## HET-HRU: SUNSET

*Het-Hru (Hathor), the Lady of Divine Love and Beauty, makes her appearance with the setting of the Sun. Our ancestors called her Het, Hert nebt Amentet or Hathor, Lady of Amentet, for Amentet is the West, where the Sun sets, and thus the place of renewal for the ancient Khamitic peoples.[3]*

## HET-HRU RITUAL

During the hours of Het-Hru, who is dwelling within you, become intimate with yourself.

Take an Epsom salts or Dead Sea salt bath that includes aromatherapy oils or essential oils to enhance your inner beauty, your gentleness, your peace (do not use any salts if you have high blood pressure or edema). Essential oils such as cinnamon, lotus, or lavender were used by the ancients for anointing and for sweetness.

While in the tub, chant your own way to Het-Hru, Lady of Amentet, or Het-Hru, Lady of the Sunset. Repeat this *hesi* over and over again as the heat and the salt water and oils melt away all the challenges you may have experienced during the course of the day.

While surrounded by the ocean of water in your sacred tub, release all stress, so that you may enter the night in serenity.

If tonight is the night you choose for divine lovemaking, allow Het-Hru's beauty to come through you.

### Nut: Nighttime

*All praise to you, Mother Nut. Help me to look to you, the Mother of our daystar, the Sun, and the stars of night as they glide through the sky, to maintain my inner cosmic clock. Help me to use time wisely, to respect the time given me, and to respect the time of others. Creator/Creatress, help me to see time as being as precious as my children. Help me to become more aware that time is to be cherished and well spent, like the good times that I share with my extended family.*

*All I have is right now, this moment, to make my life work. And this time, right now, is mine and I give thanks. Help me to think before I set time and use time, for I will never again get this time back. May I use my time to heal, to build, to love, and to reason.*

*Mother/Father Creator/Creatress, as the time of my age increases, may I be made glad, for only through many years of living does wisdom grow. Knowledge is my flower, and may my time be filled with memories of thankfulness and healthy seeds sown. Let me never waste my time, for it does not stand still even for a moment. Help me remember that cycles come and go, and no matter how hard things are right now, or how good they may be, nothing remains the same.*

*Creator/Creatress, help me remember when the sun goes down and night falls, in the hours of despair or quietude, to simply go with the flow, for time will have its way; neither grief nor sweet solitude will last forever. In time, the sun will rise again and joy and peace shall once again prevail.*

*Heavenly Mother/Father Spirit, when my time in this life is all used up and my clock finally stops, may I look back upon my life and reflect that my lessons have been well learned and that the moments of my life were filled with goodness. May I leave a legacy of time well spent, and when I step over to the other side, to the realm of the Ancestors, may I keep celestial time with them.*

Now that we have entered into the concept of Sacred Time, we are ready to establish the rhythm of the Sacred Clock throughout your twenty-one days of experience in Gateway 0: The Sacred Womb and through each of the Gateways that follow.

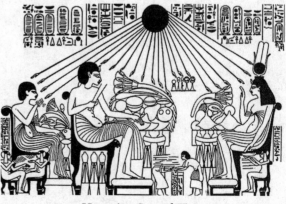

Honoring Sacred Time

## THE SACRED CLOCK

| Crossroads Times of the Day — Acknowledge with prayer and meditation each crossroad of the day | What Time Is It? | State of Consciousness | Food Time of the Day | Nutritional Times of a Woman's Age to Feed Body and Spirit | Seasons of Time through a 24-Hour Day | Phases of the Moon through a 24-Hour Day |
|---|---|---|---|---|---|---|
| 4:00 A.M. to 5:00 A.M. Nebt-Het's Hours of Power before dawn. The balance between night and day | Awaken! This is the time for meditation and giving praise, for new beginnings are about to come according to how deeply you fast and pray. | In this twilight time, the sacred nectar, my melanin, flows from my crown and taps me into Divinity. | Fast or drink herbal tea. Drink warm water or fresh wheatgrass. | Baby inside of the womb A Time for Creation | Late Winter | Waning Moon (The Coming) |
| 6:00 A.M. Sunrise/Dawn The Coming of the Day | A time for renewal and reawakening. A time for purification. This is the best time to write in your journal or do your womb dance. | No matter what has happened in the course of the previous day, dawn has returned once again to show me a greater way. | Liquid meal: Kidney-Liver Flush, fresh fruit juice | Infancy to 6 | A Time of Discovery | Early Spring |
| 9:00 A.M. Midmorning | A time for deeper and greater cleansing. | The balance of morning is flowing within me, bringing with it a spiritual state of awakening. | Lightest solid meal of the day: fresh whole fruits, soaked nuts, seeds | 7–12 A Time of Discovery | Late Spring | Waxing Moon |
| 12:00 P.M. Ast's (Isis's) Hour of Power Midday | Best time for total activity and productivity. A time for regeneration, for this is the strongest part of the day. This is an excellent time to execute your ideas. | The sun is strong in my Body Temple, which helps me to digest life with vigor, power, and vitality. | Organic fresh vegetable juice, 8–12 oz. 12–1 P.M. | 13–21 A Time of Discovery | Summer | Full Moon (The Full Arrival) |
| Afternoon | A time to follow through on your visions, to open doors, and finally make things happen. A time for fine-tuning. | The light is high in the sky, so busily I move through my day, seeking, exploring, learning, reaching, and obtaining. | Heaviest meal of the day: vegetarian protein, starch, vegetables 1–3 P.M. | 22–39 A Time for Seeking Truth | Late Summer | Waning Moon (The Retreat) |
| 4:00 P.M. 8:00 P.M. Winter Het-Hru's Sunset/Dusk } Hours of Summer Power | A time for retreating. A quiet time for relaxation and contemplation. A time for an herbal or salt bath. A time for fine-tuning. | It is time to be still and go within to reflect on what has happened on this divine day. | Organic fresh vegetable juice, 8–16 oz., to drink the first hour of sunset. Consume light dinner of fresh vegetables, whole grains, vegetarian protein during the sunset. | 40–60 A time of deep meditation and contemplation. A time for knowing truth! | Fall | Waning Moon (The Retreat) |
| 12:00 A.M. Midnight A Sacred Woman should be asleep hours before midnight to get the best from her rest. Nut's Hours of Healing and Rebuilding. | A time to recharge while in your deep, peaceful sleep, as you rest in a well-ventilated room with fresh plants hanging everywhere to purify your breath of life. A time to connect to your dreams, which will reveal to you truth that is waiting to be told. | Sleep has come to take me home to renew my body and restore my soul. | Liquid fast or dry fast. Drink the nectar of sleep To sleep is to eat from the spiritual realm. If you live well throughout your day, your dreams will reflect this. | 65–100 A time for living in absolute truth and enlightenment. | Winter | Waning Moon |

# CHAPTER 3
# THE SPIRIT OF THE WOMB

## THE SACRED WOMB JOURNAL

My sisters, we've been asleep. It's time for the womb wake-up call. Sound the alarm through Sacred Womb Journal work. It may hurt a little bit, but it's gonna be all right. Believe me, we will get safely to the other side, where self-healing dwells.

Sacred Womb Journal work is a way to demonstrate to yourself that you don't want to carry the pain anymore, that you're willing to give it up because you've allowed it to speak. There's been too much pain. Too much to bear. And the irony is that so much profound healing happens as soon as we're willing to acknowledge and listen to the voice of the womb.

The Sacred Mother's waiting hand has been outstretched as she says, "I am here. Just give your pain to me."

And you've kept saying, "No, thank you, I've got to hold on to it. I've got to hold on to it. I've got to keep holding on to it, even if it kills me."

And then it begins to—with womb cancer or hysterectomies or radiation therapy, all caused by holding on to our hurts and pains. So many things have been done to our wombs without our conscious awareness, and some things were indeed conscious acts. A lot of things that happened in our lives were just the result of pure ignorance—actions performed by those who knew no better. However, now, for us to grow and heal together, we have to be willing to

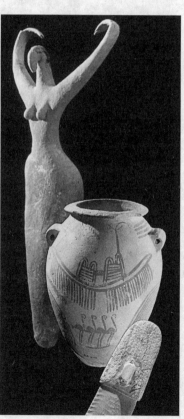

risk exposing our ignorance of ourselves and any others who share our experiences in some way, so that we can all learn by sharing our experiences with one another.

Another purpose of Sacred Womb Journal work is as a tool to ground and center you in your self. Centering into the womb means being able to look at our relationship with our body.

We must start at the center, for developing a healthy womb is the platform from which we develop a healthy body. From the center, we learn not to put our brain above our body any longer. We learn not to numb ourselves to our real physical condition any longer. We learn to use every womb experience as a medium for growth.

When we are disconnected from our wombs—for whatever reasons—then we are not fully able to have an intimate interchange with another. Then the art of sharing love from your very center is compromised. For if you cannot share from your center with yourself, then it's impossible to really share it in union with one another.

It is helpful to discuss these issues with the women in your circle, such as sisters or friends, not only for yourself, but to help prevent the suffering of others.

As medicine women born again, we must use everything as medicine. Everything in our life is here to help us, to give us strength and empowerment. Hearing other women's womb stories makes you ask yourself: "What am I going

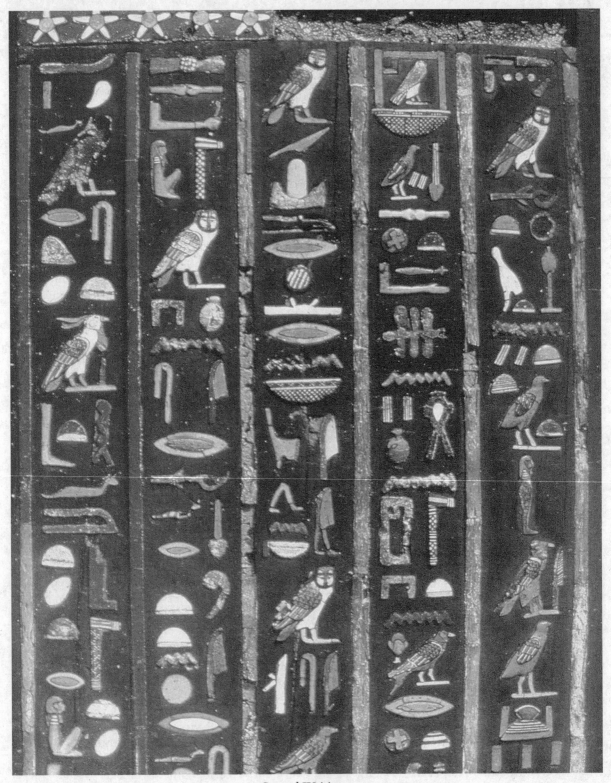

Sacred Writings

through?" That's your medicine—your story. And it's our medicine, the stories that we share. It's absolutely never too late to reconnect with your womb—your sacred center, and to become a lover and a friend to yourself.

In order to heal or rejuvenate our sacred center, we must first know what lies deep inside. The Sacred Womb Journal helps us to get comfortable with our wombs, so we can get on the road of cleansing, purging, and rejuvenation. It aids in identifying our intuitive womb concerns so that later we can assess our level of womb wellness and begin to actively heal ourselves.

For the liberation of our womb-related afflictions, let's visit that exiled part of ourselves—the "down there" part, as so many women refer to the womb center. You don't need to get a passport sometime way in the future to visit "down there." Your Sacred Womb Journal will help you take part in a daily loving womb ritual that allows you to blossom into the beautiful lotus that you are by nature.

## The Voice of the Womb

When I was discussing dialoguing with the womb in a circle of sisters, one of them asked me, "Does a womb have a voice, and if so, how does it speak?"

"The womb does have a voice," I told her. "The womb has a language all its own, and yes, it does speak."

Sisters, go within the heart of your womb in your daily meditation and listen well. Your womb desires to speak through you. Your womb will tell you what she needs. Your womb will tell you where she's going and where she's been. She will tell you how she wants to heal.

The womb misses nothing; she knows all. The womb records every event of our lives. She records all of our interactions and reactions within our relationships. She senses our misgivings and receives all of the loving. The womb never forgets the lessons or the blessings. As we enter into the depths of our wombs, we will discover that our womb remembers and is prepared to speak to us of every fear and every joy.

The womb has a language all her own. The womb sings and moans. When she speaks of

pain, tumors grow. When she speaks of pleasure from the interaction of a nurturing mate, love grows. The womb sometimes says yes. But oftentimes she says no. When she exults, babies are born. When she yells and screams, the blood clots.

Listen closely to your womb; learn her language, heed her message. Let your Sacred Womb Journal become the interpreter between you and the voice of your own womb.

It's time to go deep into our wombs. Be courageous; don't be afraid of your truth coming forth, for truth is the foundation through which healing takes place. If at any point in your Sacred Womb Journal exploration you experience blockage and are unable to hear or feel your womb, then just sit back and place your palms over your womb area a few inches below your navel. Breathe deeply and relax. Tell her gently not to be afraid. In time, the voice of your womb will be reassured and feel safe enough to speak. Never force the issue. All things come in their own right time. The more you cleanse, the better and easier the communication will get.

Begin your Sacred Womb Journal work over a three-day weekend, seven days, twenty-one days, a season, a year, or for the rest of your life. Remember, your womb is alive! And you need to stay in touch. However, if you miss a day or a week of your Sacred Womb Journal work, it's okay. Don't be discouraged. Keep right on going. The more time you put into your Sacred Womb Journal reflections, the deeper your discovery and recovery. Your womb is a treasure chest waiting to be explored. So open it up. See what intuitive gems of wisdom await you as you discover yourself by bringing what's inside . . . out!

## Waking Up the Womb

Your Sacred Womb Journal can be a tremendous aid in helping you reconnect to yourself because it awakens you to the body, mind, spirit, and womb connection. It encourages an inner dialogue that helps you examine your life in a new, deeper, way. Your Sacred Womb Journal will help you explore the life of your womb and give you a better understanding of who you are and what you have become.

In order to heal and rejuvenate your womb center, you must first know what is deep inside. Journaling helps us get on a roll of cleansing, purging, and rejuvenating the womb. It helps us to be comfortable with our wombs by helping us to identify our womb concerns so that we may actively heal ourselves. Once we identify what is out of balance, we can do something about it—until then it's just nameless pain.

Relax and let go. Close your eyes and ask your womb to tell you what she feels. Just get out of the way, and trust her to speak. Once you're connected, you might want to repeat your Nut meditation to make a deeper connection to your sacred seat (see page 29).While in this state, allow Nut, the heavenly Sky Mother who dwells within you, to pour her healing life force in your womb to revitalize her. The more you allow your womb to speak, the more light shines through.

### How the Sacred Womb Journal Work Came Through

I want to share something very intimate with you. One night I was happy and excited about a lecture I'd heard, so I kept talking about it to my mate. I talk a lot at home. It's constant talking—and he listens. Then I went to lie down, and we were still talking, and you know what he did?

He took a pretend microphone, pointed it at my womb, and said, "Now, would you ask your womb to tell me why you don't want to be touched on your womb?" And he tried to touch me there—and I laughed. "That's what you always do," he said.

I realized he was right, that whenever he would touch my womb, I would laugh. But when I started to think about it, I said, "Well, you know, at the beginning of the relationship, you would touch me, but you used to sing to me more, you used to play the guitar, you recited poetry. That would open up my heart center, and it would open up my womb, and open up my trust and all my intellect." But I knew that was only part of the truth.

Then he said, keeping the mike pointed at my womb, "Well, can the womb speak?"

I told him that she can say anything she'd like. I didn't know what she might say, but my sense was that she didn't like the way people touched her.

I took a deep breath and said to my womb, "Speak!" And she began to speak through me. She spoke through my memories of when I had my second child. That time was all a fog to me, because some of it was very traumatic. But my womb remembered it all. My doctor wasn't there when I went into labor—you know, you're in labor but your doctor doesn't report in until you're about to deliver. I'd thought she was going to be right there the whole time.

Instead, there was this male European doctor who checked me out and examined me, and I felt like dying. "Oh, God," I thought, "what's he going to do?" I didn't even want to be there because I felt like I was going to jail instead of going into the hospital. I'd been on the healing path for years, but I still hadn't cleansed sufficiently for my womb to be in a healthy enough state to have a natural birth.

This doctor made me put my feet up in those cold stirrups, and then he pushed his hand way up inside me. When I jumped back, he said, "I bet you didn't do that when you got pregnant."

The tears came pouring down my face, and I was as tense as a board. I started pulling the little band off my wrist, ready to leave. I was in my twenties then, and my family always told me I was too sensitive. I kept hearing my family say, "Listen to the doctor; he knows best."

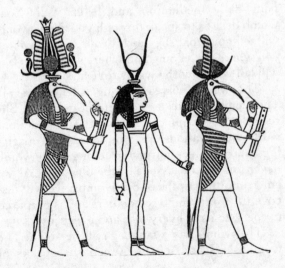

So I'm looking up at the ceiling, thinking, "I have to submit to this." I felt like I was at death's door. In order for me to relax, I had to die; I had to leave my body there for that doctor to touch. When he was finished I was never the same. The experience buried itself deep inside my womb.

And then my woman doctor came. She was a nice doctor, but she ran through all the laboring women there like an assembly line. There were all kinds of womb conditions: pain, cramping, everything going on. She got to me and said, "Okay, put your feet up. So how are you feeling?"

And I said, "Oh, gosh, I want to die right here." And she really didn't hear me. The next thing I knew, she had me in surgery for another cesarean. This is what made me so committed to healing my womb, because I told myself, "I can treat my own womb sweeter, with greater reverence, and with greater respect."

I went to study about everything natural that we can do to heal our wombs and prevent a future womb problem, or a future womb relationship that would make me shut down further. Then I realized we also have to look at our relationships and emotional responses.

I thought about my relationship with my former husband at that time. It had been a total trauma to me, and of course it had ended in a divorce.

It was all that unloving, uncaring touching of my womb that had made me so defensive and self-protective. Even now that I've finally found a man who is kind and gentle, I find I'm still having trouble when my womb is touched. But I'm laughing—I'm being nice by laughing. This time, though, I told him about my bad experiences, and we talked about it all.

Then he said, "Now I understand. For seven years I never quite understood what was happening." And then I started holding him and hugging him while he explained to me how he felt, how he had related to my sensitivity and emotions. It felt as if we had started all over again—like everything was brand-new between us, like spring. Then suddenly my husband began to rock me and sing to me like a poet, and my womb broke out into a wondrous smile. It was because he decided to interview my womb that we got so clear about the whole touching issue.

## The Unhealed Womb: Preparing for Your Sacred Womb Journal Work

As poet Langston Hughes said so powerfully in "A Dream Deferred":

> *Does it dry up*
> *like a raisin in the sun?*
> *Or fester like a sore —*
> *And then run?*
> *Does it stink like rotten meat? . . .*
> *Maybe it just sags*
> *like a heavy load.*
> *Or does it explode?*[1]

This is a good description of an unhealed womb. If we don't relate to our wombs and resolve our inner womb conflicts, the spirit of the womb dries up, and we are numbed, or the womb releases a stench because we are bitter, or it's crowded out by a tumor and destroys our creativity. Worse, it can fester and drip and create even more serious diseases that cause our wombs to rot and then be lost through hysterectomy.

To heal our wounds, we need to be willing to go deep into the memories that our wombs retain. We must be willing to return to the scene of the crime, or the pleasure, and meet the one(s) who insulted, abused, outraged, or misused our wombs—or the one(s) who have been kind, respectful, loving, and gentle to our wombs.

We need to tell ourselves, "If this is what it's going to take to heal, so be it!" The next step is to call upon our inner guidance by meditating and contemplating. We need to ask Mother Ast for her help as we find ourselves returning to the place we thought was behind us forever. As we walk through this painful place we'll discover how mistaken we were when we thought that if we turned away, it would all be over and done with. In actuality, we never leave that place inside us—not until we heal it once and for all. Otherwise the situation plays itself out in our lives again and again. The suffering may change its cast of characters or location, but it's still the same suffering.

When I first entered that place in myself, when I got to the very core of my womb, my center, I found myself in conflict. There were two of me fighting over what to do. One part wanted to run away; one part wanted to finish the work once and for all:

*"It's beginning to hurt, oh, no."*
*"Come on, girl, just breathe."*
*"It's too much, I gotta go. I don't wanna know."*
*"Girl, you've been brave to come so far. Just keep breathing in love and healing, and breathing out all that pain and fear."*
*"It's too hard!"*
*"It's a lot harder to keep carrying that load of pain."*
*"Well . . . I know have to get to the bottom of my womb dilemmas."*
*"We can do it, we can do it. We're a born-again Healer."*

The more I communed with the depths of my womb, the stronger I got. Tears rolled, but I didn't budge. This is how the answers to my questions began to be revealed to me. And I was encouraged to keep going because I could feel a blanket of soulful healing comforting me.

So I told my fearful self:

*"Come on, girlfriend, don't shut down, don't quit. Let's explore those deep dark hidden places in our womb that we haven't wanted to look at."*
*"But it hurts too bad. I feel so sad."*
*"Come, I'll hold your hand."*
*"Okay. If I go within, can you help me soothe the hurt? 'Cause my womb just might lose control and shout and scream because of what is locked down there."*

*"That place is a mystery, even to me. Come, I'll help. If we do it together, it won't be so hard. Our womb/body/mind/heart has been longing to help us heal ourselves so we can return to our natural state of wellness and wholeness."*

## THE WOMB AS SPIRITUAL CENTER

The physical womb (or uterus) is located in the pelvic region, and is sheltered by the ovaries and fallopian tubes. The most sacred female organ of reproduction is hollow and pear-shaped, and lies on top of the bladder. The uterus is composed of three layers. Beginning at the innermost layer, we have the endometrium, the myometrium, and the parametrium. The uterus also has two parts—a body and a cervix. The body of the uterus extends from the top of the organ to its narrow outer end, the cervix.

To find your own womb, sit quietly, with your eyes closed, on cushions on the floor, tailor fashion, or upright in a comfortable chair, with your feet on the floor, legs uncrossed. Relax and just be for a minute or two.

- Now, rub your palms briskly together, and when you have built up continuous heat in your hands, press them right over your womb. You will find it between your navel and your pelvic girdle, between your fallopian tubes and your ovaries—remember, the womb is not the vagina.
- Let your hands feel the presence of your womb, the spirit of your sacred seat. Allow the inner heat to pass from your hands to your heart and into your womb. Be still, focus your attention within, and feel your womb energy.
- Now, open your eyes, and sit quietly within your Divinity. Sit with yourself as a Sacred Queen. Know that we are all divine.

The spiritual aspect of the womb in the body is seen as an *arit,* the original Khamitic word for "spiritual energy center" or "gateway." The *aritu* (plural) are also referred to as the chakras, the seven basic subtle energy centers of the body. The womb *arit* corresponds to the second chakra, representing the aspects of procreation, inspiration, and family.

If a womb is damaged in any way—if it has experienced heavy menstrual bleeding or PMS, if it has sustained numerous infections, fibroids, or tumorous growths, if the womb area has been cut or bruised, irradiated, or chemically sprayed, if it has experienced invasion or abuse by a sexual partner, if it has been harmed by abortions or a hysterectomy—then a woman's level of creativity and inspiration, stability, success in relationships, fertility levels, and joy are potentially impaired.

The womb *arit* is governed by the Moon and thus the ocean tides, representing the element of water, which so deeply affects our emotional tides. This is why, as women, we're so positively affected by all water rituals and healings. In the *Sacred Woman* teachings you will learn that you can bless and drink one glass of water, and transform your negative disposition back to balance. Try it; you'll be surprised.

You can shower under your bathroom's waterfall, inhaling the blessed negative ions from a cool shower spray, or you can bathe in the ocean, walk in the rain, take a salt bath in your private hydrotherapy room (do not use any salts if you have high blood pressure or edema), fast on live juices and water, or wear shades of blue and white, the colors of water—any one of these water works will amazingly reconnect you with your Sacred Woman self, and restore your beautiful, natural, forgiving, "overstanding" womb state. This in turn will spin the energy of your womb chakra in the natural clockwise motion of an *arit* in NTRT Maat divine right order.

### Meditation and Prayer for the Womb

Let's begin the following meditation by sitting upright in a chair, feet flat on the floor, palms facing up. Now close your eyes and relax.

Take a deep, deep inhalation into your womb, and a long exhalation out through the nose.

Inhale again, reaching into your womb deeper and deeper, sending love and light to your sacred seat. Now exhale all stress from your womb. Inhale deeply once more, and this time as you breathe out, exhale all negativity—everything that blocks you from your blessings and keeps you from your good.

Take another deep inhalation into your womb and a long exhalation out. Breathing into the womb and out again allows her to open to this prayer:

*My womb decrees protection and peace. As I inhale deeply into my sacred seat—the gateway of all life on earth, the gateway of all creativity and power, the gateway for all transformation and change—I release all that is blocking me from your message, your strength, your energy, your balance, your harmony.*

You must always be open in your spirit because, as women, our strength is the spiritual realm. You know we always feel things from our wombs. We make our decisions from there. When your womb is shut down, you're cut off from your intuition, your Mother Wit. We have to keep our womb wisdom wide open or we get lost. How many times have you said, "Something's telling me . . ." or "I've got a gut feeling . . ."?

This is one of the reasons *Sacred Woman* came to be, so that as we heal our sacred seats, we heal our knowing. That's the power of being a woman. You know it all. It's inside of you. And the more that you cleanse and acknowledge your Divinity, the more that truth begins to come out.

You have all the medicine in you to heal yourself. You're made up of five key elements that rule the universe: spirit, air, fire, water, and earth. Those are the elements that are inside your holy Body Temple. Those are the elements that are outside in the world. Those are the elements that are in your kitchen laboratory, where you heal the womb of your mind, the womb of your heart, and the womb of your sacred seat.

### The Emergence of the Sacred Womb Journal Questions

The questions for the Sacred Womb Journal came through intuitively, but not until I'd done a lot of cleansing. It took me a month of baths and putting on clay packs. Then some days the questions would come, but they'd be disjointed. Finally, it all started to take on a form and a shape, as if somebody were actually working through me. I believe the spirit of Nut saw me and said, "This is how I want you to do it as you create your Womb Profile. This is how it's going to work for you."

So what I ask of you is to be as honest with yourself as you can. Some womb questions you might not want to share with anyone. There may be some things in your womb life that are just between you and your Most High. That is your privilege and your honor. Just try to be at peace with yourself, with whatever you're feeling, with whatever hurts your feelings. When you share this with yourself you can become closer to yourself and begin to flush out, and wash out, and start all over again in contact with the higher spirit of your womb.

This is waking up the womb!

When we disconnect from our wombs for whatever reason, then we're not fully able to have an intimate relationship with another person. This compromises our ability to share love from our very center, for if we cannot share from our center with ourselves, then how can we share it in a union?

It's absolutely never too late to recapture your womb and become a lover and a friend to yourself. Unpin those blocked, painful emotions. Forgive yourself. Bless your womb. Let go from the depths of your womb. Listen to the voice of your womb throughout your meditation and throughout your day's activities. You may get a message during the day just by drinking your womb tea. You may get a message when you wake up because the First Mind, the First Spirit that comes through you in the morning, is the answer to your womb question that you put into your mental computer earlier. You might have asked, "Why am I so angry about my vagina?" Or "When I looked at my womb in the mirror, why didn't I think it was beautiful?"

You don't have to find an answer when you ask the question. Just go to sleep. When you wake up, it will come to you. And although you may not yet know how to heal from that condition, you'll go ahead and take your bath anyway, you'll drink your tea, and maybe while you're in that tub, soaking by candlelight, or meditating on the four directions and the foundation, it will come to you. You'll get the idea to say this prayer, or to work with this color. You'll get an urge to talk to this Elder Mother, or to send a letter to your mother in the spirit. Then you'll burn it with sage so it can go straight into the cosmos.

Record your womb feelings as you explore the many avenues of Sacred Womb work. Really dialogue with your womb when you do your exercises. Talk out loud. Have conversations. Have funny ones or deep, serious ones. Say, "Girl, why are you always all uptight? You can't do anything when your womb is locked. Girl, why

don't you just try to relax? I'm going to work with you. Let me massage you lightly. All right. It's okay to heal."

Have a conversation just the way you'd talk with everybody else around you. You can have a conversation with your breasts or hips. You can say, "Yes, breasts, I love you. I love your soft roundness." Or "I love these hips, cellulite and all, because they're mine; I got the power to work it out."

Please remember, when your womb is in pain, particularly when difficulties or challenges or questions come up, it means your womb wants to speak to you. So begin to breathe deeply. Perhaps you won't hear anything after four breaths or ten. But by the time you get through fifty to one hundred Fire Breaths, you will truly hear her voice begin to speak. She's been trying to get your attention, so listen with care, and then write down what you hear in your Sacred Womb Journal.

You want your womb to recover? You want peace in your womb? You want to attract good men into your womb and around your womb? You want to attract healthy relationships and healthy babies and good high thoughts? Then take time for your journal. Take time for you. Your womb is a treasure chest waiting to be explored, so open it up.

You'll find that some questions are more difficult than others. So you'll say, "Okay, I'm not ready today. I might be ready by the fifth day." And then you may still not be ready. It may take you a few weeks or months to look at that issue. It may take getting away for a few days into Nature. But if you make the commitment to your womb, your wisdom will come.

### Questions and Reflections to Contemplate in Your Sacred Womb Journal Work

This is your opportunity to begin a dialogue with your womb, an opportunity to get to know all of who you really are—what you think; how you honestly feel about yourself, relationships, and events; your griefs, fears, and anger, both conscious and hidden; the condition of your womb and your sense of yourself as a woman; and fi-

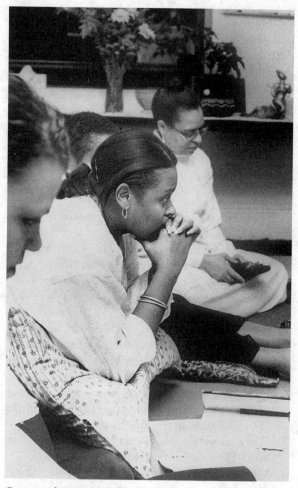

Contemplating the Sacred Womb Journal Questions

quiet breathing as you go deep within. Then simply write your initials at the top left of your journal page, and ask your womb if she will speak with you. She won't refuse, but do her the honor of asking.

For her reply, simply write "My Womb:" at the left of the next line, and then . . . write down whatever pops into your mind. When nothing more comes, ask your next question. Your exchanges may be long or short. She may have a lot to say, or speak only briefly, and the same is true for you. Each session will be different, and fascinating, and healing—for you both.

You may feel like working through all the questions here in one long session. Or you may want to focus on one or two of the questions at a time, and go deeply into what they mean for you. There is no right way or wrong way—there is only your way.

Use the questions that follow to explore your attitudes toward your womb as part of your Sacred Womb Journal work in the privacy of your home. If you choose, you may share your experiences in your Sacred Womb Circle.

### Things to contemplate:

1. Something you might want to discuss with your womb up front is why you might not have dialogued with her before.
2. Do you feel that talking about your womb is important? Why? Why not?
3. Are you friends with your womb? Why? Why not?
4. How have you silenced your womb?
5. Write about what's going on in your life and how this may affect your attitude toward your womb. What does your womb have to say about all this? Ask her; she'll reply directly and honestly.
6. Have you divorced yourself from your womb and disowned your womb pain? If so, how? What Band-Aids have you used to cover up your womb pain and your dissatisfaction— food, drugs, alcohol, work, sex, and so on?
7. How can you help yourself let go of your womb pain? How do you need to alter your life so that you may heal your womb?

nally, your hopes, plans, and visions for the future.

If this is your first womb dialogue, don't be afraid or nervous, because you're about to meet your wisest, most honest, and most loving friend, the one who will never let you down. Your womb remembers everything but does not judge. Even if she has been surgically removed, her indomitable spirit remains intact within you, ready to communicate with you and to support you.

To begin, take up your special pen and journal, sit quietly in your sacred space, preferably after you have done your sacred bath and meditations and at a time when you know you won't be interrupted for a while. Take several deep breaths, and give yourself a minute or two of

### Ask your womb about her physical condition:

1. Have you ever touched or felt your womb or vagina, beyond washing yourself?
2. What did you feel about her?
3. When you have touched the entrance to your womb or vagina, how did you feel about her? Were you embarrassed? Did you feel at ease?
4. Does your vaginal area have a clean smell? What do you feel about the touch or smell of your vaginal area and womb center?
5. Discuss what disease(s) you feel reflected in your womb. What does your womb have to say about this?
6. Do you feel you've numbed yourself out of feeling your physical condition because you're too frightened to connect? What do you think will happen when you do connect? What wisdom does your womb have to offer about your fears?
7. How many of your friends, associates, and family members have fibroid tumors or other female diseases? Discuss their conditions in detail (omit their names if you plan to share your journal with others).
8. How many of your friends, associates, or family members have had hysterectomies or mastectomies?

### Ask your womb about her emotional condition:

1. Knowing that your womb is your center, identify and record the blows that your womb has taken and absorbed.
2. How deep is your womb wound?
3. What are some of the pains you've felt in your womb since childhood, your teens, or as a young adult, mother, or elder?
4. How did you feel about your first menstrual period?
5. Describe your first experience of sexual intercourse. How did you feel about it then? How do you feel about it now? How does your womb feel about it?
6. How do you feel about sex?
7. Do you have sex or do you make love? What's the difference? Which do you prefer? Why?
8. Are you sexually aggressive or suppressed?
9. What was your experience in giving birth to your first child, and any others?

10. Think about all the men in your life—family, extended family, friends, and lovers—and ask your womb what she thinks of each of them.
11. What do you feel about your sexual orientation?
12. Are you sexually intimate with women? Why? How does it make you feel? How is it different from a relationship with a man?

### Ask your womb how she feels about your relationships:

1. How do you feel about your present relationship?
2. Who, or what, is still left inside of your womb? Give name(s) and physical condition(s).
3. How many men and what type of men have entered into your womb space? What was each experience like?
4. How were you feeling about your self, your womb, your life during each relationship?
5. How do you feel when your lover touches your womb?
6. Have you ever had a "womb crisis" in your life? Write about what you learned from it. How did you attempt to heal yourself?
7. Were your parent(s) sexually abusive with you? How has this affected you?
8. Were you ever molested? Tell your story. How has it affected your present relationship with yourself and with others?
9. Ask your womb to tell you her version of your womb "herstory." You may find it very enlightening.

As you develop an ongoing inner dialogue through your journal work, write down your real feelings. Let your written Womb Wisdom show you why you keep drawing the same toxic situations into your womb and into your life. Commit to a daily ten-minute morning womb prayer and meditation, followed by your journal work. Go into a quiet, still place within yourself and write in your journal. Give your inner dialogue time to evolve, and you'll find that it will teach you a great deal about yourself and everything you've been carrying around. It will give you an entirely new perspective and understanding of yourself and others. Allow your womb to speak on your behalf as you witness the miracles taking place inside of you and all around you.

## Womb Meditation

After you have explored your Womb Journal questions, remember to perform the following meditation.

- Sit quietly on your cushion or in a comfortable chair. Close your eyes. Take several deep breaths as you place your hands over your womb and attune to her.
- In your mind's eye, see yourself entering into your womb and walking around in her. What do you see and what do you feel now that you've been doing all this internal womb exploration? How's your body feeling? How's your womb feeling now?
- Scan yourself. Do you feel better or worse, more hurt or less hurt? What is your sense of yourself right at this moment?
- Affirm: "My womb and I are loving partners on the path of the Sacred Woman."

# FROM DEVASTATION TO SWEET INSPIRATION

My conscious introduction to my womb came when I had my first period at age thirteen. I was totally unprepared for what was to come. The hour after my first issue of blood was the beginning of hell on earth for me. The throbbing, thrashing pain in my womb was overwhelming. The throwing up, the cramping, the moaning, the rolling in my mama's bed for comfort went on and on. By nightfall I had completely lost it. I just wanted to take out my womb. I cried out and my mother gave me a painkiller that put my womb to sleep. I was numb and lifeless, but I was at least able to breathe and the pain was gone, temporarily.

I just could not believe that I—and every woman—had been sentenced to such agony and would have to learn to live with this each month for thirty-five years or more. I would have done anything never to experience again what felt like war in my womb.

I recall thinking in my young mind, "I cannot wait until menopause when all of this pain will be over." Little did I know that I had to change my entire lifestyle in order to experience peace within my womb—to discover a womb with no pain, no cramping, clotting, pulling, throbbing, or heavy bleeding for seven or eight days a month. What a mess! My personal prayer request was for a quiet womb that spoke peace.

By the time I was eighteen years old, I had stopped eating all flesh and had become a complete vegetarian. That's when I ceased passing clots of blood. At twenty-three, after the birth of my first child, came the true beginning of my journey to womb wellness. I learned to pack mud over my pelvis. The healing properties of the mud seeped into my womb and pulled out my pain. I drank bush tea of red raspberry and dandelion. I placed my legs up against the wall at a forty-five-degree angle to send healing energy throughout my womb. By the birth of my second child, I had begun drinking green juices every day to strengthen my Body Temple. And I also began to develop my inner sanctum.

Continuing on my journey of womb wellness, by the birth of my third child, I had begun to recite womb prayers for sweet inspiration.

I thank the Creator/Creatress for my renewed sacred attitude about my womb, my sacred seat. I am particularly grateful that through trial and tribulation I ultimately connected to the voice of my womb. Over the years that unfailing voice has become my divine protection and guide to a healthier, more vibrant life.

Now, you may wonder with all I was doing why I had to have three cesarean sections. When I was writing this book, that was the last thing I wanted to talk about. I was not proud of it, because I started on all this so late. When you've been living in a toxic manner for so long and you're trying to be natural, you can't really be as natural as you'd like as quickly as you'd like because your body hasn't caught up to where it should be. So my womb wasn't really ready just then. Also, at that time my body and I were part of mainstream society. I went the route of the status quo from birth to age eighteen.

But that was a blessing. I say every lesson is a blessing, and this one enabled me to go deeper and to begin to heal myself as the prelude to my

Initiation as a Sacred Woman. My experience has made it possible for me to help so many other women not to have to go through what I went through. We all learn from our past, and we grow from our past. And we learn that when we share our lessons with others we can transform them into blessings.

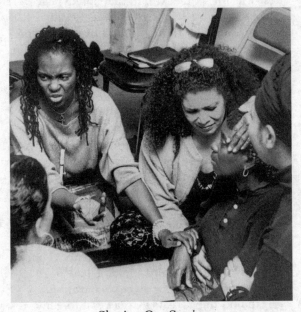

Sharing Our Stories

### Stories from the Sacred Womb Circle

#### Maria

As I began my Womb Journal work, I realized that I'd never thought about my womb. I probably was in a state of avoidance from the time my periods started. I never had a conversation with my mother because my mother never had a conversation with me except for the fact that my period started on graduation day. Mother called me at school after the nurse called her and said, "Go to the bathroom and check." And I went, and it wasn't traumatic, it wasn't huge. But it had happened. And when I came home there was a box of Kotex on my bed. My mother had anticipated this moment, but that was it.

That experience informed my teenage years at a time when one just did not talk about these things very much, or people like my mother didn't talk about them very much. She didn't even know whatever it is you should know—how not to get pregnant, nothing. So I was just sort of out there on my own. When that hap-

pens and you're a teenager, you're really vulnerable to a lot of things, especially not knowing how to handle relationships. Being someone who always read and loved words, I looked to magazines to fill me in on what I didn't know. At seventeen I was always reading those little Kotex ads. They always had questions and answers—that's about as much as I could find out.

And of course when you have relationships knowing so little, you have some pretty traumatic experiences. Mine were not abusive—they were more self-abusive, because I had to have an abortion. I remember traveling to New York from Philadelphia, because New York was the only place that you could find someone to do an abortion. When I think back to the horror of that experience, I don't know why I'm still here. No one told me what to expect. No one ever said, "Okay, you go here, and this happens, and then you go home, and this is what happens after that, which is traumatic."

Still, throughout my life, and it's now some forty years later, I've had a very positive experience with myself, and with trying to maintain varying degrees of wellness. Naturally, you get off the track. You're always going to do better, and you're always not going to have that extra glass of wine, and all of this. These are things I'd like to accomplish during my lifetime so I can pass on some wisdom to my daughter.

Ironically, my daughter called me yesterday from Tennessee to tell me that she was having this terrible flow of her period. She was just having an awful time, and what should she do? And I said, "Hang in there, we'll get you some help." She was very scared. She said she hadn't had a period for three months, and I said, "Well, why didn't you say anything?" She was afraid to. So this will be useful to me, and useful to my daughter, and useful to my other daughter, who was with me every day throughout this ordeal. So that's just a part of the story—mothers learning and sharing with their daughters in ways that our mothers could never share with us.

#### Khadeesha

I almost felt kind of stupid about the fact that I was unconscious about my womb. I started my period when I was thirteen and never had cramps or any problems, so I didn't know when it was coming. I didn't know what the cycle days were.

Then when I remarried at thirty-five, I wanted to have more children and it didn't happen right away. So I immediately thought, "It must be me. I've never had any problems in the past." So then I went to a fertility workshop and that's when I learned how many days were in my cycle. I found the whole thing so fascinating. It seems I have a clockwork cycle; I never knew that before. But it became fascinating to me to mark it on a calendar and to know what day it was coming. I think of it as an upsetting thing that I haven't had a daughter, but it's probably a blessing because I think if I hadn't had this occurrence I still wouldn't know. I've never investigated my womb or anything like that before and so that's important.

I'm a visual artist, and I'm starting to see the situation of the womb and past memory coming up in my work. I've been writing about the womb, and I've never done that. One of the things I've said is that I am the womb—I am the continuum and I am a wombman. I have within my body a memory that goes back thousands of years, and that's what I work with.

### Angela

I had been in Vermont praying that something healing would present itself to me. But I didn't expect an answer in twenty-four hours, and certainly not to be sitting here with all of you in this Womb Circle.

I'm a bodyworker—and all my life I've worked with women, and I've also been a hairdresser for forty years, and I teach vegetarian cooking. However, in the last year I have been diagnosed with a fibroid tumor, which I am not the least bit worried about because I have that much faith that I can solve it.

It's interesting that after being a vegetarian for twenty-seven years that I should have a fibroid tumor. I haven't eaten flesh, but I have eaten wrong combinations of food, and my mental state has been in trauma at different times. In Christiane Northrup's book Women's Bodies, Women's Wisdom, she spoke of problems that occur within the uterus. She said one of the things that could cause this was a poor relationship with one's mother. I did not have a good relationship with my mother, but by the time she died I had completed that karma, and it was wonderful. But I was left with unrealized creativity, unrealized relationships, unrealized many things.

I really started to look at things. I thought, "My God, I've been asleep to my womb. I've been totally asleep. I thought I was so conscious, that I could give you twenty minutes on anything to do with oriental this and that and the other. But where am I?"

I'm fifty-four years old. I got my period when I was

nine—I just looked between my legs for a few moments and said, "These tight jeans must be cutting me." I had no idea what was going on. My mom was Caribbean—Puerto Rican—and very, very strict. God forbid I should have been told about anything that was going on in my body. I had two brothers. I was the only girl child, and I was the youngest, and from there on in, no one ever told me what I needed to know.

I recalled that my mother told my dad, "Go get your daughter some Kotex, she's become a woman." I'm this little fat kid, and I'm thinking, "What am I, a woman now?" My only thought was, "Wow, now I can't kiss." I wanted to kiss. But now I couldn't kiss anymore because of course I would become pregnant. I broke all New York records; I was a virgin until I was twenty-five. I proved myself to my mother. But then I said to myself, "Let me get rid of this before it goes bad." I may have started late, but I made up for it. I was quite promiscuous for ten years. All bad relationships. Attracting all the wrong people because of my toxic condition.

Finally I heard a lecture that totally transformed my life. The speaker said that we absorb every man we've ever been with. That men want it all the time because they're cleansing themselves through us. We're the absorbers. So I'm walking around with everybody still in me. Then I got the opportunity to stop running around—I had a relationship that lasted eight years. I thought I was fine, that I'd found Mr. Perfect. I thought I could become a shaman by injection. It doesn't work.

But in the last two years, when I've had no relations, all of a sudden this part of me pulsates and talks to me. The voice of the womb. My womb talks. I've had visions. That's why I know this fibroid tumor in me is going away. I've had visions of my cave being closed off by a temporary boulder. But my womb says, no no no no no. And that's it. As we say in our affirmations: "My womb is healing, and so is my life!"

### Latitia

When my sister mentioned this Sacred Womb Circle I was surprised and happy, because I've been having a lot of womb problems. I'm definitely not close to my mother or to any of the women in my family, so I have no one to ask questions about past histories. I always had regular periods until I was twenty, and from then on it went downhill. I would have them one month, then six months would pass, three months would pass, I would bleed for one day or never.

My husband and I had several miscarriages and

there came a point where—nothing. I went to see several doctors and they said, "Oh, you're fine." I had a couple of abrasions on my tubes and they repaired them, and from then on everything, according to the doctors, was fine. "There's nothing wrong with you," they kept saying.

So a couple of months ago, probably about November, I came to this point in my life where I said, "I am going to be fine, and I know that everything is going to fall into place. I know I'm going to have a child, and I know my periods will be the way they're supposed to be, and everything in my life is going to work." Now I'm just at the point where I want to get my womb together—to let everything begin to unroll. I want to love my womb so everything that is possible happens.

## Betty

I've always managed to have a special relationship with my womb. And the thing that I've liked about my period is the rhythmicity, that it would occur at a certain time. It gave me a chance to learn what happened in that interim twenty-eight to thirty days. There were certain feelings that would let me know, and I'd say, "Aha!" I didn't need a calendar to know where I was in my cycle. I could tell by the way my body felt. And just before my period, if I started feeling real teary, I'd say, "Let me go get a book," or "Oh, God, I need to go and talk with somebody who's going to stroke me or nurture me." And I'd say, "But I can't be around so-and-so because that person's a bit abrasive, and I know I'll get my feelings hurt."

Unfortunately, I married a man who didn't have that kind of sensitivity, so I started to lose touch with some of that. It wasn't until shortly after my daughter was born that I realized I had really lost touch with my womb and I had to work at getting it back.

I don't know if any of you have been on birth control pills. Birth control pills disconnect you from feeling your rhythm. They disconnected me from being able to tell where I was in my river. Before that, fourteen days after my period I'd be horny. I'd say, "Oh, shit, I'd better make sure I have some kind of protection if I'm going to have sex, because I'm vulnerable." I knew the cycle.

Right after my period there would be this wonderful time. It was like the sun was out and everything was so clear—things that I just didn't understand before were now clear. I just loved it right after my period. Don't make decisions just before your period because you can't sort things out. Your hormones have you going all different ways. But right after your period, there's all that light.

It was a good time to study because I couldn't sleep. I'd be up the entire twenty-four hours. I learned to use those kinds of cues, and they were rhythmic, they were predictable, even to this day.

Recently, though, I've developed fibroids, and that's what made me realize I'd gotten out of touch. Then my fibroids went down. In my last examination, my gynecologist simply couldn't understand. Then I developed a walnut-sized lesion in my breast, and I've had to go inside again and say, "Something has happened. Some need is not being met." That's when a friend of mine said, "You need to go to that group I told you about." And that's how I got here.

I think that where I'm at in my own life right now is that I'm about to be reproductive—not in the biological sense, but in the spiritual sense. A giving, a birthing. So things are beginning to open up, and it requires me to get in touch not just with my uterus but with my entire reproductive system.

I'm happy to report that the lesion in my breast is now totally gone. In a visualization I saw that it was my need for nurturing that my breast was calling for, and I needed to meet that need, and honor that. And now it's gone. My doctor couldn't give me a theory. But I know how it came about. I started to go in, and I started to write. I started to talk to myself and to different parts of myself to understand what those different parts were feeling.

And a lot of stuff just started to come up for me. Then I started to do nurturing things that appealed to my sexuality, and do nice things for myself. I went out and bought a really beautiful blouse and that made me feel great. I couldn't believe how good it felt, since I usually shop for function.

That's what has begun to happen. As I dialogue with my womb, I'm getting in touch with unfed parts of myself. It's a rich discovery, but it's work. It takes a lot of time. Up front, I thought, "Where am I going to find the time?" But when you need to, you find the time. It was a good beginning, and now I think, well, there's something here for me, and I'll just be open until I find it.

## A SACRED WOMB CIRCLE HEALING RITUAL FOR THE WOMBS OF THE WORLD

It's painful to remember what your womb re-members, all the things that were said or weren't said. As the weeks go on, you may find your journal filling up with issues and feelings that you've been holding down. But who you are is made up of every one of those experiences that may have been pent up inside—until now. And now is when the pain is coming up. And now is when it needs to be felt, really felt.

Yes, it's okay to cry because tears make you whole. They're a libation to the spirit, a washing of the soul, a renewal. Whenever I hear the sto-ries the sister-Queens share, I often cry inside. And I'm never quite sure if they're my tears for my life, or their tears, or a combination of womb tears all over the earth. One of the things that's happening to this planet is that we're bleeding to death. The planet is dying. But we can restore it to wellness by just keeping our Womb Circles together and being committed to our Womb Wisdom, a wisdom that can rebirth us all.

### Strong Black Women

How often have you heard that black women have been made strong because we need our strength to carry on? Well, don't be too quick to buy into that. Recently they've done a lot of re-search on melanin and how it holds everything. It holds the good, bad, and indifferent—and the stronger your melanin, the more you will hold emotions, chemicals, toxins. When it's time to let go, other races with less melanin can release these things more easily. But our melanin holds on to all that.[2]

When things come up in your journal or in exchanges with your sister-friends, you might tell yourself, "I can share with my sisters and know I'll be safe. I'm not going to go through any of this."

But you will feel it, and feel it deeply. So I'm just going to say that I want you to rise, as often as you're able while this is going on, between the hours of 4 A.M. and 6 A.M. That's when your in-tuitive energy is flowing most strongly. That's when our power is at its peak. And within our ancient Khamitic Afrakan legacy, that is when Nebt-Het appears, the NTRU who deals with the mystery, that inner voice, that inner dream state where you're able to connect to the Source that knows all things.

## I CRY A RIVER OF TEARS THAT HEAL

One special and extraordinarily powerful cere-mony that our Sacred Circle carried out on be-half of all the wounded women of the world was a healing ritual in which we went deeply into our pain and processed it on behalf of all women, much like Ntozake Shange's choreopoem "For Colored Girls Who Have Considered Suicide When the Rainbow Is Enuf."

In this ritual, all the women in the Sacred Circle act as a chorus. Individual women tell each of the stories, but the entire chorus chants: "I cry a River of Tears that Heal . . ." You can use this basic idea, and ask the women in your circle to contribute their own special offerings, praying for deep release and deep healing.

*I cry a river of tears that heal,* for crying is good and tears are holy. Crying creates room for heal-ing to take place. Crying clears our vision so that we can see the inner desires of our heart. Crying releases and unites. Crying flushes out the un-natural and makes space for the mystical. Crying renews and restores and opens us up to all pos-sibilities. Our souls are washed by our tears. Crying humbles us to the ways of the Creator/ Creatress. When we cry from our womb so deep, we honor and baptize her, and our womb is made whole again through the libation of our tears.

*I cry a river of tears that heal* for Ankht-Ra, whose mother and grandmother, like many women of color in Trinidad, West Indies, went to the hospital for what they were led to believe was a routine surgical appendectomy, only to have their wombs removed instead. Much time passed before they found out that they were the victims of a stolen womb, a deceitful tragedy performed by physicians they had trusted with their lives. Neither will ever be the same.

*I cry a river of tears that heal* for the dear young sister who could have been my daughter.

She was sexually molested from the age of seven by her father, and her uncle, her father's brother. No one ever seemed to notice what tragedy had befallen this little girl. In the end, years of pain and grief led her to contract cancer of the womb. She died at age twenty-nine from a broken heart and a broken womb. May her soul finally rest in peace.

*I cry a river of tears that heal* for what is known as "female genital mutilation," "female castration," or "female circumcision," all terms used to describe an Afrakan tradition of cutting away the clitoris when a young girl is approaching adulthood.

In reading of female genital mutilation I wept, for the clitoris is so sensitive, like a flower. If touched with reverence, it can send you into ecstasy. But a slight blow to the clitoris can send shock waves of infinite discomfort throughout the body.

Countless women have endured this castration, where their legs are forcefully parted by the elder women who perform the procedure. This vaginal womb-crime perpetuates a tradition that causes agonizing suffering. How can women hurt women so deeply?

*I cry a river of tears that heal* for the Negro slave woman, my great-great-grandmother, who was forced to part her thighs for the entrance of a pale pink penis to fulfill her owner's demonic quest to force his way violently into her soft dark womb, leaving his . . . pardon me, I can't breathe, I'm still enraged two hundred years later. I still hurt. I still bleed. I'm outraged, feeling fear and helplessness for all my great-great-grandmothers who passed their self-hate, lack of self-esteem, their acceptance of abuse, their internal war down through the bloodline to me.

My womb still pains at the thought of the rape of all the women of my race. My grandmother's rape—I scream! My mother's rape—I shout! My auntie's rape, my sister's rape, my daughter's rape, my rape—I cry out our pain!

*I cry a river of tears that heal* for all the wombs that could not bear the pains that life inflicts. The wombs that gave up and made their transition. These losses occurred because the keeper of the womb was ignorant in the ways of healing herself. I cry because through the ages mothers lost the wisdom and confidence that they knew how to heal their own and their daughters' wombs. I cry into my cup of tea, and my tears act as a tonic and release for my soul's ascension.

When I think of women's stories of blood-filled pain, the tears from my heart fall like vast waters of the Nile. I hear the unheard voices of these women's wombs. And I cry a river of tears that heal.

*I cry a river of tears that heal* for wombs that carried on after the put-downs, the beatings, the rapes, the disrespect, the womb muggings, all causes of planetary chaos reflected in women's debilitated womb conditions.

I cry for wombs that carried on after the red flood of days and months of bleeding, and the white discharges, and the grip of the contractions. I cry for the merciful release of wombs re-birthing themselves.

*I cry a river of tears that heal* for the women who carried on after the wars and womb castration and womb scars of incest, oozing with pain, shame, and regret. I cry for wombs that carried on after babies were born, and after babies died inside of the womb. I cry for wombs that carried on after radiation and laser attacks to eliminate the tumors filled with the mucus and waste of the hate, anger, and vexation of the spirit trapped in the womb, the holy nest.

*I cry a river of tears that heal* over men and women to wash away our womb exhaustion, for although we keep on keeping on, we've had to bear so much through our wombs it's a wonder we're still standing. Holy Spirit, Olodumare, why it gotta be so hard being a woman?

I am the Afrakan Woman, crying out my pain, screaming and retching Rivers of Tears from generation to generation. My tears boil up from the bile of plantation slave life here in America the Beautiful. Here, where institutionalized sex factories were brutally imposed upon a stolen people for generations.

I cry for the soft wombs and damaged souls of my Mothers who were forced to bear babies of rage and incest. They were womb casualties in a four-hundred-year war that damaged them down to their DNA. The wounds go oh so deep within the wombs of the womenfolk of my tribe.

Our wombs still choke and stammer, fight and flee.

Mother, help me.

I'm praying without ceasing for renewed wombs to bring in a future so bright that they draw to themselves respect, gratitude, grace, and love.

To women who go on suffering from womb crimes I say, "Tighten up your loins, and purify and fast and pray until you see a change in every corner of your life, until you see light all about you." My tears honor those wombs that carried us all, that carried on after womb alienation and mutilation. Wombs that carried on even after self-inflicted and societal womb violations; wombs that carried on with only one ovary left to fend for itself due to inner toxicity.

*I cry a river of tears* that may not heal in this generation for the rape of Nanking in China during their World War II holocaust at the hands of the Japanese. Tears flowed into the lap of a woman whose soul flew away through her womb when all that made her a woman was beaten out of her as her thighs were tied to each side of a rape chair to be repeatedly attacked by Japanese soldiers.

Tears continue to flow to a joint river for the subhuman soldier who took a metal rod and rammed it through a woman's womb as she lay helplessly naked in the streets of her homeland. Somebody's daughter and somebody's mother go right on suffering, caught up in the flames of war.

And will there ever be enough tears to heal the women of Bosnia who were ruthlessly forced to sexually service the soldiers inside of rape camps, a diabolical institutionalized machinery that cranked out wounded wombs and destroyed all possibility of life?

*I cry a river of tears that heal* for our daughters who yearn for peace within their wombs. I cry soul tears of truth and vision, hope and praise for the resurrection of the sacred wombs of the first women. My tears cry a river of healing rays of lapis lazuli, emerald, and energizing malachite as they dance on the vision of newfound prayed-up, purified-up, joyous wombs, Sacred Wombs lifted up by us women and protected by our holy men, our good men.

This womb vision offers us a future so bright that it sends crystal-clear light throughout the land in a tide of deliverance.

*I cry a river of tears that heal* with all the women all over the Planet Earth. May our collective tears become pure light and transform into wings that fly our souls, like Heru the Falcon, through a global ocean of redemption to heal and baptize the earth.

My Lord! my Creator/Creatress, Mut, Ast, and Mother Mary, bless all your daughters in the whole world, especially the Dark Woman of the Womb, the Eldest Mother. Mother Ast (Isis), protect our wombs throughout our life journey so that we women may age gracefully and beautifully inside of our sacred selves.

*I cry a river of tears that heal.* Now we can roll out of the river and into the healing mud. As our womb draws the nourishment from the earth, we face the Sun and get charged. We dance by the river and wash our wombs, reborn Sacred Women, moving into our original divine womblike state.

All hail to the mothers who held and nurtured us so that we could be delivered to the planet through our constant attentiveness to the great womb.

*"Thank you, Mother/Father Creator/Creatress."* I offer these words in gratitude for keeping us and growing us like tall trees; for loving us and caring for all your ignorant children who may have been deaf to our body's plea and numb to our pain. Dearest Mother/Father Creator/Creatress, may we all be delivered, encouraged, and inspired to make a massive world womb change. If there is no change in the global attitude toward women's wombs, it will be impossible to find peace on earth. If there is no change, war and slavery and the injustices done to humans will always rule.

*So I cry tears* of praise and honor, respect and gratitude, grace and love, to those wombs that have made their transition into the next world, and to those wombs that survived.

### A Mother Nut Blessing

To all the wombs in the world, look up toward Nut the heavenly Sky Mother and listen well as she speaks from within you:

*I am Nut. I am the breath and the Womb of the Cre-
ator/Creatress, put your trust in me. I, Mother Nut,
pour down upon my daughters clouds of serenity. For
today is a new day. It is your day, and on this day
I grant you, my daughters, another chance, a higher
vision, another opportunity, a greater way, a second
coming.*

*Know this, my daughters, no matter how heavy or
hurtful your womb life, I bore you with countless illuminating stars that dwell within your being. I planted
within you a seed of womb enlightenment that will
grow as you become more conscious of my presence
within you. My beloved daughters, sit with me daily,
and I will shine light upon your womb and give you
peace.*

## WOMB RITUALS, MEDITATIONS, AFFIRMATIONS, CHANTS, AND PRAYERS

### Release Ritual to Cleanse the Womb

The Release Ritual to cleanse the womb of your
soul is to be performed after or during your
prayer work. Release helps us to purge both psychic and physical attacks on our wombs. Take a
look at all your womb experiences as lessons.
Trauma by trauma, your womb will begin to release the baggage that adds up to mental, spiritual, and physical disease.

Write a journal letter to the people in your
life who offended your womb in any way. In
your letter include self-forgiveness if you have
brought any harm or pain to your womb consciously or unconsciously. Know that there
comes a time when, to survive, we must let it all
go. Pour your feelings onto the pages of your
journal. For example, write, "I, Barbara, release
and let go of the pain Michael left inside my
womb and my life."

Wake up! Shake off and out of your divine
womb center the residue of anger or resentment
you have stored up. Come on, just let it happen.
Through seven days of fasting and prayer and
spiritual baths, release the emotional venom out
of your womb, your Body Temple. If you are
able to reach the person you have been hurt or
offended by, then send them a release letter directly.

## MY WOMB
### Queen Ife / Cassandra Battle

I commit to "Heal Myself."
I commit to healing my womb—
The womb that a nation generates
The womb that a nation penetrates.
By birth and birthing babies
Woman, woman womb that we do create,
The hard blows and trauma by what we ate.
The dairy, the meats, the rape
Of your emotional, your physical being.
The deed of you who enters my womb,
my sugar wall
Who I let enter in an angry state
Creating havoc or the lustful pleasure, I partake.
And when the baby I kill, by choice to terminate,
The cysts, the tumors, all from what I ate
Oh, womb, what a wretched state.
We kiss, have mindless sex, which stimulates
Abuse—abuse, the womb accumulates
The down note blues, pain, sickness does not relate!
Then all disorders will constipate.
My Womb communicates,
Degrading injected toxins, suffocate.
The womb from her agony expels the poisons
She regurgitates.
"Let's do spring cleaning," the doctor dictates
And the surgeons diligently wait
For the womb the doctor says, "Too late."
I fought for my womb to remain whole.
Not a fraction will you take
Not too late as the doctor states.
I then turned to alternative medicine
Now I could relate.
Especially in my state.
My womb, womb cries, out,
*I hurt, I ache*
And screams,
*the broken dreams, unloving
relationships—family and men.*
I now flush down the stool
Using the lever as my tool,
I flush, I flush away all the waste.
I take my time and not in haste
I vacate, eliminate I cleanse and cleanse
I make love to my womb.
I elevate.
I say to my womb,
"I love you, womb."
I say to my womb, REJUVENATE!

If for whatever reason you are not able to connect with the person, then once you have completed your writing ritual, burn the letter, perhaps with a little sage, and release your pent-up emotions in spirit smoke. As the letter burns, pray that your release may be taken on wings of air and that freedom may be your destination.

Then immediately go into Nature, to the ocean or the forest, and sing, dance, shout, cry, stomp. Be the queen of your Body Temple. Allow your mind and spirit to be filled with a new world of revelation, self-acceptance, and self-healing.

Working on your forgiveness or letting-go ritual is not necessarily for the person you feel may have harmed you. What it really does is ensure your own personal healing. When we release we create room to draw to ourselves the divine unions that are our birthright.

## The Feather of Maat

We need to make sacred time every day to restore our inner balance and peace and to release everything that weighs down our heart and our womb and our spirit.

One way to do this is to meditate with the feather of Maat, the symbol of truth, harmony, and balance. Think of the hours of 4 A.M. to 6 A.M. as the time of Nebt-Het. She is the Lady of the House, the Body Temple—and she is the Lady of the Heavens, the Celestial Body. Nebt-Het also represents the spirit of intuition. At that hour, your melanin is pouring out and you hear things that you could not hear during the day. You receive visions that you could not see later on, and you connect with your dreams and receive messages. You begin to understand the depth of who you are, what you are, and why you are.

It's at the hour of Nebt-Het that we drink pure water and herbal tea, such as red raspberry. It's at that hour that we take our healing bath. And it's at that hour that Nebt-Het will come and talk to us, and answer us. To welcome her, we must eat lightly to hold the light. If we're full of a dense, heavy dinner, we will not have the ears to hear.

Let's celebrate that spirit. Let's walk with a feather. All womb wellness workers must have a feather in their medicine bags, because your feather is going to be the quickest way to lighten up your heart, for illness happens when your heart becomes heavy. The ancient Khamites weighed the heart against a feather to determine the quality of one's soul. When your heart is heavy due to an accumulation of anger and pain and strife, it becomes imbalanced, and that's when tumors grow and cysts grow, and that's when you create seven days of bleeding. When the heart is heavy day in and day out, year after year, it begins to accumulate upsets that you may not even be aware of. The body begins to be deeply imprinted with distress and it becomes totally off balance. This is when the feather of Maat can bring us the clarity we need to restore our balance—inner and outer.

Recently, I had put a feather on top of my head because I was in the spirit. But I had a business appointment that morning and I got to wondering if it was okay to go to the appointment with my feather. Could they handle this? Did I have to change my look to do business? I knew the person I was seeing quite well, and when I asked her if I should put away my feather, she said, "No. Be who you really are." And then she took out her medicine bag, which every Sacred Woman must have.

So my friend opens up her little medicine bag in corporate America, and she tells me to close my eyes, and she puts a little tiny feather in my hand. I almost passed out, I was in such a state of joy. It was the most miraculous thing.

It was a blessing from Nebt-Het, for we cannot enter her house unless we come with the feather of Maat. This is because we have to come to all our decisions through balance, righteousness, truth, and harmony. Maat rules the lightness of the heart through the feather. We can check our heart daily when we come out of the bath. We don't have to walk through our day with a heavy heart.

## Maat Feather Meditation

To clear your heart, practice the following Maat Feather Meditation. Try it for just one week and see what opens up in your life. You may want to tape this meditation and play it as you relax and go deeper.

- Lie down in a quiet sacred place where you will not be disturbed. Place a white feather over your womb, close your eyes, focus on your breath, and allow yourself to slip deeper and deeper into a meditative state.
- Breathe in and out slowly as you become one with the lightness of the feather. Relax and let go of the stress and pressures of the world. Release all anxiety from your womb. As you continue to breathe deeply, let go of the pain from this life and all past lives.
- Allow your body to drift easily into a serene state of oneness with the Divine Spirit. You're becoming one with the feather resting gently on your womb as you move deeper and deeper and deeper into that quiet, safe space. Feel peace and calm flow into you as your inner balance is restored and renewed. If you're in bed and the day is done, just slip off into a sweet sleep.
- If you're starting your day and you're ready to emerge from your Maat Feather Meditation into the active meditation we call life, bring your Feather Meditation to an end by breathing like the quietly rolling ocean, deeply and fully.

Then, slowly and easily, sit up and continue your ocean breathing. When you're ready, stand up, knowing that you are filled with light and clarity, and move into your day with the same quiet balance that you achieved during your Maat Feather Meditation.

### Breathing Healing Light into the Womb Meditation

This is another excellent meditation to do at the hour of Nebt-Het to clear, balance, and nurture the womb.

Our wombs have been subjected to all kinds of trauma. We may have experienced emotional trauma. There may be vaginal discharges, clotting, cramping, and heavy menstruation. There may be physical tumors growing or removed, hysterectomies, difficult childbirth, cesarean sections, abusive sexual intercourse, abortions per-

formed, a history of scalpel or laser surgery, or radiation therapy. As we do our daily womb meditation, we can release those traumas with breath, color visualizations, proper diet, and hands-on healing.

- Sit comfortably in a chair, or better, sit on the floor with your legs crossed and your arms resting on your lap, or lie down flat on your back—whichever feels right to you. Begin to breathe deeply and slowly as you relax your face, chest, arms, hands, womb, hips, thighs, legs, and feet.
- Charge the energy in your hands by briskly rubbing them together until they're full of healing heat. Place your hands over your sacred womb, and now be very still. Breathe deeply, feel the warmth from your healing hands penetrating and filling your womb. Feel her relax.
- Continue to breathe deeply. Inhale slowly, visualizing light and peace and healing entering your womb as the air expands your abdomen and then your chest. Then, exhale slowly, visualizing all emotional and physical toxins departing from your womb as your abdomen contracts and your lungs push out the remaining air. Repeat ten to twenty times.
- Now use your breath to help feed healing colors into your womb. Use all the colors in the spectrum as color healing to charge, cleanse, and rejuvenate. Continue breathing in each successive color until your womb feels filled with that particular energy, and then move to the next color. While each color bathes your womb, say: "Womb, be still. Be at peace."
  Slowly breathe into your womb the color white, for cleansing. Now breathe in red/orange for power and energy. Next comes a deep shade of blue for peace. Breathe the color green into your womb for abundant wellness. Then breathe purple into your womb for spirituality; pink for divine love; violet for high womb consciousness; then gold for prosperity. And finally, breathe a fine clear yellow into your womb for the higher mind.
- Now recharge the energy in your hands and gently place them on your womb. Feel the peace, harmony, and well-being that fill your sacred womb.

• Finally, as you continue your slow breathing, visualize the four elements of the natural world—fire, water, air, and earth—and invite them to come and heal your womb. As you did with the color visualizations, spend as much time as you need with each element as you visualize them healing, nurturing, loving, and bringing you harmony.

First, visualize the Sun energizing your womb. Next experience the ocean washing and cleansing your womb. Feel the air caressing and bringing ease to your womb. Then feel the earth beneath you drawing out all the negativity from your womb.

Now that you have completed your meditation and have arrived at a deep state of relaxation, you might want to do as many Womb Rejuvenation Techniques (see pages 88–92) as your body requires, or your time permits. (You will find them in chapter 4.) Whatever you do, just be good to yourself, not just at this moment when you're attuned, but later in the day when things get hectic, and day after day, until your life becomes one endless meditation of peace, balance, and harmony.

## USING CHANTS AND AFFIRMATIONS TO SUPPORT THE WOMB

In addition to meditations and visualizations, try filling your womb with sacred words of wellness through daily chants and affirmations at sunrise and sunset. Feed positive thoughts, words, and attitudes into your womb throughout your day. Freely fill up your plate with these affirmations— you don't have to worry about gaining weight. As a matter of fact, if you consume enough of these affirmations, you're liable to lighten up your life.

Through mental, spiritual, and physical reprogramming and cleansing, we can change the direction of a lost womb. Let's begin by applying the affirmations I offer you as a guide to direct or redirect your ideas and conditions for a body, mind, and spiritual womb healing.

If healing your womb is the desire of your heart, then speak words of power to your womb regularly. Speak with all the fervor and love and compassion needed to strengthen the sacred consciousness of your womb.

Repeat as many of these affirmations as necessary to heal, recharge, and purify the spirit of your womb. As you speak these affirmations of empowerment, allow a flow of natural creativity to fill up your womb, to lift you up, and to inspire you to heal, to love, and to be a full woman, free!

### Twenty-Five Womb *Hesi* (Chants)

Chant your womb into wellness through these twenty-five *hesi* at sunrise and at sunset. Feed these and other positive affirmations into your womb throughout your day.

1. My womb is sacred, and so is my life.
2. My womb is precious, and so is my life.
3. My womb is divine, and so is my life.
4. My womb is love, and so is my life.
5. My womb is whole, and so is my life.
6. My womb is free, and so is my life.
7. My womb is radiant, and so is my life.
8. My womb is light, and so is my life.
9. My womb is great, it is good, and so is my life.
10. My womb is celestial, and so is my life.
11. My womb is peace, and so is my life.
12. My womb is bliss, and so is my life.
13. My womb is bright, and so is my life.
14. My womb is natural, and so is my life.
15. My womb is liberated, and so is my life.
16. My womb is full of energy, and so is my life.
17. My womb is pure, and so is my life.
18. My womb is in tune, and so is my life.
19. My womb is all-powerful, and so is my life.
20. My womb is the seat of my creativity, and so is my life.
21. My womb is full, and so is my life.
22. My womb is filled with prayer, and so is my life.
23. My womb is a dynamic force, and so is my life.
24. My womb is holy, and so is my life.
25. My womb is the gateway to heaven here on earth, and so is my life.

## Chanting "Womb"

Sound helps to harmonize the body, mind, and spirit.

- Sit quietly in a meditative pose in your sacred space, palms facing up.
- Breathe slowly in and out, coming back to your center and relaxing, going deeper each time. Now, chant "womb" twice. Chant as if you were chanting "om" or "ankh," but use the sound of the word "womb."
- Now relax and inhale. And when you exhale, you're going to exhale the sound "womb." Again, inhale. Find your note, your harmony if you're in a Sacred Circle, and chant "womb."
- Chant the sound "womb," and let it vibrate over your womb as you open up and relax even more deeply. Place your mind and sound right over your womb. Visualize the color of vitality, red or orange, which represent Ra, the Sun. Send the sound of "womb" and the color of the sun into your womb to help to resurrect her. Bring forth the sun from within your womb with color and sound and breath. Inhale. Chant "womb."
- Now you're going to baptize your womb with the color of serenity, because we carry so much stress in our wombs and our hearts and our minds. Visualize a rich, deep blue, as blue as the blue ocean, for serenity. Chant "womb," and as you vibrate with the sound, visualize the blue of the ocean filling your womb with serenity. Inhale. Exhale. Chant "womb."
- We also want to work with light, so now you're going to illuminate your womb with light. As you inhale, visualize white light all around your womb. Chant "womb." Let the sound go as high as your voice can reach, because when you welcome the height of the sound, then the womb energy goes up, so shift your voice from an alto to a soprano. Visualize white light filling your womb. Inhale. Exhale. Chant "womb."

Womb Wisdom wellness is here and present, and we're here to defend, support, and uplift the spirit of our womb so that we are free to create and birth divine ideas, divine energy, divine creativity, and divine children onto this planet. The resurrection of our wombs is the resurrection of Planet Earth. The earth's womb has been violated, just as our own wombs have been denied and forced into disharmony. But as we heal our wombs, we will also heal the womb of our Mother Earth.

---

### Womb Affirmations: Revelation to Regeneration

Put on or play beautiful music—flute, piano, or tambour (finger piano). Or be silent as you do your womb meditation and recite your litany of womb regeneration affirmations.

*I love my womb, she pleases me.*
*My womb's in perfect harmony.*
*My womb is disease-free.*
*There are no tumors, cysts, discharges, or PMS in my womb.*
*My womb is happy and whole, free of any and all disease.*
*I send love to my womb. I send peace to my womb.*
*I send light and breath to my womb.*
*My womb is the seat of my womanness, my power as a woman rests within me.*
*I release and let go of all hurts and disappointments as I affirm:*

I will turn every lesson into a blessing.

*I receive the lessons through my prayers and meditations.*
*I release all baggage from my womb's memory.*
*I replace the whirlwind of negativity with truth and divine love.*
*My womb will never again get stuck in the ignorance of womb disease, for I commit myself to womb wellness.*

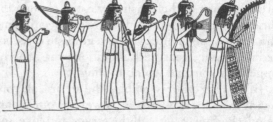

## A Womb Song

*Queen Afua and Hru Ankh Ra Semahj*

Sound coupled with breath can heal. The ringing of your voice in melodic tones inside your Body Temple can put your *aritu* (chakras) into a state of Maat. Feel free to be creative and sing your own womb song. Observe as your womb becomes more attuned and harmonious.

> *Khat-A M khu*
> (My womb is of light.)
>
> *Khat-A M Nut*
> (My womb is of Heaven.)
>
> *Khat-A M Ast*
> (My womb is of the Divine Mother.)
>
> *Khat-A M Maat*
> (My womb is of harmony.)

## Womb Purification Ritual and Prayer

Here is a ritual exercise for intense spiritual purification of your sacred womb.

Place a small round disk of charcoal used for smudging (available in botanicas) in a cast-iron or other fireproof pot. Light the charcoal disk, and when it is hot, sprinkle a handful of rock frankincense and myrrh onto it. Place the pot on the floor, on a stand or on a metal trivet so you don't burn the floor. Spread your legs and stand over the pot of frankincense and myrrh, as ancient Khamitic women used to do. As it smokes away all the negative vibrations, add a pinch of cinnamon to the charcoal to sweeten your womb.

If you need further blessings, protection, and cleansing, anoint your outer womb with the oil or essence of frankincense and myrrh, lavender, or sage. (You may follow the master Gateway chart on pages 130–135 to choose your anointing oils.) Also anoint the crown of your head and your heart *arit* for high thoughts and a pure heart.

Recite the womb prayer given here or your own affirmations:

*Creator/Creatress, I open my womb to thee for healing. I release all disappointment, tumors, infections, pain,* *resentment, PMS, hurt, and sadness. My prayer request is for a healthy, whole womb.*

*Creator/Creatress, I offer my womb to you for complete healing; I accept the womb that you have placed within me as being sacred, holy, and divine. Therefore, I submit to and accept your natural laws of purity and of cleanliness in each and every way.*

*Today I release all blockages that may dwell within my womb because of an unsettled mind and spirit. Without reservations, I accept and send healing energy to my sacred seat. On this day I celebrate the rebirth of my womb. I give praise and thanks in advance for the anointing and the healing of my blessed womb.*

*My Beloved Creator/Creatress, guard my mind, my womb, and my soul from the unrighteousness of the world so that my sacred womb may be protected and filled with perfect peace and my soul with the light of love. May my womb speak and know health and healing as a natural state of being.*

Now go about your day in a high, holy spirit. Look forward to becoming stress-free and empowered because your womb is now spiritually free.

## Prayer Work

Do some or all of the following. Listen to the Voice of your Womb and let your spirit guide you.

1. Smoke your womb with frankincense and myrrh.
2. Anoint your womb with sacred oils.
3. Give praise to the Creator/Creatress (Tua NTR) for the many blessings that have already manifested in your life and the lives of your blood and extended family.
4. Give praise to the Creator/Creatress for your womb.
5. Release through prayer. Let go of all negativity and toxic emotional feelings that may be trapping your womb and causing disease and upheaval.
6. Make prayer requests for the healing of your womb.
7. Offer up affirmations or womb prayers to Nut. Use the ones in this book as a model, and let the spirit in you flow so that you begin

to create your own womb prayers. Use them regularly for inspiration and illumination.

8. End your prayer work with several minutes of deep breathing as you move into your womb meditation.

## Creating and Wearing Your Waist Beads

Wearing waist beads is another loving, spiritual activity that has been handed down to us from the women of my culture, who were the first to wear waist beads for protection and adornment. Beads were worn around the waist for the physical and spiritual healing of the womb.

You can purchase waist beads from markets where Afrakan products are sold. Or you can lovingly make your own. Use clear quartz crystal beads for cleansing and purification, or rose quartz crystal beads to represent Divine Love.

Have an Elder Mother or mentor bless your waist beads before you wear them, so the love, blessings, and healing of the generations fill and protect your womb.

## Womb Rituals for the New Moon and Full Moon

Women's emotional and spiritual lives reflect the ways of the Moon and its cycles. As the Moon is renewed through its waxing and waning and fullness, so, too, are the states of women. Tune into the Moon through conscious meditation and ritual.

Go out into Nature under the New Moon; create a Sacred Womb Circle if you are working with a group of women. Play your sacred instruments (drums, sistrum, bells, etc.).

Begin your purification ritual using air (sound) and fire (smudging).

The Woman Elder, Spiritual Guide, or High Priestess guiding the ritual is to smudge everyone present with sage from head to toe.

The Woman Elder is to call out the Name of the Divine in gratitude. Then she calls out the name of Khonsu Nefer Hetep several times. As the son of Amon and Mut, Khonsu crosses the sky every night in the heavenly Moon boat. He is an ancient deity of healing and regeneration. Khonsu aids women with fertility problems and

the conception of a child or the conception of ideas.

Then call out Tehuti's name several times. Tehuti is the guardian and the protector of the Moon.

Now call upon the Guardians of the Directions:

Adoration to Mother Mut Nebt-Het, from the East. *Tua NTR.*
Adoration to Mother Mut Serket, from the South. *Tua NTR.*
Adoration to Mother Mut Ast, from the West. *Tua NTR.*
Adoration to Mother Mut Nt, from the North. *Tua NTR.*
Adoration to our Heavenly Mother, Nut.
Adoration to our Earthly Father, Geb.
Adoration to Shu (breath, atmosphere).
Adoration to Tefnut (water, moisture).

Drink Sacred Women's Herbal Tonics in honor of the womb. Choose the tonic according to your need. For example, if you have tumors, use goldenrod; if you have heavy bleeding, use shepherd's purse; if your womb needs toning, use raspberry; if your womb needs strengthening, use dandelion.

If your Sacred Womb Circle is honoring the Full Moon, all the women are to dance in a clockwise circle, echoing the Full Moon in their dance with flowing movements like the ocean of Nun. The dance is to move and lift the spirit, and to acknowledge our ebb and flow that is cosmically expressed in the Moon. Give praise for the visions that have come from the light of the Moon.

If your Womb Circle is having a ceremony for the New Moon, pray for what you desire, what you want to build on, to manifest—a work to generate, a mission to unfold, a project to begin, a happening to take place. New thoughts, new visions, new beginnings are what we bring to the New Moon Ritual. Dance for new beginnings that the New Moon brings forth. Dance for the New Moon, to acknowledge our visions coming of age.

The New Moon is also a powerful time to ask for forgiveness and to forgive wrongs done, to rise to a new state of mind. It is a time for cleansing. Breathe deeply as you hold a clear quartz crystal or moonstone over your womb, flushing out the old hurts and pain, clear back to your beginnings.

Give thanks for what has already manifested, the gifts that have already been received, the journeys that have come to an end. Give praise for the help that you have received.

Close the circle by giving thanks and praise under the Moon, under Mother Mut, by dancing to drums, bells, shekere, and so on. Let the spirit move you. Give praise to Nebt-Het, the Guardian of the New Moon.

Together say, "Adoration to heavenly Mother Nature for holding the Moon and the Sun in the sky!"

Keep a moonstone on your altar of Nut to support the harmony and healing of your womb.

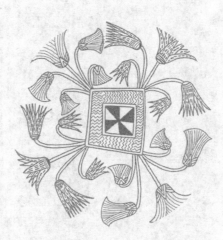

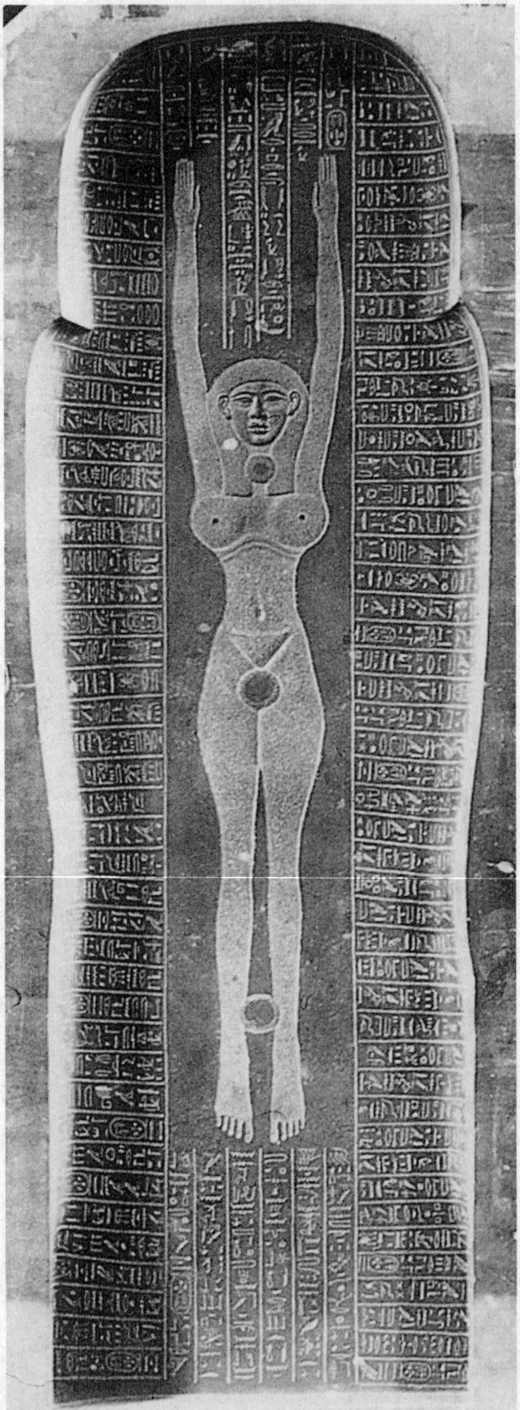

# CHAPTER 4
# THE CARE OF THE WOMB

I've been on the Natural Living path for more than forty-five years, and for at least thirty-eight of those years I've been helping women. It was not necessarily my intention to focus on women. My commitment was to healing families. Nevertheless, I kept seeing a lot of women with health concerns, and they would inevitably have a problem with the womb. Their challenges ranged from high blood pressure to diabetes, from heavy menstrual bleeding to cysts and tumors. But I discovered with each of them that there was always some level of blockage in the womb.

My clients' womb challenges led me to study womb herbs and womb foods, womb affirmations and womb meditations and womb colors. To my amazement, what all this taught me was that you could transform your whole Body Temple by healing just one part of your body.

As a colon therapist, I've come to truly honor that our miraculous bodies are made up of many worlds, and that we can focus on one world and see what's going on with all our other worlds. Take reflexology, for example. Your foot is a map of your whole body, from the big toe (representing your brain) to the arch of your foot (representing your spine), the heel (the lower extremities), and the ankles (your reproductive organs). And if you've done any delving into iridology, you've discovered that when iridologists look into your eyes they can identify where all the blockages are and how they correspond to the rest of the body.

All of my explorations into Natural Living and the healing arts have led me to one conclusion—the womb is the foundation of a woman's whole self. It is the defining sacred center of our bodies, minds, and spirits.

Over the years many women have come to me when they're facing a health crisis, such as having their womb removed. Rather than telling them not to schedule surgery, I would simply ask, "How much time is the doctor giving you?"

"Well, the doctor said in the next two months, or maybe even the next month."

And then I'd offer another possibility: "Let's see how much work we can do now. Perhaps there are alternatives worth exploring rather than just accepting hysterectomy as your only option."

What grew out of my work is the concept that there is a nonviolent approach to womb wellness. It comes through being conscious of the womb's own wisdom and utilizing natural therapies that honor our whole being, including:

- Juice therapy
- Live foods
- Nature's herbs
- Water therapy
- Movement and breath
- Essential oils
- Clay infusions and applications

## EAT TO LIVE

There is a toxic lifestyle that actually feeds tumors in the womb, breasts, and other parts of the body. However, if we change to a natural, flesh-free, and limited-starch diet, we can prevent growths and diseases found in the womb, in the breasts, and throughout the Body Temple. For example, mango, papaya, coconut water, ginger, sorrel, honeydew, celery, parsnip, and cucumber, plus all the many kinds of greens, make our wombs supreme.

In *Heal Thyself for Health and Longevity*, I say

that it takes love to feed a child, water to feed a plant, and milk, eggs, cheese, and flesh to feed a tumor. What this means is that we have control of the destiny of our wellness. When we, as women, practice the principles of "eat to live," rather than "live to eat," then we will eat ourselves into good health.

The methods of natural eating presented in this chapter will support your womb as you recover from the poisonous nonlive foods that contribute to disease. Study these principles and techniques of natural living and become transformed.

Wherever you start off with your womb concerns, whether it's PMS, fibroids, heavy menstrual bleeding, infertility, or menopause, within twenty-one to twenty-eight days of applying the Natural Living approach, you will begin to see changes. Our monthly cycles offer us a perfect form of measure. You will see how your life will change from one period to the next when you become conscious of your womb and her wisdom. You will see how the rest of your life changes when your womb changes. Your attitudes will change—how you look at men, how you look at your children, how you look at your work, how you look at your life—and you will begin to truly comprehend just how much is held inside your womb and how her state affects everything in your life.

## THE SACRED WOMB WELLNESS APPROACH

To begin our journey into the care of our physical wombs, I offer you the following womb wellness visualization and affirmations:

### Sacred Womb Wellness Affirmation

Meditate on womb wellness. Visualize a well womb daily, upon the rising and setting of the sun, for what you see and breathe into your soul you become. Affirm:

*My fallopian tubes are clear and clean. My ovaries are rich and filled with life. My vagina is a channel of purity. My uterus is radiantly healthy, for my womb is a sacred part of me.*

### The Sacred Ancient Mirror

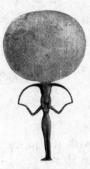

The mirror was first developed thousands of years ago in Khamit by polishing a metal surface to a high reflective shine. Mirrors were important, for they symbolized fertility, beauty, and protection. In ancient times we didn't just use the mirror to see how we looked. When we gazed into a mirror we knew that it not only reflected our physical body and beauty, but also reflected our spiritual condition and offered us an opportunity to view our very soul looking back at us. This power is embodied in the Egyptian word for mirror, *ankh*, which is also the ancient Egyptian word for life. The mirror reflects and symbolizes childbirth, fertility, and protection.

The Khamite people also used mirrors to banish negative forces and to draw in positive right energy—as the ancient Chinese practice of Feng Shui still does today. Everything the ancients did was spiritually inspired; even the faces of mirrors were shaped round like the sun to reflect its penetrating power and vitality.

### Exploring Your Womb: Womb Mirror Self-Reflection Exercise

From an art museum shop, purchase a copy of the ancient Het-Hru (Hathor) mirror, or create your own Ancient Mirror of the Spirit. Take a simple small round mirror with a handle and beautify it. Paint it artfully, or glue cowry shells on it, or glue on silver, gold, lavender, or green sparkles—all while you're in the spirit of Het-Hru, the spiritual guardian of beauty.

To begin to get to know your womb, take your spiritually charged Het-Hru mirror with you to a quiet private space in your sacred sanctuary, preferably where some sunshine is flowing through your window. Put on some soft music, strings or flute or piano, to create the right atmosphere for your womb journey. Sit quietly on the floor and breathe deeply as you meditate on Mother Nut for inner peace.

Now, pull your dress up to the waist, or take off your slacks, and remove your underpants.

Slowly spread your legs wide and place your sacred mirror between your thighs, looking inward. Take a long, deep, meditative look at the entrance of your womb. When you're ready, breathe deeply, and gently separate the lips of your gateway to see further into your sacred garden. Meditate quietly on what you see. Stay with her for a few minutes, and give yourself a chance to become acquainted.

When you're done, bless your sacred gateway, and thank her for sharing herself with you. Remaining in your inner meditative space, sit quietly and write in your womb journal. Record what you feel about this sacred part of your womanness:

- Did you want to hurry up and get it over? Were you able to just take your time?
- How did she look—pretty, healthy, smooth, inviting, weak, dry, moist?
- Was she foaming at the mouth; did she have a drip?
- Did she smell clean, sweet, and natural? Or did she smell fishy, yeasty, or fleshy?
- Has this Sacred Womb Journey made you feel dirty or beautiful? Embarrassed or ashamed? Is your attitude positive or negative about looking at the face of your womb?

During this exercise, know that a great deal of healing is taking place on the inner, subtle planes. You might be scared or shocked or at ease. Many emotions are going to rise from you—all carrying stored-up information about yourself. Just let them flow.

Fear not, for the Most High is with you all the way through your womb healing. As you tune into your inner womb spirit, open a dialogue; talk out loud or in silence. Listen intently— your womb is speaking to you through your womb mirror about what she needs in order to heal.

## My Womb Mirror Adventure

I was reluctant to explore my inner self with the womb mirror the first time. I kept telling myself I was too busy with other things. Then I finally said, "It's time." So I went into my bedroom, sat quietly, and opened up my legs. I took the mirror, and I looked at my womb entrance.

My first thought was, "I've been here before." Then I said, "Hmmm, this looks strange. Oh, you need to be groomed. Okay, you need brushing." I got some olive oil, and a little lotus oil, and I just oiled her down. I said, "Oh, Mother Nut, I've been careless."

When I opened the lips, I thought, "Mmm, they're very pink. You two look so beautiful, let me try to think beautiful thoughts about what I'm seeing."

I also saw who came out, who was left out as I did this profound meditation—all the different feelings, the babies that came through, the pain I had experienced from periods to infections to giving birth.

You too will see different things in your womb. Some will be physical. Some will be spiritual. The Womb Mirror Self-Reflection Exercise will be your moment of truth, your moment to look at yourself in the mirror and say:

*I love you. I love you unconditionally.*
*I loved you even in my ignorance.*
*I loved you when I didn't even know.*
*I just love you.*

Send that love to your womb—even if you don't believe it in the beginning. Remember, your womb mirror reflections are also a reflection of your life.

Upon completing this part of your Sacred Womb Journey, smudge your womb area carefully with sage smoke in the ancient Khamitic way by wafting smoke over your body from a small iron pot with a small burning charcoal round from a botanica over which you have sprinkled sage leaves and twigs. Or anoint the outer surface of your womb with lotus oil as you affirm and pray for womb healing. Be careful not to get the oil on the sensitive inner lining of your vagina.

Perform this womb ritual daily for three to seven days or until you feel totally at ease with your womb, and until your womb has said all she needs to say on behalf of your womb wellness.

From time to time when you receive inner guidance, repeat this exercise to gain greater womb wisdom and insight.

# THE FEMALE
# REPRODUCTIVE SYSTEM

It's now time to explore the physiology of the womb so that we can make an inventory of what isn't in balance. By taking a long, hard look at what is not functioning properly, we can learn more about our bodies, and begin to follow the Path of Wellness as informed women of wisdom.

## The Reproductive Organs

The main female reproductive organs are the uterus (womb), ovaries, fallopian tubes, and vagina.

*The uterus* is a hollow muscular organ about three inches long, located deep inside the pelvic cavity; it houses the developing fetus.

*The cervix*, the neck of the uterus, projects into the vagina. The *vagina* is a tube, about four inches long, that receives the penis and sperm and serves as the birth canal.

*The fallopian tubes*, a pair of structures each about four inches long, join the uterus near the top. Their flared ends lie near the ovaries.

*The ovaries* are paired almond-shaped glands that produce *ova* (eggs) and female hormones. After an ovum is expelled into the pelvic cavity, it passes through a fallopian tube into the uterus. If the egg has been fertilized by a sperm, it implants in the wall of the uterus and gestation begins.

## Common Manifestations of Womb Imbalances or Illnesses

### Menstrual Health
*Amenorrhea.* There are many possible causes of primary and secondary *amenorrhea* (the absence of menstrual periods), including: *chronic absence of ovulation due to:* anatomic abnormalities, hypothalamus or pituitary dysfunction, other hormone system dysfunction, or genetic defects; excess exercise and stress; premature menopause; pregnancy.

*Dysmenorrhea* (menstrual cramps) often results from uterine contractions during an ovulatory cycle, but a specific cause cannot be determined in every case. Two common causes of dysmenorrhea are endometriosis (growth of endometrial tissue outside of uterus) and fibroid tumors.

*Menorrhagia* (excessive duration or amount of menses) often lasts five to ten days and is accompanied by pain and discomfort and can occur with fibroids, endometriosis, or hormone dysfunction.

*Symptoms and signs:* Bloating, weight gain, irritability, headache, depression, and edema.

### Sexually Transmitted Diseases
*Vaginitis.* An inflammation of the vagina, usually caused by bacterial or yeast infection.

*Symptoms and signs:* Vaginal burning or itching or discharge and yellow or white foul-smelling discharge.

*Bacterial Vaginosis.* Bacterial vaginosis results from overgrowth of particular vaginal bacteria. The prevalence of bacterial vaginosis is higher in African American women. Bacterial vaginosis has been associated with the use of some genital cleansing (douching) products. It can lead to low birth weight and preterm delivery (premature birth).

*Chlamydia.* A bacterial infection that occurs primarily in the cervix in women and the urethra in men. If antibiotic treatment is not prescribed, it can lead to infertility in both women and men.

*Genital Herpes.* A sexually transmitted virus that appears around the genital area.

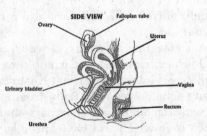

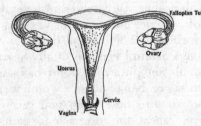

Female Reproductive Organs

*Symptoms and signs:* Include burning, itching, and the appearance of painful blisters. There is no cure; therefore, treatment is designed to relieve discomfort and prevent bacterial infection.

*Gonorrhea.* One of the most common STDs. A bacterial infection that causes inflammation of the glands. If left untreated, it can cause pelvic inflammatory disease, infertility, or ectopic pregnancy. Treatment includes antibiotics; however, there are some strains that are resistant to treatment.

*Syphilis.* A bacterial infection that multiplies rapidly in the body. It begins with a canker in the genital area. Left untreated, syphilis can result in serious symptoms, from fever and headache to bone pain, mental deterioration, and even death. Syphilis can be treated with antibiotics, but it cannot be cured. You must see a doctor for treatment.

## Reproductive System Disorders

*Endometriosis.* The endometrium is made up of cells that create the lining of the uterus. These cells can break away and grow inside the uterine cavity, implanting themselves within the pelvis, ovaries, appendix, bowels, and/or bladder.

*Symptoms and signs:* Menstrual cramps (chronic pain), pelvic scarrings, and adhesions within the womb. May be associated with infertility.

*Fibroids.* A mass of rapidly dividing cells that invade surrounding tissue. These cells rob neighboring normal cells of their nutrients.

*Symptoms and signs:* Pain and cramping, unusual bleeding or discharge, clotting, severe menstrual cramps. Can lead to miscarriages.

*Genital Prolapse (Prolapsed Uterus).* A condition in which weakened pelvic muscles fail to hold the uterus and other pelvic organs in place. Often due to a prolapsed, impacted colon or complications from labor and childbirth.

*Symptoms and signs:* Weakened vaginal and bladder muscles, frequent urination, low back pain, abdominal pain. May result in infertility, blocked tubes, and miscarriages.

## Pregnancy Health

*Pregnancy-Associated Hypertension.* Symptoms may include sudden elevation of blood pressure, headaches, visual disturbances, bloating, protein in the urine. Can result in the death of both fetus and mother.

*Miscarriage (Spontaneous Abortion).* When a pregnant woman delivers or loses a fetus before the twentieth week of pregnancy. Spontaneous abortion may result from infections, nutritional deficiency, structural or chromosomal abnormalities, diabetes, drug use, excess stress, and unknown causes.

*Preterm Delivery (Premature Birth).* Birth of a premature infant between twenty and thirty-seven weeks old. The cause of preterm delivery is often unknown. Risk factors include untreated bacterial vaginosis, poor nutrition, and previous preterm birth.

## Menopause

Menopause is not an illness or any form of disease, but rather is part of a woman's natural life processes. It is the period of glandular changes that indicate the end of a woman's menstrual cycle.

It signals a time when a woman has the privilege of keeping her "wise blood" and shifts her perspective to make her voice heard in the larger community.

Menopause is brought about by decreased production of the female sex hormones. It generally occurs between the ages of forty-two and fifty-two, but premenopausal symptoms can begin as early as thirty-five.

*Symptoms and signs:* While menopause is a natural part of our cycle, the indications that this is happening can be an easy, gentle process, or it can be a difficult time. Those women who eat poorly, do not get enough exercise, and live a stressful lifestyle may experience some or all of the following symptoms: severe nervousness, irritability, depression, overexcitability, headaches, abdominal pains, rushes of blood to the head and upper body called "hot flashes," backaches, leg cramps, night sweats, and nosebleeds.

However, we have the power to prevent or heal ourselves of these various toxic symptoms by eating live foods and fresh fruit, by drinking fresh fruit and vegetable juices and herb teas, by maintaining a clean colon, by exercising and meditating daily—and above all by healing or releasing all negative relationships and getting them out of our lives.

# WOMB WELLNESS PROFILE

The following Womb Wellness Profile has been divided into six categories of wellness that will help you assess the current health of your womb. This profile will aid you in your quest for womb wellness because it helps you keep an accurate record of your womb health over time. It is suggested that after you record your current baseline, you continue to monitor your womb wellness for a minimum of six cycles (months).

To get a clear picture of the state of your current menstrual periods, you need to consider the intensity of the flow, i.e., light to heavy, clot-free or clotting, odor-free or menstrual odor, and the number of days your menses last, i.e., optimal (1–3 days), average (4–5 days; may mean the womb is already in a diseased state), chronic (6–10 days), and beyond.

---

## WOMB WELLNESS PROFILE

Complete the following information about your menstrual cycle no matter where you are in your reproductive years (childbearing years or menopausal).

Date of first menstrual cycle _____Number of days in cycle _____
Length of menstrual flow (number of days) _____

**Directions for Rating Womb Wellness**
Use 0 to 3 to rate the items on your Womb Wellness Profile.
Use 0 if the condition never existed or no longer exists.
Use 1 if the condition occurs infrequently.
Use 2 if the condition occurs frequently.
Use 3 if the condition is a serious health challenge (i.e., endometriosis, cervical cancer, etc.), or if you have ever experienced a traumatic womb episode (i.e., rape, childhood molestation, abortion).

| Category A—Menstrual Health | Date | | | |
|---|---|---|---|---|
| Record Length of Each Cycle | Cycle 1 | Cycle 2 | Cycle 3 | Cycle 4 |
| 1. Menses flow | | | | |
| 0=1 or 2 days | | | | |
| 1=2 or 3 days | | | | |
| 2=3 or 4 days | | | | |
| 3=5, 6, or more days | | | | |
| P=Postmenopausal (indicate date of last menstrual cycle) | | | | |
| 2. Menstrual aches: head/back/legs | | | | |
| 3. Menstrual cramps | | | | |
| 4. Heavy menses bleeding and/or clotting | | | | |
| 5. PMS/mood swings: depression, anger, hostility | | | | |
| SUBTOTAL | | | | |

| | Date | | | |
|---|---|---|---|---|
| **Category B — Vaginal Health** | Cycle 1 | Cycle 2 | Cycle 3 | Cycle 4 |
| 6. Chronic vaginal itching or burning | | | | |
| 7. Chronic vaginal odor | | | | |
| 8. Chronic vaginal discharge or vaginitis | | | | |
| 9. Vaginal sores | | | | |
| 10. Medically diagnosed vaginal cysts | | | | |
| 11. Candida (chronic vaginitis) | | | | |
| SUBTOTAL | | | | |
| **Category C — Sexual Health** | | | | |
| 12. Painful intercourse | | | | |
| 13. Inability to experience orgasm | | | | |
| 14. Frigidity (averse to sexual activity) | | | | |
| 15. Sexually transmitted diseases (syphilis, gonorrhea, chlamydia, genital herpes) | | | | |
| 16. Sexual abuse (rape, molestation) | | | | |
| 17. Toxic partners | | | | |
| SUBTOTAL | | | | |

**Category D — Pregnancy Health.** Record a score of 3 in each cycle if you have ever experienced any of the following reproductive health challenges, even if you are not experiencing them in your current cycle. When you have achieved body-mind-spirit healing, you may reduce your score accordingly.

| | | | | |
|---|---|---|---|---|
| 17. Infertility | | | | |
| 18. Toxemia during pregnancy | | | | |
| 19. Difficult childbirth(s) | | | | |
| 20. Miscarriage(s) [Spontaneous Abortion(s)] | | | | |
| 21. Abortion(s) | | | | |
| SUBTOTAL | | | | |
| **Category E — Menopause** | | | | |
| 22. Hot flashes | | | | |
| 23. Vaginal dryness | | | | |
| 24. Medically diagnosed hormonal imbalances | | | | |
| 25. Irritability and mood swings | | | | |

| | | Date | | |
|---|---|---|---|---|
| | Cycle 1 | Cycle 2 | Cycle 3 | Cycle 4 |
| 26. Night sweats | | | | |
| 27. Headaches, backaches | | | | |
| SUBTOTAL | | | | |
| **Category F — Common Illnesses** | | | | |
| 28. Pelvic inflammatory disease (PID) | | | | |
| 29. Blocked fallopian tubes | | | | |
| 30. Medically diagnosed fibroids/tumors/cysts (indicate size: grapefruit, orange=3, lemon=2, pin-size=1) | | | | |
| 31. Endometriosis | | | | |
| 32. Hysterectomy | | | | |
| 33. Genital Prolapse (Prolapsed womb) | | | | |
| 34. Uterine cancer | | | | |
| SUBTOTAL | | | | |
| GRAND TOTAL | | | | |

## Interpreting Your Scores

We are striving for low scores. Low scores indicate a less toxic womb, less blockage to the womb, and thus more womb wellness. Remember, when you're measuring toxic conditions in the womb, lower scores are best. The grand total gives you an overview of the state of your womb, and helps you establish a baseline as you progress toward achieving a 0 score.

- A score of 0 indicates excellent womb wellness. Keep up your wonderful healing work!

- Scores of 1 with challenges primarily in Category A indicate occasional blockage or that a blockage is clearing. For maximum rejuvenation, continue the Womb Cleansing regimen for one to four cycles.

- Scores of 2 with challenges primarily in Category A and Category B indicate frequent blockage. For maximum rejuvenation, continue the Womb Cleansing regimen for four to six cycles.

- Scores of 3 with challenges primarily in Category C indicate constant and/or acute blockages There are no short-term or simple solutions to the challenges in Category C.

## Deep Healing Requires Deep Commitment

Many of the conditions in Categories C through F indicate the existence of long-term challenges to womb wellness. It will take a serious commitment and disciplined effort to regain maximum womb wellness. In addition to radically changing your nutritional habits and general lifestyle, it is critical to seek the help of licensed health professionals, such as a gynecologist, fertility specialist, psychotherapist, and so on. Joining a Sacred Womb Circle for support and feedback is also highly recommended.

To thoroughly rejuvenate your womb, you must be willing to commit to deep and constant cleansing. Before you begin a long-term cleansing, consider the following:

- Give your womb a rest for maximum healing during the cleansing period; abstain from, or at least limit, sexual intercourse. This would be an ideal time for you and your mate to explore alternative exercises to express your lovemaking desires.
- Women preparing to conceive a child should strive for a perfect score of zero. Beginning a pregnancy with a healthy womb reduces crises during the pregnancy and creates a more balanced environment for mother and child-in-the-making.
- Monitor your progress for a minimum of four cycles, up to twelve cycles.
- Remember, womb wellness is a prerequisite for the Gateways of Initiation.

## Womb Imbalance Stops Here!
## Healing the Wombs of Your Family

Attaining and maintaining womb wellness is a lifetime process. You will see the results of your cleansing according to your willingness to adopt the Natural Living lifestyle and your body's capacity to release the toxins that cause blockages to your wellness.

Now that you have completed your Womb Wellness Profile and know your score, keep in mind that this is just a beginning. You cannot get all the necessary work done in a couple of months when you've been carrying so much discomfort

for five, ten, or twenty years, or perhaps all your life. All conditions begin at the beginning—in the womb of your mother—and all the mothers before her. If you start checking out the womb histories in your family, passed down from your mother, your grandmother, and her mother and grandmother, you'll find that what's been going on with your womb follows some of the same patterns as with your foremothers. This is partly because of ingrained thoughts and attitudes, and partly because of the foods you've learned to eat from them, which is actually of greater importance.

This chain of womb unwellness cannot come to an end until you realize that you're the only one who can change the whole energy pattern. I can say that because in every family there are always women like you. There's always one who stands out, who looks peculiar to the family, who does things a little bit differently, dresses a little differently, wears colors a little differently. And the family is always saying, "Why are you doing that?"

In that woman there's a light that refuses to be turned down or off, no matter how the whole family has been functioning for hundreds of years. You are that light, that Sacred-Woman-in-Training. And you, sister-Queen, have probably been feeling alone because you're the one who's so different. You've been feeling insecure, feeling isolated from the family.

Remember, my sister, you are the healer. You are one of the First Mothers. You are the one who's going to show them another possibility, another way. You are one of the Medicine Women the whole planet has been waiting for— waiting for you to remember, to bring forth the earth wisdom once more.

We are the generation that must retrieve this knowledge. I couldn't ask my grandmother about her womb wisdom; she's passed on. So I told my mother I was going to go to New Orleans to check with my aunts and their friends. And my mother said, "I don't know who can help you. Maybe Aunt Sadie, she was a little bit into the herbs—and I think maybe there was a midwife."

This is when I realized that our most precious knowledge is dying out. We must catch this knowing in our generation, and then pass this knowledge down to our children so it remains alive in our daughters and our sons and our families. We must regain this wealth—the knowledge that we are Medicine Women. When we were left on these shores, when our captors would not take care of our health needs and we had to heal ourselves, what did our foremothers do? They prayed. They meditated. They tuned in to their inner voices. And then they went to nature—to the roots and the wild herbs.

I always remembered the sacred elder women who would rock on their porches, and while they were rocking they were aligning their energy centers. And they were humming, tuning in to who they were and listening to what they had to do to heal their child, their husband, or their sister-friend, or a neighbor down the road.

They would keep listening until they connected to the Source, to the Most High, and they would hear what they needed to know: "Ahhh . . . this is the clay we need to put on this person's forehead; this is the bush or leaf or flower we need to get." George Washington Carver would speak to plants, and they would hear. Our foremothers would pick up all those energies and those vibrations and heal themselves and others as well. This is part of our rich legacy.

Much of this tradition lives on today in the islands. Island people are more often in tune because they're closer to the ways of Afraka. Their culture was not dismantled or destroyed as much as ours, so they were able to hold on to a link with the Motherland.

Even though we've become more contaminated—the fast foods, the fast life—and have forgotten about the bush, forgotten about the natural way, the South still maintains that connection with the Afrakan mainland. I have memories of children being lined up for their bush teas and remedies.

I have this memory, not because I ever saw anyone actually standing in line, but because my DNA holds all these memories. As a result, I raised my children the urban Medicine Woman way. I wake them up every morning and say, "Here's your drink. Here's your herbs." In the afternoon I'd check them out and say: "Oh, you have an attitude. Well, take this purge."

That's our power—to know all things, to

know how to connect, how to tap back into that sacred place of empowerment. We do that to heal ourselves, and to inspire other people to come to us to learn how to heal themselves.

## The Seasons of Womb Wellness

The first rule of being a good Medicine Woman, a really strong one, is that you've got to heal yourself!

That is why we began with the Womb Wellness Profile. It will help you chart the map of your growth. You may want to make copies of it so you can use it for an entire year. I believe that in four seasons you can resurrect and heal anything, because each season leads us to do a different kind of healing work.

To give you an example: When you go into spring, you feel it's a time of renewal. Like a budding flower, you open up and let go. You'll be doing more exercise and dancing and singing because it's one of the best times to open the womb.

Then, when the summertime comes, if you're healthy, you don't get wiped out by the heat. Heat energizes, and you really grow to your fullness then. In summer your healing work can take you to a higher level. It's a time when the sun's rays can heal you. The sun purges, cleanses, and recharges the physical and the spiritual body.

In the autumn, your revitalized Body Temple will go into a state of rest. All that activity you completed in the summer will bow to the crisp chill of autumn. In the cooler weather you'll be moved to meditate on the good that you've done for yourself.

And when the winter comes, you deepen and extend your stillness. You'll write down your visions, your dreams, your thoughts, in your Sacred Womb Journal. You won't be inclined to go out as much. It's a good time to make full use of that quiet inner time, because the spring will come again. And when it does, you're really on home ground, ready to achieve higher and higher levels of womb wellness.

## Reviewing Your Cycles

Let's look at Cycle 1 on your Womb Wellness Profile. Make a note of how long your menstrual flow lasts, because you may flow half a day less or more from one cycle to another, and you need to know what's really going on. The initial change may not represent a big jump—it may be one day less, it may be half a day less, even a quarter of a day. Or you may have a cycle in which you may go from eight days of bleeding down to four days. Although there isn't usually such a big jump in such a short span of time, don't forget that a commitment to healing makes all things possible. It takes a while to heal the womb. Make a note of your current womb status on the chart, and make additional notes about conditions you are experiencing in whichever issues apply to you in the first part of the Sacred Womb Journal questions.

For example, if there is vaginal discharge—if it happens every single day—it's chronic. If you have a vaginal discharge that occurs two or three times a week, then it's there, but it is not as chronic. If you have a discharge once a week, then you have a lower score. Again, the goal during each cycle is to get to zero, which means the womb is whole and well. The lower the score, the healthier the womb. While you may start off with higher numbers, a new cycle begins every twenty-five to twenty-eight days (although the normal length of your cycle may vary). As you start to apply the Heal Thyself techniques, your scores should become lower and lower.

## Womb Wellness Profile Q & A

*My menses have stopped. How do I record that?*

Make a note of that and put down the year that it happened. I've seen a few menopausal women who ended up getting their menses again. So the date is important. How long you've been menopausal will be an indication of whether you might be able to reverse it. The reason women would want to reverse menopause is that the hormonal shift can cause serious health problems for postmenopausal women.

*When you tell us to keep track of our periods do we put down the dates between periods, or from beginning to end?*

I mean the cycle of time from beginning to end. You may spot for two days, but that's still part of your menses, so you have to add up the entire time. You may have a heavy flow for two days and then spot for three days. Include all that, and make a note of the heaviness or lightness of the flow.

Let's say you used to have kidney or low back pain, or you had bloating, or your skin was breaking out, or you had mood swings, and you were eating a diet that was feeding your toxicity. But when you changed your diet and started detoxifying your system, you moved out of that realm. Your Womb Wellness Profile will show you your progress. That's why we need to keep a record of our previous cycles.

For example, I have a history of asthma, and if I eat a certain way, it can recur. If you go back to the same old unnatural lifestyle, then the same womb problems are going to recur. If you've had a tumor removed, it will be more likely to grow back in a year or two if you continue consuming dairy products or if you're living in a highly stressed emotional state.

*Do you fill out all of the questions again in Cycle 2 after you've monitored your womb for one month?*

In each cycle you should fill in all the questions that apply to you. That way you have a personal record of your womb history. The important facts of your Womb Wellness Profile can also be part of your Sacred Journal work. If you find something that is not a simple yes or no for you, that's a strong signal to explore it further. You have to get more information. And this is the perfect time to turn to your Sacred Womb Journal.

For example, you might write: "I had my menses for ten days and then a clot came out, so I went back to the doctor." Or, "For three or four months my menses went down to four days and I was having no clotting. I didn't have any more PMS. And I remember I was drinking Womb Works Tea. I was doing clay packs and castor oil packs, and made other changes, that's why I had a different reading." That's the kind of information you want to start to record in your Sacred Womb Journal. It will demonstrate to you that as you begin taking more responsibility for your womb wellness, your healing starts to take place.

# THE SACRED WOMAN'S WOMB WELLNESS DIET

The more you cleanse the body, the easier it is to make healthy changes. As you look over the Sacred Woman's Womb Wellness Diet, you'll see that this womb diet is basically vegetarian. While you don't have to be a vegetarian to get on board with your womb wellness, you do need to start cutting back on flesh foods.

## Going Vegetarian

*Beginning:* If you are able to make a change now and you've been eating all levels of flesh, graduate to fresh fish (not shellfish) for the next twenty-one days. Just fish—as fresh as you're able to find. It is the least toxic of all the flesh foods. Keep in mind all the chemicals—all the antibiotics, steroids, and other hormones—that are injected into our meat supply. They completely disrupt our hormonal balance. Don't forget that the more you take in something that bleeds, the more you will bleed. So you want to come off the beef right now. You want to come off the chicken. If you crave that taste, then work with the flesh food alternatives. Work with soy proteins—try soy chicken, or soy turkey. There's even soy bacon. We want this first stage of purification to be a painless womb process, and so your protein source will be fish or soy.

*Advanced:* If you're ready to take the plunge into the deep cleansing work and go vegetarian, the protein sources in your diet will be beans, peas, lentils, and limited amounts of nuts and seeds. Just don't overindulge in the nuts and seeds because you'll bleed as heavily as you do on flesh foods. Don't forget that overindulgence in any proteins feeds tumors.

The Womb Wellness Diet calls for vegetarian proteins. So if you're having fish, then on Monday have fish, Tuesday black beans with brown rice or millet and vegetables, Wednesday fish with vegetables, Thursday kidney beans, and so on.

There are primary enemies that attack the womb on a dietary level. One is flesh foods. One is dairy. Another is white-flour products. Milk, cheese, ice cream, eggs, and flesh foods feed a tumor. Tumors grow on something inside of you—they don't come out of the air. When you add all the intense emotions you're feeling—anger, pain, frustration—to meat, dairy, and white-flour foods, you're giving your tumor a banquet.

Every time you find yourself eating heavy foods, you're giving your body negative affirmations. You're saying, "I'm angry," because eating that flesh is an expression of anger or rage. You're tired, because when you eat heavy foods you get tired, you feel lifeless, and so your body is not able to assist and support you.

But when you cleanse, your body literally wakes up when something foreign enters it. Your body will automatically begin to expel toxic foods, just as it will begin to expel toxic thoughts or toxic attitudes. That's what we're striving for. So work on those principles as you follow your womb diet as closely as you can.

## Natural Herbs

Begin to work with nature's bounty—herbs. All of the herbs I mention can be purchased at a good health food store. One outstanding womb toner is red raspberry tea. Or if you experience heavy bleeding, try dandelion tea to replenish your iron. If you're suffering from tumors or cysts right now, get goldenrod tea.

On pages 134–135 I suggest specific teas for different womb-healing projects. But right now you want to work with one particular tonic first—Womb Works Tea, available from Heal Thyself (see the product list in the appendix).

### Womb Tea
Boil 4 or 5 cups of water in a stainless steel, glass, or other pot (never aluminum) at night before going to sleep.

Turn off the water and add 2 to 3 tsp. each of dried red raspberry, dandelion, and goldenrod. Cover, and let it steep overnight. In the morning, when you're up between the hours of 4 A.M. and 6 A.M., strain the tea.

Sip Womb Works Tea before or after prayer time, during your soul fast, in your meditation, in your womb state, in your rebirthing process. What you're doing is allowing those herbs to become a part of your womb, and to begin to flush the toxins out.

## The Benefits of Celibacy During Womb Renewal Work

During this time, if you're able, celebrate yourself by being celibate. This is the time that you are clearing the way for womb restoration—a womb celebration and a womb renewal. So commit to holding on to yourself so you can receive the spiritual wisdom that is now coming through and is so soul-cleansing for you. When your partner wants to mate, offer gentle affirming kisses and warm, cuddly hugs. Offer herbal tea. And if your mate really wants to be with you, run an Epsom salts or Dead Sea salt bath and put some herbs, bubbles, and rose petals in it (do not use any salts if you or your lover have high blood pressure or edema). That's how you make love to your mate when you're being celibate, because there are many different ways of loving someone.

In our renewal work the Most High Womb Presence begins to connect with us and to speak to us. That's why we often feel as though we are hearing a voice. And you're going to say, "Wait a minute, what's going on here?" If you tell your sister-friends what you're hearing, you'll discover that we're all hearing some of the same messages because we're all having some of the same cycles. We're all the children of the Blessed—children of the Most High. We've all gone through many of the same things, so we don't have to be ashamed of any of it, whether we speak about it or not.

Always remember that it's in the releasing that the healing takes place. Even if you think you don't have the strength, just go into your bathroom—your hydrotherapy room—and light a candle. Put some fresh flowers in there, create a divine altar in that bathroom, because that's where you're going to do your cleansing. Let your bathroom become your healing sanctuary. That's where you can turn the lights off and tell yourself, "No one is here but me and the Most High. It is the Mother Principle who's here. It is Ast. It is Nebt-Het. It is my aunt. It is all the angelic forces of the Most High. It is me and my Divine Self."

The Creator/Creatress is an expression of femaleness as well as being an expression of maleness, and we have every right to anoint our sacred female space. How could it not be sacred when we women create all life? The whole world comes from our wombs. As we create better thoughts and ideas, more creativity will flow through our wombs and out into the world.

I may not have another human child, but *Sacred Woman* is truly my child, for I have gone through true labor to birth her. For me, birthing a child, a book, or a dance is part of the same cycle of creativity. The "births" are the culmination of a period of growth and the expression of the life force.

I remember my mother saying, "Where are you going now?"

And I'd say, "I've got to go to dance class! I must dance to save my womb." When I dance, I connect with spirit, and I feel my womb release, and I feel my womb being restored, and I feel my heart empty out those relationships that need to be flushed out so I can claim a new body, a new mind, and a new heart.

It's not that we have to do so much, or that we have to change so much, but we can't afford to have our wombs working against us. We don't want our wombs to hurt us any longer. We don't want to be angry that we've used our wombs to strike out at another sister because we're having PMS or in our pain manipulate a lover. We don't even have to have PMS. We don't have to let our menses be a painful experience. One of the joys I experience when women go through their womb healing is hearing them say, "Wow, my menses just came discreetly. It didn't come as an irritant. It didn't call me out and make me tighten up two or three days before." That's not who you truly are—the pain, the tightening, the fear. Womb work is not based on the attitude that you're going to do all this hard labor; rather, it's based on loving experience, on self-love. And it's going to be the greatest love relationship that you've ever had in your life.

## THE WOMB WELLNESS CLEANSING FOOD PLAN

Green foods will help to connect you to your spiritual essence. The more green you take in, the more forgiveness comes through. The green represents the gateway to your spiritual life. It helps you communicate on a higher spiritual plane. That's where the significance comes in. (You can also infuse your being with the color green by visualizing it filling your womb when you meditate, or when you take your salt bath.)

Flesh foods and mucus-forming foods destroy the life of the womb, allowing disease to set in. Avoid mucus-forming foods, such as all white-flour products, pasta, white bread, white rice, white potatoes, and dairy foods. Use grains in moderation, even whole grains. The ultimate goal is to eat them only when the sun is at its highest point in the sky (midday).

The following dietary recommendations are designed to help you eliminate congestion and mucus, which comprise tumors, fibroids, and cysts, especially in the vaginal and breast areas.

*Note:* At the onset of this cleansing regime, please fast from all starch, because it causes congestion throughout the body, along with constipation and stagnation. If you can also fast from all protein for at least seven days, you will give your body a much-needed rest.

### Before Breakfast: Kidney-Liver Flush

The Kidney-Liver Flush lasts for seven to twenty-one days. Colon Ease and Liquid Kyolic can be purchased in a health food store. Mix together in a blender:

2 tbsp. Colon Ease or cold-pressed extra-virgin olive oil with equal parts of castor oil
12 drops Liquid Kyolic garlic, or 2 fresh garlic cloves, crushed
Juice of 1 lemon or lime, or 1–2 tbsp. organic apple cider vinegar
1 pinch cayenne pepper (do not use if you have high blood pressure)
8 oz. warm water (purified or distilled)

Blend and drink up.

## What You'll Have for Breakfast

Gone are the days of cereal for breakfast—eat fruit instead. You can have one to three pieces of fruit, for example, apples or pears; blend them with ½ to 1 cup of strawberries, depending on the size of your appetite. You can have ½ cup of mixed blueberries and raspberries. Foods in the berry family, including cranberries, are all very good for cleansing the womb and the bloodstream. Their vital red energy detoxes and cleanses. And this will lead to a very healthy menses.

Do not eat bananas during the first month of your cleansing, as they can cause constipation, gas, and bloating, particularly if not well ripened.

Juices are also terrific for breakfast, such as fresh-pressed grapefruit, pineapple, orange, apple, or unsweetened cranberry. Use 4 oz. juice to 4 oz. water (distilled or purified).

If your disposition is a little evil, and you need extra sweetness that day, then add a pinch of cinnamon or nutmeg to your juices or fruit sauces. Cinnamon's also good if you're feeling deprived and can't hear your inner voice, and you're thinking, "Oh, this regime is too much, I want to eat what I want to eat when I want to eat it." That's when you put the cinnamon in, and that will keep your rebellion in check. Remember, the more you can stick with your healing womb work, the more energy you will have!

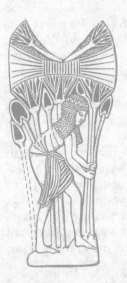

Do a little bit more than you think you can do—every day. It would be ideal if you're able to prepare everything fresh. Even if that's not possible in the beginning, at least try to stick to your fresh juices and fresh fruit. Don't let your devitalized insides talk you out of your wellness. So do what you can. If you make apple or pear sauce at night, you can take a nice jar of it to work for dessert.

So that you eat the best-quality products, when possible purchase organic fruits and vegetables, or soak produce for a few minutes in a bowl with distilled water with ½ cup of organic apple cider vinegar. After soaking, rinse off if you have a water purifier attached to your sink, or use the best possible water you have available to work with to cleanse your food.

### What to Have for Lunch and Dinner

Lunchtime will consist of a large, delicious, and vital raw salad.

For dinner you'll make another large salad. And you can add a grain to the salad, such as tabouli, couscous, or bulgur wheat (unless you are allergic). These are wonderful because you don't cook them, so you'll have live wheat.

*To prepare wheat grain:* First, put 2 cups of the grain into a large bowl—this will last you for a few days. Next pour 2 cups of water over the grain, cover the bowl, and let the grain soak 7 minutes, or up to 15 minutes for the coarser grains. Then taste a teaspoon of the grain to see if it's still hard. If it's not soft, then add a little more water. In 3 or 4 minutes your live grain should be done. Refrigerate your leftovers.

While the grain is plumping, chop up all the various vegetables you want to add to the grain. Then fluff up the grain with a fork, add the vegetables, and marinate these ingredients together for another 10 minutes.

A very special healing herb to add to your grain dishes is sage. The sage I mean is *Salvia officinalis,* the herb your grandmother stuffed into the Thanksgiving turkey, not the wild desert sage you burn for sacred smudging—although both kinds of sage are powerful herbs for women. *Salvia officinalis* provides a wonderful cleansing for the womb (unless you're breastfeeding, because it stops the milk flow).

*Base of salad.* Avoid iceberg lettuce; it is devoid of nutrients. Work instead with grated purple or green cabbage, or both. Also experiment with adding live, fresh vegetables like red and green bell peppers, celery, and/or grated carrots to your grain medley.

*Okra.* Another vegetable that is an essential for maintaining womb wellness is okra. Have okra every day as a purge. For those of you who have never enjoyed cooked okra, let me tell you that fresh, raw okra is never slimy. Just chop it up in small pieces and add it to your bulgur or whatever grain you're preparing. It's delicious.

However, if you still don't like okra, use flaxseed. At bedtime, just put 2 tbsp. of flaxseed in purified water to cover. It will gel up overnight and then you blend it into your fruit sauce or your fruit juices to help purge your system.

*Protein sources.* During your cleansing diet use alfalfa sprouts, mung bean sprouts—anything from the sprout family. (See "Do Eat" on page 74.) I'm reluctant to suggest nuts because experience has shown me that we tend to overdo the nuts, rationalizing them as substitutes for everything we're sacrificing as we begin to develop conscious eating habits. Try seeds instead of nuts, but don't overdo them, either. Just sprinkle over your finished salad a few raw, unsalted sunflower seeds that you've soaked for half an hour in pure water.

*Tofu.* Also watch your consumption of tofu, as you can get just as clogged up on tofu, which is produced from soybeans, as you can with cheese. So if you want to use tofu, take a fourth of a big cake, chop it up into little cubes, and let it marinate with your bulgur or vegetables. You can also let it sit by itself and put Bragg seasoning (available in health food stores) on it; or you can use cayenne pepper or garlic or kelp as a seasoning, or a little cold-pressed extra-virgin olive oil. You want to use the cold-pressed olive oil because it's untreated and contains chlorophyll.

You can use 2 to 3 tbsp. of hummus as you make your transition into live foods, but as you progress, keep in mind that we're trying to get away from dependency on cooked food.

Your lunch and dinner menus are the same, with variations that you will begin to enjoy more and more. You will discover over time that your taste buds become increasingly sensitive, and you will begin to relish the subtle differences in taste of each ingredient in your live salads.

If you have a food processor, then you can

really work—you can put in broccoli, turnips, and cabbage, and all those different greens, and grate them all together. Then spread this over your salad as a lush live-food dressing.

*Herbs.* Be creative and think of all the fresh herbs you can get from your health food store. You might even try growing your own in a pot or window box. Be sure to check all bottled herbs to make certain they have not been irradiated. If you need more taste, put the herbs in your food processor with the vegetables. You can also use a blender, but you have to add water for the blender.

If you want to have a full feeling, a sense that you've eaten a starch, the grated vegetables served over the grain will give you that full feeling. You can experiment with broccoli, celery, and green and/or purple cabbage. Or try green onions, or some red bell peppers, and you'll really feel full.

*Kelp.* A sea vegetable is another terrific addition for your salad meals. Kelp is high in iron and minerals, which are good for your thyroid and your immune system. It's even available in a convenient kind of saltshaker for your dinner table. If you crave fish, try using kelp in your vegetables instead. It will help you feel satisfied.

*Added nutrients.* To increase the nutritional value of your salad meals, you'll want to add such ingredients as spirulina, wheatgrass, vitamin C. Lecithin helps to open up your arteries, so that the blood and the oxygen can flow through. Routinely add a tablespoon of lecithin to 8 oz. of live juices at least twice a day to build your immune system.

## Juices to the Rescue

Use vegetable juices for rejuvenating and building. Use prune juice for detoxing. If you take double the amount of prune juice, you will be more emotional and more sensitive, and you may start breaking out, which is a symptom that detoxification is going on.

Don't get lazy with the juices. And don't complain that they don't taste good. We're trying to rise above the taste and elevate into the heal-

ing. As time goes on, you'll like the effects so much that taste will cease to be the issue. Besides, the cleaner your Body Temple, the better everything will taste.

Vegetable juices are for building and rejuvenating, and they keep your emotions calm. You'll feel as though you're on top of things. As you open yourself up, greater prosperity and greater riches will be able to come into your life—riches of the body, mind, and spirit. That's all part of our true wealth.

Adding spirulina or wheatgrass to your live juices will help cut down the desire to eat so much. You won't want to eat because you'll already have most of the vitamins that your body needs. Spirulina has vegetarian protein in it, and calcium for the bones and the nerves. It has B vitamins, too. If this is your first time using spirulina or wheatgrass, begin with 1 tbsp. in your juice. If you've been cleansing for a while, add 2 tbsp.

If you find you're having difficulty drinking a lot of vegetable juices, drink dandelion or alfalfa tea. Steep it for 2 hours, and you will still have that wonderful healing experience.

## Do Eat

Lentils, sprouts, soybeans, tofu, peas, nuts, soy-based meats, TVP (texturized vegetable protein). *Beware:* Read labels. Many soy meat products contain egg whites and MSG.

Soak all beans, seeds, and nuts overnight, in water to cover, for better digestion. However, if you want a faster snack, soak nuts and seeds for at least 10 minutes, but don't make it a habit.

## Do Not Eat

Clams, oysters, lobster, shrimp. (These are all "brooms" that clean up the ocean by gathering the toxins—which you then eat!)

Avoid pork, lamb, beef, chicken, and MSG.

If you must have a transition period from eating flesh, eat only baked or steamed fish (not shellfish), no more than two or three times a week.

Eat starches (carbohydrates) no more than three or four times per week—the less the better. The easiest complex carbohydrates to digest are millet, couscous, tabouli, bulgur wheat, or toasted sprouted bread.

Abstain from heavier starches or eat them in moderation, such as baked sweet potatoes, raw or cooked carrots or raw or cooked corn on the cob, and whole-grain bread (toasted or dried in the oven).

Make your own bread by grinding down to a powder sunflower and pumpkin seeds or almonds and other nuts and use them in place of whole wheat flour. The texture will be denser than wheat flour breads, but tasty. Consult a good vegetarian cookbook for recipes.

### Nutritional Supplement Choices

These formulas are nutritional foods. So just as you eat fruit and vegetables, incorporate them into your nutritional lifestyle. They should be taken two or three times a day:

- Formula I: 1–2 tbsp. Heal Thyself Super Nutritional Formula; normally 1 tbsp., but if stressed take 2. This formula contains all the vitamins and minerals the Body Temple needs in order to be rejuvenated and nourished. (See the product list in the appendix.) Or . . .
- Spirulina, 1–2 tbsp. (powdered form). Or . . .
- Wheatgrass, 1–2 tsp. (liquid or powdered). Or . . .
- Blue-green algae, spirulina, or chlorella, 4–6 tablets.

Take the following nutrients once or twice a day.

- B-vitamin complex (25–50 mg tablets). These are powerful antistress vitamins.
- Vitamin C with bioflavonoids (500–1,000 mg). Helps to arrest bleeding and infections, builds the immune system, and calms emotional outbursts and quarrels.
- Vitamin E (400 mg). Can increase oxygen-carrying capacity of blood and stimulate circulation.
- Lecithin (1–2 tbsp.). Lecithin is a brain food. It also brings oxygen to the cells by clearing clogged arteries throughout the body. Use leci-

thin to clean and reawaken the blocked tubes in the womb.
- Flaxseed oil (1–2 tsp. unrefined, expelled, or cold-pressed). Flaxseed is exceptionally high in alpha-linoleic acid and prevents essential fatty acid deficiencies. It is useful in the treatment of chronic degenerative diseases.

### Internal Cleansing

Develop colon wellness for a lighter womb. Our elders believed in cleaning out the colon for every problem. Women should do the same to promote womb wellness.

Take an enema one to three times weekly for up to twenty-one days or as many as twelve weeks if there is a chronic problem (see directions on page 90). Work toward Natural Living as you help yourself to colon wellness.

### For Intensive Womb Rejuvenation Work

For every womb affliction, drink 1 pint of fresh green juice daily. This is a combination of any green vegetables pressed in a juicer. Also take some form of chlorophyll, such as alfalfa tablets or 1 to 2 oz. of wheatgrass, spirulina, or blue-green algae diluted, in vegetable juice or water. These green juices help to strengthen and rejuvenate the womb.

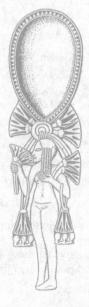

# RECIPES FROM THE KITCHEN HEALING LABORATORY

## Warrior Queen Juice

Helpful for women suffering from heavy blood flow and/or anemia. Run through juicer:

¼–½ cup kale
½ cup broccoli
2 stalks celery (omit if you have edema or high blood pressure)
¼ cup mustard greens
1–2 cloves garlic

## Water Rush Juice

Recommended for relief of menopausal "hot flashes." Run through juicer:

¼ cup parsley or organic watercress
½ cup brussels sprouts
½ cucumber (remove skin if not organic)

## Garden Green Juice

Run through juicer:

½ cup string beans
¼ cup spinach
½–1 cup mung or alfalfa sprouts
½ cup green or purple cabbage

## Red Womb Fruit Julep

For rejuvenation and purification of the womb.

¼ cup raw cranberries
½ cup strawberries, hulled
¼ cup blueberries
¼ cup raspberries
2 cups organic apple juice

Mix all ingredients in a blender.

## Garden Green Womb Salad

½ cup mung or alfalfa sprouts
1 cup chopped raw okra
½ cup chopped red bell pepper
3 cups mesclun salad greens
¼ cup soaked sunflower seeds (optional)

Mix all ingredients together. If you like, you can sprinkle your greens with sage seasoning, kelp, herbal seasoning salt, or Liquid Aminos.

## Salad Dressing

½ cup cold-pressed extra-virgin olive oil (keep refrigerated)
2–3 tbsp. organic cider vinegar

Blend together and pour sparingly over your greens.

## Womb Delight Fruit Shake

"The blacker the berry, the sweeter the juice," goes the Elders' wisdom. This delicious shake creates a sweet womb and a sweet disposition—just ask your mate.

½ cup blueberries
½ cup raspberries
1 cup strawberries
½ cup cranberries, sweetened by soaking with ¼ cup dates in distilled water to cover
½ cup organic apple juice

Blend all ingredients together in a blender.

## Seaweed and Okra Salad

Include seaweed—such as kelp, dulse, nori, arame, kombu, hijiki, or wakame—in your diet for vitamins and minerals. Seaweed is especially recommended for women who are trying to conceive or who are already pregnant. Once you have progressed to a live-food diet, vegetables are the *only* foods you should eat from the sea. You can dice, slice, chop, or grate your sea vegetables, or create a fresh salad, or freely add them to your soups, salads, and steamed green veggies. (Some come in dried form, and need to be soaked before use.)

Chopped raw okra
Soaked seaweed
Salad dressing (see recipe above)

## Womb Wellness Soup

Especially recommended for women with a displaced womb as the result of an impacted colon, or following childbirth.

2 cups sliced raw okra
¼ cup sliced scallions
Pinch each of sage, kelp (seaweed), and dried red raspberry leaf

Simmer okra and scallions in 3 cups of pure water for 5 minutes, then turn off flame. Add remaining ingredients. Cover and allow to steep for 20 minutes. Then pour into your favorite soup bowl and enjoy.

## Okra Popcorn

2 cups raw okra chopped into bite-sized pieces

Toss with a little tamari sauce and olive oil. Put in plastic bags and eat as a snack.

## THE MUCUS TRIP

As I've mentioned, mucus-forming foods include devitalized white-flour products such as white bread, muffins, bagels, and pasta, as well as white rice, white potatoes, and dairy foods (such as cheese, milk, and ice cream). In fact, the flesh of animals is a major cause of mucus accumulation. Daily consumption of mucus-forming foods can debilitate you and put you to sleep, psychologically, physically, and spiritually. Also, tumors and cysts are basically mucus that has solidified into a mass.

- *If mucus has accumulated in your brain*, you may develop headaches, poor memory, possibly even tumors in the brain.
- *Mucus in your eyes* causes cataracts, poor vision, and red eyes.
- *Mucus in your ears* causes loss of hearing and wax in the ears.
- *Mucus in your nose* causes sinus congestion, colds, and hay fever.
- *Mucus in your throat* causes thyroid problems, colds, and loss of voice.
- *Mucus in your lungs* causes asthma, influenza, bronchitis, and low endurance.
- *Mucus in your colon* causes constipation.
- *Mucus in your breasts* causes tumors or cysts in the breasts.
- *Mucus in your womb* causes fibroid tumors in the uterus, cysts in the vagina, vaginal discharges, heavy bleeding, and clotting. The larger the quantity of mucus-creating foods eaten, the longer mucus-related bleeding continues (five to eight days). The level of mucus trapped within the womb is indicated by how long and how heavy your monthly blood flow is.
- *Mucus generally* causes swelling of neck, hands, knees, and ankles.
- *In men, mucus in the prostate* causes tumors, cysts, impotency, and even cancer.

### How to Break Down Mucus Throughout the System

The Womb Wellness Cleansing Food Plan and internal cleansing can clear away all the symptoms of mucus.

Follow these Womb Regeneration Techniques:

1. Kidney-Liver Flush (see page 72).
2. Colon wellness kit. (See the product list in the appendix.)
3. Flush body out with the juice of lemons, limes, oranges, grapefruits, pineapples, and watermelon. Keep in balance by eating a diet high in raw green vegetables (as salads and as fresh green juices).

**Mucus Clearing Drink**
Take 2 grapefruits, or 3 oranges, and juice them. Grapefruits are known to bring down mucus. This fresh juice will help purge out the womb. You can mix the juices too; have 1 grapefruit and 2 oranges.

If your skin has a tendency to break out, it means your blood is impure and your colon is impacted. You may want to slow down your cleansing regime a bit. You may have one day of grapefruits and oranges, and the next day you may have pure, fresh apple juice and pear juice. This is because apple juice and pear juice are alkaline and purify the blood. When you alternate them with stronger juices such as fresh orange or grapefruit juice, you won't have a heavy detox coming out through your skin. However, if your skin is breaking out, try a mixture of lemon juice, cold-pressed extra-virgin olive oil, and fresh grated ginger as your morning drink (see Fire Element Morning Drink, page 80).

Another wonderful alternative to the citrus juices is cranberry juice, which has a lot of fire. Use the unsweetened kind you get at the health food store, because the sweetened kind has been treated in addition to having sugar in it. Sugar deteriorates the brain, the bones, and the nervous system.

## THE COLON AND THE WOMB

If you're taking in three meals a day, which adds up to twenty-one meals in a week, and you've had only one bowel movement a day, that means fourteen meals are backed up in your colon. You have fourteen meals turning into gravel, or lining the colon like smooth leather. All of that weighs us down. With all the added weight, the colon, which belongs above the navel, sinks below the navel and presses down on the womb. Visualize your ovaries dancing, happy to be free, and your fallopian tubes in place. Now visualize how a heavy colon would come crushing down. How does your womb feel about this?

Colon problems come from dense living, from the solid mass that you bring into your body. This includes holding on to angry thoughts and not forgiving. It's all density building up. And who's it hurting? Maybe the person you're angry at. But the person who's really suffering is you. So if you don't want to hold on to anguish, if you don't want to hold on to the pain, drink at least six 8-ounce glasses of pure water a day—and call in the angels. They're the living representatives of Het-Hru. Ask the angels to come and save you, to resurrect you. Something as simple as getting in a bath can open you up to healing and allow you to let go.

### Enemies of the Womb

If you just keep holding on to where you are, you're going to want to eat more and more starch. For example, new vegetarians moving from eating less meat to no meat often double up on the starches in their diet. Think about all that denseness, and you'll begin to understand exactly what constricts and holds you down.

The same thing happens when we hold on to anger. When we're distressed, do we eat apples and pears? No. When we're stressed out and angry at the world, we eat starches—and the more the better. When we're really mad, we want to crunch. And the crunch is usually something that's going to be heavy and dense.

### Menses and Elimination

Beginning when I was thirteen and for a decade after, my menses were my monthly nightmare. I also remember that I was having a hard time with elimination. I was extremely constipated, and I would sometimes go days without elimination.

Today, I understand that there's a definite connection between menses and elimination. When we examine the colon of a woman with

womb challenges, we frequently see a condition where the colon is pressing down on the womb because of constipation. And because of this stress, and because of the burdensome emotional state that so many women are carrying, all that weight is bearing down on our wombs like a ton of bricks. These colon "bricks" block what we would like to release—both physically and emotionally.

My personal experience with constipation, and my discovery of how it leads to womb afflictions, would be the beginning of my mission.

I also remember that during my years of womb disconnection, bleeding for seven and eight days every month, the only reason I didn't grow a tumor is that at the age of eighteen I was blessed to learn how to radically change my lifestyle.

The more time you spend unconscious of your womb, the more likely you are to have womb problems in your future. The way our society eats—fast foods, processed foods, eating on the run, feeding ourselves all kinds of toxic combinations of foods, from white-flour products to contaminated flesh foods—all adds up to devastating womb and colon problems.

### Is Your Womb Under Attack from the Weight of Your Colon?

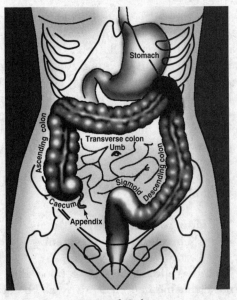

Normal Colon

A normal, healthy colon is the result of Natural Living.

A normal colon is maintained by consumption of vegetable proteins, an ample amount of fresh fruits and vegetables, small amounts of whole grains, and plenty of purified drinking water, coupled with exercise and a positive mental outlook.

A healthy colon allows the womb to function freely. It allows space for the fallopian tubes and ovaries to function in an unhampered way.

*Note:* For every meal you eat, a bowel movement should follow, particularly before the next meal is consumed. If you consume two or three meals a day, you must have at least two or three bowel movements daily. That would indicate that you have a vibrant colon, and thus a vibrant womb.

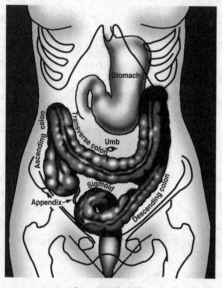

Abnormal Colon

An abnormal, unhealthy, prolapsed, constipated, constricted colon is the result of a toxic lifestyle, including toxic eating patterns.

A prolapsed, constipated, constricted colon can cause a prolapsed womb. If the colon is prolapsed, it clamps down on the womb, causing poor circulation within the womb, blocked fallopian tubes, cramping during menses, irregular menstrual flow, and constricted ovaries. You are more susceptible to womb-infecting growths and womb pain.

An impacted, prolapsed colon can cause miscarriages because the womb becomes crowded and suppressed, with little space for a fetus to grow to full term. That is one of the reasons why it is so essential to purge the colon well before conception. Adopt the Natural Living lifestyle presented in *Sacred Woman* for at least four months to a year before conception.

An unhealthy, prolapsed colon is the result of late-night eating, inappropriate food combinations, not drinking enough water, lack of exercise, and finally, suppressed, depressed thoughts.

Be mindful! If you have only one bowel movement a day and you consume two or three meals a day, or worse, you eliminate only a few times a week, and the waste is hard and you are gaseous, then know that you have a prolapsed and impacted colon. This means your womb is debilitated and crying out for help.[1]

### Creating Colon Wellness

Since the condition of the colon affects the wellness or disease of the womb, one of our first priorities is to regain a normal, balanced, and healthy colon. In a twelve-week program of colon wellness you can restore a prolapsed or impacted colon to its normal state.

Try the following regimen to provide relief to your colon:

- Eat fresh vegetables and fruits.
- Drink fresh juices, particularly green juice.
- Drink six 8-oz. glasses of distilled or purified water daily.
- Take enemas and herbal laxatives (1 tbsp. soaked flaxseed or 2 to 4 cascara sagrada tablets two to three times a week).
- Massage your abdomen from right to left with olive or castor oil.
- Do abdominal exercises such as leg raises, leg swings, and sit-ups. Or do Dance of the Womb exercises in Gateway 3.

*Leg raises:* Lying flat on your back so there is no stress on your spine, raise your left knee to your chest and raise your leg seven times. Repeat with your right knee and leg seven times. Do for one or two rounds.

*Breathing rule for all body movements:* As the body goes upward, inhale; as the body goes downward, exhale. Breathe in rhythm with the flow of the movements.

*Leg swings:* Standing, with your right hand hold on to a chair or a table for balance. Keeping your neck long, your back straight, your shoulders down, raise your left leg behind you. Swing it forward and back seven times. Turn around and hold on to the table or chair with your left hand. Raise your left leg behind you and swing it forward and back seven times. Do for one or two rounds. Follow breathing rule above.

*Sit-ups for beginners:* Lie down, back flat, knees up, hands behind your head. Gently sit up, moving toward your knees. Exhale as you come up, inhale as you slowly lie back down again. Do seven to twenty-one times. As your stomach muscles get stronger you can increase the number of sit-ups.

### Fire Element Morning Drink and Bath to Clear Colon

Most of us have prolapsed colons. Why? Because we've been eating late at night. And we've been eating cooked starches and proteins—a lot of them. Plus, we haven't been taking in enough water and greens.

So we want to clean out the colon, break down the fecal stones and hard matter that may be in the colon so that they can pass out. Then that lovely colon can come off the womb and begin to breathe. Right now she's feeling a little stressed out, and this drink is just what she needs to help her out.

### Fire Element Morning Drink

For seven days, start your day with this drink. The chlorophyll in the cold-pressed olive oil really helps your colon.

    Juice of 1 lemon
    ¼ teaspoon cayenne pepper
    2–4 tbsp. cold-pressed extra-virgin olive oil
    8 oz. pure warm water

Mix all ingredients together and drink.

When you start drinking the lemon juice and olive oil mixture, you'll often find that a lot of gas starts coming out. We have a lot of gases in our bodies, and these gases also affect our emotional bodies. Once all that toxic wind comes out, you'll start to feel much better. You'll feel lighter and you'll have a more positive outlook. So after you've done this morning cleanse for a few days, try this addition: Juice or grate a 3-inch piece of fresh gingerroot and add it to the lemon juice and olive oil.

This gives you a wonderful deep cleansing for your whole system. The womb is going to feel it because ginger is fire and the womb represents your fire element. The womb's aura is red and orange, so the ginger fire cleanses your auric field as well as your physical body.

### Ginger Bath

After you begin adding ginger to your drink, add ginger to your bath. Use a piece of fresh gingerroot the size of your hand. Run it through your juicer or grate it. If you juice it, add the juice to your bath. You may want to run a little water through your juicer to get all the ginger out, and then put the juice in your bath. Or if you're using grated ginger, put it in a clean washcloth, fasten the washcloth with a rubber band, and drop it into the bath—it makes a good scrub for your skin as well, to help remove the toxins. While you're soaking in the bathwater with a pound of Dead Sea salt, you can also add a few drops of your favorite essential oils (do not use any salts if you have high blood pressure or edema).

The Fire Element Morning Drink opens you up and you'll start feeling flushed. This is because all the mucus is coming out of your lungs. Some may come out through the womb as well. With the ginger drink and bath you're getting an internal cleansing as well as an external cleansing.

## MENSES: TO BLEED OR NOT TO BLEED

A woman's menstrual period is a very sacred time, for this is when a woman is most spiritually in tune and most sensitive to her surroundings. She is more open and able to receive messages from the Most High Creator/ Creatress that will aid her in living a more harmonious existence. And a womb in tune has a peaceful time during the menses. However, this advanced monthly spiritual state can exist only if a woman is truly purified.

This healthy state is unlike the so-called normal woman who bleeds four or more days coupled with excessive womb pain and the passing of blood clots. Such a woman is prey to toxic thoughts, eats toxic foods, and is less spiritually in tune. As a result, she is in opposition to her true divinity. This "normal" woman is environmentally, socially, and dietarily poisoned. Her unnatural lifestyle causes her to suffer from PMS, depression, anxiety, mood swings, tumors, cysts, and so on. This is why, during her menses, she experiences more acute womb conditions.

So it's no surprise that a woman who continuously defiles her Body Temple by eating pork, beef, lamb, turkey, chicken, and fast foods will encounter suffering in her womb. In addition, the level of uncleanliness shows up in both men and women—as jealousy, greed, depression, and overpowering ego. And in men, a toxic lifestyle can render the sperm toxic as well; women receive these poisons during intercourse.

The health of the womb indicates what is going on in the rest of a woman's body. Once all flesh foods, their by-products, and cooked starches are removed from your diet, your menses will begin to reflect total wellness, and you will bleed for one or two days, or even just a few hours. A pure diet creates a pure womb, filled with love, light, and wellness. With purity comes a menses that is much shorter and no longer plagued with PMS, pain, cramping, red blood clots, or exhaustion. As you dedicate yourself to womb wellness, bear witness to the fact that your menses will flow less and less each month as you drain disease out of your womb.

## THE BREASTS

Precious breasts so big and round.
Precious breasts small and profound.
You are the mountains and the great hills of my world.
I shall meditate on top of my world
and visualize my breasts filled with
vibrant sun energy.

*Sacred Woman* could not be complete without some mention of breasts. The breasts represent a woman's capacity to mother, and they're also one of the areas of powerful sexual attraction. Why is it that men judge a woman by the size and fullness and uptilt of her breasts? This is because the breasts represent our gift of nourishing and maintaining life. They are the sacred foundations of our divine energy for both our children and our lovers. Just as our babies suckle at our breasts for comfort and nourishment, so our lovers reenact this desire to partake of the breast's sacred nectar.

The state of the breasts is inextricably related to the state of the womb, and the hormones that affect the functioning of our womb interact with those that affect our breasts. This is why the same care and feeding plan presented in the Womb Wellness Cleansing Food Plan for the revitalization and purification of our wombs can also have a profound effect on our breasts. What may affect the size of a tumor in the womb is just as likely to work in a tumor in the breast. Of course, given the epidemic occurrence of breast cancer today, it's equally important for you to consult your physician as well as to maintain your Sacred Woman approach to Body Temple wellness.

The following suggestions for natural breast care are the perfect complement to our approach to womb wellness.

### Breast Facts

October is National Breast Awareness Month. The American Cancer Society reports in its 1999 publication *Cancer Facts & Figures for African Americans* that "Overall, African Americans are more likely to develop cancer than persons of any other racial and ethnic group. . . . African American women are more likely to die of breast (31.5 per 100,000) and colon and rectum cancer (20.1 per 100,000) than are women of any other racial and ethnic group.

"Although the incidence of breast cancer is lower among African American women than in the general population, we have a higher rate of breast cancer deaths. For African American women with breast cancer, the five-year survival rate is 70% as compared with 85% for white women. At the time of diagnosis, 58% of the breast cancers found in African American women have spread beyond the breast." The overwhelming conclusion is obvious. Early diagnosis in African American women can significantly reduce breast cancer mortality rates. Consequently, it is very important to perform a monthly breast self-exam, and to have your doctor perform a yearly breast exam, and between the ages of thirty-five and forty.[2] If anything comes up, be sure to continue to consult with your doctor on a regular basis.

Also, researchers have long been aware that the disease kills African American women at double the rate of European women.

Afrakan women, we must get busy with Mother Nature to heal ourselves. Within her we can heal ourselves naturally.

### Gentle, Natural Care of Healthy Breasts

Caring for your breasts is not just for breastfeeding and not just for beauty, although those are important. You care for your breasts primarily for the sake of your personal health.

To relieve non-cancerous lumps and cysts or tumors, avoid all flesh foods, dairy products, and white flour. Live naturally, and follow the steps below.

1. When you arise, let your hot shower run over your breasts to stimulate and detoxify them.
2. After a hot bath or shower, gently massage your breasts for ten minutes with olive oil, almond oil, or peanut oil. Do this nightly or at least three times a week for chronic problems, twice a week for maintenance.
3. Place castor oil packs over your breasts three to four times a week (see page 92 for instructions).
4. Place clay packs over your breasts for seven nights, then every other night. Use Queen Afua's Rejuvenation Clay, or use powdered green or red clay, or black mud from the health food store. Mix two parts powdered clay with one part water. Spread clay over several lengths of household gauze wide enough to cover both breasts. Place gauze clay-side down over breasts and tape in place with surgical tape. Keep on overnight. In the morning remove and discard pack, and rinse off any remaining clay in a hot shower, which will provide further breast stimulation and detoxification.
5. Rest on a slant board daily, or prop your feet up against a wall at a forty-five-degree angle to draw toxins out of the breasts and to improve circulation. Do this for fifteen to twenty minutes, or take a nap in this position. If you have heart problems, do this for only fifteen minutes.

6. Do arm rotations, arm swings, and breast contractions and releases daily. Do all your exercises to music if you like.

*Arm swings:* Stand up straight, head up, neck long, shoulders down; take a few deep breaths and relax. Inhale, and raise your arms in front of you, all the way up toward your head. Exhale, bringing your arms back down and behind you, and swing them back and forth seven to twenty-one times.

Next, cross your arms in front of you, palms facing you. Raise your arms to the ceiling, then open them wide, making a full circle as you bring your arms back down. Do this seven to twenty-one times. Inhale as you raise your arms, exhale as you lower them. Now reverse direction and do another seven to twenty-one times.

*Breast contractions:* Stand or sit, back straight, shoulders down, arms at your sides. As you exhale, bring your chin to your chest, and contract your chest inwardly, allowing your back to curve into a C. As you inhale, open your chest as you straighten up. Feel your chest expand as your head goes fully back to upright.

*For more advanced students:* Hold your arms out in front of you, gently curving inward. Open your chest as you bring your arms behind you, relaxing your head back. Then contract as you exhale, bringing your arms forward again.

*Breastfeeding:* Breastfeed your child if you have the opportunity to do so. Breastfeeding is highly recommended for the sake of the child—and for the mother as well. The nutrients in human breast milk (the only natural milk designed for consumption by human babies) help to build the baby's immune system, while the process of breastfeeding creates a mother-child bond that lasts a lifetime. Finally, the sucking action of the baby during the breastfeeding process helps to expedite the return of the uterus (stretched during pregnancy) to its prepregnancy shape and placement.

This kind of loving care and attention given to your breasts will bring forth a beautiful, fulfilling level of pleasure to you and your mate and all your future children.

As you travel throughout the temples of Khamit, you will witness Ast (Isis) feeding Hru. These paintings symbolize the mother nourishing and supporting her child so that he/she may one day soar high spiritually, like the Falcon Hru.

## A RADICAL RECOVERY PLAN FOR HEAVY BLEEDING, TUMORS, AND CONSTANT MENSTRUAL PAIN

The following womb wellness plan promotes the rapid drainage of toxins from the womb.

- Over a period of twenty-one to eighty-four days (three to twelve weeks), maintain a diet that consists of 50 percent green juices, purified or distilled water, and herbal teas specific to the symptoms your womb experiences (see pages 134–135).
- The remaining 50 percent of your diet should consist of green vegetables, preferably raw and/or lightly steamed. It can also include light vegetarian protein sources such as sprouts, lentils, and peas. For maximum results, fast from starches of all kinds during this period.

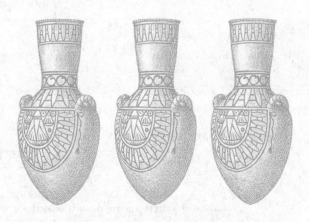

# HOW TO FEED AND GROW A TUMOR OR CYST
# AND CREATE HEAVY MENSTRUAL BLEEDING

**Foods That Feed a Tumor or
Cyst into the Womb or Breast
of a Woman**

**Emotions and States That
Feed a Tumor or Cyst into the
Womb or Breast of a Woman**

**BEWARE OF THE
WAR ON THE WOMB**

**BEWARE OF THE
WAR ON THE WOMB**

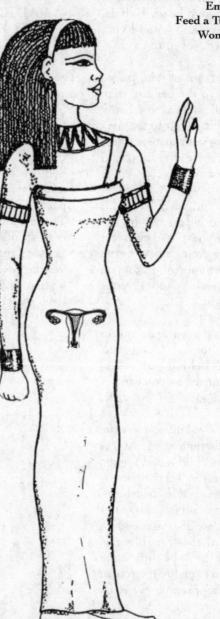

Flesh
(pork, beef, chicken, fish)

Anger

Cow or Goat Milk

Worry

Cow or Goat Cheese

Resentment

Milk- and Sugar-Based
Ice Cream

Lack of Forgiveness

Eggs

Lack of Love

Devitalized Starches

Depression

Fried Foods

Acid Sperm
(produced by your mate if he eats
the foods listed above)

**The more you consume dead foods, the greater the emotional and physical imbalance**

# HOW TO STARVE AND RELEASE A TUMOR OR CYST AND HEAVY MENSTRUAL BLEEDING

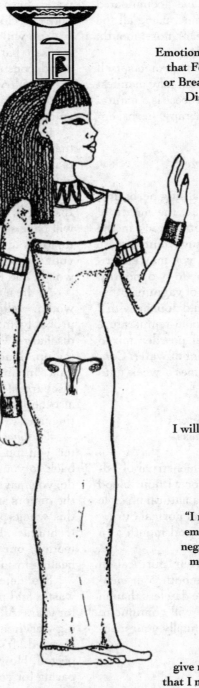

**Foods that Feed Wellness into the Womb or Breast of a Woman and Create a Disease-Free Body Temple**

**Vegetarian Proteins:**
Nuts, Seed, Beans, Lentils, Sprouts, Spirulina

Soy, Nut, or Seed Milk

**Green Vegetable Juices**
(calcium sources)

**Fresh Fruit Juices**

**Fresh Vegetables and Fruits**
(organic is best)

**Alkaline Sperm (acid free)**
Feed your man pure foods as listed above for maximum vibration of your love.

**Natural Food Consumption Creates a Balanced (Maat) Consciousness**

**Emotions and States and Affirmations that Feed Wellness into the Womb or Breast of a Woman and Create a Disease-Free Body Temple**

*Affirm Daily: I am*

Joyful

Loving

Patient

Peaceful

Whole

A Shining Being

"I affirm on this day that I will no longer feed a tumor or cyst to my Body Temple."

"I release and let go of all foods, emotion, and people that have a negative affect upon me, so that I may be free of the tumors that dwell within me."

"Beloved Creator, give me the strength to change so that I may be free of all that ails me!"

Artist: Rashida Art World

# WOMB DETOXIFICATION: WHAT TO EXPECT AS YOU CLEANSE

Once you begin to purify the Body Temple, your body will drain toxins that have accumulated over long or short periods of time, using all the openings in your body—eyes, ears, nose, mouth, vagina, and the pores of the skin.

Detoxification is how the body protects itself from accumulations of poisons that may manifest in disease. The detoxification process is a natural outcome of fasting, live juice therapy, herbs, enemas, and so on.

## Womb Discharge

Once you begin to consume cleansing herbs, live juices, whole foods, and the like, the mouth of the vagina begins to purge out poisons in the form of discharge. If you have any womb disease and begin to detox in this way, you may experience a vaginal discharge for one to two months, especially if you have a history of vaginitis.

During this period, you should douche with 2 oz. of wheatgrass in a pint of room-temperature water, or ¼ tsp. of goldenseal powder mixed with the juice of 1 lime and a pint of water. Continue to douche two or three times a week until the discharge ceases.

## Menses as a Barometer of Disease or Wellness

If you have a history of heavy menstrual bleeding of five days or more, with or without blood clotting, once you begin to live a natural lifestyle you may bleed more heavily than normal during your menses for the first or second month as a cleansing reaction.

If you remain steady on your purification regimen, by the third to fourth month your menses will last half a day to a whole day less than in the previous month. Your flow will continue to decrease month by month until finally your menses lasts only one or two days.

## Tumors

Dissolving a mucus-based tumor or cyst requires you to diligently liquefy your diet with distilled water, herbs, live organic vegetables, and fruit juices specifically formulated for womb cleansing.

You will also need to employ enemas, colonics, salt baths, and castor oil and clay packs; avoid consuming flesh and dairy foods (meat, fish, poultry, milk, cheese, ice cream, yogurt, eggs); get more rest; meditate; do journal work; and perform the Dance of the Womb.

If you stick to this regimen, you may notice that after one to three months the tumor or cyst that was once solid and immobile, once locked within a particular spot within your womb, should begin to move from one spot to another. Instead of being hard to the touch, the tumor will have softened. This is an indication that the tumor is in the process of dislodging itself from your womb. Nature is winning on behalf of your womb, and the tumor is losing the war.

As the months proceed and you grow in your womb wellness and consciousness, you will probably find that you experience bouts of womb discharge. This means the tumor or cyst is breaking up, liquefying, and draining out of your vagina. In time, there will be less to no vaginal discharges, and fewer days of menses. There will also be less or no vaginal odor and blood clotting, and PMS will have been eliminated.

*Warning:* At this point, now that you are better, you must remain aware that you cannot go back to your old stressful toxic lifestyle. If you do, you may regress and experience the return of the tumors and other vaginal disorders. After all, this whole process is not about a diet or a few techniques. It's about an entire lifestyle transformation, one that will ultimately bring about a healing inside your womb.

The detoxification process will get rid of wastes and poisons that have been in your body for years. All of those who fast experience cleansing reactions when they begin, so don't be alarmed. It's a natural reaction and to be expected. However, the more time you spend preparing for your fast—eating more raw fruits and vegetables—the less pronounced your "detox reaction" may be.

You may experience anywhere from one to three different cleansing reactions. Here's a list of some of the things you may experience during the first few days of fasting:

Headaches
Heavy breathing
Flatulence
Weakness
Fever
Shortness of breath
Fatigue
Skin eruptions
Rising blood pressure
Nightmares
No patience
Mood swings
Mental confusion
Aches and pains
Heavy bleeding during menses—first two
   months
Depression
Dizziness
More menstrual clotting
Vaginal discharges
Blurred vision

## General Detoxification Tips

These reactions are the result of years of a poor diet, nighttime eating, ingesting too much starch and too much sugar, and heavy meat intake, along with consuming a lot of fried foods and dairy products. The reactions you may experience can last from an hour to two or three days.

The best way to help your body adjust to these changes is to first discontinue drinking all fruit juices until the symptoms subside. However, do continue taking your vegetable juice combinations. Drinking only vegetable juices will stabilize and strengthen the body before deeper cleansing continues when you resume taking fruit juices.

Take enemas immediately, using only warm water in a quart-sized enema bag. Discontinue taking salt baths for two days and take warm showers instead. Give yourself a vigorous massage starting at your feet and working upward toward your heart, or have a professional massage.

Discontinue taking your Kidney-Liver Flush. If you have not already done so, replace it with the Fire Element Morning Drink (see page 80). Also drink a mixture of dandelion and alfalfa tea: 2 tsp. of each herb to 2 cups of boiling water, steeped for 2 hours.

Above all—get more rest and sleep!

If you follow these instructions, your cleansing reactions should be over within one to three days. If the symptoms persist, please contact your fasting consultant or get an emergency colon cleansing. Fasters who were on a light vegetarian diet before fasting usually don't experience the reactions listed above.

One key thing to remember throughout fasting is to constantly give yourself intense prayer treatments. Call on the Most High with all your heart and soul for your restoration and healing.

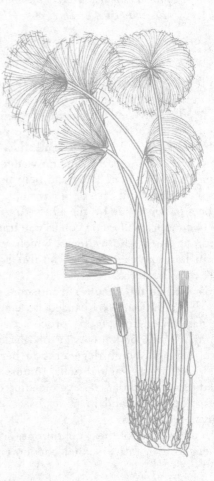

## TWENTY-FIVE NATURAL-LIVING WOMB REJUVENATION TECHNIQUES

*As a Sacred Woman,
I strive to follow the Natural Living
approach so that I will be able to
avoid the use of drugs, surgery,
and/or radiation therapy.*

*Mother/Father Creator/Creatress
has not
abandoned me without means, for in
nature I can find what I need to
Heal Myself.*

*I claim my womb and all of me and
I put my trust in Thee.*

I offer these Womb Rejuvenation Techniques to you in the spirit of the ancient Afrakan priestesses, Medicine Women, Sacred Women, ju-ju women, grandmothers, mothers, and aunties from Afraka, the Caribbean, and the South. These power women carry the knowledge of the Original Wise Women. They can help us claim divine ownership and care of our wombs, which have been given to us by the One Most High. These techniques will guide you as you travel the road to wholeness and wellness, which includes living in harmony within the Natural Laws of the Creator/Creatress.

Most women today suffer from some sort of womb degeneration. It is caused by emotional stress, devitalized, toxic foods, processed liquids, and, finally, lack of knowledge of the laws of Natural Living. Womb degeneration begins as vaginal discharges, vaginal boils, tumors, cysts, blocked tubes, candida, massive bleeding during menses, and PMS, and in many cases it ends with hysterectomy.

If you have any of these conditions, or if you experienced a negative sexual encounter, then follow these simple techniques to cleanse and rejuvenate your womb.

These techniques are also excellent to purify and strengthen the womb if you are striving to conceive a baby, or simply trying to stay in tune with your sacred womb.

### Healing Drinks

#### 1. Water
Increase your intake of water. Drink at least six 8 oz. glasses of room-temperature distilled or purified water daily to wash all your inner organs.

- Drink warm water to release growths that cause stress on the womb.
- Drink cool water if your womb is prolapsed or if you're experiencing frigidity or low energy.

#### 2. Herbal Tonics
Drink precious herbal tonics for a precious womb. Try Queen Afua's Heal Thyself Woman's Life Formula (see the product list in the appendix), which contains red raspberry, goldenrod, blue cohosh, dong quai, dandelion, and red clover, or your favorite herbal teas.

#### 3. Wheatgrass
This is one of the foods that best absorbs the sun's energy, which is why wheatgrass is a naturally high source of vitamins and energy. Wheatgrass contains all the vitamins and minerals that the human body needs, except vitamin C. It has strong rejuvenation qualities to strengthen nerves, cells, tissues, and bones as it cleanses the blood.

*Note:* Wheatgrass is a very potent detoxifier. If your system is congested with toxic foods, drinking large doses of wheatgrass may cause nausea and/or dizziness. The cleaner your system, the more wheatgrass you will be able to consume comfortably.

Wheatgrass Drink
Take 1 or 2 oz. of wheatgrass juice daily, mixed with 8 to 12 oz. of room-temperature water. For deeper cleansing, build up to 3 to 4 oz. of wheatgrass juice a day.

### 4. Ginger Drink

Gingerroot is a fire root that burns toxins out of the body. It's like drinking the healing fire of the sun.

---

### Working with Herbs

Generally, these are the rules of thumb, especially for those who are new to working with herbs for womb wellness.

- When working with herbs in the form of roots, bark, leaves, and flowers, use 1 tsp. per cup (8 oz.) of boiling water. Steep all herbs for teas at least 30 minutes to 1 hour.

- When working with herbs in powdered form, use ¼ tsp. to 8 oz. of water.

- When working with herbal extracts, use 10 drops to 8 oz. of water.

#### How to Make Womb Wellness Teas

The way you make a pot of real medicine tea is to boil 5 cups of water at night in an enamel or nonmetallic pot, turn off the flame, then add 2 or 3 tsp. of the tea or herbs, and let it steep overnight. In the morning, strain it into a dark bottle and then drink it until midday. Don't reheat it and don't refrigerate it. It's got to be natural.

This will help to rejuvenate and tone the womb, and also to flush it out at the same time. The reason why this is important is that we're not just rejuvenating the womb to create babies, but also to create ideas and birth them into the world. You know what your ideas are, your visions, your hopes, your art, your business. Whatever you need comes out of your womb center—the womb of your mind, the womb of your heart, the womb of your sacred seat. That's why we must purify these centers and fill them with spirit.

#### Advanced Herbal Preparation

Add 3 to 5 tbsp. of herbs to 3 to 5 cups of purified water in a large glass jar. Place jar outside in the sun or on a sunny windowsill and allow the sun and time to steep your herbs. Let sit for 24 to 48 hours. Enjoy!

For tea, slice pieces of fresh gingerroot into 8 oz. of boiling water and let steep 30 minutes to an hour. For a drink, juice ¼ cup of fresh gingerroot, and dilute it in 8 to 16 oz. of fresh vegetable or fruit juice or purified water.

### 5. Clay Drink

Bentonite clay or volcanic clay can be taken internally. Take 1 tsp. from Sonne's Formula #7 or 1 to 2 tbsp. from Sonne's Formula #9 three times a day with fresh fruit juice (see the product list in the appendix). Don't forget to take some form of chlorophyll along with the clay formula. Also take daily enemas along with laxatives that are enclosed in the formula package.

### Showers and Baths

### 6. Shower

Use a handheld shower massager over the pelvic area. Alternate temperature from hot to cold, and repeat.

### 7. Salt Bath

Use 2 to 4 lbs. of Epsom salts or 1 lb. of Dead Sea salt in a tub of hot water. Drink at least ½ to 1 qt. of purified water or herbal water (tonic) while in your bath for internal and external flushing. (Do not use any salts if you have high blood pressure or edema.)

### 8. Sitz Bath

Sit in a cold sitz bath for three to five minutes; it will energize and awaken your pelvic wall.

### 9. Ginger Bath

For increased circulation, add 8 oz. of ginger juice to a hot whirlpool bath or plain tub of hot water. Soak for 30 minutes.

### 10. Earth Bath

When you go to the Caribbean Islands, or any ocean beach area, dig a large, deep hole in the sand at high noon. Cover your head with a hat. Cover your pelvic area with gauze or a cabbage leaf, and climb into your earth "womb" and allow the earth to drain out toxins. When you come out of your sand sauna, take a bath in the ocean with the mother spirits, Nu (Khamitic), Yemaya (Santería), etc.

### 11. Steam Bath
Take a steam bath (moist heat) one to three times a week to release toxins from your pores.

### 12. Sauna
Take a sauna bath (dry heat) one to three times a week to release toxins from your pores.

### 13. Sun Bath
The skin is the largest elimination organ in the body, so try to bathe in the Sun's rays one to three times a week to release toxins from your pores. For twenty to thirty minutes, expose your abdomen to the Sun by resting in a beach chair as your womb faces the Sun. For increased healing, massage castor oil into your abdomen.

## Douches

### 14. Cleansing Douche
To 1 pint of purified water in a douche bag, add *one* of the following ingredients:

- ¼ tsp. goldenseal powder with the juice of ½ lemon or lime
- 2 cups red raspberry leaf tea
- Juice of 1 lime or lemon
- 3 tbsp. organic apple cider vinegar

### 15. Wheatgrass Suppositories and Douche
When you go to the health food store for your wheatgrass juice (if you don't have a juicer), you'll see the pulp coming out of the machine. Put that pulp into a plastic bag and take it home to use as a suppository. It acts just like a sponge, breaking up all that mucus. If you have a discharge of vaginal toxins or odor, the wheatgrass suppository should clear that up.

*To use the suppository:* Soak the pulp in some of your wheatgrass juice. Insert the pulp into your vagina, just a few inches up. Let it sit for an hour, then take it out. It's easy to remove—just put your hand gently into your vaginal area

and pull on the pulp. It will slip out easily. Then douche with the rest of your wheatgrass juice—1 or 2 oz. in 1 quart of water will draw out even more toxins.

### 16. Internal Cleansing
To a quart-sized enema bag add the juice of 1 lemon and 1 lime. Or you can add 3 to 4 tbsp. of organic apple cider vinegar. (This is especially good if you have a lot of gas, indigestion, and bloating.) If you have an ulcer, which should clear as you keep doing your womb healing, then use chlorophyll in the water—either 1 or 2 oz. of wheatgrass or 2 to 4 tbsp. of liquid chlorophyll. Then fill the bag with warm water, making sure the clamp is shut.

Now lie on the floor on your left side to take the enema. (You might want to lie on a towel and have another one handy.) Put your hand up against the wall. Wherever your hand is, put a nail or hook there, because that's where you'll hang your enema bag.

A healthy colon is related to a healthy womb. Remember, if the colon is impacted, then the womb will also be affected.

When the transverse (middle) colon is prolapsed due to late-night eating, or the eating of heavy, indigestible foods such as meats (flesh) and white denatured starches, the colon can drop down below the navel. If you're carrying ten to thirty pounds of excess waste, it can press down on the womb, causing many womb problems.

### 17. More Cleansing Techniques
Use a natural herbal laxative. Cascara sagrada is the gentlest one I know, and you won't feel any griping. Take 3 tablets with a glass of warm water before you go to sleep.

If you snore in your sleep, or you have breathing difficulties, or if you wake up with mucus in your head or bags under your eyes, then before you go to bed take 3 tablets of your laxative with the juice of a lime or 2 tbsp. organic cider vinegar diluted in 8 oz. of warm water, to open up your lungs and your colon. This will help to flush you out while you're sleeping. While you're cleaning out the colon, you're also flushing out the mucus above and below.

## How to Take an Enema

- Fill a 1- to 2-quart-sized enema bag with warm water, making sure the clamp is shut. At this point you may add ingredients listed in #18 in the list of techniques. Note that using oil in the enema helps to loosen waste impacted within the colon.

- Now, before inserting the enema bag nozzle, open the clamp up a little bit and let some of the water out so that any excess air in the tube can be cleared; this way, you won't get any gas backup in the colon with your first intake of water.

- Close the clamp. Then put a natural cream lubricant on the nozzle of the tube of the enema bag and ease it into your anus.

- Lie on your left side and open the clamp and release a little of the water. Then take in as much water as you can, while massaging or vibrating the left side of the colon with your hands. If you've already had some experience with enemas, turn over on your back for a little bit. Then turn to your right side and repeat the same step.

If you feel very advanced, then you can let all the liquid inside of you and hold it. If not, no problem; simply let in all the water that you can hold. If your colon's impacted, you probably will use only a quarter or half of the water. In a week, though, you might be using the whole quart if you've done a lot of cleansing and have taken your okra or your flaxseed.

- Next, sit on the toilet with your legs raised on a footstool or phone books so you're in a semi-squat, and release the water and waste.

- Now that you've flushed out as much as you can, go back to the enema bag and finish the rest of the quart, if you're able. Or you can simply lie on the floor for a while, which is very relaxing; try raising your legs at a forty-five-degree angle. Begin to massage your colon in a circular motion, which creates a balance. Then move down to your womb area and massage the right ovary, and breathe deeply. Massage both fallopian tubes, and breathe. Massage the left ovary, and breathe.

- After you're completely through with your enema, you might want to lie on the floor for a while and meditate on how good you feel, how cleansed and purified.

### 18. Garlic, Castor Oil, or Olive Oil Enema

Follow directions for taking an enema. Add one oil and one astringent from the following suggestions:

*Oils*

¼ cup castor oil
¼ cup cold-pressed olive oil

*Astringents*

Juice of a lemon
Juice of a lime

12 drops of Liquid Kyolic
¼ tsp. goldenseal powder
2 tbsp. aloe vera gel directly from the plant (first mash pulp until it becomes a liquid)

### 19. Clay Pack—Internal

Wrap 1 tbsp. of Queen Afua's Rejuvenating Clay or Fuller's Earth in cheesecloth. Place in the vaginal entrance and leave in for 30 to 60 minutes. Remove clay by gently washing and rinsing with warm water. The clay helps to draw poisons such as discharge, cysts, and odors out of the womb.

You may substitute a clove of fresh garlic for the clay.

### Clay Suppositories
You can also take 1 tbsp. of Queen Afua's Rejuvenating Clay or Fuller's Earth and put it up your vagina. Then pull it in like a suction pump. It's not about neatness. Just do it. Just be natural. Leave the clay there for about an hour. Then wash it out with your shower spray or spray bottle of purified water. The clay will start flushing and cleansing you out. Do this to keep the womb healthy, to keep it cleansed, to keep it purged.

## Packs and Poultices

Clay represents the Great Earth Mother. In Her honor and to empower your womb, apply a clay pack to your womb overnight on every new and full moon for a profound revitalization.

### 20. Clay Pack—External
A very good way of beginning to heal the womb is to use clay packs. This is especially useful if you have PMS, or if you suffer from bloating or heavy bleeding.

You will need some kitchen gauze (cheese-cloth). Fold over several layers of gauze, and spread the top layer an inch thick with Queen Afua's Rejuvenating Clay or Fuller's Earth. Place it over your womb with the clay against your skin, and tape it in place with paper tape (the kind you get at the drugstore). Go to sleep.

While you're sleeping, the clay will do two things: It will pull the poisons out, and allow your skin to absorb minerals. It's a healing food for the skin, but it also goes underneath the skin and begins to nurture and heal.

### 21. Ginger Clay Pack
Mix 1 tbsp. of fresh ginger juice with ½ cup of clay, then apply clay pack over pelvis. Keep on overnight. Shower off in the morning.

### 22. Leaf and Clay Poultice
This is especially beneficial after surgery. Do not apply clay until at least six weeks after surgical stitches have been removed. See your doctor first to be sure the wound is completely closed and that this is safe to perform.

Fill a large leaf of a dark green vegetable, such as spinach, cabbage, kale, or collard greens, with ½ to 1 cup of Queen Afua's Rejuvenation Clay. Lie down and place the clay-filled leaf on wounded area. Cover with gauze and secure ends with paper tape. Allow poultice to remain on overnight.

By morning the clay will have absorbed toxins and begun rejuvenating the womb. Remove gauze and greens. Take a warm shower, concentrating the shower spray on the pelvis. In the daytime apply raw cold-pressed castor oil or liquid vitamin E oil (25,000 IU) over the pelvis; cover area to avoid staining clothing with oil.

### 23. External Castor Oil Pack
Boil some water, and then dip a clean flannel cloth or white washcloth into the water. Wring out the cloth, then saturate it with cold-pressed castor oil, and place over pelvic area. Cover top of cloth with plastic wrap, then apply a heating pad for one hour. Remove castor oil pack and apply thick clay pack overnight.

## Massages

### 24. Pelvic Massage
Briskly rub hands together to heat them up. Rubbing your hands together brings forth the magnetism of healing power that flows through them. Massage the pelvic area, particularly from right to left, several times. Use olive oil, vitamin E oil, or almond oil as you massage.

### 25. Learn Reflexology Massage
There are several books on the market for self-training. In a circular motion, massage the inner ankles, which contain the reflex point that corresponds to the womb. Also review and massage the points that correspond to the colon, reproductive organs, and breasts. *Warning: Do not massage the ankles if pregnant.*

## Rest

One of the most vital ingredients for the restoration and balance of the divine, sacred, healthy womb is rest. Set aside moments on a daily basis to rest yourself and relieve your womb of the pressures and responsibilities you handle each day, just because you are a woman.

A few more words about rest: We women work hard to birth, lift up, encourage, support, nurse, and nurture everyone else. As mothers, we breastfeed, prepare meals for, and rear our children. As wives and lovers, we care for our mates. We are on the job as counselors and friends. We wash, cook, clean, manage, and organize at home, and we work in our places of business. We are members of the PTA and block associations. We raise funds, preach, perform civic work, and lift our voices in the political arenas for the good of our communities, locally, nationally, and internationally. Some of us are actual midwives who assist other women in giving birth to their babies. But all of us are, in some way, the "midwives" who help our families, employers, and friends give "birth" to their goals, plans, and dreams.

Don't we deserve a rest? Of course we do! So sit down. Put your feet up. Allow your loved ones to serve and care for you. And rest!

## Just Do It!

There will be times when your spirit flags and you'll tell yourself, "My life isn't together enough to follow the womb wellness regimen." But the whole point is to start right where you are. Just work with what you have—don't ever be discouraged about that. You'll find your own way, your own timing. Just begin!

For example, take making orange juice. Everyone has a different way of making their orange juice—by hand, or with a hand-operated or electric juicer. And everyone will have a different time at which they do it. They'll say, "I can't get to it in the morning. I'll get to it in the afternoon." Or "My schedule is so different—I sleep during the day and I go to work at night." Take in the information, let it go through your energy path, and then say, "Okay, this is what works with my time and my life." The goal is simply to do it!

The other key thing is to make a prayer to create the space in your life to do this healing work, because without the prayer it's hard to do. You might want to say:

*I know this isn't going to be as easy as I'd like it to be, but I know I can do it because the Ancestor Mothers are supporting me. So I'm just going to do it!*

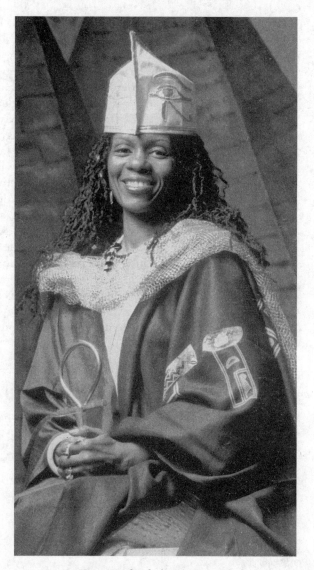

Queen Afua believes in you!

## WOMB WELLNESS, BREAST WELLNESS:
## THE CO$T OF NOT KNOWING

Below are "price tags" for six surgical procedures regularly performed on women. Some patients argue that these expenses do not come out of their pockets because they have adequate insurance coverage. But what about the price the human body pays during and after the surgical procedure? Many medical doctors agree that the better the body is prepared prior to surgery, the more favorable the outcome and the more rapid and complete the recovery will be. Ultimately, prevention of surgery would be the most cost-effective to both the human body and the pocketbook; although you cannot always avoid surgery, it is always beneficial to prepare your body, mind, and spirit with holistic wellness tools and strategies. Health care is self-care.

Whatever procedure you decide to administer, be it allopathic or holistic, remember that *you* get to choose. Some will choose both systems of medicine, merging medical and natural systems according to the severity of their womb state. Wherever you find yourself, get several opinions and know that the Sacred Prayers from the Global Sacred Woman Village go with you as you seek your womb and breast care recovery.

# TAKING CARE OF YOURSELF

Now that you've been using the Womb Rejuvenation Techniques, have changed your diet, and have begun to take your salt baths and herb baths, I'm sure you've started to feel the healthy changes in your body.

Recently I was working with a Sacred Womb Circle, and I asked them how they felt after their morning bath. They had a range of replies that may enlighten your own experience.

*Queen Afua: How did you feel after your bath?*

*Victoria:* I felt really tired.

*Queen Afua: You need to rest. You know, you have to have soulful rest. Because you're wiped out. You actually need to take a nap during the middle of the day, or tell yourself, "I'm going to leave work early today." And do it! Or tell yourself, "I'm going to take an hour to give myself a cup of herbal tea in my favorite mug, light my divine candle, and rest my body and my soul." That's a much deeper kind of rest, when you actually give yourself permission to rest your soul. We get exhausted because we push ourselves too hard all the time.*

*Victoria:* I'm like that every day. I'm so exhausted that I just pass out. I don't even do the teas because I'm so exhausted. I think that's what happened when I took the bath. It just took so much out of me.

*Queen Afua: That means you're dealing with years of toxic buildup. You have to ask yourself what your womb is doing. What has to be released in order for you to get better?*

*Victoria:* It's hard when you're the caretaker of the family. I've always been the person who carried all the weight for everybody and did everything, so even when I get up to meditate at four o'clock in the morning I always feel guilty. I think I'm doing something wrong, that I should be doing something for someone else.

*Queen Afua: Stealing time?*

*Victoria:* Yeah, I'm stealing time.

*Queen Afua: But you'd just give that time away to someone else. That's the mother syndrome. We have a problem with the mother syndrome. We overdo the mother. Don't you think that mothers are entitled to be served, too?*

*Victoria:* I do. But I also know all this sounds good and we can say it to each other. It's a matter of actually doing it and changing how we feel about it.

*Queen Afua: You just have to train yourself to do that. It takes some relearning time.*

*Victoria:* I took the bath and I was just so tired. I thought, "Maybe I made the water too hot." You know how sometimes when you take a really hot bath you're light-headed when you get out? I felt so tired and sad that I just sat there.

**Queen Afua:** *That was your healing, that was you saying, "I'm tired and I need a rest. My whole soul needs a rest." Now you have to incorporate caring for yourself into your life.*

*Think about it. If you went on a retreat, would you be picking up the phone? So why don't you take some time for yourself in the next two weeks? Tell yourself, "I will take a two-day retreat this weekend. I'm not going to go and help anyone. I'm not going to be available. I'm going to put my answering machine on. I'm going to take those two days all for me. And even if I feel guilty, I'll get over it."*

*And you will, because in a matter of twenty-four hours you'll feel better than you've felt in years, simply by giving yourself the same attention that you give to the world. Just stop the world and say, "This time belongs to me."*

*We have to train life to work for us; otherwise we just keep beating ourselves up. We're always planning to do things in the future, when things get better. Well, what about this moment right now? Get up right now and go get yourself a cup of herbal tea. Let some people wait for you. As a matter of fact, put people on hold. Tell them, "I'll get back to you in a couple of days, or a week. Because right now I have a patient I have to work on." So who's the patient? You. And you deserve the time and attention and care. Because you know what will happen if you don't — you might land in a hospital because you didn't take care of yourself. That's no way to get a rest.*

**Victoria:** My husband said that, too. He says that to me all the time: "Take an hour to yourself." But I say, "I have to do this, I have to do that, and the kids . . ." He is the most supportive person I've ever met. He keeps telling me, "Take a minute for yourself." I haven't been able to do it, but maybe I'll give it a try now.

**Queen Afua:** *More baths will help — trust me on this. Take more baths. Use more sea salt. Take one moment extra in the bath if that's all you can do. Start drinking green juice, start drinking more water. Start getting up a few moments earlier just to pray and rest your soul.*

**Mary:** I was totally the opposite with my baths. I took one yesterday — and took a day for myself. I sat home. I didn't wash clothes. I didn't do anything I was supposed to do. I did what I needed to do for me. I just sat and had a day to myself.

I got up this morning and I took a bath and I was awake — I mean totally awake. And I was going to take today off, too. I called in last night and said, "I think I'm going to take the day off tomorrow. I'm not going to come to work." But I got up with so much energy after this bath, I went to work because I was awake. I felt like my whole soul was alive and awake, and it was just a miracle. It was just like heaven. It felt so good.

**Demetrie:** After my first couple of baths, I started developing hives on my face. Usually I break out a lot. But this wasn't acne, this was actually hives on my cheeks, different sorts of bumps that I'd never seen before. But when I walked into work, my friend said, "Your face looks so different, your face looks so clear." I just felt like everything just started coming out of my pores, everything started releasing.

**Lauryn:** I had to go to an out-of-town conference and I took my bath stuff with me. Now, I'm not a bath person. I just can't lie back like people say they do. But this was a really nice hotel and the room had a big tub, and I got in and I said, "Oh, God, just sit here." And then I said, "No, you don't want to sit here. Okay, give yourself five minutes. You'll just lie in the water."

So I lay there and I felt really good. Then I said, "Something is missing. Oh, the candle. I didn't light my candle." But I thought, "Well, I missed the candle tonight. I'll do it tomorrow."

And then I slept so good. I usually have lower back pain, but this week has been great for no back pain.

Then the next day I said, "Okay, this is going to be the best bath because I've got my candle now." I had to find some matches because they didn't allow smoking in this hotel. So I got some matches. This time I stayed in for five minutes. I didn't resist it.

The next morning, I woke up with this dream that I gave birth, and it was so effortless. There was no pain and there was so much support around me. I was in this house and everybody knew that I was going to do this, but they were waiting around for me to do it. And I reached down and I pulled this baby out and our eyes met and there was this sense of knowing. The baby gave me this look, and the eyes, they were so old. And I had this sense—I felt so safe, I felt supported, I felt protected.

I've been kind of in a daze with that feeling. And I said, "Whew, okay, I'm not going to interpret that yet. I'm just going to ride with the feelings. I'm just going to enjoy the feelings."

*Queen Afua: New beginnings, renewal—your whole soul is going through a birthing.*

*Anna:* I did my baths and everything, and I started eliminating my starches because most of my starch eating is emotional. Basically I've been going through a whole rebirthing for the last couple of weeks. And I was having PMS. You know, PMS just started happening for me six or seven months ago. It's not that I'm having a lot of mood swings, but I get very hungry for heavy food around that time, and I want sugar and stuff like that. I'm not happy when that happens to me, so I have this whole struggle that goes on inside, and that's what was going on with me this week.

I usually have a lot of messages on the phone and a lot of people calling all the time, but this week my phone hardly rang. Everything was just very quiet for me, and I didn't do anything. I just pretty much hung out at home and just relaxed all week. I did my baths and wrote a lot in my journal. I generally do it at night because after I come out of the bath I'm really sleepy. Sleep is just pulling me down, so I can't do it during the day because then I wouldn't get anything done, you know?

*Ruth:* I'm a little disoriented right now. I've been feeling some sort of anxiety about something going on. I don't know what that's about, but generally during the week I was feeling pretty good. Not too long ago I came off the fast. Usually every year I do this juice fast, and every year I have a terrible time breaking the fast. I never break it properly.

But this year food has not agreed with me. It just seems like everything I eat goes to the wrong place or something. If I eat a piece of bread I can immediately feel it; that's never happened before. So this time I was really trying to be disciplined about doing the right thing.

This is the third or fourth week since I've been off the fast, and I figured by now my old self should kick in. I should be able to eat whatever I want and be all right, but it's not happening. So I'm still keeping disciplined because I know that whatever I eat, it's going to hurt, it's going to do something. I had some white rice and I had cramps so bad I could hardly walk home.

*Queen Afua: What happens is, you start to evolve. But when you evolve in your dietary laws and regulations, and you want to go back to what used to be comfortable, you discover that your body has actually left that level. A certain level of numbness had been going on in you before. Now your body has awakened. That's what's actually happening to you.*

*It's like when somebody stops eating meat for a week and then they go back to eating the meat and they start to feel sick or nauseous or have headaches. If you try to go back to the old ways, you start to feel the true response of what that food has been doing.*

*Evidently you have ascended past eating rice. Why don't you try couscous or bulgur or millet? Then you'll stay balanced and less congested.*

**Sheryl:** I still have to watch every little bit. I mean, I still cheat—just trying it out to see what's going on. But the wellness approach is a blessing. I'm doing the baths. I've been trying to get up between four and six—another thing I've done for years is try to be on time. I may not make it exactly at four, but I'm getting up earlier. I've even gotten to work half an hour earlier.

I go to school full time and I work full time and I'm a single parent full time, but I'm still making the effort. I'm just saying this because I know all of us have packed schedules, but I've pretty much been able to get up at four. I haven't felt good, no energy, but it's been okay. I didn't think I'd be able to get up at that hour, so I'm very thankful.

*Queen Afua: Well, everyone is a little different. Some of you might want to take your baths during the hours of Het-Hru, which is when the sun goes down. After sundown is the time of the divine angel of love and beauty, the time when you go into your inner self and start to beautify your inner self in your baths. And you start to bring out the more beautiful spirit of heart, beautiful tones. Your expression, everything, becomes softer, gentler. You're in a state of repose, you're in a state of retreat, and that's a really wonderful time for you to take your baths. And then what happens is you sleep deeper, so you wake up more rested. It really works.*

*Life works; you just have to find your way and what really works for you. At different times in your life you may go through new phases where you want to change your routine. You just have to find your way instinctively as you do your healing and cleansing.*

*It takes many months, years, to break down your system, and you've developed a lifestyle to maintain it. However, in order to get past being in the middle of the road—in order to have all this extra access to power, an exuberant amount of energy and vitality so that everything you do is from a place of power—you have to move away from your old toxic lifestyle. Wouldn't you like to be totally awakened? This is the wake-up call.*

*Life is a bowl for us to fill. The more good we put into it, the greater the results. So try to clear some things off your schedule and refocus your attention on you. You're still feeling helter-skelter? You're not feeling divine yet? Remember, you've only just gotten here. If you continue to do the work, then you'll start to be more relaxed. You'll be moving with grace. You'll be moving with poise. It takes time. You've been going one way for years and it's hard to reroute. Use the Gateways of your sacredness and watch how life begins to work for you. I know you can do it!*

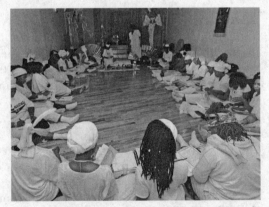

Growing Together in the Sacred Womb Circle

## THE SACRED WOMAN WOMB SCROLL

**The Womb is the Divine Lotus from Great Mother Earth Ta-Urt to Great Heavenly Mother Nut.**

### Sacred Woman Womb Scroll

*As we the womenfolk, the caretakers of the heart and the healers of humanity, bravely proceed through Geb's earthly realm to ascend to Nut's Heavenly Realm, may the natural world and the hearts of all humankind awaken with respect and honor to the power of the Sacred Womb. As it was in the beginning, may we collectively come to balance, defend, support, protect, and hold up high the wombs of womenfolk everywhere. Boldly we must return to the ways of the ancient Afrakan, where civilization was born, where the Garden of Eden originated, where women were held in the highest esteem physically and spiritually, where the Creator/Creatress was also She. The Sacred Woman Womb Scroll will guide you as you reach for the heights of womb consciousness for the survival and continuation of life, and to evoke a peaceful, nonviolent world.*

As I have observed my clients and my own growth process through the years, I have come to know that everything that has ever happened to us as women is related to our wombs. Our womb's life experiences leave an impression or wombprint etched on our womb's memory. The Sacred Woman Womb Scroll is an all-inclusive blueprint for emptying out, cleansing, and washing clear the many negative womb impressions that our wombs have absorbed.

As you conscientiously apply and activate the principles of the Womb Scroll, you will journey from Zone 0 to wholeness in the ninth womb zone. There you will be free of womb disease physically, spiritually, and psychologically, and the womb may return to its original state of womb wellness.

If each woman on earth were to apply the teachings of the Womb Scroll, then our whole planet would heal and be reborn through healthy children reflecting harmony with themselves, with their relationships, and with nature, creating a peace-filled earth.

### Benefits of Using the Sacred Woman Womb Scroll

The Sacred Woman Womb Scroll teachings are presented here to give you a systematic approach to the lifelong delights of womb wellness.

You will experience the Great Womb Purge once you regularly and actively maintain your daily practices as you travel through the nine womb zones.

The Womb Scroll teachings can help you

- release physical, mental, spiritual, or emotional womb pain.
- regenerate and strengthen the physical womb.
- prevent or eliminate physical womb afflictions and disease.
- create a protective energetic field around your womb consciousness that can help you deflect aggressive acts directed to your womb.
- create self-esteem and self-love.
- attract a more divine mate, who will offer you the utmost respect, love, and kindness.
- become more spiritually empowered by recon-

necting you to your ancient guardians and midwives for womb rebirth.

- reconnect to the natural elements of indwelling power zones through colors, food, oils, candles, and meditation by realigning you with spirit, air, fire, water, and earth.
- tap into and receive the celestial and earthly healing power contained within the womb.
- heal from womb attacks such as rape, incest, and other sexual abuses.
- make childbirth easier and aid in the elimination of all womb disease.
- evolve from having sex, which is mundane, to making love, which is Divine. The Womb Scroll teachings fill a woman and man with the spirit of Maat.

We birth and rebirth our lives with breath. The Womb Scroll helps to restore your breath, to balance the wholeness as it was in the beginning, before you were dismantled through generations of pain. *Beloved Mother/Father Creator/ Creatress, bless the rebirth of my lotus womb that she may be made whole. Bless my womb that she may become as radiant as the light of Nature, that my womb may breathe fully again and so reflect the pure essence of supreme love as wombs were in the beginning.*

### Four Ways to Approach the Womb Scroll Teachings

1. Work through one womb zone a day, over ten days. Take thirty minutes to one hour to perform that particular ritual. Doing this will allow you to become one with that womb zone. Start with Womb Zone 0, Ta-Urt, and keep going for ten days until you reach Womb Zone 9, Nut.
2. Plan a three-day retreat and perform all the recommended work in each level, from Zone 0 to Zone 9.
3. Always begin your Womb Scroll work on the New Moon as it moves toward the Full Moon.
4. Maintain your Womb Scroll work as long as needed over several twenty-eight-day Moon cycles.

*Note:* Our Western conditioning, which leads to compartmentalized thinking, would have us place the NTRU in categories. But the truth is that the Divine Aspects of the NTRU sometimes overlap and blend into one another. Consequently, if you compare, say, the Sacred Womb Scroll and the Gateway 0 practices, you will find that they don't always correspond in stone, color, or function. Don't worry. Khamitic consciousness mandates a broad vista where it is *Nebu Nefer* (All Good). When combining meditation with colors, stones, essential oils, and the invocation of spiritual guardians to heal yourself, be very creative. Allow yourself to be guided by your inner healer to discover your own natural flow and your own way of interpreting the Womb Scroll.

### Womb Scroll Meditation in the Sacred Womb Circle

- Sit on the floor or in Nature in a cross-legged position. This posture helps to open up your womb seat to Divinity. You may also lie down, or sit in a chair comfortably.
- Anoint yourself with the oil over the seat of your womb, the womb of your heart, the womb of your throat expressing your first eye, and the womb of your crown for Higher Womb Consciousness. Hold the stone of the zone you are in, reflecting your womb challenge, over your heart or your womb.
- Call out for your Spiritual Guardian to come forth through you, as you work through one womb zone to the next.
- Place before you, or visualize, or speak out, or write in your Womb Journal what it is that you want to release.
- Then visualize, speak out, or write down what you desire to bring forth in your body/mind/ spirit womb wellness.
- Visualize the colored cloth or colored candle in the womb zone you're working in.
- Now close your eyes and breathe deeply into your womb several times. Once you are feeling fully centered, go into your nature womb meditation. Take as long as you need to so that you can receive your healing and be at one with Nature.

The member of the womb circle who is acting as guide at the beginning and the end of your meditation will speak out loud the words of the particular higher womb consciousness to help the members of your group fulfill their individual and collective purpose.

- Open your eyes now and speak your truth as you commit to performing Womb Action indicated for the zone you are working in.
- Contemplate the state of higher Womb Consciousness presented for the zone you are working in.
- Offer your thanks to the Sacred Guardians.

## Daily Womb Realignment

- Drink your womb tea and eat the womb foods appropriate for the womb zone you're focusing on.
- Cover your womb with mud wrapped in gauze.

**NUT'S HEAVENLY REALM OF THE WOMB WOMB ZONES 8 AND 9**

| | | 1. Female NTRU/ Guardian Ruling | 2. Spiritual Womb Blockage Indicators | 3. Spiritual Womb Liberator | 4. Candles/Cloth Colors and Symbols of the Guardians |
|---|---|---|---|---|---|
| | ENERGY CENTERS OF THE WOMB ZONES 0–9 | Each of the womb zones represents aspects of Divine Female Principles and Affirmations. The following NTRU, all of whom are indwelling, signify the Afrakan Deity midwives who spiritually aid you in the rebirthing of your womb. | Causing physical and spiritual imbalances. Menses: 4–7 days or more. For elder women, menopausal symptoms are chronic. Each reflects that the womb is in a state of chaos and disease. Womb hemorrhage or acute menopausal symptoms indicate the womb needs to be rescued. Womb contains one or more afflictions. | General menses: 1–3 days. Menopause is gentle and nonintrusive. Womb is free of disease. Womb has overcome womb traumas. | Visualize your inner light with the use of your candles. During Womb Meditation, coordinate color of attire, sacred cloth, or shawl to charge the spirit of your womb center. |
| | WOMB ZONE 9 | **NUT** The Great Mother of the Heavenly Air Realm who represents total spiritual peace, expansion, ascension. Nut helps you to view your womb as sacred. | Unaware of womb's light and inner message. Womb shut down. Chronic womb pain. Prolapsed womb, physically and spiritually. Overly masculine/lacking femininity. Womb numbness and womb shame from previous hurtful experience. | You are able to have vision dream recall. The Ancient Khamites used dream recall as a healing therapy. From the darkness of the womb enlightenment is revealed. | White by day. Black by night. |
| | WOMB ZONE 8 | **MAAT** The Great Mother of Harmony is Balance. She rules harmony, illumination, and wholeness. Take flight on Maat's wings of spiritual womb freedom! | Feeling a heaviness, a pulling down of the womb. Womb despair, deep life disappointment, feeling trapped, and emotionally abused. Total womb trauma. | Totally healthy womb environment. A clear cleansed womb aura. Balanced womb. Womb contains clarity and lightness, emotional calm. Profound emergence of your feminine personality. A sense of safety, trust, and openness is established in your womb life. | White |

ONCE YOU REACH THIS STATE OF WOMBWELLNESS, YOUR LOTUS WOMB STRETCHES TO LIKE THE

| 5. Oils and Incense | 6. Stones (Spiritual Batteries) | 7. Meditative Nature Vision | 8. Higher Womb Consciousness | 9. Womb Action Nature Therapy | 10. Womb Foods |
|---|---|---|---|---|---|
| Anoint the womb of your mind, your heart, and your sacred seat with these sacred scents and incense as you meditate or when inspired. The following oils were used in spiritual rituals by Ancient Afrakan Khamites. | While in meditation, place specific stones around you or on top of womb, heart center, or crown, or use as waist beads. Have an elder Mother-Mentor bless your waist beads before you wear them. (The Ancient Afrakan Khamites used and wore stones to assist them in their spiritual healing.) Stone drinking: Allow the various stones to sit in purified drinking water for several hours to charge water. | Nature inside of us and outside of us has the power to heal and restore us to balance. Meditate outside in the open air or in the quiet prayerful space in your home that has been charged for meditation and prayer. | As we resurrect our spiritual mind, our womb centers merge as one filled with womb light. Proper attitude raises the vibration of your womb consciousness. A renewed womb attitude strengthens within you as you purify, fast, and meditate for the salvation of yourself and the inhabitants of Planet Earth. | Womb actions are various modalities used to transform the womb. Womb Action Nature Therapy activates your womb wellness. | Consume the following foods predominantly. As you cleanse and fast on these foods, your body will be able to release flesh foods, fast foods, artificial sweets, and congesting starches to heal your womb. |
| Lotus. An ancient Khamitic Egyptian plant whose oil is extracted from the lotus flower. This oil brings about mental, emotional, and spiritual harmony and is useful for mothers and during labor. | Moonstone. This sacred stone is connected to the moon It helps to open up the feminine and emotional nature. Cools and calms overreactions to our personal interactions. | **Sky Meditation** Meditate on Mother Nut to elevate your thoughts and spirits to the highest level. | Spiritual womb liberation is the key in this zone. | Fasting at the change of seasons. Womb *Hesi*/chanting of sacred sounds. | **Fasting on live juices and water.** You may charge the water with a crystal or moonstone as your foundation to fasting. Organic liquids from all fruits and vegetables listed from below. |
| Frankincense. Obtained from the bark of the tree. Comforts those who find physical contact difficult. Eliminates fear and anxiety. | Clear quartz crystal. This stone reflects our true nature, causing clarity to take place. It protects, balances, and harmonizes the aura and your energy field. | **Moon Meditation** Meditate on uniting yourself with the new and full Moon as purity gently emerges from your revitalized womb. All is well inside of you and your Sacred Womb space. This meditation is done best at nightfall or before dawn as you sit meditating on the Moon. | Ability to gain enlightenment from your wombniverse. Life's lessons and experiences create the potential for absolute illumination as we ascend past our apparent womb limitations. Balanced thoughts and clarity are the keys to this zone. | Form a Womb Circle with other women to pass on the Global Womb Healing Movement. | |

FEATHER OF MAAT, REJUVENATING AND RESTORING YOU TO TOTAL WOMB HEALING AND HARMONY.

| | | 1. Female NTRU/ Guardian Ruling | 2. Spiritual Womb Blockage Indicators | 3. Spiritual Womb Liberator | 4. Candles/Cloth Colors and Symbols of the Guardians |
|---|---|---|---|---|---|
| | WOMB ZONE 7 | *SESHETA* Guardian of Secrets, the Unknown. *TEHUTI* The Knower, the Guardian of Wisdom and Divine Intelligence. | Womb ignorance on how to treat her, be with her, or care for her needs. Unaware that the Divine purpose of the womb is that she's a force for life and creative ideas to support the emergence of a highly evolved planet. | The Divine secrets of your womb are revealed to you along with suppressed emotions and thoughts. Ability to use the mind and the will to create womb healing. Cleanses mental imbalance. | Yellow |
| | WOMB ZONE 6 | *NEBT-HET* The Great Mother of the Divine Temple, rules the Divine Home Space of the Body Temple that houses the Divine Womb. Lady of the Breath. | Blocked or disconnected to the womb mentally, spiritually, and emotionally; i.e., a woman may look at her womb as "down there," a distant and foreign space, lacking womb care. | Unification of Womb Oneness with Spirit. Ability to view the womb as a spiritual entity, a Divine Sacred Space of celestial beauty. Taking care of the womb. | Indigo |
| | WOMB ZONE 5 | *AST* The Great Mother of Divine Wisdom, rules teaching and communication. Ast with her husband brought Khamit to a state of high civilization. Allow Ast to communicate through Hru, the divine warrior in your higher mind. | Unable to verbally speak from your womb center. Lack of creativity in matters of life. An inability to communicate and express messages from your womb to self and others. | Ability to express, communicate, and interpret messages from your womb. Acquiring the skills to protect your womb and to heal her. Ability to speak from the Voice of the Womb for womb ascension. | Blue |
| | WOMB ZONE 4 | *HET-HRU* The Great Mother of Compassion, Love and Beauty. She allows you to view your womb as beautiful. | Lacking love for the womb; disrespect for the womb. Womb anger, womb hate, womb guilt, broken heart, and sexually abused. | Womb love, harmony, ease, and serenity. A womb that is stabilized, fully rejuvenated, and healthy. | Green |

YOUR MEDITATION HAS LED YOU TO THE GREEN HEART OF KHEPERA
THE GATEWAY BETWEEN THE HEAVENLY

| 5. Oils and Incense | 6. Stone (Spiritual Batteries) | 7. Meditative Nature Vision | 8. Higher Womb Consciousness | 9. Womb Action Nature Therapy | 10. Womb Foods |
|---|---|---|---|---|---|
| Rosemary. Part of the herb has a powerful stimulating effect on the mind and clarifies the thoughts. Sage. Relieves mental exhaustion; improves memory and the ability to concentrate; cleanses the mind. | Amethyst. Inspires meditation and the serving of humanity through the trials that one has overcome. Dispels all forms of emotional pain, such as anger, hostility, and fear. Balances and stabilizes sexual challenges. Excellent for treating impurities of the blood. | **Autumn Field Meditation** Meditate on Autumn field. Focus on Autumn leaves richly adorning a tree. Feel the brightness-glowing from your womb. | This is the greatest of discoveries: Think before you act on your womb's behalf, so that you don't create shai (karma) that you may regret. "Think before you act" is the key to this zone. | Write in your Womb Journal for attunement, particularly during the predawn hours of Nebt-Het, when your melanin or spiritual fluids are most activated. | **Yellow Foods:** Papaya, mangoes, pineapple, yellow apples, ripe bananas, goose-neck squash, ackee, grapefruits. |
| Lavender. Distilled from the fresh flowers of the plant; relieves mental tension (massage into forehead and temples). Helps to balance emotions due to stress, shock, and worry. | Sapphire. Helps to relieve mental disorders stemming from womb abuses and afflictions. Develops intuition, causing one to see the truth and so gain wisdom on womb issues, past and present. | **Clay Meditation** Meditate on your womb as she sits on the purple mystical mount an illuminating light and power into your womb. | Filled with high mental awareness. Devotion to womb harmony. Devotion to your sacred space of earth, radiating is the key in this zone. | Bathe your womb. Go to Nature to perform your water womb purging (i.e., fasting, bathing, soaking, etc.). | **Purple Foods:** Plums, grapes, eggplant. |
| Eucalyptus. Oils extracted from the fresh leaves of trees. One to two drops to any blend. Aids in thorough detoxing, so assisting in greater expression of suppressed emotions and feelings. | Lapis lazuli. Helps relieve depression and painful menstruation. Instills high idealism. Turquoise. Has the ability to absorb negative feelings. Purifies the spirit of wounded wombs. High copper content opens healing of the Body Temple. Aquamarine. Balances and stabilizes the emotional, mental, and physical bodies. | **Waterfall Meditation** Meditate on a waterfall as you are bathed in nature. Allow the water to flow from your womb as you fly freely, high in Nut's blue sky. | Peaceful, open communication with the womb. Motherly communication is the key in this zone. | Tap into the voice of your womb, the Great Mother, as she speaks through you, giving you divine guidance through your womb meditation. | **Blue Foods:** Blueberries. |
| Cinnamon. Oils distilled from the bark of the tree. Promotes the opening and the strengthening of the heart center. (Those with sensitive skin, be careful.) | Malachite. Symbol of creativity and transformation. This stone is used for protection during pregnancy. Green tourmaline. Healer of the heart, the blood, and asthmatic conditions. Emerald. The birthing stone. It helps to reveal heavenly and earthly womb experiences. Rose quartz. Allows for clarity of the womb and heart centers. | **Green Meadow/ Field Meditation** Meditate on a meadow filled with grass and wildflowers. Rest and rejuvenate, breathe in the abundant healing energy that resides inside your womb. | Healing rejuvenation, love, compassion, and patience for your womb's lesson. Forgiveness is the key in this zone. | Perform Dance of the Womb from Bes, the Gate Keeper of Dance and Art, through the loving spirit of Het-Hru. Breathe, dance . . . let go of that pain so that love can flow. Master the twenty-five rejuvenation techniques to physically and spiritually tone and rejuvenate the womb. | **Green Foods:** Green vegetables, green grapes, wheatgrass, sprouts, avocados, parsley, watercress, kale, etc. |

(TRANSFORMATION), THE WOMB ZONE OF POTENTIAL BLISS AND SERENITY, AND EARTHLY REALMS. WELCOME, BELOVED!

| | 1. Female NTRU/ Guardian Ruling | 2. Spiritual Womb Blockage Indicators | 3. Spiritual Womb Liberator | 4. Candles/Cloth Colors and Symbols of the Guardians |
|---|---|---|---|---|
| WOMB ZONE 3 | **RENENET AND MESHKENET** The Great Mothers of birthing, the head spiritual midwives who rule the house of Birthing and Rebirthing. | Unable to tap into the needs of your womb. Unable to hear her or respond to her call. Inability to rebirth your womb. Fertility and creativity blocked; blocked birth; infertile ideas and creativity and overdue labor. | Enhances both trust within your womb and intuition. The ability to rebirth your womb. Fertile in mind and spirit. | Yellow |
| WOMB ZONE 2 | **SERKET** The Great Mother of Water, who cleanses, soothes, and washes the womb and flames of pain and hurt blocking out sexual energy and disrupting our family relationships. | Debilitated, weakened womb in relationship to self and to others. Inability to deal with relationship(s) and challenges. Sexually impotent. Lacking support. | As Keeper of your womb, you make Divine intelligent decisions on behalf of womb-self in relationship to others. Ability to deal with relationship(s). Sexually balanced. | Orange |
| WOMB ZONE 1 | **SEKEMET** The Great Mother of Fire. The Female Destroyer of Evil rules the healing Flames of Vitality. Allow her fire to purge and recharge your womb. | Womb abuse by self or other(s). Womb wounded. Infertile creatively or physically. Lacking the ability to defend your womb. Heavy menstruation. | The ability to defend your womb wellness. Womb protection and high energy established. Womb center is strengthened and courageously centered. A fertile womb allows you to cleanse your emotions. | Red |
| WOMB ZONE 0 | **TA-URT** The Great Mother of Earth feeds and nurtures us through her herbs, vegetables, and earth (soil), giving us what we need to survive in a harmonious way. | Sometimes up and sometimes down. Unstable womb life compounded by tears. Infertile womb, barren. | Womb stability; no womb problems. Womb empowerment and womb trust. Fertile. | Black. All colors are born out of black. All people originated from the Dark Womb Race. |

NUT'S HEAVENLY REALM OF THE WOMB
WOMB ZONES 0-3

| 5. Oils and Incense | 6. Stones (Spiritual Batteries) | 7. Meditative Nature Vision | 8. Higher Womb Consciousness | 9. Womb Action Nature Therapy | 10. Womb Foods |
|---|---|---|---|---|---|
| Fennel. Oil extracted from seed of plant. Expectorant, diuretic; relieves constipation; helps one to spiritually release oneself to assist in emotional rebirth. | Yellow amber. Cleans and purifies the whole system. Helps to open and raise up the kundalini energy. Warms the womb. Clears constipation, which takes the pressure off the womb. | **Spring Sun-Ra Meditation** Meditate on Spring Sun as the Sun's rays shine brightly from your womb, draining out physical and spiritual womb poisons. As you sit in a squatting position between two birthing bricks, one to your left and one to your right, place your hands on the birthing bricks, bear down, and allow the Sun to assist you in the down-pouring of your blocked womb experiences. | Spiritually evolved and charged womb. Trusting your rebirth and fearlessness are the keys in this zone. | Renenet will celebrate the coming of your womb rebirth with cobra-like, vibrating, reawakening dance movements. Perform a Birthing/Rebirthing Ceremony for yourself or with a group of women who have journeyed with you through womb work wisdom once you have mastered or fully activated the womb work in the Gateways within the womb zone. | **Yellow Foods:** Papaya, mangoes, pineapple, yellow apples, ripe bananas, gooseneck squash, ackee, grapefruits. |
| Rosemary. The oil is distilled from the leaves of the plant. Has a tonic effect on the womb center; helps one to digest emotions. | Orange or reddish gold carnelian. Helps against poisoning, creates grounding, helps to digest and assimilate. | **Ocean Meditation** Visualize yourself resting in a calm, still ocean as the water drains out from the center of your womb and all throughout your Body Temple. Rejoice as the ocean washes out your sexual pain and debilitated womb state. | Healing relationships in relationship to your womb self. The key in this zone is to have the skill to work with others. | To achieve closure, release past and present blocked womb matters within relationships. Write letters, make phone calls, sit in the present and release. Let go of your pain. Perform a series of womb baths, baths, showers, ocean rituals, etc. Drink a large amount of water. | **Orange Foods:** Oranges, carrots, apricots, kumquats, cantaloupe. |
| Juniper oil. Oil is distilled from dried berries. Pregnant women should avoid, as well as those with kidney disease. Juniper has a cleansing effect on the emotional and physical plane. It relieves emotional crisis. | Jasper. Supports strength, vitality. Stimulates the sacred center and the solar plexus. Bloodstone. Works on the four elements to balance out iron deficiencies in the blood. | **Summer Sun-Ra Meditation** Meditate on summer Sun-Ra Vision as the hot Sun purges and energizes your womb. | Womb energy radiates for the survival of your womb. Protection and energy are the keys in this zone. | Burn up womb poisons. Go to the flames of nature to perform a womb purge (i.e., sweat lodging, Sun-Ra bathing, eat and drink red fire foods). Consume fire foods (i.e., berries, ginger, cayenne, and garlic). | **Red Foods:** Raspberries, cherries, strawberries, cranberries, ginger, cayenne, red grapes, sorrel, beets, red cabbage, radish, watermelon. |
| Frankincense. Obtained from the bark of the tree. Emotionally lightens up one's inner trauma, causing great calm and stillness. | Black tourmaline. It handles negativity by reflection. It acts as a protective shield against negative energy. | **Cave Meditation** Go into the stillness and serenity of the dark inner cave of your mind and soul to heal and reflect. From the black of Earth, all the colors of the spectrum are born. From the soil of your womb, all healing emanates. In your inner cave, focus on the black dot in the center of your inner vision. | This is the center where your melanin power center is, where all creative and spiritual genius arises, womb power and stability from where all life germinates, where all hope, dreams, and life are born. Building foundation, pruning, uprooting, and planting are the keys in this zone. | Believe in and activate your intuition as you plant womb-healing seeds through womb affirmations and healing visualizations. • Laying of hands over the womb • Womb clay packs and castor oil packs over the womb • Wafting the smoke from a pot of burning herbs to begin your purification womb rites | **Womb Herbs:** Womb mud packs. |

# HOW TO USE THE SACRED WOMAN'S WOMB SCROLL

1. *Call upon the Spiritual Guardians/NTRU.* As you open up to perform the Womb Scroll work from Zones 0 through 9, or if you choose to focus on one of the womb zones, begin by calling on the particular Guardians or NTRU ruling that particular womb zone to energize your spiritual womb work.
2. *Identify Your Spiritual Womb Blockages.* When a womb is disconnected in some way from its source of life, the result is the creation of a womb burden, which often manifests as a disease on a spiritual, physical, and mental level.
3. *Identify Your Spiritual Womb Liberator.* The quality or qualities manifested in each womb zone that confirm the womb has mastered the teachings of that zone and is in a free, well-balanced state spiritually, physically, and mentally.
4. *Light Your Candle and Drape Your Cloth.* Use colors, candles, and sacred cloth or shawl to set up your Nature Womb Meditation. These are tools of light that can be used to maintain this light within you, or used to turn on your own inner light. Some of these tools are live foods, light thoughts, and wholesome company and relationships; other tools are candles, stones, and essential oils. Our Body Temple, when cleansed, emanates pure light, reflecting womb wellness and the perfect health of body, mind, and spirit.

## Womb Meditations and Visualizations

Meditation is about centering and stilling the mind, body, and spirit. It is the yoking and the unifying of our upper region of the spirit to our lower region of the physical. It is, as our ancestors believed, a unification—a *smai tawi*—of our Divine Selves for the purpose of spiritual ascension, so that we may have full access to our true divine nature.

Meditation helps to unblock our lives and assists us in becoming united with our higher selves, allowing us to live and to love from an illuminated place. Meditation unites us with the light of the Creator/Creatress by igniting our own inner light. It was through meditation that our ancient Afrakan ancestors created a spiritual way of life that was so highly evolved that it has proved a resource for all the peoples of Earth. Stilling the mind stills the entire Body Temple. In that stilling we have greater access to the infinite power of the One Creative Energy, the Source of peace and divine wisdom.

Meditation allows for deep concentration on the breath and so brings you unlimited joy and grace, relaxation, and greater awareness of everything in your life. From daily meditation we receive a tremendous amount of energy, which awakens our intuition and brings us the inner information we need to heal all our conditions, however minute or vast. Meditation reduces stress, increases circulation, detoxifies our body, and purifies our soul.

The spirit/mind of the womb has an awareness, a divine memory, a storehouse of self-knowledge that allows a woman to tap into higher wisdom and higher consciousness at will through the art of meditation and contemplation. Daily practice of meditation allows us to release poisons from our wombs. It recirculates regenerative healing energy into our sacred seat, which allows us to rebirth our womb into its true state of divinity, no matter what challenges our wombselves have endured from our past shai (karma).

### Breath
Throughout your meditation, focus on your breathing. As you inhale and exhale, breathe your life back together again, breathe your womb into a higher existence. As you proceed in your Womb Scroll work, breathe into each organ from your womb to your crown. As you breathe into the womb of your mind, heart, and Sacred Seat, purge out all toxic womb conditions and/or experiences through your womb meditation.

### Meditating in Nature
The womb center is healthiest, happiest, freest, and most expansive when exposed to the beauties of the natural world—particularly under the Sun's rays in the open air, on the earth, before the open sea, upon a mountaintop, or surrounded

by a rain forest. You may perform your meditation in a quiet, clean space inside your home or temple. But whenever possible, perform your Womb Color and Womb Stone Meditations outside in Nature to reap the full benefits. Nature is composed of the same elements that we human beings possess. When we actively use Nature to heal ourselves, we become whole, harmonious, balanced, and recharged. The greater our communion with Nature, the more spiritually at one we are with the Most High Creator/Creatress.

Nature is composed of four main elements: air (oxygen circulated through our lungs), fire (Sun circulated through our blood), water (ocean circulated through our kidneys and the 60 percent of us that is water), and earth (soil and vegetation deposited in our bones)—the foundation that our bodies rely on and grow from. Nature is full enough to heal all mental, social, emotional, and physical disease. Nature purges and eradicates disease-filled toxic thoughts and bodies. The more we learn how to access and become one with Nature, as emerging Sacred Women, the greater access we have to our power as healers of self and others seeking wellness. As you heal your Earthly Womb Elements, so your Heavenly Sky Elements will have the capacity to heal.

## Nature Womb Meditation: Healing Your Womb
Use your intuition as you listen to the Voice of your Womb. Read your womb condition using a crystal pendulum before and after your meditation to measure your progress. (See pages 273–274 for suggestions on using a pendulum.)

- Close your eyes and begin by affirming the purpose of your meditation.
- According to your womb need, place the appropriate stone over your womb center.
- Visualize the healing taking place as you meditate on the color of your candle in relation to the healing of your womb.
- If you are indoors, visualize yourself surrounded by a beautiful scene in nature. Just flow with your inner vision to receive healing in the womb of your mind, heart, and sacred seat.
- Become one with Nature as you breathe into your womb and as you visualize one beautiful scene in Nature after another. Feel your womb fill with joyous healing energy.

## Higher Womb Consciousness
Moving up to a higher womb consciousness is our salvation as women. It is heaven on earth. When we are balanced and healed, our womb speaks to us from on high, from the most evolved aspect of our womb consciousness. The progression of ever-higher womb states of being are depicted in the Womb Scroll. This is the true nature of our wombs, once we have purified our Body Temples from past and present karma.

Living in the higher realm of womb consciousness draws the most advanced life situations (people, places, things) to us. As we learn to maintain this, we are assisted in living in the heights. This helps us heal all our wounds and hurts and ushers us to our inner light and divine space.

Our years of collecting pain, mistrust, fear, and stress have left us so crowded inside—filled with misery, destroying our inner serenity, and tying us up in knots—causing us to die inside or explode. Once we begin to shift our focus to on high, we witness our womb self transform as we flush out the toxins of that inner war. We become a lighthouse of pure inner space, attracting to ourselves over time only the Divine Spirit that is in us by nature.

## Color Work for Womb Zones: Color Breathing Visualization

Light rays of color in the form of candles, natural cotton or silk clothing, stones, and visualizations radiate tremendous unlimited power and energy on the physical and subtle spiritual levels of our Body Temple. Colors radiate light that helps the body to heal and become whole. They also have a profound effect on our mind and emotions. Certain colors affect specific energy centers in our Body Temple, which helps our inner world and *aritu* (chakras) to flow freely and unhampered. This then allows us greater access to higher mental, emotional, and spiritual knowledge. Use your breath to ignite the colors recommended in each Womb Zone.

## Womb Color Chart

*Zone 9 — White/Black:* This is the zone of the Great Celestial Mother, Nut. Her indwelling energies open us up to our greater inner space and put us in touch with true *hotep* (peace).

*Zone 8 — White:* Purifies the womb.

*Zone 7 — Yellow:* Helps us think clearly about the womb, her condition, and her surroundings.

*Zone 6 — Indigo:* Raises the spiritual womb vibration to the heights of wholeness.

*Zone 5 — Blue:* Calms and soothes the womb; mothers our heart.

*Zone 4 — Green:* Rejuvenates the womb.

*Zone 3 — Yellow:* Helps you fully communicate with your womb.

*Zone 2 — Orange:* Helps the womb digest life challenges.

*Zone 1 — Red:* Energizes the womb and burns away womb poisons and toxins.

*Zone 0 — Black:* Centers the womb. All colors are born out of black; all people originated from the Dark Womb Race.

## Color Breathing Visualization

- Inhale deeply into your face, lungs, and breasts, and down into your womb.
- Then exhale, releasing all toxins and negativity from the womb up to the face. Make it a full, long exhalation of relief.
- Every time you inhale, the color you are working with becomes more vibrant within your womb. As you take in energy or healing, observe your womb recover with each and every breath.
- Perform your Color Breathing seven times or more as the light of candles, sunlight, or electric light shines on you and gives you ease, greater self-awareness, and serenity.

## Womb Zone Guardians

All the female NTRU Guardians appear at the birthing ceremony of our renewed, whole selves. As midwives in the spirit they help us achieve our lotus status as Sacred Women. Summon their help as you meditate on their qualities within your womb. Work through the various aspects they represent so your womb will be reborn and healed.

*Zone 9 — Nut:* Through meditation and visualization she helps you evoke the spiritual liberation of your womb.

*Zone 8 — Maat:* Through meditation and visualization she helps evoke womb clarity, enlightenment, and illumination from your wombniverse.

*Zone 7 — Sesheta:* Through meditation and visualization she helps you think before you act on behalf of your womb.

*Zone 6 — Nebt-Het:* Through meditation and visualization she evokes mental awareness, devotion to womb harmony, and Sacred Space.

*Zone 5 — Ast:* Through meditation and visualization she evokes protection and nurturing and a direct line of communication into your womb.

*Zone 4 — Het-Hru:* Through meditation and visualization she evokes harmony and love into your womb.

*Zone 3 — Renenet and Meshkenet:* Through meditation and visualization they evoke spiritually charged wombs, fearlessness, and trust in your process of rebirth.

*Zone 2 — Serket:* Through meditation and visualization she evokes relationship healing through your womb self and helps you develop the skills you need to work with others.

*Zone 1 — Sekhmet:* Through meditation and visualization she evokes protection and charges your radiant womb energy for survival of your womb.

*Zone 0 — Ta-Urt:* Through meditation and visualization she evokes the melanin powers, the origin of all your creative and spiritual genius. She evokes womb power and stability, where all life germinates, where all hopes, dreams, and creativity are born. She builds the foundation — pruning, uprooting, and planting.

## Womb Zone Oils and Incense

Use oils and incense to anoint your womb in the spirit of each womb rejuvenation zone, using the specific essential oils listed below.

Order of anointing:

- Anoint your Womb, your sacred seat.
- Anoint your Heart center, the Heart of your Womb.

- Anoint your Throat, the Womb of your Expression.
- Anoint your First Eye, the Spiritual Eye of your Womb.
- Anoint your Crown, the Crown of your Womb.

*Zone 9 — Lotus:* An ancient Khamitic (Egyptian) plant whose oil is extracted from the lotus flower. This oil brings about mental, emotional, and spiritual harmony and is useful for a mother during labor.

*Zone 8 — Frankincense:* An ancient Khamitic remedy obtained from the bark of the tree. It comforts those who find physical contact difficult. Eases fears, nervousness, and neuroses.

*Zone 7a — Rosemary:* An herb that has a powerful stimulating effect on the mind and clarifies thoughts.

*Zone 7b — Sage:* Relieves mental exhaustion; improves memory and the ability to concentrate; cleanses the mind.

*Zone 6 — Lavender:* Is distilled from the fresh flowers of the plant; relieves mental tension (massage into forehead and temples). Helps to balance emotions due to stress, shock, and worry.

*Zone 5 — Eucalyptus:* Oils extracted from the fresh leaves of trees. One to two drops to any blend. Aids in throat detoxifying, so assists in greater expression of suppressed emotions and feelings.

*Zone 4 — Cinnamon:* An ancient Khamitic remedy. Cinnamon oil is distilled from the bark of the tree. It promotes the opening and strengthening of the heart center. Be careful if you have sensitive skin.

*Zone 3 — Fennel:* Oil is extracted from the seeds of the plant. Fennel is used to promote release both physically and spiritually and so assists in your emotional rebirth.

*Zone 2 — Rosemary:* The oil is distilled from the leaves of the plant. It has a tonic effect on the womb center; helps you digest emotions.

*Zone 1 — Juniper:* The oil is distilled from dried berries. Pregnant women should avoid it, as should those with kidney disease. Juniper has a cleansing effect on the emotional and physical plane. It relieves emotional crises.

*Zone 0 — Frankincense:* Obtained from the bark of the tree, it eases emotional inner trauma; creates great calm and stillness.

## Womb Zone Stones

Place the prescribed Sacred Stone by or on your womb or wear a set as waist beads. This meditation tool purifies, charges, speeds up, and awakens dormant states of awareness. The various stones send our energy centers profound healing. Healing stones can be worn to facilitate wellness throughout your day and at all times. Each color helps vibrate a certain illuminated state of being, as illustrated below. Also allow stones to sit in your purified drinking water for several hours to charge it — then drink.

*Zone 9 — Moonstone:* This sacred stone is connected to the energies of the moon because it helps you open up your feminine and emotional nature, while it cools and calms overreactions to events and personal interactions.

*Zone 8 — Clear quartz crystal:* This stone creates clarity. It protects, balances, and harmonizes the aura, your energy field, and reflects your true nature.

*Zone 7 — Amethyst:* Inspires meditation and the serving of humanity through the trials that one has overcome. Dispels all forms of emotional pain, such as anger, hostility, and fear. Balances and stabilizes sexual challenges. Excellent for treating impurities of blood and venereal disease. For some it is known as the Mother of Healers.

*Zone 6 — Sapphire:* Helps to relieve mental disorders in relation to womb abuses and afflictions. This stone has the ability to help you develop your intuition. This in turn helps you see the truth and so gain wisdom on womb issues past and present.

*Zone 5a — Turquoise:* Has the ability to absorb negative feelings and purify the spirit of wounded wombs. Its high copper content opens the healing of the Body Temple.

*Zone 5b — Aquamarine:* Is a balancer and stabilizer of the emotional, mental, and physical bodies.

*Zone 5c — Lapis lazuli:* Relieves depression and painful menstruation. Instills high idealism.

*Zone 4a — Emerald:* This is a birthing stone.

It helps reveal heavenly and earthly womb experiences so that we can grow and transform.

*Zone 4b—Rose quartz:* The color rose enhances the clarity of the womb heart centers. Rose quartz builds and restores your love and compassion for self and others. It heals through the release of loving energy.

*Zone 4c—Malachite:* Symbol of creativity and transformation, this stone is used for balancing and harmonizing, and for protection in pregnancy. It also helps you move from the physical into the spiritual, allowing your depressed womb state to become spiritually charged. It heals through the release of loving energy. It brings up relationship issues so they can be healed.

*Zone 4d—Green tourmaline:* A healer of the heart, blood pressure, and asthmatic conditions. This stone enhances serenity and brings about wisdom by easing conflicts.

*Zone 3—Yellow amber:* Cleans and purifies the whole system. Helps to awaken and raise the serpent power, Kundalini Energy of the Body Temple. It warms the womb. Clears constipation, which takes physical pressure off the womb.

*Zone 2—Carnelian:* Grounds, helps you digest and assimilate on every level.

*Zone 1—Bloodstone jasper:* Creates strength and vitality in the Body Temple; stimulates the Sacred Center and the solar plexus.

*Zone 0—Black tourmaline:* Disperses negativity by reflection. It is a protective shield against negative energy.

## Stone Meditation

- Place the appropriate stone on or next to your womb.
- Breathe into each organ from head to toe, as well as the womb center.
- When you are relaxed, breathe into each *arit* (chakra).
- Breathe into the heart *arit*, the heart of the womb. Focus all of your attention on the color green.
- Now focus on the color of the womb zone you are working through.
- Embrace deeply divine love and compassion into your womb center as you visualize your Nature Meditation.

- For beginners, meditate five minutes; for advanced womb workers, meditate on womb wellness up to thirty minutes.
- Be creative when combining meditation, colors, stones, and essential oils. Allow your inner healer to reveal what you need to heal yourself.

## Womb Action Nature Therapy

Womb Action Nature Therapy consists of various techniques and methods that appear throughout Gateway 0, the Sacred Womb Wisdom Gateway of Nut. They will support your body, mind, and spirit in your Womb Transformation. Follow your Womb Scroll as your guide.

## Womb Foods

Womb foods support, nourish, detoxify, and balance the womb. Womb foods are to be incorporated into your food intake on a daily basis to prevent or eliminate a diseased womb. Nature cures. Instructions on womb herbs, mud packs, fasting, and nutrition are offered throughout Gateway 0. Eat the following foods once or twice a day for womb wellness.

*Zones 9 and 8—Fasting:* Fast on live vegetable juices for rejuvenation of the Womb and fruit teas for detoxifying with 1 quart of purified water daily and womb wellness herbal teas.

*Zone 7—Yellow foods:* For wisdom, the assimilation of food and situations. Some yellow foods are papaya, lemons, squash, and grapefruit.

*Zone 6—Purple foods:* Purple food, such as purple grapes and purple cabbage, stimulates the higher mind.

*Zone 5—Blue foods:* Blue food, such as blueberries, relieves bleeding and stress.

*Zone 4—Green foods:* Green vegetables, such as cucumbers, parsley, watercress, wheatgrass, spirulina, and kale, calm and balance the emotions that prevent us from rejuvenating and restoring our womb center.

*Zone 3—Yellow foods:* As outlined in Zone 7.

*Zone 2—Orange foods:* Orange foods, such as oranges, kumquats, cantaloupe, and apricots, relieve menstrual cramps and gas and toxins that press down on the womb due to constipation.

*Zone 1—Red foods:* Red raspberries, beets,

cranberries, strawberries, watermelon, and pomegranates govern the physical body and womb body circulation, and warm the body.

*Zone 0—Womb herbs:* For the Gateway of the Heavenly Mother Nut, use womb herbs according to your daily needs. Use 2–3 tsp. of herb to 2–3 cups of boiled water. Steep overnight, and drink with your morning meditation.

## Womb Work Wisdom: Hands-On Wellness Techniques

Use wellness techniques to release womb trauma. Allow one and a half hours. This procedure should be done at least three times a week.

*Location:* Womb room, bedroom, or altar room.

### Step 1: The Sacred Womb Prayer

- Face the East. Offer a prayer at your womb altar.
- Identify womb concern.
- Call forth the womb solution.

### Step 2: Drink Charged Stonewater to Charge the Womb

- Drink crystal- or stone-charged water. Follow the stone chart to identify womb needs. Place a Healing Stone in a cup of distilled water for a few moments, or have a bottle of stonewater and place it under a pyramid for further charging.
- Drink Women's Womb Herbal Tonic to flush the womb. Use the specific herb you need to bring your womb to balance. Use 2 tsp. of herb to 2 cups boiled water. Steep 30 minutes for womb circulation, or for a potent tonic, steep 4 hours or overnight.
- Make a ginger drink for internal fire. Juice ¼ cup of fresh gingerroot; add to 1 pint of distilled water and the juice of 1 lemon.

### Step 3: Ginger Womb Sweat with Sauna/ Steambath or Salt/Seaweed Bath to Externally Burn Up and Draw Out Toxins; Rest Under Light

*Ginger Womb Sweat*
- Sweat 15 to 20 minutes in and out of sweat room. Take hot and cold shower over pelvic area in between sessions.

- Take hot bath for 30 minutes to 1 hour. Add 2 to 4 lbs. Epsom salts or 1 to 3 lbs. Dead Sea salt with 1 cup of seaweed. Pour water into a bowl to soak seaweed for 30 minutes or overnight. Add to hot bath.
- Now lie down and rest over crystal-charged bed. Place crystals under the mattress or at the four corners of the bed and one in the very center to purify your spiritual bodies, which are direct reflections of your physical body. If you are working with a group of women, place clear quartz crystals around the four points of your meeting room to honor the four directions—north, south, east, and west.

*Body Temple Rest*
- Rest under light over womb center.
- Place specific stones from the Womb Scroll over your womb area to further charge your Body Temple.
- Use aromatherapy and resting under a light positioned over your womb center. See the Womb Scroll to choose proper essential oils to burn or spray into the atmosphere for emotional and spiritual healing.

### Step 4: Womb (Khat) Breathing to Release Blockages and to Energize the Womb with Breath and Sound

- Breathe deeply into and out of your womb several times using the Maat Feather Meditation as your guide (see Gateway 0).

### Step 5: Use Affirmations to Empower

- In your group use the call and response from healer to healee based on the Twenty-Five Womb *Hesi* (Chants) listed.

### Step 6: Call on the Neterutu (midwives, healers) to Aid You in Prayer for the Healing of the Sacred Womb

- For emotional balance, take California Essences or Bach Flower Remedies that apply to your womb concerns, fears, hurt, resentment, and other womb traumas.

### Step 7: Guided Womb Meditation Using Nature Visualization and/or the Maat Meditation

- Allow the voice of the womb to speak to you at the closing of your meditation, 5 to 30 minutes.

### Step 8: Use Hot Castor Oil Packs on Womb

- Keep compress on for 30 minutes to 1 hour (see Gateway 0).

### Step 9: Use Womb Clay Pack and Leave on Several Hours

- Use a slant board or place legs against wall at a 45-degree angle for 3 to 5 minutes of clay application (see Gateway 0).

### Step 10: Drink a Green Drink

- Consider green vegetable juice, liquid chlorophyll in distilled water, or adding 1 to 2 tbsp. wheatgrass or spirulina powder to vegetable juice.

### Step 11: Womb Journal Work

- Do womb journal work at home each morning after your bath and herbal tea between 4 A.M. and 6 A.M., the hours of Nebt-Het.

### Womb Chamber: Setting Up a Womb Therapy Work Space

To uplift the vibration of your womb chamber, the color of the room, sheets, and your gown should be white, lavender, pastel blue, or green to psychologically, emotionally, and spiritually balance your Body Temple.

Your Environmental Healing Room is a tool to purify, charge, speed up, and awaken dormant states of awareness. This vibrates you into an illuminated state of being.

*Plants.* Place plants in all corners of your Womb Therapy Room to send negative ions to purify the atmosphere and enhance your breathing capacity.

*Music/Sound Healing.* Use music from harp, finger piano, zither, chimes, bells, light drums, shekere.

*Candles.* Use particular candles on the chart as needed to charge your womb center.

*Pyramid.* Lie down on a floor mat or a slant board throughout this session, under a pyramid if possible.

*Stones/Crystals.* Place stones in the four directions as well as on your crown, womb, and feet for specific harmonizing and balancing of the womb. Place crystals under the four corners of the mattress. You can also place various stones over your womb according to blockage.

*Lights/Colored Light.* Use red or orange or yellow light to charge the womb. Lie under colored light for 30 minutes. Then for the next 30 minutes use green, blue, and purple light to ease and soothe the womb.

*Aromatherapy and Burning of Essential Oils.* Burn or anoint oils according to womb blockage for emotional and spiritual health, inner balance, and harmony. Add a few drops of oil to a hot pot of boiling water.

*Ventilation.* The room should be well ventilated, for fresh oxygen facilitates self-healing.

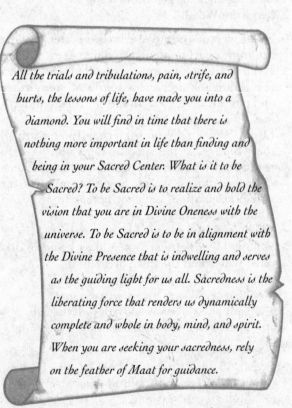

All the trials and tribulations, pain, strife, and hurts, the lessons of life, have made you into a diamond. You will find in time that there is nothing more important in life than finding and being in your Sacred Center. What is it to be Sacred? To be Sacred is to realize and hold the vision that you are in Divine Oneness with the universe. To be Sacred is to be in alignment with the Divine Presence that is indwelling and serves as the guiding light for us all. Sacredness is the liberating force that renders us dynamically complete and whole in body, mind, and spirit. When you are seeking your sacredness, rely on the feather of Maat for guidance.

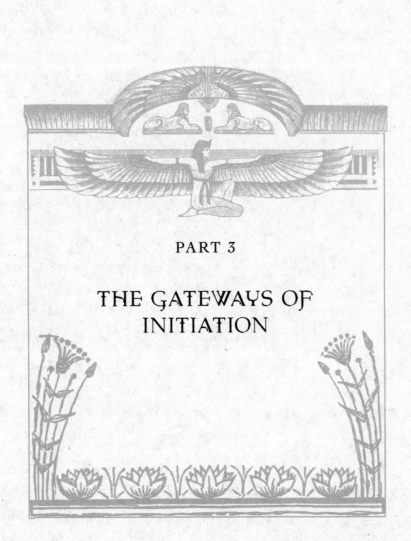

PART 3

# THE GATEWAYS OF INITIATION

# CHAPTER 5

# THE COMMITMENT: FOR ALL WOMEN WHO ENTER THE GATEWAYS

## FROM THE ANCIENT AFRAKAN VOICE OF NEBT-HET

*I, Nebt-Het, as a Sacred Guardian and Midwife, shall be with you as a guide through all the Gateways of Sacredness.*

*I, Nebt-Het, am the divine principle—NTRU—of the Lady of the House, the house of the Body Temple and the home in which the Body Temple resides.*

*I, Nebt-Het, am also Lady of Heaven, and like Maat, I bring forth truth, balance, justice. I am synonymous with order within and without.*

*It was I, Nebt-Het, who worked with my sister Ast (Isis), who reunited the scattered pieces of the first martyred savior, Asar (Osiris). I revived Asar with the spirit of breath. I helped Ast to reconstitute Asar's organ of regeneration, which caused Heru (Horus), the warrior Sun, to be immaculately conceived and born.*

*I, Nebt-Het, teach Afrakan women and men the divine art of cooperation, not competition, which is indispensable for the rebirth of our Maatian civilization.*

*In my right hand I hold the Ankh, the symbol for life. I raise my left hand with its palm facing you to represent the healing presence that I, through the Most High, will radiate across the land; my raised left hand will also block negativity and prevent it from poisoning the righteous ones.*

*On my head I wear the Crown of Nebt-Het, the Divine House in which I live in consciousness. In my room of meditation is the Maat feather I carry so that peace, harmony, and balance will always follow me. At the top of my Divine Temple is a bowl of water. This represents complete healing of the Body Temple through purification of the body, mind, and soul, all of which I grant to you, beautiful representative of the Creator. My natural Nubian locks crown my head to*

*keep my spirit in tune with NTR, the Most High Creator/Creatress, who dwells within each and every one of us providing guidance, protection, and illumination.*

*My healing spirit shall always be with you, just as the spirits of the elders, ancestors, and other spiritual guardians are always with you to guide you through the Eleven Gateways of Sacredness. Their presence wards off any fear or apprehension that might block you from your ascension. We are the gatekeepers who represent the Most High within you. We will guide you to your Divinity.*

## YOUR SPIRITUAL GUARDIANS SPEAK

Blessed be the journey you have taken through Gateway 0: The Sacred Womb Circle. It is the foundational training that has prepared you to enter the High Spiritual Initiation of the Gateways of the Sacred Woman. With the spiritual guidance of Meshkenet, Ast, Nebt-Het, and Aunt Iris, you have arrived at the entrance to the Gateways.

As you proceed, you will receive sacred tools along the way that will empower you to do great works, to awaken the divine healer in you, to anoint you into sacredness, and to liberate your Sacred Woman spirit.

### The NTRU—Guardians of the Gateways

The terms "Gods" and "Goddesses," when applied to the Deific Forces and Principles of Afrakan Khamitic cosmology, are grossly misleading. Western thought has imposed a patriarchal theory of a far-off, jealous God on the world. Therefore, to Westerners, all Afrakan

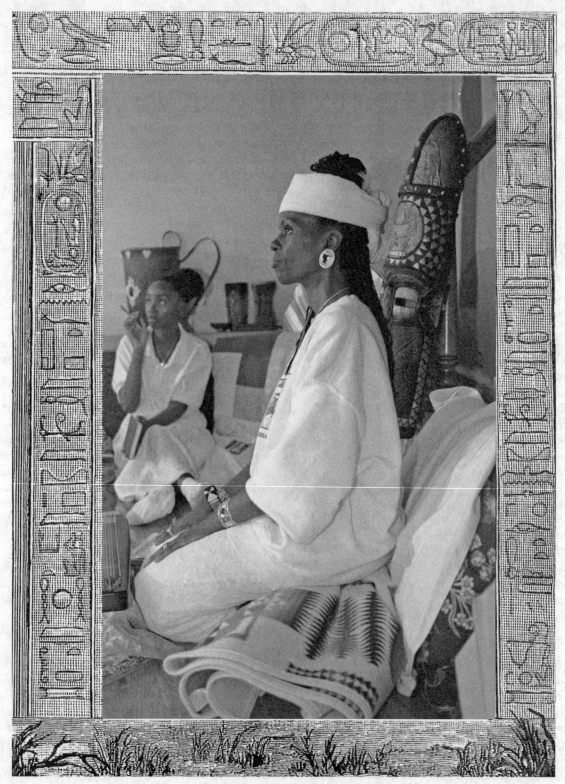

Entering the Gateways

thoughts on things divine are reduced to pagan and heathen polytheism. Khamitic people call the One/All Divine by the Nubian Heirophonic name NTR (pronounced *Ntur*). They called the collective, differentiated attributes or aspects of NTR the NTRU. As Khamites in resurrection today, we do the same because NTR was from the beginning seen by our ancestors as the Great Cosmic Mother/Father Divinity, never solely a Father God. In fact, the word "God" comes from the Teutonic "Got," which invokes a patriarchal entity. We speak English, but our name for the Divine must be in harmony with our most successful Hapi (Nile) Valley Khamitic ancestors.

The NTRU (pronounced *Neteru*) are indwelling differentiated zones of consciousness within the cosmic realm of Nun, the primordial mother mind, which we have the privilege, and in these times, the need, to call forth at will. For example, you can rebirth yourself into a new condition or circumstance as you desire, with a meditation and *hesi* (chant) of the name Meshkenet. Meshkenet is the rebirth NTRU. The NTRU are expressed in female/male complementariness. Our Khamite ancestors drew from the realm of Nature those animals, birds, reptiles, insects, and even plants whose habits or behavior best described or represented the specific aspects or attributes of Divinity. This was not animal worship. The signs, symbols, or types of implements that appear with each NTRU are tools that aid in the invocation of their forces or powers during meditation. The names in parentheses after the Khamitic names of the NTRU are the foreign, Greek-derived names that most people are more familiar with.

### Gateway 0 — Sacred Womb

**Spiritual Guardian: Nut**
Nut is the cosmic womb—the Sky Mother of Heaven who births all the fiery orbs—stars, planets, and constellations. Nut "swallows" the Sun each evening and rebirths it each morning. Nut is your brain, where ideas are processed, giving birth to action. Geb, the Earth NTRU, is consort to Nut. Western thought reversed the process so that God, the Father, dwells in the sky and the Mother was brought to Earth and reduced to a ghost—albeit Holy.

### Gateway 1 — Sacred Word

**Spiritual Guardian: Tehuti**
Tehuti is the guardian attribute of the word, and the patron of scribes. The inscribed glyphs on temple, tomb, obelisk, or *sesh* (papyrus) are the collective product of the NTRU Tehuti. Two animals, the ibis and the cynocephalus, the dog-eared ape, are used to indicate this deity. Tehuti is present at the judgment scene and records the condition of the heart being weighed against Maat's Feather of Truth. Tehuti's association with Mercury indicates that he has a messenger status. Tehuti is also associated with the Moon. Tehuti is the indwelling wisdom word that Hru (the spiritual warrior) consults in the war against Set (Challenge). A priest or priestess wearing the mask of an ibis is present at the celebration of Wep Renput, which marks the New Year in the Hapi (Nile) Valley. In addition, the ritual of "Stretching the Cord" is used to orient the foundation of temples, which is presided over by Tehuti and Sesheta, the NTRU of letters.

### Gateway 2 — Sacred Food

**Spiritual Guardian: Ta-Urt**
"Ta-Urt" means Earth—Ta, and Great—Urt. She is the NTRU Great Earth Mother Principle called Thouris by the Greeks. Ta-Urt is the provider of plenty; source of food and abundance. Her sign is the hippopotamus, known for its fierce protectorship and nurturing of its young calf. Ta-Urt is associated with the Great Bear constellation in the northern heavens. The crocodile and the hippopotamus are her emblems.

### Gateway 3 — Sacred Movement

**Spiritual Guardian: Bes**
Bes is a Twa Annu (miscalled "pygmy") and is often depicted as a bearded, homely, comical

dwarf. He is revered as the NTRU of household pleasures such as music, dance, good food, and relaxation. Bes is associated with the protection of women and children during childbirth. As a protector and entertainer of children, Bes is represented in figures placed around a child's room to ward off evil spirits and misfortune.

## Gateway 4 — Sacred Beauty

**Spiritual Guardian: Het-Hru**
"Het-Hru" means House of the Face. The NTRU of beauty, joy, nurturing, and protection, she presides over the unification of the two lands. Het-Hru is the sensual aspect of all women. She is cosmically in place in the western sky, which embraces the souls of the departed on their star journey through eternity. Het-Hru activates the Menu (Min) procreative principle through the art of sensuous dance.

## Gateway 5 — Sacred Space

**Spiritual Guardian: Nebt-Het**
"Nebt-Het" means Lady of the House or Lady of the Hut. In the Legend of Asar, Nebt-Het (Nephthys) is the sister of Ast (Isis) and is midwife to Heru (Horus), the Child Hero. Known as the Lady of Shadows, she is associated with the Black Star (Sirius B). Her orbit around her sister star Ast Spdt helps to maintain Ast Spdt in her orbit. Both are harbingers of the rising of the Nile. Nebt-Het teaches the sisterly art of cooperation, as she assisted Ast in the reconstruction and reconstitution of the body of Asar (Osiris, the world's first crucified savior on record).

## Gateway 6 — Sacred Healing

**Spiritual Guardian: Sekhmet**
Sekhmet's name means vital force. This NTRU manifests as the scorching summer heat. She is the daughter of Ra and consort of Ptah. She is mother of Nefer Atum, the Khamitic Adam—the perfected being who was born on the petals of a lotus. Sekhmet is the patron of all healers. Her activity manifests as the heat in fevers, which purges impurities. The Khamitic Sunnutu (physicians) all invoked her healing powers.

## Gateway 7 — Sacred Relationships

**Spiritual Guardian: Maat**
Maat represents divine balance, cosmic order, the law, the truth, the measure, the weight, propriety. With her symbol, the feather, Maat presides over the weighing of the heart on judgment day, which Khamitically speaking is every day. All are expected to live according to the Divine Maatian Principles in order to be in spiritual harmony. The Forty-Two Laws of Maat were the foundation of Khamitic morality. The Mosaic Decalogue, the Ten Commandments, can be found within this first body of Afrakan Khamitic moral law.

## Gateway 8 — Sacred Union

**Spiritual Guardian: Ast**
Thousands of years before the Shemite story of Eve or Mary (Mother of Jesus), Ast was history's first Madonna with her suckling child, Hru. As such she is the warrior's first teacher. Her name means throne, and she is portrayed with a throne on her head. Ast is associated cosmically with the star Spdt (Sirius), whose helical rising ushers the inundation of the River Hapi (Nile). As such she is seen as the nurturing mother who feeds her earthbound progeny through her impact upon the river. The legend of Ast and Asar shows her to be the prototype of the loving wife and mother, along with her sister Nebt-Het. She reconstituted the body of her husband Asar after he was dismembered by his jealous brother, Set.

## Gateway 9 — Nefer Atum:
## Sacred Lotus Initiation

**Spiritual Guardians: Sesheta and Nefer Atum**
Sesheta's name literally means secret. This NTRU of letters is, with Maat, consort to Tehuti. Initiates in Temple service studied the books of Sesheta to unlock the secrets of the Divine Life. "Sesh" is also the Khamitic word for

papyrus, which makes her, along with Tehuti, the Patron of Scribes. Sesheta is associated with mathematics. She counts the years on her palm frond. Her emblem is a seven-leafed blossom, coupled with a pair of upside-down horns. She also carries the scepter of the Lotus Flower of Rebirth.

Nefer Atum is the child of Ptah (the foundation) and Sekhmet (the healer). Nefer Atum is the Guardian of all essential sacred oils that are used for aromatherapy to heighten and sweeten one's body, mind, and spirit. Nefer Atum represents spiritual illumination, divinity, purity, radiant beauty, and grace. Nefer Atum is symbolized by the lotus, the essence of supreme oneness with the Divine.

### Gateway 10 — Seshat, Sacred Time

Seshat, the Scribe: the Lady of Mathematics who presided over the House of Life. Seshat's most prominent task was to assist the king in stretching the cord for the layout of all temples and other royal buildings. She is a Magician carrying a wand with its seven-pointed star, a symbol that presents the course of all creative ideas and consciousness. Her powers of cause and effect were legendary before the founding of Egypt. She was the feminine aspect of Thoth and the essence of cosmic intuition, creating the geometry of the heavens alongside Thoth. She became a goddess of writing, astronomy, astrology, architecture, and mathematics. Her title of "Mistress of the House of Books" indicates that she also took care of Thoth's library of scrolls. She is the patron of libraries and all forms of writing, including census, accounting work, and record keeping.

### Gateway 11 — Meshkenet, Sacred Work

Meshkenet was a goddess of childbirth and destiny, a divine midwife, and the protector of the birthing house. She was also a goddess of fate who could determine a person's destiny. She had the power to protect newborn babies and their mothers. Her name means "birthing place," and she was generally depicted as a birthing brick with a human head, or as a woman wearing the headdress of a cow's uterus. She is the one who breaths *ka* (spirit) into a child as it enters the world.

### Guardians and Protectors of the Gateways of Initiation

At the entrance to each Gateway, we will be there for you: your Spiritual Guides, your Ancestors, your Elders, and your Contemporaries.

- *Spiritual Guardian.* The NTRU is an aspect of the Mother/Father Creator/Creatress NTR, an indwelling spirit that lives in all of us to help guide us through life. Each of us has the power to connect with our guide in prayer, in meditation, and while performing sacred songs and dances.
- *Ancestor.* This is a blood- or extended-family member who has died and made the transition into the spirit world. This person is now in a position to render service to those who call out his or her name for spiritual guidance in the material world.
- *Elder.* She is an older member of your blood or extended family who carries the wisdom of the family. She may be someone you go to for advice, direction, and knowledge. The greater the respect you show toward your Elders, the greater your blessings will be.
- *Contemporary.* In *Sacred Woman*, a Contemporary is a woman from your peer group who inspires others by being a living example of a highly charged life in a particular arena. A Contemporary in this context is one who has mastered a particular skill, attitude, profession, spiritual level, and the like.

### RITES OF PASSAGE: THE GATEWAYS

Our people have experienced many kinds of lifestyles born out of disharmony and shaped by our heritage of slavery. A healing is needed to return us all to our innate divine order. A healing is needed to usher in Afrakan power and harmony.

We ask ourselves why the Afrakan people in

America and the Caribbean and various parts of the world are in such a state of disunity. It started more than two thousand years ago when foreigners made war on us and stole our homeland. It continued four hundred years ago when millions of our people were stolen away and sold into slavery. The result of the incomprehensible trauma, carried through our blood into the present day, has been astronomical divorce rates between mates and war among sisters, mothers, daughters, brothers, fathers, and sons.

Before we were stolen—separated from our home in Mother Afraka, and our people, our traditions, and our way of life—we were a whole and healthy people. We had traditions that provided us with balance and harmony.

The holocaust that we Afrakans endured left us as Negroes without our Afrakan land, culture, language, music, dance, customs, foods, religion, dress, and above all, without our Creator/Creatress. It left us without our Rites of Passage, from childhood to adulthood. It left us without a way to heal our scars. It left us without a healthy family life, for we were constantly being separated from parents, children, husbands, and wives, to be sent to faraway plantations as property—as slaves. Self-love was almost wiped out of us by an inhumane, imbalanced aggressor. Yet, through it all, we were never separated from spirit. So we rise today as the undefeatable dark people we are. We ascend, as surely as the sun rises and sets.

Traditionally in Afrakan tribal society, a systematic training was provided for entering womanhood or manhood. This training began at puberty and lasted from two to four years. These were our Rites of Passage. You did not go through life in a hit-or-miss fashion, unsure of your direction, role, and purpose within the community. You were groomed to be a responsible, intelligent, and productive person. You were given the skills required for the collective success of your people.

Today, however, when a woman and man come together in matrimony, they often experience misunderstandings because they have not experienced their Rites of Passage training. In traditional Khamitic life, when conflict arises between a married couple, the Elders come together to support the couple, and to help them work out or heal any and all disturbances they may have.

In this way, the problem is resolved by both sides of the family, and this helps to prevent divorce, fathers not caring for their children or their youth, or mothers or wives not being able to live up to their marriage vows. Both the man and the woman may then be given further guidance and instruction on how to be a productive family, because the family is the foundation for a strong tribe, nation, and society.

Without going through our Rites of Passage—our guidance on how to be upright women and men—there can be no healthy future. Without our Rites of Passage we, both men and women, are lost. Life, productivity, direction, healing, cannot go forward. So let us all strive to bring back our Rites of Passage, for young girls just coming into their womanness and for mature women in need of deep reconnection with their sacredness.

The *Sacred Woman* initiation is my effort to re-create our ancient rites from my perspective as a contemporary Healer. I pray that what I share with you will add riches to your pot. Please draw from these teachings what you need to move into your wholeness. Move into a greater love and respect and appreciation of your beautiful Afrakan self, as you unfold through the Healing Gateways of Sacred Womanhood.

## CREATING THE SACRED WOMAN'S FREEDOM SHAWL

As you prepare to enter Gateway 1, undertake the following ritual project.

Our grandmothers and great-grandmothers made quilts in a private mind, heart, and hand meditation, or in a circle of women friends and relatives. But it was always a women's ritual. Making these quilts took pieces of cloth of different patterns and colors and unified them into one tapestry. Each piece was perfectly measured and sewn together in meditation or over interesting conversations that created a spirit of togetherness and joy and laughter. Such quilts became monuments to our history. Today, quilts of unity become garments of freedom for Sacred Women that can be worn as shawls or placed over your bed to protect you as you make your spiritual journey.

Since ancient times, the working of cloth has been used not only for clothing and cover but also to mark special occasions, or to announce information. Cloth art, like clothing, provided a fine place for social messages. It has also been used as a mnemonic device to record events or other data. Too, it was used to invoke "magic—to protect, to secure fertility and riches, to divine the future."[1]

The spinning, weaving, and wrapping of cloth by women is an ancient practice dating back to our Khamitic origins, as early as the fourth millennium BCE. The women typically sat on low stools or the floor to spin. The loom was pegged out to the ground and two weavers squatted on either side, moving the shuttle back and forth.

As we Sacred Women in the making work our own cloth, we are stitching ourselves into a tapestry of liberation, and healing ourselves with each thread we spin and each piece of cloth we sew. As we embrace new pieces of consciousness in our entry to each Gateway, we are gathering ourselves into a cloth of unity.

## Sewing Your Freedom Shawl/Quilt

Honoring the tradition of working cloth together is a reflection of our growth into our sacredness as liberated, empowered women. Another name for such a cloth is *senab*, the Metu NTR (Khamitic) word for "health," for this shawl represents everything that is healthy and whole within a woman. It can be a shawl, a quilt, a blanket, a robe, a drape, or a wall hanging—a piece of art.

The cloth represents Gateway 0—The Sacred Womb and all the Gateways of Initiation. The gold thread we use to sew these pieces of cloth as we make our journeys through the Gateways ties together the lessons of what each Gateway offers to us. We will sew together the pieces of cloth that embody our wisdom, hope, visions, prayers, rest, and joy, as we mend the

fabric of ourselves and our lives from one Gateway to the next. Into our *senab* we incorporate all that we have learned from studying and mastering our lessons, building upon the knowledge of our Sacred Circle, receiving and sharing all that is needed to become a Sacred Woman. Our sacred quilt or shawl is composed of ten pieces of cloth. It will be a design of beautiful, enlightening, life-giving colors that represent our hard-won wisdom.

During our initiatory journey through *Sacred Woman*, we keep weaving or sewing together the various pieces representing the stages of our development as a whole woman. When we are done, we will have a quilt or shawl that will keep us warm from the cold, and will spread over our life to protect and to comfort us in spirit when needed. It will soothe us when healing is taking place, shield us when it's too hot in life's kitchen, and wrap around us like a skirt to bring out our regal beauty. We drape it over our shoulders as a shawl when calling for strength to take care of the serious business at hand. We wear it as we walk the land or place it around our shoulders as we go to and fro in the world, or rest it at the edge of our bed, when we need to contemplate what direction to take next.

These ten pieces of sacred cloth are all born out of and inspired by the wombs of the first mothers. Once each piece is joined to another through the gathering of our sacred selves, a rich and color-filled tapestry will emerge, a legacy of our true womanhood for all times. And we may pass this cloth on to our daughters as a powerful legacy for them, just as our first mothers passed on the legacy of the original Sacred Woman to all other women seeking wholeness.

## Prayer Shawl

As you enter Gateway 0, you may receive the Ast/Nebt-Het (Sister-to-Sister) shawl. You don't have to wait until the end of your Initiation to wear this shawl. You may pray with this shawl, and wear it particularly during your morning and evening prayers and purification rituals. Wear your shawl during your studies into Sacred Womanhood. As you approach each Gateway, anoint your shawl with the particular essential oil of that gate. You can also use the Ast/Nebt-Het shawl to support you through your Gateways as you work on creating your woman-made Freedom Shawl or Quilt.

## Making Your Freedom Shawl or Quilt

### Step 1: Mind
Become familiar with the *Sacred Woman* text. Read each Gateway. Be ready to apply what you are learning as a Sacred Woman to the preparation of your Freedom Shawl. Observe what signs and symbols appear in your life. Reflect on how these symbols represent what you and your shawl will become.

### Step 2: Spirit
As you sew, meditate on this ritual as a means of gathering all the pieces of your woman self together into one beautiful unified tapestry. Visualize thoughts of wellness into your life, and stitch them and your highest vision of yourself into your design.

### Step 3: Body
Collect swatches of cloth using the ten colors symbolic of each Gateway listed in the Spiritual Observances Road Map Through the Gateways chart (see pages 130–135). In each of Gateways 0 through 11, you will complete sewing a swatch

every seventh day. Remember to put Gateway 0 in the center and to let the 11 Gateways surround your sacred womb. The last thread will be sewn as you, the Sacred Woman in the making, are about to leave that particular Gateway.

This process continues at the beginning and ending of each subsequent Gateway. This is the ritual of beginnings and endings, linking one piece of cloth, one piece of self, to the whole by hand and by spirit.

After you've finished sewing the pieces of your shawl together, sew a white, blue, or silver strip of cloth completely around the edges of your quilt or shawl as a border. You may then choose to appliqué a patch of silver or blue cloth on one or all of the Gateways to represent the overarching divine spirit of Nut, our heavenly Celestial Mother. As a sacred artist, feel free to paint stars on your shawl as well.

From the silver or blue cloth, cut out the shape of the throne (the seat) of Ast (Isis). Then appliqué this symbol of Ast onto the very center of your shawl or quilt. Now cut out the shape of a lotus from white cloth and sew it above the seat of Ast. As you stitch, think of this ritual as a means of gathering together all the pieces of your woman-self into one beautiful unified design showing a rich life embodied in cloth.

Since there is no limitation to your creativity, you may now want to sew or glue a sacred stone that corresponds to each Gateway (see your Altar Work chart) onto your shawl. If you

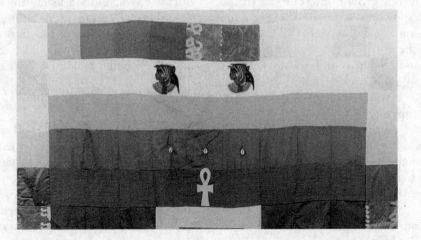

choose, you may paint images of yourself and the Guardians, Ancestors, and Elders of your choice on your cloth. Finally, anoint your cloth with the essential oils of each Gateway. Let your cloth speak of your sacred life.

## Mounting Your Collective Freedom Quilt

There is a third project you might wish to undertake. Collectively, the women who are studying and becoming Initiated as Sacred Women may choose to make a Freedom Quilt together to symbolize the unity of their Sacred Women's Circle. When it is completed at the end of your journey through the Gateways, the Freedom Shawl may be mounted on the wall in a common, shared area for all to enjoy, along with a dated

picture of the members of your Sacred Women's Circle. This display helps to keep the history of your Sacred Woman clan ever visible, and may encourage other sister-initiates to do likewise.

## Challenge of the Sacred Woman

If at any point you feel your creative energy or your life force being challenged, call on Ast and Nebt-Het, the original Sister-to-Sister pair. Call on the spirit of your Freedom Shawl as you drape it over your shoulders or over your crown. When you wear your Freedom Shawl, think of your Spiritual Guardians, Ancestors, and Elders, and ask for their help to make a breakout or breakthrough. They will always be there to guide and to comfort you.

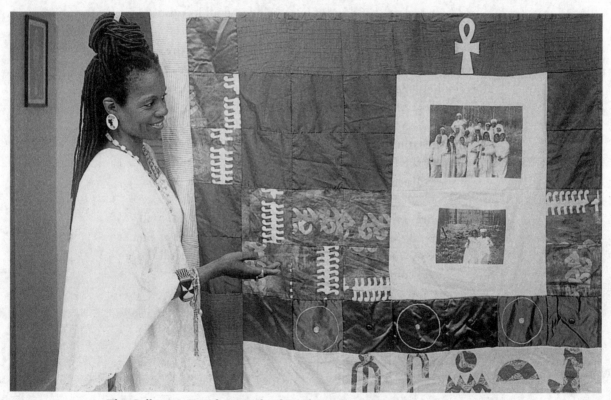

The Collective Freedom Quilt of Washington, DC's Sacred Woman Circle

# ENTERING
## THE GATEWAYS

The voice of your womb is calling you to step
forward to reawaken and continue the healing
legacy and traditions of our Afrakan past. Your
work in parts 1 and 2 of *Sacred Woman* has equipped
you to experience, share, and live the path of the
sacred ancient Medicine Woman. She still lives within us
in this present age, as we become whole, healed, and
empowered women. The Planet Earth exists within you
and around you, and is ready to bring you all its wisdom
of wellness and healing.

Let us Afrakan womenfolk, the original healers of the earth,
now set forth. Let us prepare for ourselves a wellness table of
flowers, herbs, garden vegetables, sun-ripened fruits, and good
vibrations. Let us attract to ourselves all the joy
and happiness that is our due.

Communicating with the voice of the womb has prepared us
to enter the Gateways of Luminosity, with the guidance
of the Ancestors, Elders, and Afrakan Guardian Angels,
our beloved NTRU.

The work we do in the Gateways of Transformation will
equip us to take on our work as the Medicine Women of Planet
Earth. As we empower ourselves as Sacred Women, all those
who come in contact with our visions, prayers,
and our sacred touch will be lifted to their
heights. For within ourselves we will
have discovered the indwelling powers of
NTR, the Most High Creator/Creatress
of all healing.

# SACRED WOMAN DAILY NATURAL LIVING OBSERVANCES FOR ASCENSION

During your journey within the Global Sacred Woman Village, please honor the following intentions:

**Observe Nut:**

• Abstain from sexual activity. Be celibate during your Sacred Woman Initiation Training. Ask your partner to honor your commitment of abstinence, but if there is intimacy between you and your mate, be sure he does some degree of cleansing for two to three days with you to adequately prepare himself for holistic lovemaking.
• Fast every New Moon and Full Moon period and during your menses.

**Observe Tehuti:**

• Observe silence for one to four hours daily.
• Limit conversation both on the telephone and in person. No gossiping.
• Watch your words. No cursing, judging, or criticizing. Avoid putting yourself or anyone down. Use words as medicine.
• Record your experiences—lessons, tests, and blessings—in your Sacred Womb Journal as you travel through each Gateway.

**Observe Ta-Urt:**

• Follow a total vegetarian diet. If you are still a meat eater, you have a seven-day grace period to make your transition into a vegetarian lifestyle. All the information you need to begin is in part 2 of *Sacred Woman*.
• Study the *Heal Thyself Kitchen Power* video course on natural food preparation or read *The Heal Thyself Cookbook* by Dianne Ciccone.
• Fast one day a week on vegetables and fruit juices, distilled water and herbal tea.
• Welcome transformation. Allow toxic conditions, people, things, food, and work to be flushed out of your life.

**Observe Bes:**

• Perform sacred movements, exercises, and dances daily.

**Observe Het-Hru:**

• Beautify body and spirit in words, deeds, and appearance.
• Commune with Nature once a week. Go to the park or to the beach for healing Nature meditations. Nature is the mirror of your sacredness. Harmonizing with Nature will keep you in tune.

**Observe Nebt-Het:**

• Rise at 4 A.M. daily for prayer and meditation.
• Purify your home in some way daily.
• No television or video viewing unless the program is of the highest vibration, that is, uplifting and inspirational.
• Release old hostilities, malice, anger, resentment, hurt, or depression out of your Body Temple by consistently using the purification techniques found in part 2 of *Sacred Woman*.
• Keep your Body Temple, your home, and your work space purified and clean.

**Observe Sekhmet:**

• Be totally honest, loving, patient, and supportive of your woman-self. Give yourself the time you really need to heal.
• Focus on your healing purpose. Do not waste precious time.

**Observe Ast:**

• Emanate a healthy reflection and example of your Divine Self daily.

**Observe Maat:**

• Give thanks and praise for lessons learned, and pray for the courage and strength to face the ones to come as you maintain your balance.

**Observe Nefer Atum:**

• Perform a good deed to others through words and actions daily.

**Give thanks and praise for lessons learned.**

## Sesheta Journal Work for Each Gate

The Spiritual Guardian Sesheta, Keeper of Secrets, is found throughout all Gateways. When she is asked, she will unveil herself so that we may purge those well-kept secrets about ourselves that block us from entering into our true divine nature and fullness as women. She will guide.

Sesheta will guide you as you come face-to-face with your secrets within each Gateway. This may be the bravest and most difficult thing you've ever done. The following Sesheta questions help to bring information to the surface of your mind, body, and spirit from the depths of your being. Once these secrets are revealed and you have seen yourself in the raw, real healing can begin to take place. It is puzzling, but by revealing the hidden, the protected, we can receive greater clarity, power, and peace.

We often protect ourselves through Sesheta out of fear that we ourselves or others won't accept us, won't love us, won't comprehend us. We're afraid to lose. As Sesheta reveals the secret of each Gateway to us or to others, we are given an opportunity to "wash our dirty laundry" so that we will gain healing. Sesheta's process of unveiling gives us the gift of purifying ourselves through each Gateway.

*Sample Sesheta Questions for Gateway 1, Sacred Word, Guarded by Tehuti.* Intuitively use this system for each Gateway. Hold an inner conversation with yourself, or an outer conversation with your sacred sister of support.

*Question #1: What is my hidden truth? What words am I afraid to speak to people?*

*Question #2: Why am I afraid to express hidden truths to others? Am I afraid to lose a friend? What would happen if I lost this friend? Am I afraid to be alone?*

*Answer from the Guardian Tehuti, who is indwelling:* First, the truth is that you're never alone. And second, truth will set you free. So if you keep purifying and rejuvenating through the Sacred Woman work, just as you appear to lose a friend

from the lower realm of being, you are also gaining and growing into new friendships from the higher realm who mirror your growth back to you.

In each Gateway ask your spiritual guardian to reveal to you, directly or through your journals, who you are, what you are, why you are. Ask Sesheta to reveal your secrets to you. Know that Sesheta within will allow you to bring the answer to the surface. If you find it difficult to receive the answers to your secrets, then ask Sesheta to allow you to be willing to ask the Gateway Guardians to speak through your voice or journal on your behalf. Record your questions and the answers you receive in the journal work for the Gateway that you are in. Repeat:

*Tua NTR* (thank you), Sesheta, for revealing my secrets. I give thanks and praise for the kingdom of the truth that you had opened to me.

## SEVEN-DAY TRANSFORMATIVE WORK

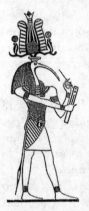

The Sacred Gateway Transformative Work is the most important work you will do in part 3 of *Sacred Woman*. It integrates everything you're learning in each Gateway, and gives you an overview of the whole plan.

The Transformative practices offer powerful daily spiritual and physical exercises, important reminders about diet and cleansing techniques, useful lists of dos and don'ts, and uplifting visualizations, meditations, affirmations, and prayers. Above all, they help you create appropriate new priorities and integrate these practices into your daily life as you continue on your journey of Sacred Womanness.

As you spend seven days traveling through each Gateway, remember to keep transforming the words "I can't" into "I can," "I won't" into "I will," "I'm unable" into "I am able," and watch your life transform before your amazed eyes!

# BLESSING OF THE FIRST SACRED WOMAN

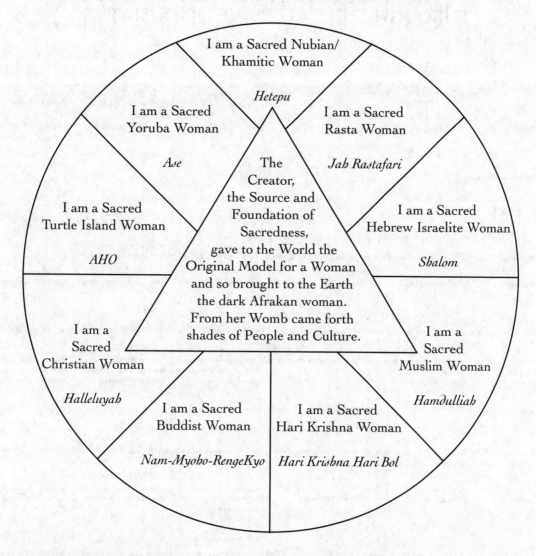

I am a Sacred Nubian/Khamitic Woman

*Hetepu*

I am a Sacred Yoruba Woman

*Ase*

I am a Sacred Rasta Woman

*Jah Rastafari*

I am a Sacred Turtle Island Woman

*AHO*

The Creator, the Source and Foundation of Sacredness, gave to the World the Original Model for a Woman and so brought to the Earth the dark Afrakan woman. From her Womb came forth shades of People and Culture.

I am a Sacred Hebrew Israelite Woman

*Shalom*

I am a Sacred Christian Woman

*Halleluyah*

I am a Sacred Muslim Woman

*Hamdulliah*

I am a Sacred Buddist Woman

*Nam-Myoho-RengeKyo*

I am a Sacred Hari Krishna Woman

*Hari Krishna Hari Bol*

Sacred Women of the world, I come to you with greetings and peace as you come together in *smai tawi*, in unity, to spread healing to all corners of the earth.

I am the First Woman, the Nubian Afrakan woman, mother of all other women within the rainbow of colors, traditions, and cultures that now cover the globe.

As the Original Woman, every aspect of my existence was spiritually directed—in government, work, marriage, family life, foods, healing, ceremonies. Life and transformation (death) were directed by the Most High NTR (Creator/Creatress). There was no separation of spirit and state in my time. All was one, coming from the One Creator/Creatress, the Divine Spirit. As an Afrakan Nubian woman I lived and breathed, even dressed and adorned myself in, the Holy and Living Spirit of the Great Mother and Great Father Spirit.

From me, the Original Woman, the Afrakan woman—every woman—every language, culture, religion, was born. Every tradition was inspired by the First Woman. Give honor, praise, and adoration to the First Mother, the sacred Afrakan woman.

# SACRED WOMAN'S DAILY SPIRITUAL OBSERVANCES ROAD MAP THROUGH THE GATEWAYS OF INITIATION

| GATEWAY 0 | GATEWAY 1 | GATEWAY 2 | GATEWAY 3 | GATEWAY 4 | GATEWAY 5 |
|---|---|---|---|---|---|
| SACRED WOMB | SACRED WORD | SACRED FOOD | SACRED MOVEMENT | SACRED BEAUTY | SACRED SPACE |
| **Gateway Element:** | | | | | |
| WATER AND AIR | EARTH | EARTH AND AIR | EARTH | | AIR |
| **1. The Spiritual Bath:** Add 4–6 drops of essential oils to bathwater along with 1 lb. of sea salt. Fill tub with warm water. | | | | | |
| Frankincense Oil | Eucalyptus Oil | Thyme Oil | Bergamot Oil | Rose Oil or Cinnamon Oil | Lavender Oil |
| **2. Setting Up Your Altar:** Set up your Sacred Gateway Altar according to the outlined Gateway Altar Work. Also place the following spiritualized objects | | | | | |
| Place a tantric quartz crystal egg on altar. | Place a rolled up papyrus with ribbon and pen on altar. | Place a bowl of fruit on altar. | Place a tambourine, drum, or ankle or waist bells on your altar. | Place a sacred instrument on altar and play it daily as you pray. | Place a small broom by your altar (a cinnamon broom preferred) |
| **3. Anointing with Oils:** Before your altar, anoint your crown, forehead (the Body Temple Gateway of supreme spirituality), heart (the Body Temple Gateway of compassion and divine love), womb area, palms, and bottoms of your feet to spiritually align yourself (for stepping out in power, promise, | | | | | |
| Frankincense Oil | Eucalyptus Oil | Thyme Oil | Bergamot Oil or Frankincense and Myrrh Oil | Rose Oil or Cinnamon Oil | Lavender Oil |
| **4. Opening the Gateway:** To invoke each Gateway's Spiritual Guardian, offer a sincere prayer that pours spontaneously from your heart. For example, here's a prayer that might be modified to use at each Gateway: *Sacred and Divine _____, Spiritual guardian of the Gateway of* | | | | | |
| As you offer your prayer, simultaneously shake, ring, beat, or rattle a sacred instrument (drum, shekere, sistrum, or bells) | | | | | |
| **5. Libation:** Pour a libation for the Sacred Guardians, Ancestors, Elders, and Contemporaries. | | | | | |
| Sacred Guardian *NUT* | Sacred Guardian *TEHUTI* | Sacred Guardian *TA-URT* | Sacred Guardian *BES* | Sacred Guardian *HET-HRU* | Sacred Guardian *NEBT-HET* |

| GATEWAY 6 | GATEWAY 7 | GATEWAY 8 | GATEWAY 9 | ELDER GATEWAY 10 | GATEWAY 11 |
|---|---|---|---|---|---|
| SACRED HEALING | SACRED RELA-TIONSHIPS | SACRED UNION | NEFER ATUM Sacred Lotus Initiation | SACRED TIME | SACRED WORK |
| | | | | | |
| FIRE | AIR | WATER/MOON/ FEMALE FIRE/SUN/ MALE | ETHER | AIR | EARTH |
| | | | | | |
| Frankincense and Myrrh | Lavender or Ylang-ylang | White Rose Oil | Lotus Oil | Rosemary | Fennel, to release, to let go |

upon your altar.

| | | | | | |
|---|---|---|---|---|---|
| Place a bowl of garlic and an aloe plant on altar, both of which are ancient Khamitic sources that were used for healing. | Place a diagram of your blood and extended family tree on altar. | Create a picture collage of harmonious relationships and place on altar. | Place one white flower in a crystal bowl, add a drop of lotus oil, and place on altar. | Knotted cords to measure, hourglass | Vision Quest, Business Plan |

and faith), and use your hands to make everything you touch become more sacred (use only essential oils).

| | | | | | |
|---|---|---|---|---|---|
| Frankincense and Myrrh | Lavender or Ylang-ylang | White Rose Oil | Lotus Oil | Rosemary | Fennel, to release, to let go |

*Sacred _____, please accept my deepest gratitude for your healing presence on my altar and in my life. Thank you for your guidance and inspiration and for your love and blessings in return. Hetepu.*

to awaken the Most High that is indwelling.

| | | | | | |
|---|---|---|---|---|---|
| Sacred Guardian *SEKHMET* | Sacred Guardian *MAAT* | Sacred Guardian *AST* | Sacred Guardians *AST AND NEFER ATUM* | Sacred Guardian *SESHAT* | Sacred Guardian *MESHKENET* |

| GATEWAY 0 | GATEWAY 1 | GATEWAY 2 | GATEWAY 3 | GATEWAY 4 | GATEWAY 5 |
|---|---|---|---|---|---|
| SACRED WOMB | SACRED WORD | SACRED FOOD | SACRED MOVE-MENT | SACRED BEAUTY | SACRED SPACE |
| Ancestors<br>*Biddy Mason*<br>*Queen Mother Moore* | Ancestors<br>*Zora Neale Hurston*<br>*Margaret Walker* | Ancestor<br>*Ast* | Ancestors<br>*Josephine Baker*<br>*Pearl Primus* | Ancestor<br>*Queen Tiye* | Ancestor<br>*Queen Nefertari*<br>*Aab-mes* |
| Elders<br>*Aunt Iris O'Neal*<br>*Dr. Josephine English* | Elders<br>*Maya Angelou*<br>*Toni Morrison*<br>*Camille Yarbrough*<br>*Nikki Giovanni* | Elder<br>*Amon d Re A* | Elder<br>*Katherine Dunham* | Elders<br>*Lena Horne*<br>*Kaitha Het Hru*<br>*Nekbena Evans* | Elder<br>*Barbara Ann Teer* |
| Contemporaries<br>*Dr. Jewel Pookrum*<br>*Nunkeleko Lychessia* | Contemporaries<br>*Edwidge Danticat*<br>*Jessica Care Moore* | Contemporaries<br>*Cher Carden*<br>*Dianne Ciccone* | Contemporaries<br>*Carmen Delavallade*<br>*Judith Jamison*<br>*Debbie Allen*<br>*Queen Esther* | Contemporaries<br>*Erykah Lauryn Hill* | Contemporary<br>*Queen Afua Mut*<br>*Nebt-Het* |

Softly play a sacred instrument—drum, sistrum, shekere, or bells—to awaken the indwelling angelic host at the beginning and endind of prayers

**6. Sacred Spirit Prayer:** Sacred Spirit, hold me near, close to your bosom. Protect me from all harm and fear, beneath the absolute perfect light. Anoint me in your sacred purity, peace, and divine insight. Bless me, truly bless me, as I share this Fire, Water, Earth.

**7. Sacred Prayer:**

| | | | | | |
|---|---|---|---|---|---|
| Sacred Womb Prayer | Sacred Womb Prayer | Sacred Food Prayer | Sacred Movement Prayer | Sacred Beauty Prayer | Sacred Space Prayer |

**Chant (*Hesi*):**

| | | | | | |
|---|---|---|---|---|---|
| | | | | | |

**8. Fire Breaths:** Prepare your Fire Breaths by slowly inhaling four times and exhaling four times and exhaling four times; then, when totally at ease,

| | | | | | |
|---|---|---|---|---|---|
| 100 times a day | 200 times a day | 300 times a day | 400 times a day | 500 times a day | 600 times a day |

**9. Sacred Woman Gateway Meditation:** Increase the length of your meditation every seven days. The longer you are in meditation, the deeper your inner peace and the more solid your spirit (*ba*). The cleaner your Body Temple, the easier it is to go into and live in a state of meditation.

| | | | | | |
|---|---|---|---|---|---|
| 5 minutes | 10 minutes | 20 minutes | 30 minutes | 40 minutes | 50 minutes |

**9a. Color Visualization:** Visualize the color of the Gateway you are in. As you perform your meditation, you may wear a

| | | | | | |
|---|---|---|---|---|---|
| White or blue for purification and serenity. | Yellow for divine wisdom, high intellect. | Brown or green for grounding or regeneration. | Reddish brown or orange. | Green for regeneration, fertility, and growth. | Purple for spiritual liberation. |

**9b. Sacred Stone Meditation:** While in meditation, place a sacred stone on the body part that is symbolic of the Gateway

| | | | | | |
|---|---|---|---|---|---|
| Moonstone, turquoise, or black tourmaline—womb | Aquamarine—throat | Gold carnelian—stomach | Carnelian and fire agate—spine | Green malachite—heart | Indigo sapphire—lungs |

| GATEWAY 6 | GATEWAY 7 | GATEWAY 8 | GATEWAY 9 | ELDER GATEWAY 10 | GATEWAY 11 |
|---|---|---|---|---|---|
| SACRED HEALING | SACRED RELA-TIONSHIPS | SACRED UNION | NEFER ATUM Sacred Lotus | SACRED TIME | SACRED WORK |
| Ancestors *Dr. Alvenia Fulton* *Ankh Hesen Pa* *Aten Ra* | Ancestors *Sojourner Truth* *Sarah and Elizabeth Delany* | Ancestor *Betty Shabazz* | Ancestors *Queen Hatshepsut* *Mary McLeod Bethune* | Ancestor *Harriet Tubman* | Ancestor *Mary Ford* |
| Elder *Berlina Baker* | Elder *Queen Nzinga Ratabi-sha Heru* | Elders *Ruby Dee* *Coretta Scott King* | Elders *Nana Ansaa Atei* *Empress Akwéké* | Elder *Michelle Obama* | Elder *Aturah Bahtiyah* *Maxine Waters* |
| Contemporaries *Dr. Sharon Oliver, M.D.* *Earthlyn Marselean Manuel* | Contemporaries *Oprah Winfrey* *Iyanla Vanzant* *Lady Prema* | Contemporaries *Camille Cosby* *Susan Taylor* | Contemporary *Anukua Atum* | Contemporary *Michelle Obama* | Contemporary *Lauren Von Der Pool* |
| | | | | | |
| Sacred Healing Prayer | Sacred Relationship Prayer | Sacred Union Prayer | Nefer Atum Sacred Lotus Initiation Prayer | Sacred Seshat Prayer | Sacred Meshkenet Prayer |
| | | | | | |

begin your Fire Breaths.

| 700 times a day | 800 times a day | 900 times a day | 1000 times a day | 1000 times a day | 1000 times a day |

Meditation time can be joined with your journal work.

| 60 minutes | 70 minutes | 80 minutes | 90 minutes | 90 minutes | 90 minutes |

colored scarf that reflects the Gateway.

| Red for vitality, health, power. Limit or avoid if hypersensitive. | White for purification. | Royal blue for inner peace. | White with light blue for purification, illumination, and devotion. | Time is on your side. Visualize your life in a golden light that radiates brighter and more brilliant over time. | Squat as you press down on two brown bricks with right and left hands, breath as you birth out your vision. |

resurrecting and purifying each area.

| Bloodstone—solar plexus | Pink tourmaline and rose quartz—heart | Lapis lazuli—first eye | Amethyst | Topaz—attunes one with inner abundance of the alignment to sacred time offers. | Clear Quartz—enhances clear vision. |

| GATEWAY 0 | GATEWAY 1 | GATEWAY 2 | GATEWAY 3 | GATEWAY 4 | GATEWAY 5 |
|---|---|---|---|---|---|
| SACRED WOMB | SACRED WORD | SACRED FOOD | SACRED MOVE-MENT | SACRED BEAUTY | SACRED SPACE |

**10. Herbal Tonics:** Drink herbal tea during spiritual writing work and throughout the week. Drink 1-4 cups daily.

| | | | | | |
|---|---|---|---|---|---|
| Heal Thyself Woman's Life Tea or Dandelion to detox and strengthen the womb | Eucalyptus to expel word congestion | Parsley to rejuvenate | Gingko Biloba to unblock the mind | Aloe Vera to purify | Gotu-kola to enhance intuition |

**11. Flower Essences:** To deepen your experience of each Gateway, choose up to three of the following flower essences,

| | | | | | |
|---|---|---|---|---|---|
| Alpine Lily, Pomegranate, Star Tulip, Black-Eyed Susan, Angelica | Calendula, Cosmos, Trumpet Vine, Snapdragon, Larch, Heather | Crab Apple, Iris, Pink Monkeyflower, Goldenrod, Self-Heal, Walnut | Dandelion, Star of Bethlehem, Self-Heal, Manzanita, Hibiscus | Pomegranate, Iris, Indian Paintbrush, Pretty Face, Pink Monkeyflower | Indian Paintbrush, Mountain Pennyroyal, Iris, Canyon Dudleya, Star Tulip, Sagebrush, Shasta Daisy |

**12. Diet:** Follow Sacred Woman Natural Living Dietary Laws presented in each Gateway.

| | | | | | |
|---|---|---|---|---|---|
| 60% cooked (steamed), 40% raw (live/uncooked) foods | 60% cooked (steamed), 40% raw (live/uncooked) foods | 60% cooked (steamed), 40% raw (live/uncooked) foods | 60% cooked (steamed), 40% raw (live/uncooked) foods | 50% cooked (steamed), 50% raw (live/uncooked) foods | 50% cooked (steamed), 50% raw (live/uncooked) foods |

**13. Sacred Journal Writing:** Write in your journal the significant thoughts, realizations, activities, and experiences that present themselves. Journal

**14. Senab Freedom Shawl:** Choose a new piece of cloth that corresponds to the Gateway color to add to your Senab Freedom Shawl or Quilt. The cloth will serve as a mini-canvas to represent your experience in each Gateway. Also collect meaningful symbols, such as natural objects,

**15. Sacred Woman's Tools:** Supplies and special objects needed to support the work of each Gateway.

| | | | | | |
|---|---|---|---|---|---|
| Wooden table or raised platform to establish the foundation for your Sacred Altar. Materials needed to set up Gateway 0: The Sacred Womb Altar. | Tape recorder or video camera to observe how you use words. | Kitchen Laboratory tools: juice extractor; blender; stainless steel pots; glass or nonmetallic pot for brewing herbal teas; jars for herbs; strainer for herbs; wheatgrass extractor | A Body Temple willing to transform Womb Yoga Dance Yoga mat | Four yards of cloth to practice wrapping and draping your Body Temple. Beads for waist beads and ankle bracelets. | Sacred Cinnamon Brooms. A small one to place by your Altar and a large one to place by your front door. Portable cast-iron pot for burning sacred oils. |

**16. Sacred Reminder:** Throughout the week, observe closely the wisdom presented for the Gateway you're in. For maximum results, harmonize with

**Closing Sacred Words:** Close your daily altar ceremony with sacred wods honoring the NTR—Mother/Father Creator/Creatress—

| GATEWAY 6 | GATEWAY 7 | GATEWAY 8 | GATEWAY 9 | ELDER GATEWAY 10 | GATEWAY 11 |
|---|---|---|---|---|---|
| SACRED HEALING | SACRED RELATIONSHIPS | SACRED UNION | NEFER ATUM Sacred Lotus Initiation | SACRED TIME | SACRED WORK |
| | | | | | |
| Ginger to energize | Chamomile to harmonize | Lemon Balm to align | Solar Water to purify | Angelica to clarify | Alfalfa for creativity and courage |
| take 4 drops 3 times per day. | | | | | |
| Self-Heal, Love Lies Bleeding, Shasta Daisy, Pink Yarrow, Black-Eyed Susan | Calendula, Fawn Lily, Mallow, Violet, Pink Yarrow, Forget-Me-Not, Poison Oak | Evening Primrose, Chamomile, Forget-Me-Not, Sticky Monkey Flower, Snapdragon, Penstemon | Star Tulip, Pomegranate, Mugwort, Iris, Angelica, Alpine Lily, Lotus | Rosemary helps one to overcome the stagnation that blocks forward movement in time. | Chlorophyll-rich green vegetable juice. |
| | | | | | |
| 50% cooked (steamed), 50% raw (live/uncooked) foods | 25% to 40% cooked (steamed), 60% to 75% raw (live/uncooked) foods | 25% to 40% cooked (steamed), 60% to 75% raw (live/uncooked) foods | 100% raw (live/uncooked) food or Sacred Woman Fast; 100% Liquid Fast on vegetable and fruit juice, herbs and alkaline H2O | 60% cooked (steamed), 40% raw (live/uncooked) foods; 100% Liquid Fast on vegetable and fruit juice, herbs and alkaline H2O | 60% cooked (steamed), 40% raw (live/uncooked) foods |
| work is best done after meditation or internal or external purification. If your journal work is blocked, consult Sesheta. | | | | | |
| family heirlooms, collectibles, etc., to be added to your shawl or quilt. | | | | | |
| | | | | | |
| Crystal pendulum and pendulum charts. Oracles such as the Black Angel Cards, Sacred Woman Divination Cards. Materials for Sacred Woman's Healing Medicine Bags (see pages 279–281). | Beautiful white ostrich feather to be your Maat feather to create a feather fan. A sacred scale that resembles the scale of justice. | A special Ankh to symbolize the union of the masculine and feminine. Sacred Union Dialogue Journal. | White ceremonial cloth and garments required for Initiation. Special sacred objects required for all participants in the Sacred Lotus Rebirthing Ceremony. | Knotted cords to measure. | Join pen and papyrus (paper) wisdom at 4 A.M. to channel and to write your most powerful life. |
| the various systems of wellness presented, and perform the Seven-Day Transformative Work presented at the conclusion of each Gateway. | | | | | |
| and express deep gratitude for the blessings received. | | | | | |

# CHAPTER 6
# GATEWAY 1: SACRED WORDS

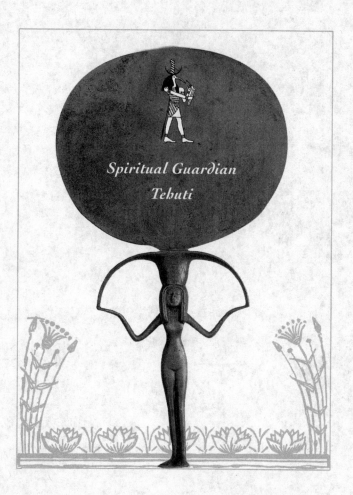

Spiritual Guardian

Tehuti

**Ancestors**

Zora Neale Hurston

Margaret Walker

**Elders**

Maya Angelou
Toni Morrison
Camille Yarbrough
Nikki Giovanni

**Contemporaries**

Edwidge Danticat

Jessica Care Moore

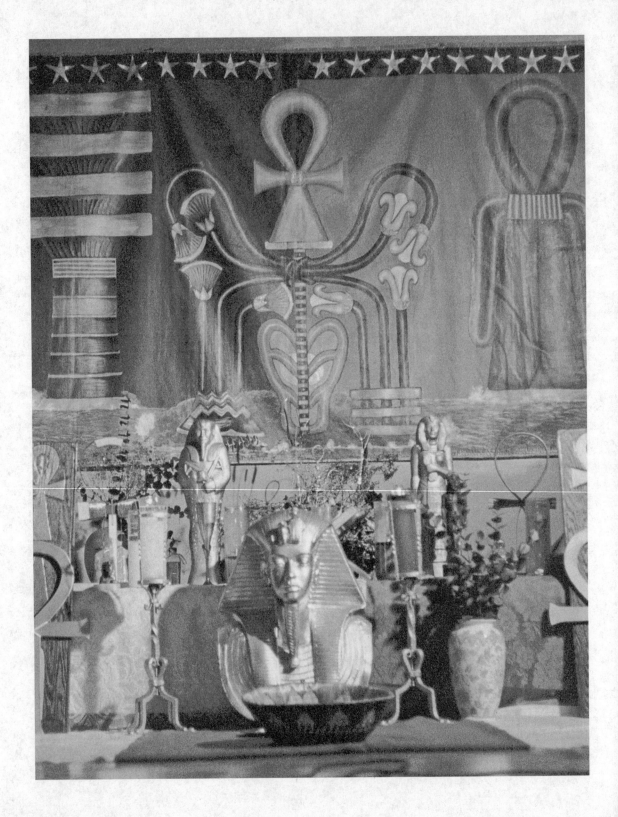

# SACRED WORDS ALTAR WORK
## Face Your Heart to the East—to the Rising Sun
*(Layout from top view)*

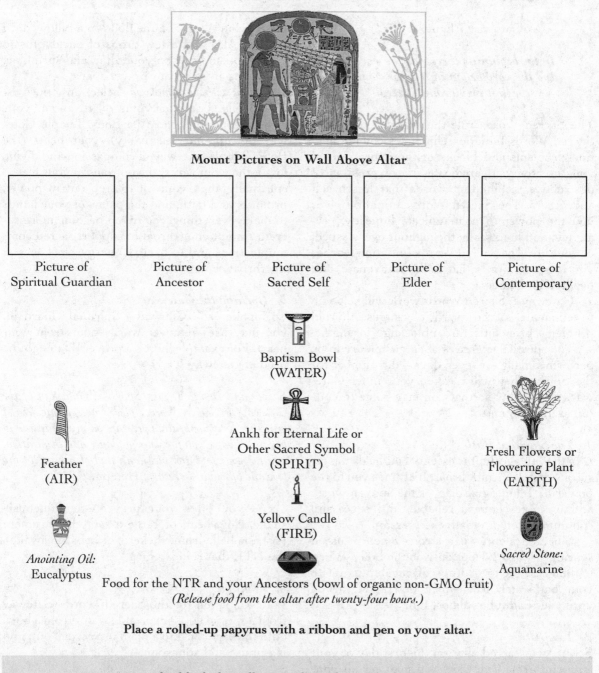

**Mount Pictures on Wall Above Altar**

Picture of
Spiritual Guardian

Picture of
Ancestor

Picture of
Sacred Self

Picture of
Elder

Picture of
Contemporary

Baptism Bowl
(WATER)

Ankh for Eternal Life or
Other Sacred Symbol
(SPIRIT)

Feather
(AIR)

Fresh Flowers or
Flowering Plant
(EARTH)

Yellow Candle
(FIRE)

*Anointing Oil:*
Eucalyptus

*Sacred Stone:*
Aquamarine

Food for the NTR and your Ancestors (bowl of organic non-GMO fruit)
*(Release food from the altar after twenty-four hours.)*

**Place a rolled-up papyrus with a ribbon and pen on your altar.**

Sacred tablecloth (yellow) and scarf to wear during prayer.
Sacred color cloth to lay before altar. Sacred instruments to be played as you pray.

# GATEWAY 1: SACRED WORDS DAILY SPIRITUAL OBSERVANCES

### Gateway Element: Air

*In the beginning there was the word,*
*and the word began in Nu, the womb,*
*the first primordial waters.*

The Sacred Words rule the throat center. The Sacred Words Initiation eliminates communication problems and blocks in the expression of your creativity. It eradicates the expression of destructive, debilitating words that lessen self and others. The Sacred Words Initiation gives you the power to communicate honestly, creatively, and holistically throughout every aspect of your life. The Sacred Words Initiation teaches you to speak words that build, rejuvenate, and heal self and others.

Gateway 1: Sacred Words work will help you to eliminate sacred word blockages: thyroid problems, bronchitis, throat blockage, laryngitis.

The spiritual exercises of ascension are to be performed daily for seven days—the number for the Spirit. They will awaken your inner Gateways of Divinity so that you may come to your full sacred center.

### 1. The Spiritual Bath

A bath with eucalyptus essential oil heals the respiratory system and throat. It attunes you to the power of Tehuti, guardian of the spoken word, and promotes honest, reliable, and successful communication or creative expression.

Since eucalyptus is a strong essence, use it sparingly—1 to 2 drops only on the body. When bathing, add 4 to 6 drops of eucalyptus oil to your bathwater. Remember, don't add the oil until your bathtub is almost full.

### 2. Your Altar

Set up your sacred altar on the first day of your entry into this Gateway. You may set up your altar according to your own spiritual or religious beliefs (see page 18). Sit quietly and meditatively before your altar—on the floor on a pillow, or in a chair. Also add a few drops of eucalyptus to your baptism bowl on your altar, and sprinkle a few drops around your prayer space.

*Anoint with eucalyptus oil.* Select only pure essential oils. Use eucalyptus oil to anoint your crown, your forehead (the Body Temple Gateway of supreme spirituality), your heart (the Body Temple Gateway of compassion and divine love), the womb area, the bottoms of your feet to spiritually align yourself to step out in power, promise, and faith, and the palms of your hands to make everything you touch become more sacred. Anoint your throat to support sacred communications and to heal all energy blockages at the throat center.

### 3. Opening the Gateway

To invoke each Gateway's Spiritual Guardian, you may use whatever words pour from your heart. For example, here's a prayer that might be used at Gateway 1:

*Sacred and Divine Tehuti, Spiritual Guardian of the Gateway of Sacred Words, please accept my deepest gratitude for your healing presence on my altar and in my life. Thank you for your guidance and inspiration, and for your love and blessings, and please accept my love and blessings in return.* Hetepu.

As you offer your prayer, simultaneously shake, ring, beat, or rattle a sacred instrument (sistrum bell, drum, shekere, or bells) to awaken the NTR that is indwelling.

### 4. Libation

Pour a libation for the Sacred Words Gateway from a special cup, or sprinkle water from a bowl onto the earth or into a plant as you call out, giving praise and adoration.

- *Pour a libation* as you say, All praise and adoration to the Spiritual Guardian, Tehuti, the

Protector of the Sacred Word and Divine Intelligence.

- *Pour a libation* as you say, All praise and adoration to the Ancestors, Mothers of the Sacred Word, Zora Neale Hurston and Margaret Walker.
- *Pour a libation* as you say, All praise and adoration to the Elders of the Sacred Word, Maya Angelou, Toni Morrison, Camille Yarbrough, and Nikki Giovanni.
- *Pour a libation* as you say, All praise and adoration to my Divine Self and my Contemporary Divine Sisters, Edwidge Danticat and Jessica Care Moore, who honor the Sacred Word.

## 5. Sacred Woman Spirit Prayer

Ring a bell or play another sacred instrument at the beginning and end of this prayer. As you open your palms to the Sacred Spirit, or gently place them over your heart, recite:

### Sacred Woman Spirit Prayer

*Sacred Woman in the making,*
*Sacred Woman reawaken,*
*Sacred Spirit, hold me near.*
*Protect me from all harm and fear*
*beneath the stones of life.*
*Direct my steps in the right way as I journey*
*through this vision.*
*Sacred Spirit,*
*surround me in your most absolute*
*perfect light.*
*Anoint me in your sacred purity, peace,*
*and divine insight.*
*Bless me, truly bless me, as I share*
*this sacred life.*
*Teach me, Sacred Spirit, to be in tune*
*with the Universe.*
*Teach me how to heal*
*with the inner and outer elements*
*of air, fire, water, and earth.*

## 6. Sacred Word Prayer

Ring bells, beat sacred drums, or play another instrument at the beginning and ending of this prayer.

*Divine Creator/Creatress, assist me in speaking* hekau, *words of power. May my words be anointed. May my words not damage a soul. Divine Mother, help me to speak words that heal, words that empower, words that build, words that transform. Help me guard my words so no venom passes my lips, and no destruction results from my speech. Rather, may my words impart light to souls who are seeking Your face. If my words show me to be out of divine right order, may my mind and mouth be cleansed. Help me to not speak words that break down the divine in me or in my sister or my brother, my mate, my child, my Elders, or my Ancestors.*

*Divine Creator/Creatress, place words upon my lips that make my voice disperse sacred medicine. May my words be lotus blossoms that encourage all the souls I meet to reach for greater heights. May my words speak with your breath, and sing your sweet song of life. Because of the words and the evolved tones that I utter, may goodness follow me all the days of my life.*

## 7. Chanting Hesi

Chant this *hesi* from the first language, Mtu NTR, four times:

*Nuk Pu Ntrt Hmt* — I am a Sacred Woman.

## 8. Fire Breaths

Prepare for your Fire Breaths by slowly inhaling four times and exhaling four times. Then when totally at ease, begin your Fire Breaths. Inhale deeply like a pump through your nostrils (mouth closed) as you expand the breath down into the abdomen, then back up to the chest, and then exhale fully out as your abdomen contracts in and your lungs release your breath completely. Repeat this breath rapidly, releasing your breath completely in and out.

Allow each deep Fire Breath — rapidly inhaling and exhaling through your nostrils — to represent the opening of the thousand lotus petals of illumination and radiance that lead to Nefer Atum — the ultimate Afrakan lotus station of Divinity. We began with fifty to one hundred breaths in Gateway 0. We move to two hundred breaths in Gateway 1. At each new Gateway, you will add a hundred more Fire Breaths until you are performing a thousand breaths of power and light.

### 9. Gateway 1: Sacred Word Meditation

Increase the length of time you spend in meditation every seven days. The longer you remain in meditation, the deeper your inner peace will be, and the more solid your *ba* (spirit) will become. The cleaner your Body Temple, the sooner you will be able to live permanently in a state of peace and inner balance in your meditative state.

- Breathe Tehuti, the Guardian of Sacred Word and Divine Intelligence, into your mind and your heart, and purge out mental chatter, toxic speech, and word blockages that create confused speech.
- Now breathe in for four counts and out for four counts seven times, so that the power of the words you speak may heal yourself and all others as you meditate on the color yellow.

*Maat Feather Meditation.* Our ancestors placed a feather on the scales of Maat, to weigh the tongue against the heart, so that our words may always be balanced and in harmony. While performing your morning spiritual observances, and before you begin your Tehuti meditation, take your feather of Maat and place it over or in front of your mouth for a few moments in quiet meditation. Visualize Maat on your tongue, guiding your every word. After your meditation with the Maat feather, speak this prayer in your sweetest tones:

*I am pure of heart, and pure of tongue.*
*My life is created through my words.*
*May Tehuti bless and keep me.*

*Color Visualization.* Visualize the color yellow at the Gateway. As you perform your meditation wear yellow and/or place a yellow cloth on your altar. Yellow is the color for divine wisdom and high intellect. It carries positive, magnetic currents that strengthen your nerves and brain.

*Sacred Stone Meditation.* While in meditation, hold in your palm over your mouth the Sacred Healing Stone of Gateway 1, the aquamarine, which aids in unblocking throat congestion. It also promotes clarity and purity of vision, and the ability to express truth through the power of the spoken word.

### 10. Herbal Tonics

Drink eucalyptus herbal tea. Parts used: the oil of the leaves. Helps to open up the throat center to enhance clear expression and creativity. Use your eucalyptus tea or tonic for seven days to receive the full benefit of tuning into Gateway 1. Drink your herb tea in your favorite mug during or after spiritual writing.

*Preparation.* Use one teabag to 1 cup of water. Boil water in a glass, clay, or stainless steel pot, turn off flame, and add tea to steep before or after your morning bath or sacred shower. Strain herbs from water, then drink with joy and peace as you breathe between sips and settle into easy contemplation and reflection.

### 11. Flower Essences

To deepen your experience of Gateway 1, choose from the following flower essences.[1] Take 4 drops four times per day directly on or under the tongue, or add the same amount to a small glass of purified water and sip. For instructions on how to choose flower essences, see page 23.

- *Calendula:* Contacting the healing power of the word, using words as a positive healing force.
- *Cosmos:* Speaking with clarity and depth when speech tends to be too rapid or inarticulate.
- *Trumpet vine:* Clarity and vitality in verbal expression.
- *Snapdragon:* Addresses issues of lashing out, using biting or cutting words; supports emotionally balanced communication.
- *Heather:* Addresses problems of self-absorption, excessively talking about one's problems.
- *Larch:* Confidence in self-expression. Heals the throat; communication and creativity chakra.

## 12. Diet

Follow the Sacred Woman Transitional Dietary Practices presented for Gateways 1–3.

## 13. *Sacred Word Journal Writing*

This is best done after internal cleansing (enema) and/or meditation. When you are cleansed and centered, you can receive spiritual messages from the One Most High with grace. When you are in the spirit, messages travel down through your spirit mind, to your heart, into your hand, and onto the paper. (This is how I do all my writing.)

The best time to receive your spiritually inspired written work is after you have completed your altar work, between the hours of 4 A.M. and 6 A.M. Keep your journal and a very special pen by or on your altar to work with the power, force, and stillness at the coming of dawn, the hour of Nebt-Het.

Affirm your daily life. Write in your journal at this time any thoughts, activities, experiences, and interactions that present themselves. You can also write down your visions, desires, dreams, and affirmations so that you will be able to draw on these resources when help and support are most needed.

*Consult Sesheta.* If you find that you are unable to contact your inner voice during your journal work, call Sesheta, the keeper and revealer of secrets (who is indwelling), to assist and speak through you.

To inspire your journal work, place on your altar a rolled-up piece of papyrus tied with a ribbon. Slip a pen under the ribbon.

## 14. *Senab Freedom Shawl or Quilt*

Choose a new piece of cloth that corresponds to the Gateway color (indicated in exercise 9 of your Daily Spiritual Observances or in Sacred Altar Work) to add to your Senab Freedom Shawl or Quilt. This cloth will serve as a mini-canvas to represent your experience in the Gateway you're working in.

Also, collect meaningful symbols that can be added to your shawl or quilt in appliqué or patchwork style. You can add stones, other natural objects, collectibles, family heirlooms, photographs that have been reprinted on fabric, or any other significant items that embody the essence of your experience. Give your imagination free rein and let your craftswoman spirit tell your story. For more information about the Senab Freedom Shawl or Quilt, see pages 122–125.

## 15. *Sacred Tools*

Use a tape recorder or video camera to observe how you use your words (see page 151).

## 16. *Sacred Reminder*

Throughout the week, observe closely the wisdom presented for the Gateway you're in. For maximum results, live freely and harmonize with the various systems of wellness and practice the Seven-Day Transformative Work at the end of the Gateway.

## *Closing Sacred Words*

*Mother/Father Creator/Creatress, help me to speak sacred words to myself and to all others.*

# MAKING THE WORD SACRED

Thousands of years ago, on the walls of their temples, our ancient Afrakan Nile Valley Ancestors summed up who we were and who we are by nature in the language of Mtu NTR (the Words of the Divine), revealing to us the depths of our sacredness.

> *Nuk pu nuk khu, ami khu qemam xeperu em*
> *NTR hau*
> *Nuk ua em ennu en khu amu khu.*

*I am a shining being and a dweller in light who has been created and who came into existence from the limbs of NTR (the Creator/Creatress). I am one of those lights dwelling in the Light.*[2]

Repeat these words throughout your day to become one with your sacred self. As you speak the sacred words, know that no one can ever take your light away from you, for the source of your light is NTR, our Blessed Eternal Creator/Creatress.

If we embrace our true sacredness and allow our light to shine, then this suffering earth on which we live shall be healed. With the clarity and the strength of the Creator/Creatress from which you come, let no place, person, or thing prevent your sacred light from coming forth.

*Note:* For those who would like to speak in the original language of our Ancestors as you read through the Gateways, the words for "Sacred Women" are *"Ntrt Hmt"*; "I am a sacred woman" is *"Nuk Pu Ntrt Hmt."*

A Sacred Woman is a spiritual woman who relies completely and absolutely on the Creator/Creatress for all things. A Sacred Woman is spirit moving. She is natural and pure in all her actions, thoughts, ways, and words. She resides in the House of Healing and Transformation, inspired by Nebt-Het. All who enter her aura are healed by her presence.

When a Sacred Woman enters a room, the vibrations of the people and the room are raised and filled with light. Due to her sacredness, wherever she walks, the ground becomes sacred. She holds no anger, revenge, rage, or strife. In her spirit she carries the ancient Afrakan feather of Maat, which symbolizes truth, justice, and righteousness, indicating that her heart is as light as a feather.

Free of malice and disease, the Sacred Woman feels no pain. Her developed spiritual wisdom means that she allows absolutely nothing to disturb her peace, calm, and grace. She moves in confidence, unfazed by earthly confusion, illusion, or madness because she is certain that the Most High moves and breathes through her being. Throughout this Sacred Woman's journey of life she heals all things.

A Sacred Woman is a holy woman, a whole woman. A Sacred Woman is a spiritual woman who is NTR conscious, God conscious, Allah conscious, Olodumare conscious, Jehovah conscious, Krishna conscious, Yeshua conscious, Grandmother/Grandfather Spirit conscious. A Sacred Woman is filled with the light and love of the Most High Supreme, and she shares this love brilliantly with whoever enters her life walk.

A Sacred Woman's love is so fierce, so deep, that she can reclaim a man from jail, a homeless person off the street, a man who is high and dry, and wrap him up, pack him with clay, scrub him, soak him, steam him, feed him, and pray him into being his true self, a High King.

This is the natural power and skill of the Sacred Woman. No one can compare to her.

## Sacred Word Affirmations

*As a Sacred Afrakan Woman, I stand firm and empowered by my ancestry; with the guidance and blessings of my Elders, Ancestors, and Guardian Spirits, my divine sacred NTRU, I speak myself into power.*

Recite these principles aloud daily and claim the power of the word to strengthen your divine role as a Sacred Woman as you bring a healing spirit forth on every plane of existence.

> *I am a Sacred Woman filled with the Spirit of the*
> *Most High Supreme.*
> *I am a Sacred Woman full of love and grace.*
> *I am a Sacred Woman pure in state.*
> *I am a Sacred Woman spreading healing across*
> *the land.*

*I am a Sacred Woman radiant and bright.*
*I am a Sacred Woman bringing forth the light.*
*I am a Sacred Woman moved only in the Spirit.*
*I am a Sacred Woman standing tall and strong.*
*I am a Sacred Woman healthy, wealthy, and all-wise.*
*I am a Sacred Woman working magic from my Kitchen Healing Laboratory.*
*I am a Sacred Woman, a natural beauty in all ways.*
*I am a Sacred Woman holding no malice for man or woman.*
*I am a Sacred Woman empowered with freedom and harmony.*
*I am a Sacred Woman working skillfully with Nature's four elements, calling air, fire, water, earth: "Come journey with me as we work, restoring harmony upon the earth."*

## Charging Your Power with Sacred Words

Think about the affirmations you say daily for your womb, because you can speak yourself into wellness just the way you can speak yourself into sickness. Always remember that. So even if you had a traumatic day, you can change the words around to make your life work for you. Take the higher road. Say, "That was a very challenging day, but I am victorious because I am still standing!"

We choose the words we say, and we must recognize the real power they carry. There could have been a fire in your house, but you choose to say, "I still have my life. I have the lives of my children." Give praise that there's something to still give praise about.

Suppose you had your womb removed. What words of power could be affirming? "I still have my womb spirit." "I still have my life." "I still have the ability to create."

Always look for the higher road. Always look for that word that will help to recharge your spirit. That's the sacred word. You choose and create your world through the words that you speak. So if you're constantly saying words like, "I don't have any . . . I am tired. I can't make it. My needs aren't being met. I don't have anybody," then you carry all that energy in your aura. Words like those weigh your spirit down

and wear you down. When you are worn down, disease can enter into your energy field and attack your sacred womb.

So we have to protect our sacred womb, our sacred seat, by watching our minds. We have to keep our minds up on high, watch the words we speak, and feed our Body Temple the right words, higher thoughts, and higher food. One way to do this is by being in communication with high Queens who are going in the same direction we are. We can change ourselves, but it will take some time. It takes learning to change your words to reflect the Spirit. It takes your continual prayers and your affirmations and meditations.

Think of the martial artists. How do they become black belts? Through discipline. Through consistency. Through constantly working it out and mastering themselves. If they get knocked down, they learn how to fall. When I was studying martial arts it took me months and months and months just to learn how to break a fall. That was so important—how to break a fall with grace so you don't break your arms or legs.

You may drop down, but there's a positive way to drop down and a negative way. Instead of just falling down, or out, you say, "Oh, I'm falling, it's time to rest." That's a message of sacred words telling you it's not time to break down and fall apart. It's a good message from our body, telling us it's just time to go and get some rest. It may take fifteen minutes to talk to your spirit, and another fifteen minutes to do a womb meditation or a womb affirmation. It is golden time that will come back to you a hundredfold.

When we speak conscious words we are speaking ourselves into power, into wellness, into healing. Whenever we think of our womb being whole, we are actually rebuilding it. We are healing our wombs from all of the traumas we have gone through. That's why our words and thoughts are so powerful.

We are always growing from our lessons, our experiences, and every day is a new beginning. There is always a new healing opportunity to look forward to. We are divine by nature. We have been divine from the beginning of time, and we will be for all eternity.

## Sacred Silence

Sometimes we as women can talk too much. Let us be mindful of our words. Some talk uplifts and encourages; other talk can destroy one's spirit and bring harm to one's soul. Nevertheless, healing talk coming from healthy whole beings can take you on high and heal your world and everyone in it. There will come a time in your sacred development when you will have purified your soul so much that you will become quiet and still. You will rest from talking. You will have purified your heart, your feelings of jealousy, judgment, anger, rage, guilt, bitterness, wickedness, and other negativity that separates you from the Creator/Creatress, and keeps you agitated and in a state of "toxic talking." With time and healing all this will wash away in a bath of silence.

There is a cosmic conversation going on within you, but you have to be quiet to hear this sweet language of the unspoken. In the stillness of your inner silence, your purity will allow you to hear the language of the trees, the grass, the wind, the healing rays of the sun. Spirit and Nature speak the same language, the language of the Creator/Creatress.

As your sacredness fills you more and more, you will step into a world of peacefulness. A place where the life energy is just waiting to answer your questions and help you attain your full magnificence.

Enough talking! Do a talk fast. Go within, pray, and meditate. In this way you will ignite your spiritual powers, and they will quietly impart answers you may be seeking.

When you find yourself quiet in a world of so much activity, the world may see you as detached or aloof. But in reality you're within the sweet, quiet state that comes from inner listening and deep purification.

Through silence, you will discover that when you do need to speak, your words will carry more weight and be more profound because you have gathered energy from your power source— that silent place of inner peace.

As your quiet sacredness unfolds, you will come to know and understand the blessings of detachment. Through detachment comes purity.

When you experience a loving state of detachment, it is to your advantage, and to the advantage of others, for then you have the capacity to love unconditionally—the ability to allow love to flow into you and through you uninterrupted. That is freedom! The freedom to love, no matter what. When you are in a loving, detached, quiet state, know that the magical peace that you are experiencing is undisturbed by conditions, circumstances, people's utterances, or mood swings.

There are many blessings that being in your quiet state of detachment can bring.

When people are in your life actively, and you are interacting in a good way, you feel blessed. And when it's time for them to move on, you feel equally blessed. You are able to release them to go and grow. The gift of peace is that nothing disturbs your inner stillness. If someone says, "I love you," it's good. And if they say the opposite, it's still good, because you trust in the Most High living within you, and you know that all that happens to and through you is good. You have faith that things are working out on your behalf, and this makes you stronger and wiser and gives you spiritual muscle.

Use every experience to lift you up as you advance spiritually on the path of purification and sacredness. Keep peace at the center of your life as the quiet state of loving detachment flowers from your "talk fasts."

## A Talk Fast Experience

1. Go into Nature and sit within her profound quiet. Breathe in that green meadow of grass and trees, or listen to the sound of the mighty ocean, absorb a running brook, or simply lie back and view the beauty around you.
2. Try to be quiet from one to four hours a day. Go within and experience the joy and peace of quietness. Fast from talking. And when you see a brother or sister in your travels, bow to him or to her in your silence, and from your heart send absolute quiet and love. If they are tuned into their own quietness, they will feel your unspoken love, for they are deep enough to respond to the voice of the heart.
3. Go about your life undisturbed as you move

within the sweet silence. Be ever so quiet. This is a place, and a state, where heaven on earth truly dwells.

4. At the end of your day, sit in silence, sipping a cup of Quiet Herb Tonic and ask yourself, "Did I bring harm to anyone with my words?" If so, clean it up! Then go within and be quiet once again.

5. Write down in your Sacred Womb Journal the whisperings and inner knowings that come to you in your sacred silence.

## Quiet Herb Tonic

This is a tea to quiet and still the soul. Enjoy it during your talk fast.

1 tsp. dried chamomile
1 tsp. dried hops
5–10 drops valerian extract

Boil 2 cups of water in a glass, clay, or stainless steel pot, turn off the flame, then add herbs. Steep 20 minutes. Drink as you quietly sit back to contemplate.

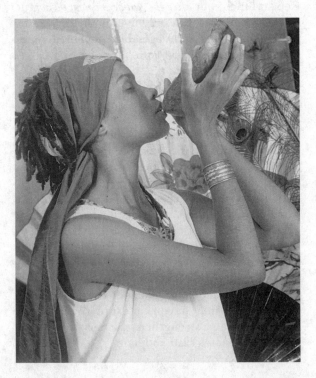

### Journal Entry for Sacred Words
*Rha Goddess from the NTRU Cipher*

*Sacred words manifest in the silence.*
*Daughters of Divinity, chant the libations*
*of surrender*
*as the Creator/Creatress channels forth*
*universal truth.*

*Sacred words live in the spirit,*
*the essence of "self," which journeys from*
*land to land*
*gathering pearls of wisdom and healing*
*along the way.*

*Sacred words dance in the temple of the*
*Goddess, surrounding Ra-filled auras with*
*infinite blessings,*
*guiding purposeful steps that build*
*upon destiny's path.*

*Sacred words bear the seeds of organic fruit,*
*nourishing weary souls with the nectar*
*of upliftment,*
*filling empty vessels with love, abundance,*
*and joy.*

*Sacred words play upon the lips of Sacred Women*
*And hold the potency of ancestral ways*
*with enough mystical magic to heal the world.*

*Sacred words unfold in courage,*
*speaking the unspeakable with clarity, vision,*
*and purpose,*
*sending messages of honor and protection.*

*Sacred words rest in the heart,*
*and awaken to the joyful sounds of promise*
*radiating light channeled from above.*

Yolanda Tribble drinks from a purified gourd.

# TRANSITIONAL DIETARY PRACTICES FOR GATEWAYS 1–3

In Gateways 1 to 3, you will eat 60 percent cooked (steamed) and 40 percent raw (live/uncooked) food.

## Before Breakfast

Kidney-Liver Flush (see page 72).

## Breakfast

Freshly pressed fruit juices, 8 to 12 oz. (dilute with 8 to 12 oz. of pure water), with Heal Thyself Green Life Formula I, 1 to 2 tbsp.

*Fruit Juice Rule:* Eating fruit and drinking fruit juices is done one hour before each meal for greater digestion.

*Fruits:* Acid fruits: grapefruit, lemons, limes, oranges, tangerines. Sub-acid fruits: apples, pears, plums, cherries, berries, peaches. No bananas. *Do not mix acid and subacid fruits together.*

Include cooked whole wheat, dairy-free pancakes with maple syrup one to three times a week, or rice, soy, sesame, or almond milk.

## Lunch

Freshly pressed vegetable juices, 8 to 12 oz. (dilute with 8 to 12 oz. of water), with Heal Thyself Green Life Formula I, 1 to 2 tbsp.

Large raw salad. Use red and/or green cabbage as a base, adding okra, kale, cauliflower, turnip greens, mustard greens, broccoli, or seaweed in any form (i.e., kelp, dulse, hijiki, wakame, nori). No tomatoes, but include plenty of sprouts, such as alfalfa and mung bean.

*Proteins:* Choose one only:

- Sprouts
- Beans
- Peas
- Avocado
- Lentils
- Texturized vegetable protein (TVP)

If you are a flesh eater in transition, prepare baked fish, soy chicken, or organic chicken one to three times a week. You can also include raw soaked nuts (almonds, filberts, walnuts, pecans; avoid cashews and peanuts, including roasted peanuts) and seeds (sunflower, pumpkin).

*Starches:* You may eat grains four to seven tmes a week. These foods must be eaten in moderation. Choose one of the following:

- Millet
- Bulgur
- Brown rice
- Couscous
- Baked white potato or yam
- Corn on cob (steam or eat raw)
- Whole wheat and sprouted bread (dry toasted)

## Dinner

Repeat lunch, but *after the sun goes down, do not eat proteins or starches.* Eat only live foods, for example, salads, fruits and vegetables, steamed vegetables, vegetable soup/broth.

## DIETARY SUPPORTS
### Nutritional Supplements

- Heal Thyself Green Life Formula I. This formula contains all the vitamins and minerals the Body Temple needs. Take three times a day with juice or take some form of chlorophyll, such as powdered wheatgrass (1 tsp. to 1 tbsp.) or liquid, 1 to 2 oz., with distilled water; powdered spirulina (1 tsp. to 1 tbsp.) or liquid (1 to 2 oz.), with distilled water; powdered blue-green manna (1 tsp. to 1 tbsp.) or liquid (1 to 2 oz.), with distilled water.
- If stressed, take 25 to 50 mg of vitamin B complex or you may have skin eruptions. Vitamin B complex also strengthens the nervous system and rejuvenates skin and hair.

- For poor memory and poor circulation, take 1 tbsp. of granulated lecithin. Helps to clear out the arteries for increased circulation.
- Take 500 to 1,000 mg of vitamin C daily, to build immune system and fight colds and infections. Ester C is easier on the digestive system.
- Heal Thyself Breath of Spring (optional), 3 drops twice a day with warm water, particularly during hay fever season. (See the product list in the appendix.)

## Internal Cleansing

Take enemas three times a week. Begin by taking enemas seven nights in a row, then continue three times a week throughout the weeks you are journeying through Gates 1 to 3. Also take 3 tablets of cascara sagrada with 8 oz. of water before bedtime every other day.

For deep cleansing, take one to three colonic irrigations during a twenty-one-day fasting period.

## Physical Activity

Do your Dance of the Womb exercises fifteen to thirty minutes daily (see Gateway 3: Sacred Movement). Do Fire Breath Meditation 5 to 15 minutes daily.

## Rejuvenation Baths

Put 1 to 4 lbs. of Epsom salts in your bath, seven nights straight. Or use 1 lb. Dead Sea salt with the same routine.

Time for soaking: fifteen to thirty minutes, then shower off all salts. (Do not use bath salts if you have high blood pressure.)

## Heal Thyself Master Herbal Formula II

Boil 5 to 6 cups of purified or distilled water, turn off the flame, and add 3 teaspoons herbs. Strain in the morning, and drink before 2 P.M. (See chapter 3 in part 2.)

## Queen Afua's Rejuvenating Clay Application

Follow instructions in chapter 3 of part 2, and Gateway 4: Sacred Beauty.

## Other Nature Cures

Drink 2 to 4 quarts of distilled water daily. You may add the juice of 1 lemon or lime and/or a sacred crystal to the water. (Caution: Do not swallow the crystal.)

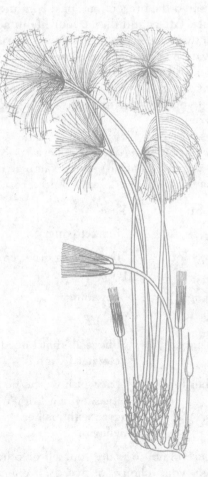

# SACRED WORDS: SEVEN-DAY TRANSFORMATIVE WORK

• *Identify and write down words or phrases that block you from your blessings.* How frequently or infrequently do you think them or speak them? Toxic words and ambiguous words can set you up for a painful, nonproductive life.

• *Identify and make two lists in your journal: one for words or phrases that disempower you, and another list for words or phrases that empower you.* How frequently or infrequently do you think them or speak them? Observe how your use of words has created the present and past conditions of your life. Affect and direct your life in a more productive way by practicing power words. By observation and reflection homework, you will get a clearer picture of why your life is in its current state. You will witness how you have created your world with each word spoken or unspoken.

• *Khepheratize your words.* ("Khephera" is Khamitic for transformation). For example, rather than saying, "I'm tired," say, "I need rest."

| Instead of: | Say: |
| --- | --- |
| "I'm sick." | "I'm detoxing." |
| "I hate my job." | "I'm seeking other employment." |
| "I'm trying." | "I'm doing." |
| "I can't." | "I can." |
| "I don't have . . ." | "I have all that I need to get what I want." |
| "I hate her/him." | "I accept how she/he behaves, even if I don't agree with his/her behavior." |

Be careful not to make yourself or others ill through your choice of words. When you transform and restore the healing power of your words, you will transform and restore harmony in your life.

• *Experiment with other ways to purify your words:*
— Perform a toxic word fast and avoid gossip, backstabbing, and empty, wasteful words spoken to self and others.
— Fill your mind with divine thoughts by reading spiritually charged healing material; highlight the most healing words.
— Commune with individuals who speak from the heights.
— If you must watch TV or videos, make sure your viewing is filled with food for your soul. At all costs, avoid violent, aggressive TV that feeds poisonous thought forms and expressions.
— Eat live, organic vegetarian foods that feed the mind.
— Avoid sugar in all forms unless it's natural sugar from fruit. Sugar deteriorates and eats up the brain tissue like lye, and so it deforms your words over time.
— Drink two quarts of water daily to help flush negative thoughts out of your system and energy field.
— Daily for the next seven days, flush out old, impacted waste and gases from your colon with enemas, herbal laxatives, okra, flaxseed, or freshly prepared apple juice. If you have a clean colon, you have a clean mind that expresses itself by speaking Sacred Words.
— Avoid cursing yourself or others in the open, or in silence.
— Be truthful at all times. Avoid lying. Partake of spiritual conversations with others. Speak of spiritual development, of ascension, of self-healing, and of the release of one's condition. Encourage others in conversation to release poisonous word ways and toxic habits out of daily life.
— Avoid intoxicants and toxins (drugs, alcohol, sugar, table salt, flesh, and fast foods).

• *Remember, words are like* hesi *(sacred chants).* The words you choose dictate the condition of your soul. Transform your life by speaking spiritually charged words.

- *Write nine empowering affirmations in your journal to build your new lifestyle.* Speak these words of power every day in silence and out loud, and see how your life begins to heal and improve. Also, be aware of your quiet thoughts—they too are words. Remember, unspoken doesn't mean not heard.

- *Be observant of how your friends or associates talk about you.* As you reevaluate your world of words, decide whether you should continue the relationship, limit it, or eliminate it. Are the words spoken about you defeating you or strengthening you, losing you or improving and empowering you?

- *Words can heal, soothe, or hurt.* What about the words you speak to your associates, family, or friends? What are your words doing to them, or what are their words doing to you?

- *Wash your words the way you wash your walls and floors.* Scrub your words until they are clean, each and every one of them. Make them sacred. If someone is cursing you or you are cursing another, then you need to change your existence by cleaning your own word house and the way you have responded in the past.

- *To master your words, work with the following tools:*
  - *Tape recorder.* As a tool for developing a golden tongue, you'll find it helpful to record your speaking voice. Read a poem into the tape recorder. Or speak your feelings on an issue. Then play the tape back and listen to yourself with a conscious mind so you can begin to purify your words and modulate your tone.
  - *Video camera.* We speak with our bodies, so it's wise to study ourselves on video as we communicate with others. Observing how you speak and how you move will give you a full picture of your communication gifts and blockages. Be sure to include others in your video presentation so that you can witness how the world views you and interacts with you. Be up for change: create your video presentation on day one of Gateway 1, and then again on day seven; compare the results.

- *Honor yourself as an Afrakan being.* Charge yourself culturally and spiritually by studying your ancient Afrakan Nile Valley language, Metu NTR. Experience the healing and the high consciousness of our ancestors and their use of words. Throughout *Sacred Woman*, I will share with you some ancient power words for your ascension. Use them often to strengthen you as you grow through each Gateway.

- *Slow down your life enough to observe and record your words in these next seven days.* Begin your word surgery as you diligently correct what you say and think. All words have the power to break down or re-create. With the right words, backed up with a pure heart and correct intentions, you can start a new world order of divinity. It's all in the word. Make it your mission to choose Sacred Words to create a sacred life.

  As you continue to purify your life daily through sacred words, thoughts, and deeds on a physical, mental, emotional, and spiritual plane, the words coming out of your mouth and back to you will be words of power, light, and healing. You will speak Sacred Words to sacred souls.

- *Perform a talk fast over the next seven days.* Speak only when necessary, watch each word spoken, don't talk for hours, watch your words, become pure and organic. Observe a seven- to twelve-hour talk fast, alone or with others who are doing the same practice throughout the week.

- *Choose the appropriate flower essence* from those listed on pages 134–135 to support your Sacred Word Transformative Work.

• *Sacred Word Affirmation.* Finally, speak the following affirmation daily, particularly after morning and evening prayer and meditation to begin to reclaim your natural and sacred self through your words:

*My life reflects the levels of the words I speak. Today I am transforming my life to express my higher good through energizing, healing words.*

**My Sacred Word End-of-the-Week Commitment:**

I commit myself to establishing and continuing the wisdom of Tehuti and the power of Sacred Words in all the areas of my life.

Signature: _____

Date: _____

# CHAPTER 7

# GATEWAY 2: SACRED FOOD

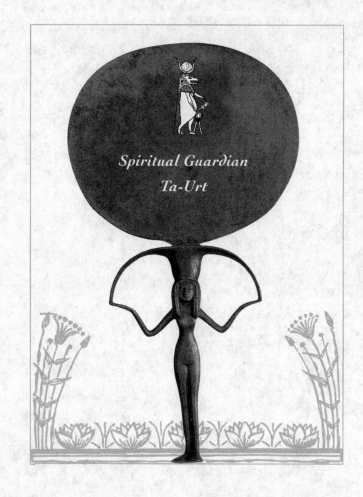

*Spiritual Guardian*
*Ta-Urt*

**Ancestor**

Ast

**Elder**

Amon d Re A

**Contemporaries**

Aturah Bahtiyah

Cher Carden

Lauren Von Der Pool

Dianne Ciccone

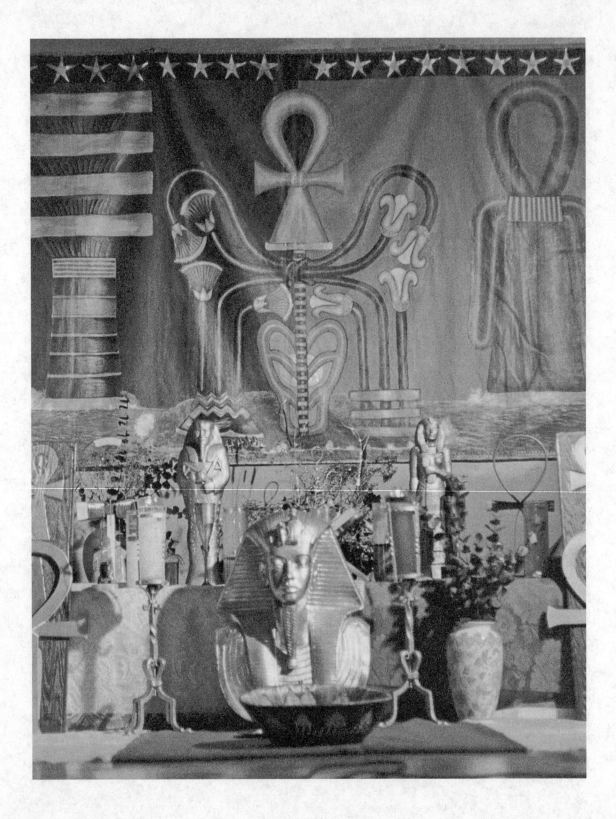

# SACRED FOOD ALTAR WORK
## Face Your Heart to the East—to the Rising Sun
*(Layout from top view)*

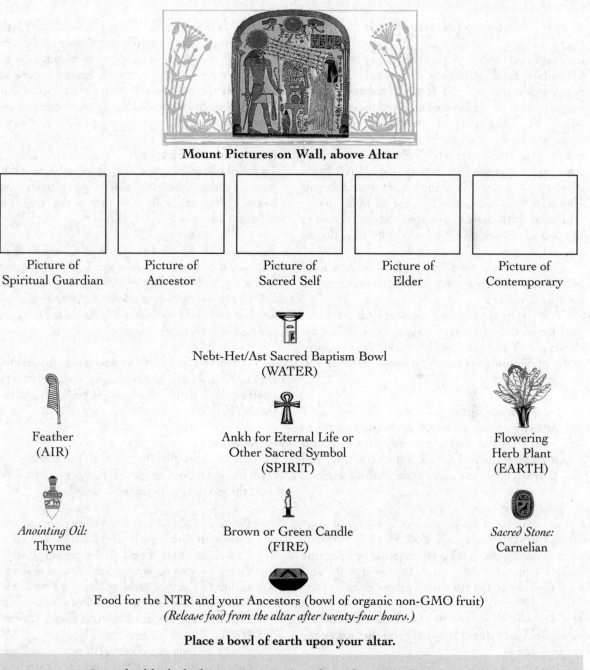

**Mount Pictures on Wall, above Altar**

Picture of
Spiritual Guardian

Picture of
Ancestor

Picture of
Sacred Self

Picture of
Elder

Picture of
Contemporary

Nebt-Het/Ast Sacred Baptism Bowl
(WATER)

Feather
(AIR)

Ankh for Eternal Life or
Other Sacred Symbol
(SPIRIT)

Flowering
Herb Plant
(EARTH)

*Anointing Oil:*
Thyme

Brown or Green Candle
(FIRE)

*Sacred Stone:*
Carnelian

Food for the NTR and your Ancestors (bowl of organic non-GMO fruit)
*(Release food from the altar after twenty-four hours.)*

**Place a bowl of earth upon your altar.**

Sacred tablecloth (brown or green) and scarf to wear during prayer.
Sacred color cloth to lay before altar. Sacred instruments to be played as you pray.

# GATEWAY 2: SACRED FOOD DAILY SPIRITUAL OBSERVANCES

## Gateway Element: Earth

Sacred Foods will give you the ability to eat and assimilate food and ideas that heal. Through consumption of holistic foods, you are taught how to achieve a healthy, well-balanced, nourishing life. Eating flesh, fast food, and junk food will destroy a woman's vitality. Vegetarian, vegan, fruitarian, and live-food eating will strengthen and heal a woman's body. Live foods give the Sacred Woman longevity and will eliminate fear, hate, and a sense of being overwhelmed with life's challenges. Sacred Food is the foundation of the Body Temple of a divine Sacred Woman.

Gateway 2: Sacred Food will eliminate food blockages, such as obesity, compulsive eating, or compulsive starving.

The spiritual exercises of ascension are to be performed daily for seven days—the number for the spirit. They will awaken your inner Gateways of Divinity so that you come to your full sacred center.

## 1. The Spiritual Bath
A bath with thyme essential oil helps you regulate your appetite and eliminates bingeing and emotionally triggered eating. When bathing, add 4 to 6 drops of thyme oil to your bathwater.

## 2. Your Altar
Set up your sacred altar on the first day of your entry into this Gateway. You may set up your altar according to your own spiritual or religious beliefs (see page 18). Sit before it quietly and meditatively on the floor on a pillow or in a chair. Place a bowl of fruit on your altar. Also add a few drops of thyme oil to your baptism bowl on your altar, and sprinkle a few drops around your prayer space.

*Anoint with thyme oil.* Select only pure essential oils. Use thyme essential oil to anoint your crown, your forehead (the Body Temple Gateway of supreme spirituality), your heart (the Body Temple Gateway of compassion and divine love), the womb area, the palms of your hands to make everything you touch become more sacred, and the bottoms of your feet to spiritually align yourself to step out in power, promise, and faith.

## 3. Opening the Gateway
To invoke each Gateway's Spiritual Guardian, you may use whatever words pour from your heart. For example, here's a prayer that might be used at Gateway 2:

*Sacred and Divine Ta-Urt, Spiritual Guardian of the Gateway of Sacred Food, please accept my deepest gratitude for your healing presence on my altar and in my life. Thank you for your guidance and inspiration, and for your love and blessings, and please accept my love and blessings in return.* Hetepu.

As you offer your prayer, simultaneously shake, ring, beat, or rattle a sacred instrument (sistrum bell, drum, shekere, or bells) to awaken the NTR that is indwelling.

## 4. Libation
Pour a libation for the Sacred Food Gateway from a special cup, or sprinkle water from a bowl onto the earth or a plant as you call out.

— *Pour a libation* as you say, All praise and adoration to the Spiritual Guardian, Ta-Urt, Protector of the Food of the Sacred Earth.
— *Pour a libation* as you say, All praise and adoration to the Ancestor of Sacred Food, Ast.
— *Pour a libation* as you say, All praise and adoration to the Elder of Sacred Food, Amon d Re A.
— *Pour a libation* as you say, All praise and adoration to my Divine Self and my Contemporary Divine Sisters, Cher Carden and Dianne Ciccone, who honor Sacred Food.

## 5. Sacred Woman Spirit Prayer

Ring a bell or play another sacred instrument at the beginning and end of this prayer. As you open your palms to the Sacred Spirit or gently place them over your heart, recite:

### Sacred Woman Spirit Prayer

*Sacred Woman in the making,*
*Sacred Woman reawaken,*
*Sacred Spirit, hold me near.*
*Protect me from all harm and fear*
*beneath the stones of life.*
*Direct my steps in the right way as I journey*
*through this vision.*
*Sacred Spirit,*
*surround me in your most absolute*
*perfect light.*
*Anoint me in your Sacred purity, peace,*
*And divine insight.*
*Bless me, truly bless me, as I share*
*this Sacred Life.*
*Teach me, Sacred Spirit, to be in tune*
*with the Universe.*
*Teach me how to heal*
*with the inner and outer elements*
*of air, fire, water, and earth.*

## 6. Sacred Food Prayer

Ring bells, beat sacred drums, or play another instrument at the beginning and ending of this prayer.

*Divine Creator/Creatress, help me to break my food addictions that cause me disease. Help me to avoid eating foods that cause cancer, high blood pressure, tumors, anxiety, and premature aging. Help me discern angelic foods over foods that create demonic action. Give me the power to eat foods that build my body into a temple of wellness, radiance, and health.*

*May I be blessed to be of the mind to feed my Body Temple meatless, vegetarian, and fruitarian foods made to perfect and sustain my sacred Body Temple. May my debilitated taste buds be transformed and revitalized so I may take pleasure and delight in eating foods that your divine spirit has prepared for my healing.*

*May I find solace in consuming sacred organic fruits, vegetables, nuts, whole grains, sprouts, and pure water. May all these gifts of true nourishment make me into a Holy Light Being—a Sacred Woman.*

## 7. Chanting Hesi

Chant this *hesi* four times:

*Nuk Pu Ntrt Hmt*—I am a Sacred Woman.

## 8. Fire Breaths

Begin by slowly inhaling four times and exhaling four times; then when totally at ease, begin your Fire Breaths.

Inhale deeply like a pump through your nose (mouth closed) as you expand the breath down into your abdomen, then back up to your chest. Completely exhale out through your nostrils from your abdomen as it contracts and the lungs release your breath completely. Repeat this breath rapidly, in and out, in and out.

Allow each deep Fire Breath to represent the opening of the thousand lotus petals of illumination and radiance that lead to Nefer Atum—the ultimate Afrakan lotus station of Divinity. We move to three hundred Fire Breaths in Gateway 2.

## 9. Gateway 2: Sacred Food Meditation

Increase the length of time you spend in meditation every seven days. The longer you remain in meditation, the deeper your inner peace will be, and the more solid your *ka* (spirit) will become. The cleaner your Body Temple, the sooner you will be able to live permanently in a state of peace and inner balance in your meditative state.

### Ta-Urt, Mother Guardian of the Earth Visualization

- Sit comfortably as you breathe in the life force—the nourishment from the earth.
- Begin by inhaling spiritual earth food through the soles of your feet all the way up into your crown.

- Then exhale out from your crown back into the earth the essence of your nourishment: four counts as you breathe in, and eight counts as you breathe out. Continue inhaling and exhaling the spirit of the Mother Guardian of the Earth, Ta-Urt.
- Visualize the color of brown and/or green earth energy coursing through your blood. Breathe into your cells, into your joints, and then out.
- Now breathe deep into your bones, then out again. Breathe into your nerves and then out. Breathe into your skin and then out again.
- Breathe the nourishment into your muscles, then out again. Breathe nourishment into your organs and your lungs, then out again. Breathe nourishment into your brain, then out again.
- Now that you are filled with the *prana* (breath) from the earth, rest and be *hotep* (at peace).

*Color Visualization.* Visualize the Gateway colors of brown or green. The brown/black soil brings forth the green grass and leaves to feed and nourish us; the green represents regeneration. As you perform your meditation wear brown or green and/or place a brown or green cloth on your altar.

*Sacred Stone Meditation.* While in meditation, hold in your palm over your stomach the sacred Healing Stone of this Gateway, the carnelian. Carnelian regulates the intake of food and assists in assimilation and circulation. It also helps the digestive system filter out impurities effectively.

## 10. Herbal Tonics

Drink parsley tea. Parts used: roots and seeds. Parsley regulates the menstrual cycle, and is high in iron and chlorophyll. (Because it helps to dry up the milk in lactating mothers, do not use while nursing.) Drink your parsley tea for seven days to receive the full benefit of tuning into Gateway 2—enjoy your herb tea in your favorite mug during or after spiritual writing.

*Preparation.* One teabag to 1 cup of water. Boil water in a glass, clay, or stainless steel pot, turn off flame, pour over teabag, and steep. Drink before or after your morning bath or sa-cred shower. Drink with joy and peace as you breathe between sips and settle into easy contemplation and reflection.

## 11. Flower Essences

To deepen your experience of Gateway 2, choose from the following flower essences. Take 4 drops four times per day directly on or under the tongue, or add the same amount to a small glass of purified water and sip. For instructions on how to choose flower essences, see page 23.

- *Crab apple:* Supports release of toxins during cleansing or fasting regimens.
- *Iris:* Helps suppress craving for sweets and general hypoglycemic tendencies; promotes body awareness, feminine consciousness.
- *Pink monkeyflower:* Addresses issues of using food as a buffer for emotional oversensitivity, stuffing oneself to "dull out" or numb feelings.
- *Goldenrod:* Addresses issues of overweight used to hide one's true Self.
- *Self-heal:* Confidence in body's ability to digest and assimilate food; being nourished and energized by what one eats.
- *Walnut:* To break habitual ties to old patterns of eating and to develop new relationship to nourishing foods.

## 12. Diet

Follow the Sacred Woman Transitional Dietary Practices presented for Gateways 1–3 or perform the Sacred Woman Seven-Day Fast, page 175.

## 13. Sacred Food Journal Writing

This is best done after internal cleansing (enema) and/or meditation. When you are cleansed and centered, you can receive spiritual messages from the One Most High with grace. When you are in the spirit, messages travel down through your spirit mind, to your heart, into your hand, and onto the paper. (This is how I do all my writing.)

The best time to receive your spiritually inspired written work is after you have completed your altar work, between the hours of 4 A.M.

and 6 A.M. Keep your journal and a very special pen by or on your altar to work with the power, force, and stillness at the coming of dawn, the hour of Nebt-Het.

Affirm your daily life. Write in your journal at this time thoughts, activities, experiences, and interactions that present themselves. You can also write down your visions, desires, dreams, and affirmations so that you will be able to draw on these resources when help and support are most needed.

*Consult Sesheta.* If you find that you are unable to contact your inner voice during your journal work, call Sesheta, the keeper and revealer of secrets (who is indwelling), to assist and speak through you.

### 14. Senab Freedom Shawl or Quilt

Choose a new piece of cloth that corresponds to the Gateway color (indicated in exercise 9 of your Daily Spiritual Observances or in Sacred Altar Work) to add to your Senab Freedom Shawl or Quilt. This cloth will serve as a mini-canvas to represent your experience in the Gateway you're working in.

Also, collect meaningful symbols that can be added to your shawl or quilt in appliqué or patchwork style. You can add stones, other natural objects, collectibles, family heirlooms, photo-graphs that have been reprinted on fabric, or any other significant items that embody the essence of your experience. Give your imagination free rein and let your craftswoman spirit tell your story. For more information about the Senab Freedom Shawl or Quilt, see pages 122–125.

### 15. Sacred Tools

You will need kitchen laboratory tools as outlined in this chapter: a juice extractor, blender, stainless steel pots, an enamel or heat-proof glass pot for brewing herbal teas, jars for various herbs, a strainer for herbs, a wheatgrass extractor.

### 16. Sacred Reminder

Throughout the week, you are to observe closely the wisdom presented for the Gateway you're in. For maximum results, live freely and harmonize with the various systems of wellness presented, and practice the Seven-Day Transformative Work at the end of the Gateway.

### Closing Sacred Words

*Mother/Father Creator/Creatress, guide me to choose well from the fruits of the earth, and help me to eat natural Sacred Foods that keep my Body Temple healthy and pure.*

## WE BECOME ONE WITH
## ALL WE CONSUME

What we consume dictates who we are and what we are. Whatever we consume we become. Gateway 3: Sacred Food shows us how to consume on the highest and purest level to transform ourselves into our highest possible vibration as light beings. As we study and apply the Sacred Woman philosophy, ascending toward the top of the pyramid (*merkut*), we are consuming greater purity, self-knowledge, peace, healing, and wholeness. We are consuming the knowledge that supports the lifestyle of an evolved woman, consuming our fill of light until we are fully enlightened and empowered. With each tasty bite of self-awareness, we cast out the thoughts, foods, situations, and people that starve our sacredness. As Sacred Women in the making, we are increasingly sustained by the illumination of the Most High Divine. As this inner light grows, we begin to express our true glorious nature for all to witness.

We consume and become the company we keep. We consume and become our environment. The lye and dye we put on our scalps seeps down into our brain, flooding our sacred crowns with toxicity, dementing our minds. We become the visions we consume. We become the sounds we consume. We become the smells we consume.

We become the men we allow to consume our wombs—in the heat of the night as he flows through our veins, and even after he's gone. If it tastes good, we keep needing a fix, even if it ain't in the mix. Girl, watch out who you eat and who's eating you. Don't let that man become a drug and ruin you, because for a Sacred Woman that just won't do. Our vaginas drink in his essence, and we reflect his nature, good or bad, toxic or pure. Oh, but when a woman consumes the essence of a pure man, her soul is filled and fulfilled as she dances in the crescent of the moon.

We must also beware of the television programming we consume, for what we watch creates who we become. Our psyches become overwhelmed by the constant violence, blind consumerism, and fear. As we consume the countless subliminal suggestions, who knows what it creates in us. As we consume righteous, inspiring visions for our soul's ascension, we grow wiser.

For us to ascend upward and outward, to become a reflection of the Divine, we must be especially mindful about raising the vibration of the

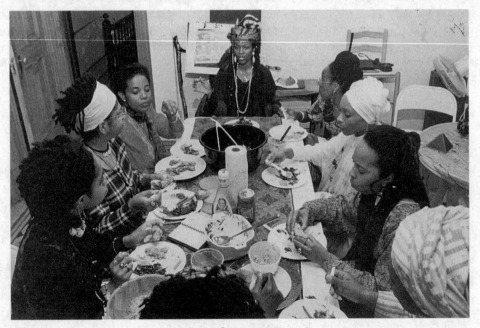

A Sacred Woman Feast

foods we consume. As we systematically ascend through the various Sacred Woman Gateways, we need to consume a higher ratio of live foods, foods that are filled with living enzymes and that contain more oxygen and nutrition.

Because we become the foods we eat, the thoughts we think, and the emotions we feel, when we consume life-giving, organic, uncooked vegetarian foods, our Body Temple reawakens from the grave of flesh. We are no longer tired and worn. When we drink freshly pressed green vegetable juices (such as cucumber, watercress, parsley, broccoli, and kale) daily, our cells rejuvenate. When we consume beets and cranberries, our blood is purified and our circulation improves, leaving us with healthy, radiant skin and a cleansed disposition. When we consume okra and vegetable salads with a bit of garlic, our colon cleanses out old toxins, waste, gases, and worms. As we consume gotu kola tea and spirulina, the algae from the sea, combined with fresh juices, our brain becomes activated, our memory improves, and our senses focus and become sharp once again. When we drink ginger tea and put leeks and scallions in our soup, our lungs expand and detox, giving us greater vitality and vigor as we eat away our hay fever, asthma, and stagnation.

On the other hand, if you find yourself without energy and cancerous cells have taken over your body, or if you are sexually aggressive and have become desperate for just any man to fill your bed, or if you have a damaged immune system and you easily get infections, you're probably experiencing a meat-eating overdose. If you've had tumors surgically removed from your womb or breast, you'll find they grow back with each piece of flesh consumed.

If you are experiencing shortness of breath and a lot of mucus, check to see if milk, cheese, and ice cream are a key portion of your dietary consumption.

If your joints are in pain and you're stressed out and on the edge, or you suffer from a quick and out-of-control tongue and you're sorry because you keep hurting folks due to loose lips, then check your diet for sugar, white flour, or cocaine—it's all the same. All of these substances have the same debilitating, addictive content.

If you are sluggish, heavy, and out of tune, if you think all those fat-filled pastries, cookies, cakes, and french fries are fulfilling and chilling you out, then the next time you take a mouthful, check to see if starch is becoming your lover.

If you're experiencing premature aging and cellulite thighs, maybe you're not taking enough exercise.

Come on, sister-friend, get busy. If you keep attracting negative people into your life and emotional pain is your domain, then you're probably consuming four square meals a day with an overload of fatty meats, fried foods, fast drinks, junk foods, and morning coffee breaks, all of which lower your vibration and drain away your sacred powers. Child, you better check your plate. Is she friendly or is she girlfriend-destructive? Is she turning out your lights with each bite? Time to change your plate to some greens, whole grains, and freshly prepared beans.

The Sacred Woman really evolves as she is healed by consuming the right things, becoming one with the elements of nature—earth, air, fire, and water. As she masters her inner and outer environment, she receives supreme access to her body as a universe complete unto itself. She will discover that she has dominion over the heavens and the earth. Say a volcano is threatening to erupt; a Sacred Woman in her full radiance can talk to the elements and ask the volcano—or earthquake, or hurricane, or other phenomenon, on a human level or an environmental level—to please be still, and it is done.

By the time you reach total Natural Living and fasting (eating 100 percent live uncooked foods) at the very top of the purification pyramid—with weeks or months of purification wrapped around you like your lappa—you'll find that you've been made over into a Divine Sacred Queen. You will be an angelic force to reckon with—a mover, a shaker, a maker of pure light.

As you are sitting on your seat of power, positioned to transform your world and everyone in it, always remember:

*If you want to ascend on the Sacred Woman path, know that you become one with all that you consume.*

## THE KITCHEN HEALING LABORATORY

We must make our home a Healing Center, a Sanctuary, a Temple. By doing this, we become our own healers. The more informed we become about working with the principles of Natural Living, the more naturally equipped we will be as a spiritual advisor, a Healer. We will become our own psychologist, our own herbalist, and our own spiritual counselor, for ourselves and our family. Strive to arrive at the Divine Principle of "Heal Thyself."

Sacred Women, once realized, are doctors of the home. Sacred Women contain the wombniverse. The original healers on this earth were the "bush women." Today, we must transform our mundane, modern-day, toxic-filled, microwaved kitchen that creates disease, mental and physical ill health, and shortened lives into a Kitchen Healing Laboratory. Within this laboratory we must create disease-free Body Temples full of wellness, power, and genius. Our tools are freshly pressed juices, and whenever possible live, organic fruits and vegetables, soups, salads, herbs, and spices.

Our Kitchen Healing Laboratory is a sacred place where we dry our sister-friend's tears with a steaming pot of mint tea as we smoke the air with jasmine for peace.

Our Kitchen Healing Laboratory is where we protect our children from illness and prevent unnecessary childhood disease. We actively feed our children correct substances from our Sacred Lab, where food is our medicine.

Through proper food education we can single-handedly heal our mates from such afflictions as high blood pressure, strokes, and negative health situations with live juices and soups. We deal with strokes through herbal tonics; we help heal prostate conditions and depression with greens from the fields. When things don't go smoothly in your relationship, don't blame him. Just clean up from within. There's nothing wrong with him as a man or you as a woman. You are a divine couple by nature, wholesome, loved. What's wrong here is the fried chicken, spare ribs, and candied yams—the meat, the fat, the sugar that have us acting outside of our natu-

ral state of Divinity. Toxic thoughts and attitudes are created by the poisons on our plate.

The place where we heal all of our afflictions is in the "old way," in the kitchen of our ancestors, where foods contained the power to nourish bodies, minds, and spirits. Our grandmother's kitchen was a place where women sat around the stove and worked out and balanced their lives and relationships as they passed around red raspberry and goldenrod tea. They were just being natural women. They came together as sisters around food. They worked with their bare hands and compassionate spirits to heal their families.

We must imitate these Sacred Women. We must heal our families during meals, reunions, and family outings as we pass around the food. We've come to a time where we must once again heal our families through the wisdom of the "old kitchen." Make your Kitchen Healing Laboratory a place where you and your family can experience inner freedom.

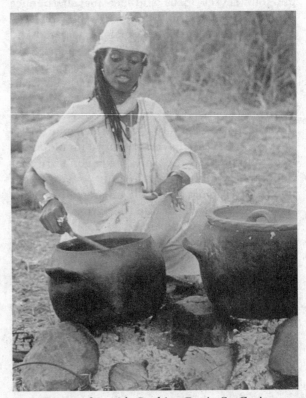

Queen Afua with Cooking Pot in St. Croix, Virgin Islands

# Basic Equipment for the Kitchen Healing Laboratory

We do not want kitchens with microwaves—places to eat flesh, fried food, or fast food on the run. We do want a Healing Laboratory used to heal yourself and your family with juices, live foods, and herbs. Here's the basic equipment that you will need to create a kitchen of the twenty-first century, one that has been resurrected from an Ancient Afrakan Healing Perspective.

Juicer
Cast-iron pot
Food processor
Herbal jars with labels
Sprouting
Sprout jar
Wheatgrass juicer
Blender

Clay cups
Stainless steel knife
Nut/seed grinder
Strainer
Stainless steel pots
Wooden cutting board
Inspirational posters and images

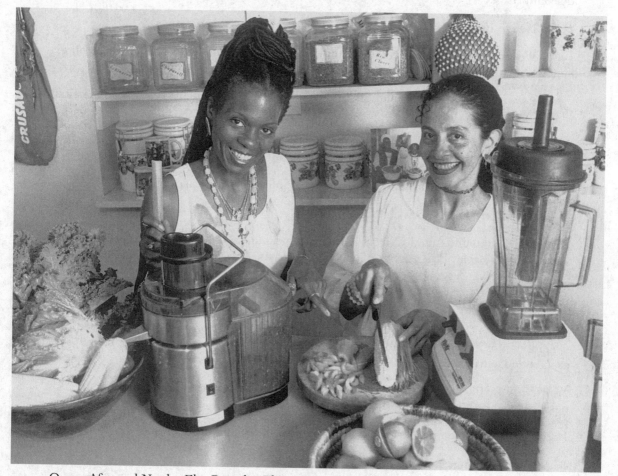

Queen Afua and Ntrelsa Elsa Bernal, a Thirty-Year Holistic Guide and Natural Food Specialist, in the Kitchen Healing Laboratory

# Herbs and Spices for the Kitchen Healing Laboratory

*Alfalfa:* A valuable source of chlorophyll. Alfalfa may also speed the elimination of toxins from the body.

*Cascara Sagrada:* Acts as a laxative and promotes colon cleansing.

*Cayenne:* Checks profuse menstrual bleeding; improves circulation and low blood pressure.

*Chamomile:* Antispasmodic that is a wonderful digestive aid and calmative. It relaxes not only the digestive track but the uterus as well.

*Cinnamon:* Stimulates the uterus; decreases menstrual flow; acts as an aphrodisiac.

*Dandelion:* A diuretic and digestive aid, dandelion is very helpful with PMS and bloating discomforts.

*Dulse:* Is high in iron and minerals (as are kelp and other sea vegetables).

*Garlic:* Produces oxygen; builds the immune system. Acts as an aphrodisiac; wards off evil spirits.

*Fresh Gingerroot:* Improves circulation; breaks up cellulite and mucus; relieves congestion; brings on menses.

*Goldenseal:* Calms the stomach and the uterus. It may also aid the body in the treatment of bacterial and fungal infections.

*Mint:* Acts as an aphrodisiac and a treatment for infertility; increases virility.

*Nutmeg:* Is a germicide; eases childbirth.

*Parsley:* Has vitamins A and C, iron, iodine, magnesium, and copper. Good for the kidneys and nervous system. Dries up milk in swollen breasts. *Do not take parsley while breastfeeding.*

*Sage:* Aids digestion; helps bring on delayed menses; promotes menstruation. *Do not take sage while breastfeeding, because it can stop the flow of milk.*

*Shepherd's Purse:* Contains substances that hasten the coagulation of blood. The dried herb is helpful in reducing nosebleeds and heavy menstrual flow. Externally it can be helpful as a wound astringent.

*Sweet Basil:* Invokes protection; increases fertility; cures menstrual pain and morning sickness; expels afterbirth.

*Valerian:* A calmative for intestinal cramps, nervousness, and headaches.

*Watercress:* Is high in minerals and good for the liver.

# My Kitchen Is Free from Negativity

My kitchen is free from negativity.
It's serious business, my Kitchen
   Healing Laboratory.
I sit at the crossroad, cast-iron pot
   in right hand and Bush Tea in my
   left, I check all bags and boxes for
   contents of death.
I awaken the sleeping, rejuvenate
   the living, energize and purify
   with soups and tonics, live foods,
   and juices.
No death in here, no chickens, no
   pigs, no cows or lambs. No fish,
   no goats, no milk, no ham.
It's plain to see that what we eat can
   make us free.
Beware, for some of what binds and
   holds us still comes in many forms
   and fashions.
It's resting right there on your plate.
Dead foods control our mood
   swings.
Family fights, husbands, wives,
   children too, we eat our war so
   violence rings.
We hold the weapons of death right
   in our hands—through forks and
   spoons, through pots and pans.
Beware of Mr. Flesh Burger,
   dripping pizza, greasy french fries
   too, diet soda, it's all sugar blues,
   stuff we simply cannot use.
Demons wrapped so beautifully,
   stopping us from who we
   really be.
It's on your plate and in our pots.

Beware the habit, beware the
   drooge, the perfect program to
   make you lose.
Putrefaction causing rot.
Demons, demons,
Get out of my healing laboratory,
   get out of my pot.
I'll wash you out and set you free
For purification is the key.
It's sunrise sausages, coffee and
   cream, it's bedtime cookies and
   cow's ice cream.
Beware the damage, the perfect
   program to make you lose.
Check your kitchen cabinets, those
   bags and boxes too. If it's not live,
   it's not coming through.
Fruits, vegetables, nuts, whole grains,
   you're all welcome to remain.
Regain your mind, your nerves,
   your flesh, your bones, your
   breast, your knees, your chest.
Regain your husband and your
   children, release the strife,
As you chase the demons from your
   life.
Restore your Kitchen Healing
   Laboratory with power, pride,
   and dignity
You hold the power within your
   hand
To raise the dead and free the land
Flesh free, drug and alcohol free,
   processed food and sugar free
Is how the kitchen becomes a
   Healing Laboratory.

# "MY KITCHEN IS FREE FROM NEGATIVITY" FOOD LISTS

For inspiration, place a list of nonfoods on the wall that are anti-life, and a list of natural foods that are pro-life.

| Anti-Life Demon Food | Pro-Life Natural Food | Nutrient Jar |
|---|---|---|
| Meats<br>Devitalized grains<br>White-flour products<br>Soda pop<br>Fried foods<br>Eggs<br>All dairy foods including milk, cheese, and ice cream<br>Old grease<br>Table salt and sugar | Fresh vegetables and fruits<br>Wheatgrass (fresh juice)<br>Sprouts<br>Beans, peas, seeds, nuts, whole grains<br>Organic apple cider vinegar<br>Lemons, limes<br>Soy-based ice cream | Green nutrients<br>B-complex vitamins<br>Vitamin C<br>Lecithin<br>Vitamin E<br>Inner Ease Colon<br>Formula<br>Wheatgrass (powdered)<br>Bowl of fresh garlic cloves |

# FOODS AFFECT OUR EMOTIONS

Over my years of experience giving holistic health consultations, I have observed the following body-mind connections.

| Flesh Foods | Emotional and Social Diseases | Alternatives | Physical Diseases |
|---|---|---|---|
| Pork, beef<br>Chicken<br>Goat, fish | Causes resentment<br>Dulls the senses<br>Creates anger<br>Brings on violence | Eat vegetable proteins<br>Cleanse with red clover and chaparral herbal tea | Cancer<br>Low energy/fatigue<br>High blood pressure<br>Swelling |
| | Causes inappropriate sexual aggression and envy | Take enemas and herbal laxatives | Prostate conditions<br>Impotence, infertility |

- Eating flesh foods indicates attempts to fill emotional voids.
- Sisters, if there is a male in your family who is inappropriately sexually aggressive, get him off flesh foods immediately! The ham, barbecue, bacon, hamburger, lamb, veal—all of it: Throw it out the window!

| White-Flour Products | Emotional and Social Diseases | Alternatives | Physical Diseases |
|---|---|---|---|
| White bread, white flour, pasta | Emptiness in your life<br>Lack of fulfillment<br>Boredom | Millet<br>Couscous<br>Bulgur<br>Brown rice | Poor circulation<br>Constipation<br>Hemorrhoids<br>Congestion |

- Eat whole grains in moderation. For easiest assimilation and digestion, eat grains only during daylight. Be sure to eat raw or steamed vegetables with your starches.

| Dairy Products | Emotional and Social Diseases | Alternatives | Physical Diseases |
|---|---|---|---|
| Milk, cheese, ice cream, and similar milk-based products | Loneliness<br>Feeling unloved<br>Unfulfilling relation-ships (sticky relations with either parent, es-pecially your mother) | Soy milk<br>Nut milk, seed milk<br>Green vegetables, juices<br>Live vegetables: wheatgrass, spirulina, alfalfa, dandelion | Tumors<br>Glaucoma<br>Colds, fevers<br>Hay fever<br>Asthma, mucus |

• Dairy products come from animal milk. This means that they are as destructive to our Body Temple as meat itself. In addition, dairy foods create mucus all through our bodies and create any number of diseases, from asthma to tumors.

## FRESH FRUITS PURIFY YOUR LIFE

Bring angelic forces into your life and the lives of those in your family with fruits such as berries of all kinds, mangoes, peaches, cherries, papaya, red grapes, pineapple, apricots and plums, melons of all kinds, grapefruit, oranges, lemons, and limes (but no bananas). Eat fresh, organic fruits in their proper seasons. Eat fruits in solid form or freshly juiced. Canned or frozen fruit is forbidden to those who want a life of ever-flowing blessings.

### Eating fresh fruits can:

Enhance love relationships
Bring forth bliss, peace, and grace
Enhance compassion
Create serenity
Purify thoughts
Purify your mental state
Sweeten disposition
Create a loving notion

Relieve the body of breathing difficulties such as asthma, colds, and sinus congestion
Cleanse skin, blood, cells, and tissues
Purify lovemaking
Eliminate vaginal discharge and growths
Bring forth a pure generation of babies
Clear out prostate blockage in men

## BREAKING THE CHAIN

In order to break the chain of hopelessness, depression, pain, and confusion, consume light-liberating foods for a more liberated state of being. If you need to be reminded, check the list below.

| Oppressive Foods | Oppressed States | Liberating Foods | Liberating States |
|---|---|---|---|
| Flesh | Anger | Vegetable protein | Able to make positive changes |
| Sugar | Depression, anger, frus-tration, mood swings | Fruits | Joy |
| Dairy | Loneliness, stagnation, resentment | Green juice, nutseed milk | Calm consciousness |

| Oppressive Foods | Oppressed States | Liberating Foods | Liberating States |
| --- | --- | --- | --- |
| Processed and fast foods | Deficient, toxic state | Whole foods | Ability to digest life |
| Devitalized foods and juices | Low energy | Fresh raw vegetables and fresh juiced fruits | High energy, alertness |
| Greasy, canned, and frozen foods | Clogged consciousness, death | Raw olive oil | Flexibility, energy |
| Coffee | Poisoned, hyperactive | Blackstrap molasses | Energy |
| Cooked foods | Confusion, tiredness, sluggishness | Live foods | Empowered |

## GREEN FOODS:
## POWER FOODS THAT BRING DIVINE ORDER INTO YOUR LIFE

| | |
| --- | --- |
| Celery | Enhances positive thinking |
| Cucumbers | Enhances forgiveness |
| Spinach | Enhances creativity |
| Broccoli, brussels sprouts | Enhances physical and mental strength and endurance |
| Spirulina | Brings forth a strong generation |
| Blue-green algae or manna | Brings forth understanding, connects you to the Creator/Creatress |
| Parsley | Enhances your spiritual life |
| Watercress, string beans | Draws prosperity |
| Sprouts | Gives you a majestic presence |
| Dill | Rejuvenates bones, removes aches and pains |
| Fresh peppermint | Restores hair, skin, and nerves |
| Turnip greens | Restores the blood, clears up eczema, boils, pimples, and acne |

- Drink green juices twice a day and eat green foods two or three times a day.
- Wear green for additional power and productivity.
- No canned, frozen, or microwaved foods permitted. They are dead, devitalized foods.

## The Poetry of Green Foods: Power Foods That Bring Divine Order into Your Life

Eat green, drink green, meditate and walk on green grass, for the ultimate in realizing maximum vitality and profound lasting beauty.

*Celery bring to me sweet serenity.*
*Cucumber, parsley, and watercress help me to release and clear the way to forgiveness.*
*Spinach build my creativity.*
*Broccoli and brussels sprouts bring to me physical and mental stability.*
*Spirulina, blue-green algae, manna, and sun chorella bring forth regeneration for a renewed Body*
*    Temple filled with Ra-sunlight.*
*Alfalfa, mung beans, and sprouts reconnect me to my Divinity, therefore enhancing my*
*    spirituality.*
*Luscious turnip greens rejuvenate my bones, remove my aches and my pains.*
*Kale greens restore for me rich hair, skin, healthy bones, and pure blood.*
*Precious dill and peppermint leaves ease my steps on this sacred journey.*
*To all the green fields in all the land, and to every blade of grass that grows, I thank you for*
*    rendering my soul prosperity.*

## Remember, Food Is Your Medicine: Eat Well for 100 Percent Wellness

- If you have a "sugar addiction," drink the juice of or eat grapefruits, limes, and lemons. Also drink goldenseal tea: ¼ tsp. powdered herb to 1 cup warm water.

- Foods to avoid while you still have high blood pressure: celery, cayenne, ginger, salt.

- Use the following as substitutes: For mayonnaise, use soy mayonnaise. For salt or Worcestershire sauce, use tamari sauce or light miso. For chocolate, use carob powder. For processed mustard, use natural unsweetened mustard and wheat germ.

- Safflower, olive, canola, or sesame oil are not to be cooked (heated) with your food. It is best to put oil on your food after your steamed or simmered vegetables have cooled down—if there is a need.

- As you become cleaner, incorporate more live foods in your diet. Eventually you may eat and drink nothing but live foods.

- For advanced devotees of purification, eat 100 percent raw (live) foods.

- Prayer is food for the soul, so please include prayer offerings and thanksgivings before and after each meal.

- Eating natural food will keep you spiritually connected to the divine sources of all that is good and holy and blessed.

# Earth Cookers
## by *Wahida Abdul Malik*

Out of our vast garden of earth comes a bountiful host of herbs, fruits, vegetables, grains, nuts, and seeds. They are all needed to cleanse, repair, build, and bring peace and tranquility to our bodies, minds, and spirits.

These are divine foods, gifts from our Creator/Creatress to nourish and heal us. Everything we could possibly require is contained within them. They fulfill multiple needs as sustenance and vital medicine to cure our ills in our developmental journey.

The Creator/Creatress has blessed us with these magnificent, miraculously fashioned bodies, and it is our divine right and duty to maintain these vessels of life with the utmost care and love.

There is tremendous joy derived from eating right because when we eat natural and wholesome foods we do our body, mind, and spirit justice, and we reap the benefits by functioning at our optimal level of productivity.

This cause-and-effect principle clearly affirms the well-known adage "We are what we eat." The Creator/Creatress, by making His bounty available to us, is telling us that this is how He wants us to eat. All that we have to do is take heed of His clear signs and accept what is good and reject what is not.

Man-made food is processed and contains unnatural chemicals that clog, slow down, and ultimately destroy our physical bodies all in the name of convenience. If the Creator/Creatress could tell us what is best for us, I believe He would say, "I have set before you all that is good and natural. Partake of it."

There is a science to eating correctly, and the key to understanding this science is to realize that the best foods are the ones that our bodies can make maximum use of in their entirety, discarding little or nothing.

When we walk into our kitchens we should visualize them as Healing Laboratories and ourselves as healing scientists for our families. Always enter this sacred domain in a highly conscious and prayerful state of mind. Be ready to unfold new miracles and discoveries that will help further the development of not only our families but our nation. Our systems must be fortified to the utmost to combat the relentless attacks waged against us in our polluted environment. We all have the divine choice of becoming "Earth Cookers," of making a conscious decision between healing our nation or contributing further to its destruction.

Earth Cookers always ask the Creator/Creatress for guidance before entering their Healing Laboratories to create healing foods and formulas. When we do this, we find ourselves truly amazed at what materializes because of our total faith and trust in God. Becoming an Earth Cooker is an essential step when one decides to travel the Heal Thyself path of liberation through purification.

## Stirring the Pot

"Stirring the pot" and "straddling the stove" are the ways a woman puts her vibrations in the food she's preparing. It's not only a pot full of celery or onions or sage, it's a pot full of vibrations. You're preparing "joy soup," or "release-me-from-bondage soup," or "I-love-my-family soup." We used to hear stories about how an Elder woman was able to feed her family on little or no money or food, yet everyone was full and in good spirits after eating her soup. This was due to the high spiritual vibrations coming from the cook—the Healer, the Mother, the Sacred Woman—as she stirred her pot.

One day my divine mate and I met in the Kitchen Healing Laboratory and out of habit he took the lid off an empty pot that was on the stove, looking for a cooked meal. I reminded him, "Honey, we are live-food eaters now. Remember, no more cooked, dead food for us. We have gone all the way I pray!"

To help him in his transition from cooked to raw foods, I grated celery, scallions, broccoli, and beets for a salad in my food processor and put it in the pot. I straddled the stove and stirred the pot in the traditional way with much love, herbs, and natural pure oils. I served him dinner from the pot, and his soul was content as he ate a plate full of live raw foods.

Pots talk! A Saramaka man may accuse his wife of divorcing him if she takes too many of her pots from his village back to her own village.[1] So, women, be mindful of your pots and what they say.

*Note:* Never cook in aluminum pots. Long-term use has been known to lead to debilitating diseases.

## Let the Spirit Move That Soup

In our Kitchen Healing Laboratory, Women Sacred and Divine, let's stir our pots to victory! "Eat my soups so I can watch another sleeping giant wake up, because I got power in my soup."

The power has always been in "the soup." Afrakan women everywhere, stir those pots, show you care, be creative, let the Spirit move

that soup! Use distilled or purified water in the preparation.

As an option, you can add vegetables steamed three to five minutes. The less you cook the food the better, for then it retains more vitamins and minerals. You, like Sister Wahida and other spirit cookers, must become an Earth Cooker by allowing your inner spirit to guide you as you prepare your sacred natural foods for nourishment of the body, mind, and spirit.

Use your intuition and your Mother Wit in measuring out the amount of water, vegetables, and seasonings required for the work intended. Prepare food in your best spiritual mood so you can tune in to the Earth Cooker within you. Here are some suggestions:

- *Inner Peace/Nerve Soup:* Dill, celery, chopped scallions, mint leaves
- *Rejuvenation Soup:* Alfalfa, dulse, parsley, chopped kale or mustard greens
- *Lovemaking Soup:* Sea moss, beets, seaweed
- *Colon-Cleansing Soup:* Okra, onions
- *Weight-Loss Soup:* Garlic, pinch of chickweed or fennel, watercress

At all costs avoid eating poisonous, devitalized foods. This is why the preparation of soup from fresh, natural, live ingredients is a must to bring peace to one in a troubled state. If lonely, depressed, or just plain stressed, try not to eat! Fast on juice instead. If you must eat, then enjoy a soup that will ensure your purity, peace, and love. Better still, go into your rejuvenation chamber (bedroom) and consume your divine mate instead.

Don't throw out your old recipe books; just replace toxic ingredients with alternatives of natural live foods. Instead of cow's milk use soy, nut, or seed milk. Instead of using white rice, use brown rice, millet, or couscous.

## Recipe for a Joyful Soup

Sing
Laugh
Hum
Pray
As You Prepare Your Soup

# TRANSITION RECIPES FROM THE EARTH COOKER

In this section, Sister Wahida Abdul Malik, the Earth Cooker, will help you make your transition from toxic flesh eating to a vegetarian lifestyle.

## Barbecued Mushrooms

| | |
|---|---|
| Firm tofu | Thyme |
| Garlic, minced | Cayenne |
| Paprika | Onion salt |
| Veggie salt | Olive oil |
| Sage | Whole wheat flour |

Cut tofu into long strips like barbecued ribs and season both sides with a light sprinkling of garlic, paprika, veggie salt, sage, thyme, cayenne, and onion salt. Grease a baking pan or cookie sheet with oil and sprinkle whole wheat flour evenly to cover the pan. Place seasoned strips on the pan and bake in oven for 30 minutes at 350° until a little crispy and brown. Then spoon natural barbecue sauce (below, or available from your neighborhood health food store) on tofu, put back in oven, and bake for 15 to 20 minutes longer. Serve hot.

*Natural Barbecue Sauce:* Blend together 1 tbsp. smoky sauce, 1 tbsp. natural mustard, 1 tbsp. honey, and 1 tbsp. Braggs Natural Seasoning Salt.

## Vegetable Stew

| | |
|---|---|
| Olive oil or 1¼ sticks cold-pressed olive oil | 1 tbsp. veggie salt |
| 2 onions, peeled and chopped | 1 tbsp. fresh dill |
| 1 green pepper, de-veined and chopped | 1 tbsp. parsley |
| 2–5 stalks celery, chopped | 2 tbsp. Braggs Natural Seasoning Salt |
| 3 cloves garlic, minced | ½ cup water |
| ½ tsp. sage | 4 bags spinach, carefully washed and chopped |
| 1 tbsp. curry powder | Pinch of cayenne |
| | ½ cup grated firm tofu |

In the bottom of a large 1- to 2-gallon pot, sauté onions, green pepper, celery, and garlic in olive oil or soy margarine. When onions are transparent, add sage, curry powder diluted to a thin paste in a cup in a small amount of water, veggie salt, dill, parsley, Braggs, ¼ stick of margarine, ½ cup water. Then add spinach. Let simmer. You can add a pinch of cayenne according to taste and ½ cup of grated tofu in place of cheese. In a blender, put 1½ to 2 packages of tofu with parsley and dill, ½ tbsp. of veggie salt, and Braggs.

*Honey Topping:* Blend together 1½ cups of tomato sauce, 1 tsp. mustard, veggie salt to taste, and 1 tsp. honey. Spread on top of the vegetable mixture. Serve over brown rice.

## TVP (Texturized Vegetable Protein) Curried Chicken

| | |
|---|---|
| 1 lb. TVP | 2 tbsp. curry powder |
| 2 tbsp. soy margarine | 1 tbsp. honey |
| 3 onions, peeled and chopped | ½ tbsp. sea salt |
| ½ tbsp. garlic, minced | 16 oz. chickpeas |
| 1 tbsp. veggie salt | 1 cup chopped carrots |
| ½ tbsp. sage | 2 tbsp. olive oil |

Soak TVP in lukewarm water until nicely textured and softened. In large pot, melt 2 tbsp. soy margarine and sauté onions, garlic, veggie salt, sage, and curry powder diluted to thin paste in small amount of water, honey, and sea salt. Then add 8 oz. of cooked chickpeas and carrots. Run another 8 oz. of cooked chickpeas through a blender, and add to mixture for thickness. Add about 2 cups of water. Add cold-pressed olive oil after the mixture has cooled for 10 minutes.

## Sweet Potato Pie

| | |
|---|---|
| 9-inch piecrust | 1 tsp.–1 tbsp. cinnamon |
| 1 5-lb. bag of sweet potatoes (will make about 4 pies) | 1–2 tsp. nutmeg |
| Approximately 4 tbsp. olive oil (for a lighter pie) | Organic maple syrup, or 3 cups of dates blended in water as a sweetener |

Prepare 9-inch natural piecrust or buy from health food store. Boil sweet potatoes. Once potatoes are cooked through, remove the skin, and return potatoes to pot. Add 4 tbsp. olive oil. Add cinnamon, nutmeg, and maple syrup or dates to taste. Blend all the ingredients together until smooth. Pour batter into piecrust shell. Place in 350° oven and bake for 30 to 45 minutes.

## QUEEN AFUA'S GREEN RECIPES

To support your dietary transformation, I offer you helpful recipes to help you clean, rejuvenate, and Heal Thyself.

### Poppin' Steam Veggies

| | |
|---|---|
| 2 cups string beans | 1 tsp. basil leaves |
| 2 cups snow peas | ¼ tsp. marjoram |
| 1 cup sweet yellow peppers, deveined | ¼ tsp. Spike (natural seasoning salt) |
| 1 cup sweet red peppers, deveined and sliced | 1 tbsp. barbecue seasoning |
| | 1 tbsp. powdered sage |

Steam for 3 minutes string beans, snow peas, yellow peppers, and red peppers. Turn off heat, then add basil, marjoram, and Spike, barbecue seasoning, and powdered sage. Mix lightly and serve.

Soak beans and nuts overnight for easy digestion.

### Green Dream

| | |
|---|---|
| 4 stalks celery | sprouts |
| 1 head cauliflower | 1 cup mung bean sprouts |
| 2 sweet red peppers | |
| 1 head broccoli | Fresh peppermint leaves |
| Purple cabbage leaves | |
| 1 cup sunflower | |

Run the celery, cauliflower, 1 red pepper, and broccoli through a food processor with the shredding blade, then place vegetables in a salad bowl. Add sprouts. Add dressing (below) and marinate for 2 to 4 hours to intensify taste. Serve on purple cabbage leaves and red pepper strips, decorated with fresh peppermint leaves.

*Dressing:* Mix together ¼–½ cup olive oil, ¼ tsp. powdered garlic, 4 tbsp. organic apple cider vinegar, and ¼ tsp. barbecue seasoning.

## Super Garden Green Salad

| | |
|---|---|
| Large bowlful of arugula or mesclun | parsley |
| 1 cup diced sweet red pepper | ½ cup diced sweet yellow pepper |
| 1 cup chopped fresh | 2 cups alfalfa sprouts |

Mix all ingredients. Add dressing (below).

*Salad Dressing:* Mix well 1 cup olive oil, 1 tsp. Dr. Bronner's Balanced Protein Seasoning, 2 tbsp. apple cider vinegar, and 1 tbsp. finely chopped parsley.

### Queen Afua's Sunflower Couscous Delight

| | |
|---|---|
| 2 cups couscous | Spike (natural seasoning salt) |
| 2 cups water | |
| 2 tbsp. cold-pressed olive oil | Paprika |
| | Cayenne |
| ¼ cup parsley, chopped | ¼ cup sunflower seeds (soak in water overnight for better digestion and absorption) |
| ¼ cup onion or scallions, diced | |
| Cumin | |

Place couscous in wooden or glass bowl—it is a natural grain that needs no heat to prepare. Slowly pour 2 cups of water into the bowl of couscous. After 10 minutes, the grain is ready; fluff up lightly with fork. Add cold-pressed olive oil, parsley, and onions. Season to taste with cumin, Spike, paprika, or cayenne. Finish by adding soaked sunflower seeds.

### Live Apple-Pear-Blueberry Crunch Dessert

| | |
|---|---|
| 4 apples, cut into pieces, stems and seeds removed | ½ cup currants (soaked in water for 1 hour) |
| 4 pears, cut into pieces, stems and seeds removed | 1 cup walnuts (soaked in water overnight) |
| 2 cups blueberries | Grated coconut |

Place first five ingredients in food processor and pulse until well blended. Pour into small serving bowls, then sprinkle grated coconut over dessert.

## Working the Sacred Calabash

Calabashes for Saramaka women, and women throughout Afraka, "are a woman's thing. The trees that they come from are owned by women, the fruits are processed by women, and the finished product belongs to women."[2] Afrakan women all over use calabashes for drinking washing, eating, serving, and carrying water, as well as for musical instruments. A net of beads is strung around them to play as a shekere. The bowls are used as decorations.

I like to use my calabash for serving my man his food. I also use it to drink my water or fresh juices. A special large gourd also serves as my spiritual washbowl when performing purification ceremonies.

Recently, I've been using my gourds not only to eat my greens from, but also to create my own shekere, which creates beautiful, soul-stirring sounds. Thanks to my mentor and teacher of this most ancient sacred instrument, Sister Queen Cheryl Thomas, it is a joy to play the calabash. It helps me to ride on and keep time with the rhythmic melodies of the universe. It is also a joy to serve the fruits of the earth in a calabash. My family and friends testify that my calabash-ware gives our meals an extra-special vibration.

My longtime friend Charlene Heyliger of Brooklyn, New York, named her boutique Gourd Chips Boutique after the gourd, and to this day her beautifully designed gourd works are part of the permanent collection at the DuSable Museum in Chicago, the Children's Museum in Indianapolis, and the Weekville Museum in Brooklyn.

*Hail you NRTU of the Temple of the Soul*
*Who weigh Heaven and Earth in the balance,*
*Givers of food to the Soul*
*Hail Tatunen*
*Creator/Creatress of Women and Men from the*
  *substance of the NTR of the south, north, west,*
  *and east*
*Give praises to the Lord of Ra.*

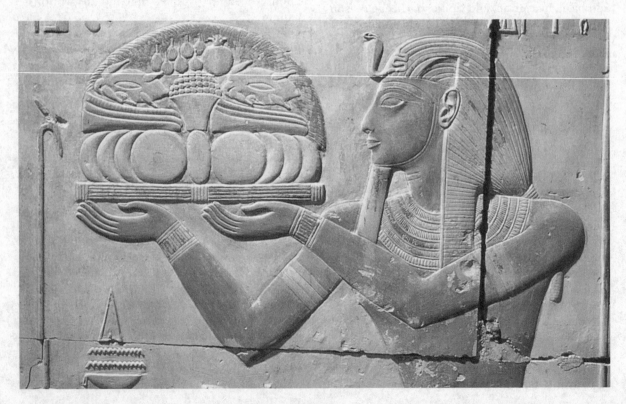

## SACRED WOMAN SEVEN-DAY FAST

*For body, mind, and spirit wellness and divine pampering, taking special time for yourself is the best thing a woman could do.*

Follow the twenty-one-day Natural Living Preparation Cleansing (pages 70–71) before taking on this fast to help avoid faster's detox. The Seven-Day Fast can be done every month. Fasting on predominantly green juices, herbs, and nutrients will aid in the prevention or decrease of bloating, irritability, PMS, heavy menses, and clotting. You will be more at ease, energetic, and emotionally stable.

*Before Breakfast:* Juice of 1 lemon and 1 to 2 tbsp. of castor oil or 2 tsp. cold-pressed olive oil.

*Breakfast:* Juice of 2 grapefruits or 3 oranges, *or* ½ cup of strawberry, blueberry, or cranberry juice mixed with 4 to 8 oz. of distilled water.

*Lunch:* 8 to 16 oz. green juice. (See page 112 for Green Foods.)

*Dinner:* 8 to 16 oz. green juice. Drink 1 pint to 1 quart distilled water at room temperature.

*Nutrients:* Alfalfa and dandelion, powdered, ⅓ to 1 tbsp. of each, *or* spirulina (powdered form), 1 to 2 tbsp., *or* wheatgrass (liquid or powdered), 1 tbsp., *or* blue-green manna, 4 to 6 tablets two or three times a day.

*Internal Cleansing:* Daily quart-sized enemas.

*Herbal Laxatives:* Heal Thyself Herbal Laxatives, 3 to 4 tablets to 8 oz. warm distilled water daily.

*Baths:* 1–2 lbs. Dead Sea salt in bath every other day.

*Exercise:* Dance of the Womb exercises, 20 to 45 minutes. Deep Fire Breaths 100 times a day.

*Heal Thyself Woman's Life Herbal Formula:* 3 tbsp. to 5 to 6 cups of water, daily.

*Womb Affirmation:* Repeat the 25 Womb *Hesi* (Chants) (page 53).

*Clay Application:* Apply clay over pelvis with gauze three times a week. If your condition is chronic, apply clay daily along with hot castor oil packs every other day.

*Douche:* 1 pint warm distilled water with 2 to 3 tbsp. of red raspberry extract and juice of 1 lime, or 2 oz. of wheatgrass.

*Sweat Baths:* Every other day for one hour; alternate showers and sweat baths.

*Attire:* Wear white each day of your fast during your early-morning prayer time, or at least when you return home after work.

### Fasting Partners

Strive to fast with another sister to establish an Ast/Nebt-Het relationship in honor of the original sister-to-sister pairing. Also, fasting with your mate is a very harmonious (Maat) thing to do together. Fasting benefits include spiritual peace, mental clarity, weight loss, more beautiful skin, burning up of cellulite, and greater womb wellness.

Establish your spiritual writing practice by creating a special fasting journal or devoting a special section of your journal to fasting only. Keep your fasting journal on your sacred altar and visit it at sunrise and sunset according to your heart's desire. Connect to the "womb" of your mind and your heart, in addition to your physical womb, by keeping a daily inner written dialogue with your womb during your fast so that you will have a record of your growth and development. As you allow the Spirit to move through you, you'll be amazed at the healing that you will receive through this divine communion.

### Celibacy: Fasting from Sexual Intercourse

Also fast from sexual intercourse during your seven-day fast. This is an appropriate time for you and your mate to explore alternative ways of expressing and making love.

Neither of you should feel unloved at this time. Continue to love and nurture your mate during the fast so he won't become overwhelmed with need or feel abandoned. Strive also to help cleanse his diet for a true unification of the relationship to take place.

Celibacy provides an excellent opportunity for your union to grow. You and your mate can pray together and develop better communication for understanding, patience, and healing. You can work on the qualities that will allow your relationship to endure and flourish.

## SACRED FOOD: SEVEN-DAY TRANSFORMATIVE WORK

- *First, scrub your Kitchen Healing Laboratory.* Wash cabinets, drawers, floors, and tabletops with natural soap and ammonia.
- *Next, put up a sign at the entrance of your kitchen* in the form of a wood carving or poster saying, "[Your name]'s Kitchen Healing Laboratory." You could also name it "Maat's Kitchen Healing Laboratory."
- *Purify your Laboratory* with a sage smudge, or burn frankincense and myrrh over heated charcoal in a fireproof pot weekly.
- *Now purge your Kitchen Healing Laboratory* of all fast food, processed food, flesh food, white sugar, and white flour products. Fill your Kitchen Healing Laboratory with foods that will heal and create wellness over the next seven days. Then vow to maintain your Laboratory in the height of consciousness.
- *Rehabilitate your taste buds.* Consume special healing foods daily to improve your health.
  - *Sour foods:* Lemons, limes, and grapefruits break up mucus and congestion. Consume these one to two times a day.
  - *Bitters:* Bitters cleanse and build up the blood. Take aloe (1 tbsp. with water), goldenseal (¼ tsp., seven days on and seven days off), woodroot (steep 1 tsp. in 1 cup water), and dandelion herb (steep 1 tsp. to 1 cup water).
  - *Chlorophyll foods:* Kale, broccoli, string beans, chard, and wheatgrass also cleanse and build up the blood. Consume 1 quart two or three times a day, coupled with 1 quart of distilled room-temperature water.
  - *Red foods:* Cranberries, raspberries, radishes, and cherries cleanse and build the blood as well. Consume these once a day.
- *Try growing a few of your favorite herbs on your windowsill or in your backyard.* After picking, hang them upside down to dry. Prepare as a tea to drink for healing, or add them to your healing soup and let them steep with your vegetables.
- Familiarize yourself with the Sacred Woman Seven-Day Fast.

### My Sacred Food End-of-the-Week Commitment:

I commit myself to establishing and continuing the wisdom of Ta-Urt and the power of Sacred Food in all the areas of my life.

Signature: _____

Date: _____

## CHAPTER 8

# GATEWAY 3: SACRED MOVEMENT

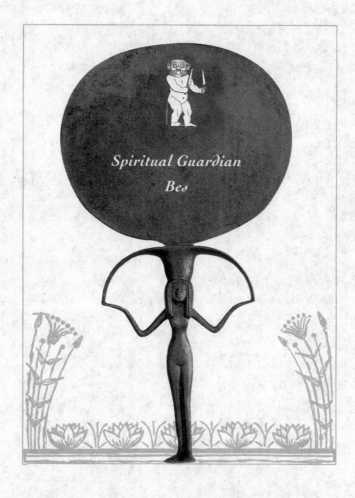

*Spiritual Guardian*
*Bes*

| Ancestor | Elder | Contemporaries |
|---|---|---|
| Josephine Baker | Katherine Dunham | Judith Jamison |
| Pearl Primus | Carmen DeLavallade | Debbie Allen |
| | | Queen Esther |

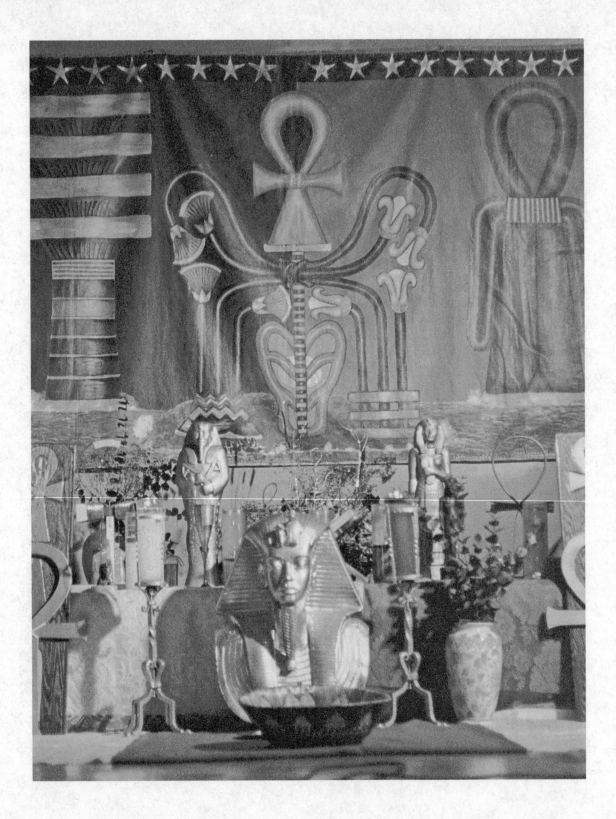

# SACRED MOVEMENT ALTAR WORK
## Face Your Heart to the East—to the Rising Sun
*(Layout from top view)*

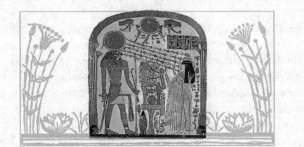

**Mount Pictures on Wall, Above Altar**

| | | | | |
|---|---|---|---|---|
| Picture of Spiritual Guardian | Picture of Ancestor | Picture of Sacred Self | Picture of Elder | Picture of Contemporary |

Baptism Bowl (WATER)

Feather
(AIR)

Ankh for Eternal Life or
Other Sacred Symbol
(SPIRIT)

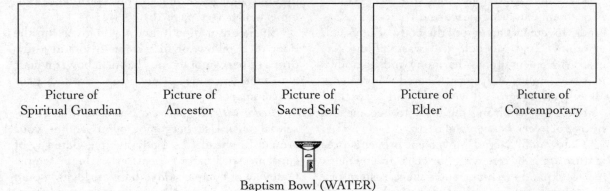

Fresh Flowers or
Flowering Plant
(EARTH)

*Anointing Oil:*
Bergamot

Orange Candle
(FIRE)

*Sacred Stone:*
Carnelian

Food for the NTR and your Ancestors (bowl of organic non-GMO fruit)
*(Release food from the altar after twenty-four hours.)*

**Place a tambourine, drum, ankle bells, or waist bells on your altar.**

Sacred tablecloth (orange) and scarf to wear during prayer.
Sacred color cloth to lay before altar. Sacred instruments to be played as you pray.

# GATEWAY 3: SACRED MOVEMENT DAILY SPIRITUAL OBSERVANCES

## Gateway Elements: Earth and Air

Sacred Movement revitalizes the physical body and teaches us how to spiritualize matter. Through Sacred Movement we learn that body, mind, and spirit are interrelated energy systems. By learning to harmonize our subtle energy systems through physical movement, we hold the key to accessing our spiritual body at will.

If you are anxious and stressed, Sacred Movement can bring peace and composure. Sacred Movement can empty the body of physical, emotional, and psychological waste. Fluid Sacred Movement creates harmony and flexibility in body, mind, and spirit. Sacred Movements allow you to ground yourself and transcend yourself by permitting the body to become the bridge between heaven and earth.

Gateway 3: Sacred Movement prevents premature aging by renewing our cells, and by helping to expand the lungs and relieve respiratory blockages, such as asthma and emphysema. If your circulation is impaired, Sacred Movement helps restore the free flow of prana throughout your Body Temple. It also helps to break up cellulite and fatty tissue. For those who are hyper, Sacred Movement calms and balances; for those with low energy, it renews and invigorates.

Spiritual exercises of ascension are to be performed daily for seven days, the number for the Spirit. This will awaken your inner gateways of divinity so that you may blossom into your full sacred center.

### 1. The Spiritual Bath
Bergamot essential oil takes you from an earth plane to a higher region. It is uplifting, refreshing, and encouraging, and increases mental alertness. Bergamot can help relieve feelings of emotional deprivation, and ease anxiety and depression, grief, and sadness. In the physical realm, it strengthens the immune system, aids in the healing of wounds and scars, and has an antiseptic effect. Essentially, bergamot fills you with energy and inspiration and makes you want to leap up and dance.

When bathing, add 4 to 6 drops of bergamot to your bathwater. Remember not to add the oil until the tub is nearly full.

### 2. Your Altar
Set up your sacred altar on the first day of your entry into each particular Gateway. You may set up your altar according to your spiritual or religious beliefs (see page 18).

Sit before it quietly and meditatively on the floor on a pillow, or in a chair. Also add a few drops of bergamot to your baptism bowl on your altar and sprinkle a few drops around your prayer space.

*Anoint with bergamot oil.* Select only pure essential oils. Use bergamot oil to anoint your crown, forehead (the Body Temple Gateway of supreme spirituality), heart (the Body Temple Gateway of compassion and divine love), womb area, palms of your hands to make everything you touch become more sacred, and the bottoms of your feet to spiritually align yourself for stepping out in power, promise, and faith.

### 3. Opening the Gateway
To invoke each Gateway's Spiritual Guardian, you may use whatever words pour from your heart. For example, here's a prayer that might be used at Gateway 3:

Sacred and Divine Bes, awaken the ancient dancer in me to allow sacred movement to set my spirit free. May sacred movement leap me into pure exhilaration, and stretch me to star Sirius in my inner galaxy. May my dance flush out my arteries, pump oxygen to my heart and my brain, detoxify my blood, lubricate my joints, and liberate my spirit.

May my sacred movements bring my soul to life, my mind to rest, my heart to balance, and my being to light. *Hetepu.*

As you offer your prayer, simultaneously

shake, ring, beat, or rattle a sacred instrument (sistrum bell, drum, shekere, or bells) to awaken the NTR that is indwelling.

### 4. Libation

Pour a libation for the Sacred Movement Gateway from a special cup, or sprinkle water from a bowl onto the earth or a plant, as you call out this prayer of praise and adoration.

— *Pour a libation* as you say, All praise and adoration to the Spiritual Guardian, Bes, the Protector of Sacred Movement.

— *Pour a libation* as you say, All praise and adoration to the Ancestors the Mothers of Sacred Movement, Josephine Baker and Pearl Primus.

— *Pour a libation* as you say, All praise and adoration to the Elders of Sacred Movement, Katherine Dunham and Carmen DeLavallade.

— *Pour a libation* as you say, All praise and adoration to my Divine Self and my Contemporary Divine Sisters, Judith Jamison, Debbie Allen, and Queen Esther, who honor Sacred Movement.

### 5. Sacred Woman Spirit Prayer

Ring a bell or play another sacred instrument at the beginning and end of this prayer. As you open your palms to the Sacred Spirit or gently place them over your heart, recite:

**Sacred Woman Spirit Prayer**

*Sacred Woman in the making,*
*Sacred Woman reawaken.*
*Sacred Spirit, hold me near.*
*Protect me from all harm and fear*
*beneath the stones of life.*
*Direct my steps in the right way as I journey*
*through this vision.*
*Sacred Spirit,*
*surround me in your most absolute*
*perfect light.*
*Anoint me in your sacred purity, peace,*
*and divine insight.*

*Bless me, truly bless me, as I share*
*this Sacred Life.*
*Teach me, Sacred Spirit, to be in tune*
*with the Universe.*
*Teach me how to heal*
*with the inner and outer elements*
*of air, fire, water, and earth.*

### 6. Sacred Movement Prayer

Shake bells, beat a sacred drum, or play another instrument at the beginning and ending of this prayer:

*Inspiring and enlivening Bes, Guardian of Sacred Movement, fill me with your joyous spirit. May I feel your divine presence in every part of my Body Temple, and coursing through my veins as I dance my gratitude for your Sacred Movement that renews my life force.*

### 7. Chanting Hesi

Chant this *hesi* four times:

*Nuk Pu Ntrt Hmt* — I am a Sacred Woman.

### 8. Fire Breaths

Prepare your Fire Breath by slowly inhaling four times and exhaling four times. Then when you are totally at ease, begin your four hundred Fire Breaths.

Inhale deeply like a pump through your nose (mouth closed) as you expand the breath down into the abdomen, then back up to the chest. Completely exhale out through your nostrils from your abdomen as it contracts and the lungs release your breath completely. Repeat this breath rapidly in and out, in and out.

Allow each deep Fire Breath — rapidly inhaling and exhaling through your nostrils — to represent the opening of the thousand lotus petals of illumination and radiance to reach Nefer Atum — the ultimate Afrakan lotus station of Divinity.

### 9. Gateway 3: Sacred Movement Meditation

Increase the length of time you spend in meditation every seven days. The longer you are in meditation, the deeper your inner peace will be, and the more solid your *ba* (spirit) will become. The cleaner your Body Temple, the sooner it will be able to live permanently in the peace and inner balance of the meditative state.

### A Moving Meditation

Visualize yourself as a glyph carved into the wall of the Great Pyramid, rooted there since antiquity. To reawaken and resurrect your Sacred Body Temple, begin to breathe deeply, fully, and slowly.

- First, breathe into your face, and then into your neck as it begins to rotate in a circular motion, bringing life to your face, and new vigor to your thyroid.
- Then reawaken your shoulders as you dance them up toward your ears and down again.
- Now open up your arms like the wings of Hru rising up toward Nut, the Sky Mother. Inhale as you soar on the breath of Maat. Relax your arms and bring them down to your sides as you gently exhale.
- Inhale into the breast of Ast as you expand your lungs, then your heart center, and down to your womb. Exhale as you release and contract your body.
- Now breathe into your hips as they begin to rotate you off the wall of the Pyramid. Breathe into your knees and legs and down to your feet, inhaling and exhaling.
- Stretch and stretch! Reach for the light of the sun as you breathe into your mind the vision of your Sacred Dance. Feel the freedom in your light-filled soul as your body dances you off the wall.

*Color Visualization.* Visualize the color of the Gateway: orange for energy, vitality, and flexibility. As you perform your meditation, wear vitalizing shades of orange and place a corresponding cloth on your altar.

*Sacred Stone Meditation.* While in meditation hold in your palm over the center of your body the sacred healing stone of the Gateway: carne-

lian or fire agate. Vibrational healing can be done by wearing and adorning your body with stones in a necklace, waist beads, or belt. You can place them under your pillow when you sleep, or at the four corners of your bed. You may also put your stone in your bathwater, as well as soak it in your drink to fill your system with stone healing. Finally, you may let the stone sit in your clay to enhance the rejuvenation and cleansing energies of your clay application.

### 10. Herbal Tonics

Drink gingko biloba. Part used: whole plant. Gingko has antioxidant properties, oxygenates the blood, and helps the body rid itself of free radicals. It increases the blood flow to the brain and relaxes and tones the muscles in arterial walls, helping to prevent heart attacks, stroke, and angina. It is helpful in eye problems resulting from decreased blood supply.

Drink your herb tea or tonic for seven days to receive the full benefits of tuning into Gateway 3. Enjoy your herb tea in your favorite mug during or after spiritual writing.

*Preparation.* One teabag to 1 cup of water. Boil water in a glass, clay, or stainless steel pot, turn off flame, pour water over teabag, and steep. Drink before or after your morning bath or sacred shower. Drink with joy and peace as you breathe between sips and settle into an easy contemplation and reflection.

### 11. Flower Essences

To deepen your experience of Gateway 3 choose from the following flower essences. Take 4 drops four times per day directly on or under the tongue, or add the same amount to a small glass of purified water and sip. For instructions on how to choose flower essences, see page 23.

- *Dandelion:* To release emotional tension in body.
- *Star of Bethlehem:* To release trauma from particular parts of body, often stored in the past.
- *Self-heal:* To arouse recuperative powers of the

body; integrating body and mind in the healing process.

- *Manzanita:* Appreciation of the body as the Temple of the Spirit.
- *Hibiscus:* Integration of libido and sexuality with soul warmth.

### 12. Diet

Follow the Sacred Woman Transitional Dietary Practices presented for Gateways 1–3.

### 13. Sacred Movement Journal Writing

This is best done after internal cleansing (enema) and/or meditation. When you are cleansed and centered, you can receive spiritual messages from the One Most High with grace. When you are in the spirit, messages travel down through your spirit mind, to your heart, into your hand, and onto the paper. (This is how I do all my writing.)

The best time to receive your spiritually inspired written work is after you have completed your altar work, between the hours of 4 A.M. and 6 A.M. Keep your journal and a very special pen by or on your altar to work with the power, force, and stillness at the coming of dawn, the hour of Nebt-Het.

Affirm your daily life. Write in your journal at this time thoughts, activities, experiences, and interactions that present themselves. You can also write down your visions, desires, dreams, and affirmations so that you will be able to draw on these resources when help and support are most needed.

*Consult Sesheta.* If you find that you are unable to contact your inner voice during your journal work, call Sesheta, the keeper and revealer of secrets (who is indwelling), to assist and speak through you.

### 14. Senab Freedom Shawl or Quilt

Choose a new piece of cloth that corresponds to the Gateway color (indicated in exercise 9 of your Daily Spiritual Observances or in Sacred Altar Work) to add to your Senab Freedom Shawl or Quilt. This cloth will serve as a mini-canvas to represent your experience in the Gateway you're working in.

Also, collect meaningful symbols that can be added to your shawl or quilt in appliqué or patchwork style. You can add stones, other natural objects, collectibles, family heirlooms, photographs that have been reprinted on fabric, or any other significant items that embody the essence of your experience. Give your imagination free rein and let your craftswoman spirit tell your story. For more information about the Senab Freedom Shawl or Quilt, see pages 122–125.

### 15. Sacred Tools

A Body Temple willing to transform.

### 16. Sacred Reminder

Throughout the week, you are to observe closely the wisdom presented for the Gateway you're in. For maximum results, live freely in tune with the various systems of wellness presented and practice the Seven-Day Transformative Work at the end of the Gateway.

### Closing Sacred Words

*Mother/Father Creator/Creatress, help me heal my life through the power of Sacred Movement.*

# SACRED MOVEMENT

Sacred Movement is the manifestation of the Divine in action. It is filled with the Divine Spirit of the Most High. The original Sacred Movement presents itself to us when a baby is in the womb and its mother and her stomach move as the little one stretches and pulls as it grows. When the new Returning Ancestor is born, we watch in fascination at the tiny one's dance of grace, at the ease, the calm stretch of movements of arms and legs and the whole body. This is truly the Dance of Life.

Whether we do or do not create Sacred Movement in our lives depends on how we think, our attitudes, our traditions, our cultural expressions, our language, our state of wellness or disease. Thoughts can birth us into Sacred Movement—which causes us to perform life as a sacred creative dance that heals. There are Sacred Movements that arise out of many cultures, such as tai chi from China, yoga from India, caperio from Brazil, and Native American ceremonial dances from the tribes of Turtle Island.

Sacred Movement ushers the breath of the Divine into us and makes our every step a prayer. So when we walk in harmony with the Divine, our walk becomes Sacred Movement. When we jog or work out at the gym with an attitude of prayer, it becomes Sacred Movement. When we climb mountains, or walk through valleys, or hug a tree, or playfully run after a laughing child in a prayerful state, we are in the midst of Sacred Movement.

Sacred Movement put to rhythm, with a spirit purpose and mission, becomes Sacred Dance. As Afrakan people we had a purpose stemming from our tradition in the form of birthing ceremonies, purification ceremonies, preparation for war, rites-of-passage ceremonies, marriages and funerals, and homecoming ceremonies. We used Sacred Dance to tell stories and give history lessons of our people's travels through time and space. Sacred Dance is used to convey spirit and emotions when words are just not enough.

Sacred Movement and Dance lift your spirit, inspire you to dance with Divinity, heal your heart, nourish your body, enrich your life, and transform your woes.

Everyone, no matter the condition of their Body Temple, can perform their Sacred Movement. Because when the legs don't work, we can dance with our arms. And when we can't move our arms, then we can dance with our head. And when we can't dance with our head, then we can dance with our eyes. And if we can't see, then we can dance with our smile. And if the smile can't come through, then we can simply dance with our heart!

## The Divination of the Body Members

The gift of the spiritual words you find in our Ancient Holy Book, the *Pert M Hru M Gbr* (*The Book of Coming Forth by Day from Night*) indicates the Divinity of our Body Temples. Every part of our temple is sacred. We are divine by nature, and we must appreciate ourselves so that our days on earth are vibrant and alive.

Learn to appreciate each member of your body as you stretch, breathe, and dance into sacred movement. When spoken aloud, these ancient affirmations for each body member will spiritually attune you to Sacred Movement. As you travel through the Gateway of Sacred Movement, these ancient affirmations will help you continue to work on self. Call out these affirmations for empowerment of the Body Temple, that you may awaken your "dry bones" and resurrect your self.

As you repeat these ancient affirmations, allow each one to become a step in your own Sacred Movement. This is Divine Choreography! Improvise and delight in the sacredness of your Body Temple, as you affirm each organ's unique dance of life.

Create your own Dance of the Body Members and share this Sacred Movement in your Sacred Circle.

This is the original text of the Divination of the Body Members, as it appeared on the ancient Egyptian (Khamitic) text of the Papyrus of Ani thousands of years ago.

Afrakan supreme melanin-charged being that you are, look deep into the signs of our language and see what messages of interpretation you receive.

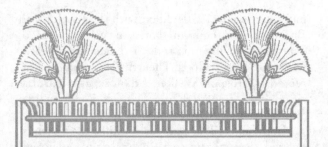

## Affirmations for the Body Members

I am the knot within the tamarisk tree, beautiful of splendor more than yesterday. My hair is of Nu [the primordial waters]. My face is of Ra [sun energy]. My two eyes are of Het-Hru [divine love]. My two ears are of Ap-uat [opener of the ways of inner standing]. My nose is of Khent-sheps [indwelling ancestors]. My two lips are of Anpu [the utterers who report to Tehuti—divine intelligence]. My teeth are of Khepera [the transformer].

My neck is of Ast the Divine. My two hands are of Khnemu [molder of form], lord of Tattu [place of stability]. My forearms are of Net [strong forearm/weaver], lady of Sau [place in the Nile Delta where Net's shrine was established]. My backbone is of Sut [stability].

My phallus/vagina is of Ausar/Ast [Divinity]. My reins [kidneys] are of the lords/ladies of Kher-aba [region in the Delta; a place of defense]. My chest inspires awe. My belly [and] my back are of Sekhmet [vital power]. My buttocks are of the eyes of Heru [watch your back]. My hips and legs are of Nut [sky]. My feet are of Ptah [grounded, solid]. My fingers and my toes are of the living Aritu [chakras, energy, forces; symbol is the cobra; feminine principle, intuition].

Not a body member of mine is without NTR [Divinity]. Tehuti protects my flesh entirely. I am Ra [solar force] every day. I shall not be seized by my arms, nor shall I be carried away by my hand, nor shall the NTRU [spiritual Guardians], shining ones, the dead [Ancestors], ancient ones, or any mortal, bring harm unto me.

I come forth, advancing. I know my name. I am light, seer of millions of years is my name. Traveling along the way of Hru the Light.[1]

## Throughout My Life, It Was Dance That Healed Me

When I was about sixteen, I went from riding my bike to studying dance in its many forms, and it became sacred medicine for me.

I find that the Divine Creator/Creatress and my Ancestors speak through me with the most power when I do my spirit dancing. When I dance, I fend off the "evil eye" and keep it from attacking me. I shake off family wars, and my children's growing pains, and my love pains, stress, and bad attitudes. When I dance, I'm filled with gratitude for having found my healing mission at such a young age.

My ancestors fill me with serenity as they dance in me. When I dance to the drum, flying through space just like a free bird, I kick and spin and jump and twirl, and reach up and grab my soul each and every time.

Dancing is my medicine. Spirit dancing is and will always be an endless sweet nectar of delight. It is delicious and fulfilling, and I do it whenever the need rises up in me. Dance heals me like nothing else.

Now, mind you, wheatgrass, spirulina, green juices, and sweat baths go very far in my book, but dance goes even farther. I can feel the Holy Spirit move through me when I'm dancing. I can feel the universe and all her stars flow through me whenever I do my spirit dance.

With dance, even if I trip over my feet and land on the floor, it doesn't matter, because when I dance, I can do no wrong. Because it ain't about the steps, it's about the Spirit that absolutely fills me. When I raise my arms, the Divine moves in me. When I kick my leg, the Divine is working brilliantly through me. When I contract and release, my world is renewed.

All the fresh new blood pumping through me carries away toxic thoughts and attitudes. Arteries clear up, opening me up to greater possibilities. My nervous system gets eased enough to release pent-up stress. My lungs expand, and I breathe in fresh experiences. Just having fun, I wash my inner ocean and become new, and clean, and whole.

I tell everybody to use dance as natural therapy, as a cultural/spiritual expression of divinity.

I tell them to take Afrakan dance, Brazilian dance, Haitian dance, every kind of dance to keep inner vibrations in tune with the cosmos.

In my past and my present, I have used dance along with natural healing to deal with all my ills. When I got married, I danced to celebrate the union. When I got pregnant, I danced to prepare to have a healthy baby. After having my baby, I danced to get my tone back. When I was breastfeeding and could not be separated from my baby, I wrapped her on my back in traditional style and danced us across the floor together. When I divorced, I danced to heal my heart. When I got a new man in my life, I danced to show appreciation and gratitude to the One Divine Spirit.

If my girlfriend hurt my feelings with some piercing words, I danced to mend my soul. If my life appeared to be falling apart, I danced it back together. When new work came through or a new opportunity opened up, I danced to rejoice. Whenever I was "off," I danced myself to sanity.

Dance, like my biking and nightly walks, has been and will always be a part of me. I dance because, like all Natural Living and healing methods available to me, it works on my body and soul.

Dance once saved my life. I was riding my bicycle home after teaching a dance class in the Bedford-Stuyvesant section of Brooklyn when suddenly a large, fast-moving car struck my bicycle. Time stood still. A voice from deep within me spoke and said: "Dance! You won't die if you just dance."

I released the bicycle, extended my arms, pointed my feet, and did a classic swan dive across the hood of the car. The driver and I stared at each other through opposite sides of the windshield.

After a few moments I climbed down off the hood, retrieved my battered bicycle, and went home. If I had tensed my body, I'm sure I would have been injured badly and probably hospitalized. I will admit I was a little shaken up, but I knew I hadn't suffered even a scratch because I had danced! I offered deep gratitude for such a lifesaving gift.

I've been dancing since my teens. I was dancing, healing, with the Sylvia Forte Dance Company in the late 1970s, filled with the rhythms of Brazilian and Haitian dance as we performed Yonvalu. During this time, I danced and acted with the Demi Gods Theatrical Company, directed by Joseph Walker. I danced at a Yoruba ritual with Baba Ishangi, a master spiritualist and teacher of African culture.

In the late 1980s and early 1990s, the Orishas danced through us to help heal souls in great need. I danced for the Grandfather and Grandmother Spirits at the Native American Sun Dance and sweat lodges in South Dakota. I danced at the Hare Krishna Temple with Hlandini Shakti Das, my longtime spiritual friend, to help raise Krishna Consciousness. I danced with my family at my grandmother and grandfather's church in Louisiana as we all shouted in praise of Jesus, the Great Healer and Light. I danced with the Olatunji Dance Company, as his Drums of Passion rocked my soul. I danced a spirit dance at a funeral (a homecoming ceremony) in Ghana, West Africa, with Joe Menza and his family.

I danced and healed through African dance classes with Professor Doris Green at Brooklyn College, and Charles Moore in Park Slope, and Chuck Davis up in Harlem, and Dini Zulu over in Queens. And there was jazz dance with Alvin Ailey, and Dunham Dance with Joan Peters, and belly dancing with Aja, and ju-ju spirit dance with Bernadine at the Smai Tawi Center. I performed the Dance of the Womb at Sister to Sister gatherings and at birthing ceremonies, naming ceremonies, and Khamitic rituals.

I dance to bring forth the Indwelling Healer to work up a divine mojo, resolve conflicts, create new conditions, or purge out negative ju-ju imposed on me by this society. I dance through my house like I'm talking with a kick, and I spin twice through the hallway to the bathroom as I run the water into my tub, then I leap into the Kitchen Laboratory and spin my arms around the pot of herb tea. I dance into my children's rooms, sending good vibes into their atmosphere.

One day my mother was not feeling like herself and she asked, "Helen, could you dance for me?" It seemed dance made her as happy as it did me.

In between writing these pages, I've gotten up off the floor, where I write most of the time, and started dancing to move and stir my creative juices so that I could go and write some more. If you're an artist or a Sacred Woman, and we're tight, I'm going to talk you into taking a dance class with me. I've shared my dancing spirit with Erykah Badu, Hazelle Goodman, and Princess. I almost persuaded my beloved client Ben Vereen to take a Dunham Dance class with me. To this day, my eldest son, SupaNova, and I dance at Alvin Ailey's School of Dance so we can summon some extra healing in our times of need. When you combine cleansing and dance, you create a blissfully charged combination that's beyond words.

Dance has always been intertwined with my healing work because, for me, there is no separation between me and my dance. You see, in Afrakan culture, our spiritual lifestyle, our rituals and ceremonies, have always been expressed through dance from the beginning of time. In my mama and daddy's day, they released their woes and expressed their joy through the jig and the Lindy Hop.

I'm just maintaining my tradition, and it continues to feed me. I've found that as long as you keep dancing and keep your body flowing and moving, diseases of the body, mind, and spirit cannot set in, and mental and emotional disturbances have no place to fester. Sickness shows up in a body that doesn't go with the flow, but if you actively purify, fast, pray, and do spirit dancing, then aches and pains, physical energy blocks, a broken heart, and even high blood pressure can be flushed out of your system.

So go forth and dance as the Ancestors that have gone before you have danced. Dance and shake off the madness and the blues of the "unnatural" society we live in, for spirit dance contains a Nature cure that modern medical science cannot duplicate.

I will never forget a particular Wep Renput festival, which falls during the month of my birth. All day our Afrakan Khamitic community celebrated our New Year through drums, tambourines, bells, *hesi* (chants), spoken word, fashion, drama, and prayers.

And then we danced! We danced led by Abdel Salaam, the Priest of Harlem's Shrine of Bes, a master dancer, choreographer, and director of the Forces of Nature, a world-renowned dance company that represents our culture at its best.

Abdel took our village through a healing dance ritual. He called forth seven brothers and seven sisters to face one another, men on one side of the room and women on the other. The dancers did as he asked, even though no one was sure what was to take place.

He then told us that we as Afrakan people used to dance in many ways, for many reasons — such as resolving conflicts, settling arguments and disputes between man and woman, between husband and wife. So dance became the conduit in our culture for resolving heated emotional conflicts between the sexes.

Then Abdel gave a sign to begin the healing ritual, and the couples paired off, ready for the duel. He reached his hands up toward the Sky, toward Mother Nut, as the drums began to roll. Then he dropped his hands down to the Earth, Father Geb, and the dance battle was on.

The first sister in the line came forward. She shook her hips in her partner's face with a lot of attitude. He then responded in kind and jumped into the air, flinging his locks wildly like a lion. She swirled at her partner like a panther. He

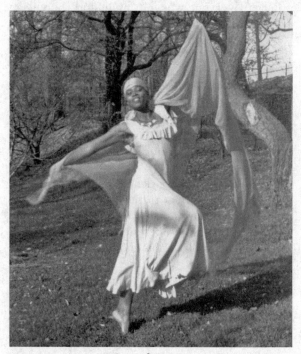

Sacred Dance

spun out on her. His leg shot up high in the air. She clasped her hands behind her, only to abruptly smack her palms down on the floor. She stopped. He looked. She stared. They smiled. We all breathed, relieved.

The drums were on fire, were all-healing. The village was gyrating in this intense atmosphere— hands flying, one couple after the next, breasts contracting, chests releasing, stomachs rolling, buttocks tightening, bodies sweating.

My sister healer Dr. Jewel Pookrum and I screamed and laughed and shouted and applauded. We flashed our Ankhs in approval and gratitude for the masterful way our Ancestors demonstrated through Abdel Salaam. It was an intense and joyful healing through dance.

When the battle was over, the couples embraced, one after the next. Abdel lifted their arms up into the air as they stood on either side of him, and we all, the whole village, clapped, for we had all won. This was a conflict that worked itself out without a curse or a slap or bloodshed. Words and emotions were expressed through movements. The language of the soul was spoken. The tension was released through the dance, and we breathed peace and joy into the atmosphere. Everyone was left intact and the village was ecstatic.

This healing dance ritual reminds me of the break dancing the young Afrakans and Latin people created and used to do battle in the 1970s without guns. Aggression, discontent, and pride were expressed, but everyone was left intact. So take the lesson, sisters and mothers—move forward and don't hold on to what's eating you. Put some music on, clap your hands, make some joyful noise, and dance!

To dance is to experience inner freedom. To dance is to reconnect to the Great Mother and Great Father. To dance is to embrace life with passion, joy, and exuberance. When you learn how to dance well to any and all rhythms, you'll find that no matter what earth or life changes are going on, you'll be able to dance with its rhythms. And you'll dance so well that you'll never be swallowed up by chaos or fear because you know how to spin around and soar above all obstacles. Dance teaches you how to leap your spirit out of confusion.

We are all spirit dancers. We know how to let the spirit move through us and flush pain or sadness away. We know how to use dance to enhance our lives. So express who and what you are through your dance. Whenever you're uptight, dance, and see what magic happens! Whenever you're lost for answers to your life, dance out a vision of your quest. Dance to commune with your inner self. Dance to commune with your Ancestors. Dance joy and peace and beauty into your life from on high. Dance a healing dance. Dance a freedom dance. Just dance! Sacred Women everywhere, dance!

## THE DANCE OF THE WOMB: SACRED MOVEMENT FOR PHYSICAL PURIFICATION AND SPIRITUAL REJUVENATION

The Dance of the Womb is a profound cycle of Sacred Movement. It was channeled through me because I needed to heal my womb and convey my love to her. When I began to do these movements and saw the results in my body, I realized that many other women needed the same Divine Sacred Movement to restore their wombs and lives. The Dance of the Womb movements are a gift from the Divine.

So, Sisters, let's dance!

The Dance of the Womb offers a series of twenty-five rhythmic movements that gently flow one into the other. Every movement is designed to create a healthy, vibrant, well-rounded womb. It may take from thirty minutes to an hour to complete the full series of dance movements.

For womb rejuvenation, these healing movements should be practiced every day. For best results, as you incorporate the Dance of the Womb into your daily life, be sure to eat only wholesome, flesh-free foods, including an abundance of fresh fruits and vegetables, and drink plenty of pure water. You will soon find that you're on the path to maintaining a disease-free, vibrant womb, and a body that is filled with light and love.

As Sacred Women, we must cleanse our wombs daily and accept that we have the power to heal so we can be healthy and radiate pure energy through our bodies. So, upon the rising of the sun, we also rise and face the east as we lovingly and gently nurture, rejuvenate, strengthen, and relax our body, mind, and spirit through the Dance of the Womb.

With each exhalation we release all forms of death as we say, "Today I shake out of my womb all tumors and cysts. Today I stretch out of my womb all signs of pain, PMS, and cancer. Today I build strength into my most sacred seat. A healthy, whole womb is my divine birthright."

Keep in mind that revitalizing the womb takes much more than a cup of herbal tea and one or two exercises. Establishing true womb wellness requires a lifestyle change. So remember to nurture yourself with Natural Living principles every day.

The fertility dances of many of the indigenous cultures around the world—Africa, China, Japan, India, Europe, Brazil, and the Caribbean—all involve rotation and stimulating movements of the buttocks, hips, and pelvis. These movements are excellent forms of womb rejuvenation. They should become a part of your daily discipline for womb wellness because they promote flexibility, strength, agility, lubrication, and joy. They vibrate out accumulated poisons from within and around the womb. When you do these movements accompanied by drums, shakeres, bells, and/or tamboras and tambourines, you'll experience a soulful healing as well.

Playing musical instruments helps you maintain inner harmony and balance. If your mate plays the instrument while you dance, a healing transformation can take place for both of you. You don't have to be professional musicians and dancers to achieve the desired goal; you need only to seek to heal and to love. Through music and dance you can create a loving male/female attunement and reverence within your earthly and heavenly realms.

## How to Breathe with the
## Dance of the Womb

In order to be as effective as possible and to achieve maximum results, each womb movement must be accompanied by proper breathing. The basic breathing technique is continuous throughout the exercises. You inhale deeply whenever the body moves upward, and exhale long breaths whenever the body moves downward. Between the movements, continue breathing—in through the nose, and out through the nose or mouth.

Accept the challenge of improving your breathing as you perform the Dance of the Womb exercises. The more slowly you do each exercise, the more effective the Dance of the Womb session will be for developing your breath and your flexibility, as well as for balancing your chakras and elevating your spiritual level.

### The Cooling (Soothing) Breath
The cooling breath soothes the Body Temple, much the way cucumbers, hops, valerian, chamomile, or lemongrass do.

1. As you inhale, breathe into and expand the stomach and chest.
2. When you exhale, contract the stomach and relax the chest.
3. Keep your shoulders relaxed at all times and your face at ease.
4. Release all tension and stress with each breath.

### The Fire Breath:
### The Spiritual Energizing Breath
The Fire Breath is like consuming cayenne, ginger, garlic, beets, or sorrel—all invigorating and energizing for the Body Temple. Perform this rapid-fire breath twenty-five to one hundred times between movements for improved circulation and internal flushing.

1. As you inhale through your nose, expand your abdominal area and lungs.
2. As you exhale through your mouth, relax the chest and contract your abdominal area forcefully.
3. Do this breathing rhythmically and with great speed—in, out, in, out.

## Turning to Nature for
## Empowerment and Release

Step out! Have courage, be confident. Your womb is your responsibility! The most powerful revolutionary activity a woman can do is to take full responsibility for the care of her womb. For some women this is an awesome and fearful encounter. They would rather place their wombs at the mercy of strangers than trust their ability to heal themselves.

Believe in yourself by trusting Nature. Nature provides us with everything we need to heal. You have been given the tools and permission to oversee and heal your womb naturally. You have been given air, fire, water, earth, and spirit. Allow *Sacred Woman* to be one of the many gateways through which you tune in to the power and the spirit of the Wise Woman, the ancient Medicine Woman, the Bush Doctor. These handmaidens of the Divine Mother live inside each one of us, just waiting to be summoned to guide us to womb wellness.

If you ever doubt Nature's capacity to heal your womb, go outdoors and sit on her soil or grass or sand or rocks, and spread open your legs and your heart as you breathe deeply. Ask Nature, "What must I do to create womb wellness?" Sit still and listen quietly as long as it takes, and Nature will speak to you. You will be given the courage you need and the direction to take as you advance on your healing journey.

So step out on faith!

### Sitting on Our Seats

When you do your meditations, visualizations, and journal work, practice sitting on the floor because it helps to strengthen your womb center. The more you sit in a chair, the more you weaken your sacred seat. The more you sit on the floor, the more you open up and exalt your sacred seat. Ancient women knew this. Modern medicine women have to learn to sit on the floor to realign our energies.

### The Dance of the Womb Is Also a Moving Meditation

Freely dialogue with your womb throughout your exercises. Pay attention when your womb is in pain; and breathe deeply through her several times, for she wants to speak through you. She's trying to get your attention, so listen and relax into the movements as the voice of your inner womb speaks to you.

As you move through your meditation in mo-

tion, your womb may weep, laugh, sing, rejoice, release her essence. This is an opportunity to get intimate with yourself. As you heal yourself, you will discover the relationship between the workings of your womb's physical or energetic life, and how your womb relates to all your experiences.

As you perform the Dance of the Womb daily, mentally and soulfully unleash your power to be used for creativity and self-healing. Unpin those blocked, painful emotions, forgive yourself, bless your womb. Let go from the depths of your womb with each movement and with each breath. Listen to the voice of your womb throughout the Dance of the Womb very closely, and she will share all of her secrets with you.

As you experience the Dance of the Womb, one movement flows into the next. Meditate on the purpose of each of the movements as they relate to your womb. For example, the first movement is about womb release. It asks you to release whatever or whoever may be blocking your rebirth. When you practice this movement, breathe from the heart of your womb-self, and free yourself from your very center.

The key vision and approach to the Dance of the Womb is to "spiritualize matter" by pouring love, light, and serenity from your mind and heart through your body and down into your womb. You do this through the power of your breath, which is the divine life force of renewal.

To create a lasting relationship, I encourage you to perform the Dance of the Womb with your mate. This will create respect, honor, compassion, sweetness, and harmony in your union. He will receive great benefits, too, for his womb—his prostate—will be purified, energized, and strengthened, giving him control and longevity.

The following pages illustrate and describe how to do the twenty-five movements of the Dance of the Womb. Each of their benefits is listed, along with appropriate affirmations to recite or meditate on as you perform the movements.

At the conclusion of this section you'll find a useful chart that summarizes all twenty-five movements, plus the key vision that empowers each one.

# THE TWENTY-FIVE SACRED MOVEMENTS OF THE DANCE OF THE WOMB

*From the voice of Mother Earth*
*Comes the voice of the Plants*
*From the voice of the Plants*
*Comes the Dance of the Womb*

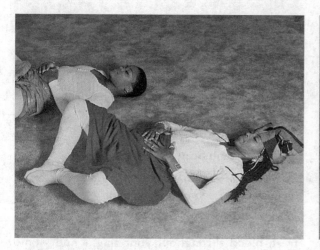

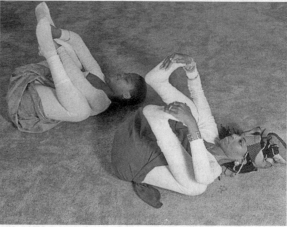

### 1. Rebirthing Pose: Womb Meditation

*Description of Movement:* Lie flat on your back and draw your knees up toward your hips. Place feet together and open thighs. Relax your back deep into the floor as your knees drop down closer and closer to the floor. Place palms gently and lovingly over your womb. Be sure to keep your elbows down. Tune into your breath and begin your womb meditation. Relax. Go deeper and deeper as you meditate.

*Benefits:* Unblocks tightness and stress within the pelvic area.

*Affirmation:* "Like a lotus blossom, I open up my womb to the Divine within me to make me healthy and whole."

### 2. Advanced Rebirth: Womb/Leg Stretch

*Description of Movement:* Continue to rest flat on your back until you are very much at ease. Then bend your knees and grasp the bottoms of your feet as you stretch your legs open and simultaneously press your thighs down toward the floor. Release all the tension in your neck, shoulders, arms, and thighs as you breathe in deeply on the inhalation and out on the exhalation.

*Benefits:* Stretches tension out of the hips, thighs, and pelvis, which allows oxygen to flow throughout the Body Temple.

*Affirmation:* "I am totally at one with my womb."

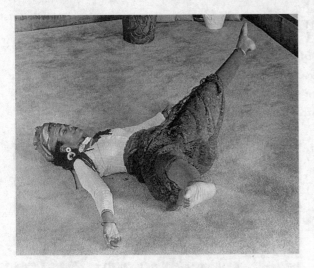

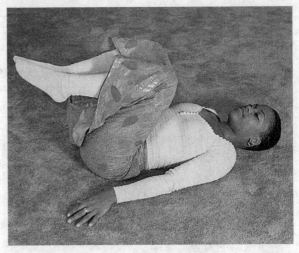

### 3. The Lotus: Legs in Stride

*Description of Movement:* While lying flat on your back with palms facing up, inhale as you raise both legs together straight toward the ceiling. Exhale, and spread your legs apart. At this time resist the urge to tighten; do just the opposite, relax. Breathe deeper and recite your affirmation. Remain in this position for one to three minutes. Then slowly inhale, and carefully bring your legs together to get ready for the next position. (If you feel any stress in your lower body, place your hands under your hips for more back and abdominal support.)

*Benefits:* Strengthens and tones the pelvis and womb. Unlocks the pelvic girdle.

*Affirmation:* "I release and let go of all the tension and stress within my womb."

### 4. The Womb Seat: Hip Press

*Description of Movement:* Still lying on your back, feel yourself becoming one in spirit with Mother Earth within you and around you. Raise your knees and press them into your chest to pump fresh blood throughout your thighs and womb area. Arms and shoulders are relaxed, hands palm down on the floor.

*Benefits:* Relaxes and stretches hips, thighs, and abdomen. Helps to wake colon in order to release toxic gases.

*Affirmation:* "My great hips are sacred mountains, full and healthy enough to house my sacred womb."

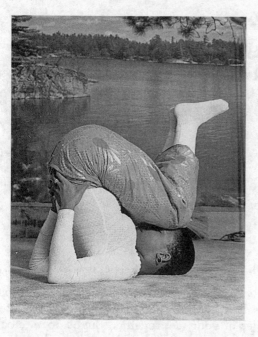

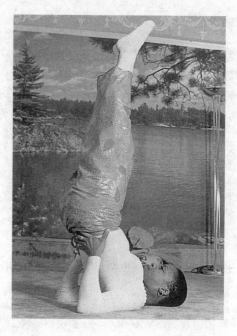

### 5. Inner Reflection: Pre–Shoulder Stand

*Description of Movement:* Still on your back, raise your hips off the floor and bring your knees to your forehead, keeping feet parallel to the floor. Place the palms of both hands securely against your back for support. Bring elbows close together to keep your body aligned.

*Benefits:* Flushes toxins out of all your lower extremities as the womb experiences relief from stress and waste. Stretches tension out of spine, hips, neck.

*Affirmation:* "I am a ball of sunlight; I radiate power from within my womb."

### 6. The Great Womb Purge: Shoulder Stand

*Description of Movement:* Supporting your body weight on your shoulders with your elbows, hands against your back, tuck your chin into your chest. Slowly raise your legs straight up toward the ceiling or sky. You are now completely inverted.

*Benefits:* All inverted movements create a grand cleansing and flushing for the entire system. It increases the circulation of the blood contained within the Body Temple. This intense motion aids in creating and maintaining a healthy womb.

*Affirmation:* "I view my world more clearly now, for my mind and my womb are refreshed and renewed."

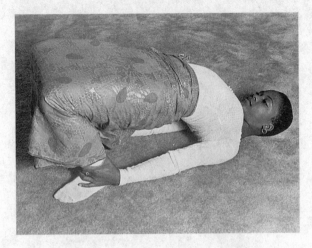

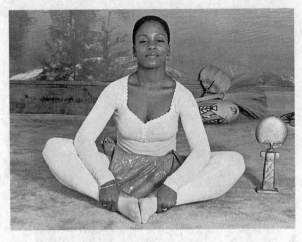

### 7. Bridge Over Troubled Water: Pelvic Lifts

*Description of Movement:* To release tension and stress, lie flat on your back, bend your knees with both feet on the floor, and press your chin into your throat to lengthen your spine. Then very slowly, to the count of four, lift your pelvis up, hold for a few minutes, then lower slowly. Repeat five to ten times.

As you lift your pelvis, keep your arms at your sides, palms flat on the floor. Lift your pelvis first, then your back. Now stretch up as much as you can, resting your weight on your arms and shoulders. While your hips are lifted, squeeze hip and pelvis muscles—internal and external—as tightly as possible, then release. Repeat four to eight times. Inhale as you ascend, and exhale as you descend. Reverse your movements as you release, bringing down the back, then the pelvis, flat on the floor.

*Benefits:* Releases tension and stress in the hips, thighs, and pelvis.

*Affirmation:* "I squeeze out all hurt and negativity from my sacred womb."

### 8. The Altar: Womb/Pelvic Stretch

*Description of Movement:* Sit up with your back straight, shoulders down, neck long, chest lifted, soles of your feet together, thighs open, elbows resting on inner thighs. Now inhale, draw knees up slightly, then exhale, and gently press your thighs open with your elbows. Do this until your legs are completely open and relaxed. Then rock slowly from side to side, from hipbone to hipbone.

*Benefits:* Opens the pelvic region, and lubricates the womb as it keeps you supple.

*Affirmation:* "I open myself and my womb to all the goodness in the universe."

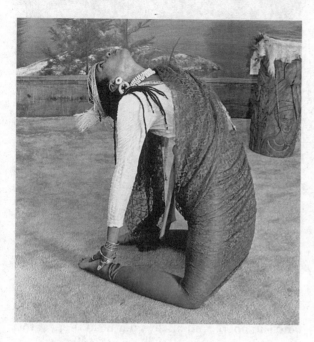

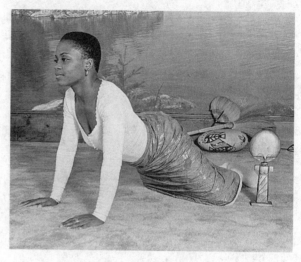

### 9. The Mountain: Womb Press

*Description of Movement:* Sit on your knees, then push your hips forward, arch your back, and reach back and hold on to your ankles as you open up your thighs. The pelvis, chest, and neck are now completely open. Allow your head to arch all the way back. Relax. Breathe.

*Benefits:* Allows for a wonderful and complete body stretch.

*Affirmation:* "I lift up my light unto the Lord, and the womb of my mind and heart are restored."

### 10. The Waterfall: Pelvic Presses

*Description of Movement:* Facedown on the floor, press up with your hands, lock your elbows straight, and keep your back flat. Press your pelvis forward, bend your knees, open your thighs, and put your feet side by side. Once in place, perform push-ups by just bending and straightening your arms several times. Next, straighten elbows and push your hips forward and backward (contract and release hips). Finally, slowly rotate hips in a circular direction clockwise and then counterclockwise.

*Benefits:* Strengthens arms, and firms hips, thighs, and pelvis. Releases tension and tightness held in your pelvic area.

*Affirmation:* "I press all congestion and heaviness out of my beautiful womb."

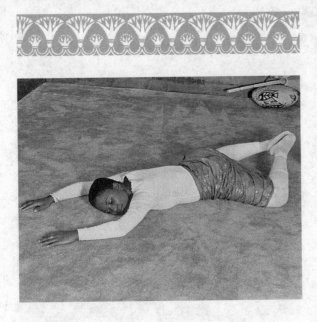

## 11. The Offering: Pelvic Release

*Description of Movement:* Lie flat on your stomach, stretch and arch upward, and turn your head to the side. Bend your knees and bring the soles of your feet together tightly. Open and relax your pelvis into the floor; breathe slowly. With each exhalation, lower legs and feet downward to the floor as you relax your pelvic area deeper and deeper.

*Benefits:* Opens the womb gently without strain.

*Affirmation:* "I submit my womb to the Creator/ Creatress and to Great Mother Earth, for I accept good health as my inheritance."

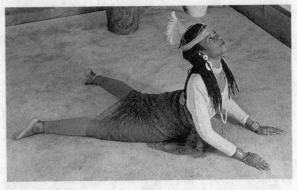

## 12. Rennenet — The Cobra: Open-Thigh Pelvic Release

*Description of Movement:* Lie on your stomach and spread your legs as far apart as possible. Place palms flat on the floor in front of your shoulders. Slowly press up, using your hands to support your upper body. Now arch your back and head backward as you inhale. Exhale as you slowly lower yourself back to the floor, bringing your abdomen down first, then your rib cage, chest, and shoulders, and finally your head. Repeat this four to seven times, slowly and steadily.

The Cobra Dance from ancient Khamit is known today as the belly dance. The snake represents women, fertility, childbirth, and the higher spiritual mind. Kings and queens wore the snake on their crowns, placed sover their third eye, their spiritual energy center, to represent the height of spiritual realization and divine union.

*Benefits:* Stretches out back and pelvis, strengthens arms, and expands lungs to circulate air fully throughout the body.

*Affirmation:* "I honor the Dance of the Womb throughout Rennenet, the Nubian Serpent Goddess, the Lady of the Fertile Land, protectress of harvest and fertility, and nourisher of children."

*Affirmation:* "I release all the coiled energies of worry, stress, and woe from my womb. I replace all stagnant energy with freedom, joy, and gladness."

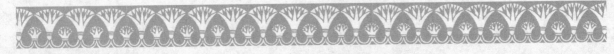

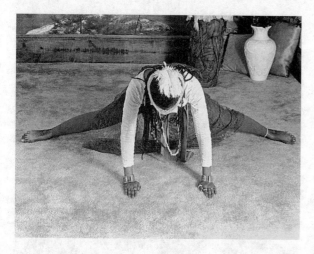

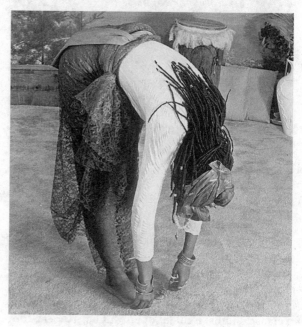

## 13. Birth: The Split

*Description of Movement:* Sit on the floor and open your legs as wide as possible. Feel yourself stretching out your very innards. Lean forward with palms flat on the floor. With your back flat and neck long, push down with arms of steel. Keep stretching open as you bend your arms to bring your chest closer and closer to the floor.

*Benefits:* Unblocks hips, pelvis, and thighs. Excellent preparation for natural childbirth.

*Affirmation:* "I salute the divinity of my sacred womb."

## 14. Nut—The Heavenly Body: Forward Bend

*Description of Movement:* Slowly and gently, bend your body from the waist, stretching the upper body down toward the floor. Reach toward your toes, tuck your chin in, and allow your body to hang at rest over the balls of your feet.

*Benefits:* Stretches out the spine to prevent lower back pain, and squeezes stress and gases out of the womb, bladder, and colon.

*Affirmation:* "I offer my omniversal womb to the womb of the earth to be renewed and revitalized."

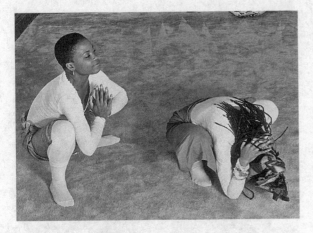

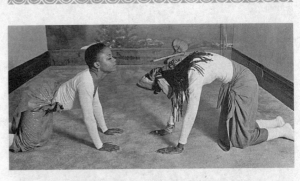

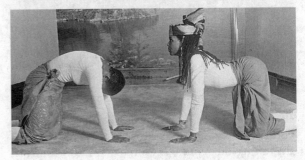

## 15. The Seat of Mother Ast: Squat

*Description of Movement:* From a standing position, separate your feet, then slowly squat down toward the floor. Hips are relaxed and both feet are flat on the floor. *Beginners:* Palms are together, elbows are bent and placed on the insides of inner thighs. Inhale slowly, then exhale slowly, pressing thighs open with your elbows. Inhale, release thighs; exhale, open thighs. Repeat four to seven times. *Advanced:* Place fingertips on the nape of your neck, chin into the chest. Place arms inside thighs and move elbows toward the floor as you arch your back completely.

*Benefits:* May help to realign the pelvis if tilted. Essentially, the squat lengthens the spine, which releases tension in the lower back and pelvis. The squat is especially helpful if you have womb stress from wearing high-heeled shoes. It's also excellent for relieving headaches. This movement is excellent for easing childbirth. Squatting is also vital for the proper elimination of waste. Squat on the toilet seat by placing a footstool under your feet while eliminating. In this position, twice the amount of fecal matter will pass from the colon.

*Affirmation:* "I open myself up to the wombniverse to restore my cosmic womb."

## 16 and 17. Bes—the Cat: Spinal and Hip Contractions

*Description of Movement:* Rest on hands and knees like a cat. Arch your back upward as you drop your head down and tuck your hips under. Allow your back to curve downward as you lift your head up and back and release your hips upward. Exhale on the arch, inhale on the release. Repeat entire exercise four to eight times.

*Benefits:* Strengthens hips, womb, and abdomen. Strengthens back and circulation around breast area.

*Affirmation:* "I move as freely as the waves of the ocean as I rotate and cleanse my womb and strengthen my breasts."

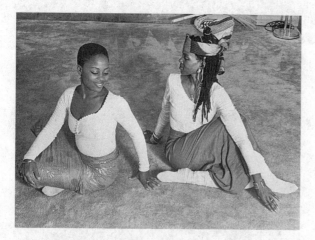

## 18. The Moon: Spinal Twist

*Description of Movement:* Sit on floor with legs crossed, tailor fashion. *Beginners:* Place right hand over left knee and left hand behind you. Your head is turned toward the right thigh as you look over your right shoulder and twist your upper body toward your left. Hold this position for one to two minutes as you breathe deeply. Repeat the exercise on the opposite side. *Advanced:* Same movement as beginners. However, bend left leg and cross right leg over the left. Reverse for opposite pose.

*Benefits:* Opens the spinal energy for deeper emotional relaxation and peace. Relaxes body, restores peace and healthiness within the womb.

*Affirmation:* "My womb, my spine, and my soul are uplifted as I twist out all doubt and negativity."

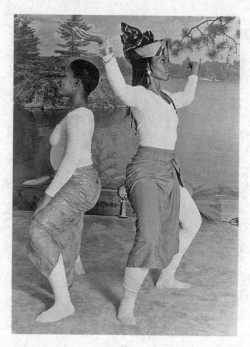

## 19. Sun-Ra: Standing Squat

*Description of Movement:* Stand up straight with feet wide apart. Move into a standing squat by going into a deep bend. Rest your hands on the inner thigh or above your shoulders in the ancient Afrakan pose of praise to the Most High for several moments. With feet flat on the floor, push pelvis forward, then to the right, back, left, then forward again, then left, back, right, forward. Do this four to seven times. Next, lift heels and do the same exercise on both sides with heels off the floor.

*Benefits:* Strengthens and stretches legs, thighs, hips, and womb.

*Affirmation:* "I affirm that power and radiance flow easily from my womb and throughout my Body Temple."

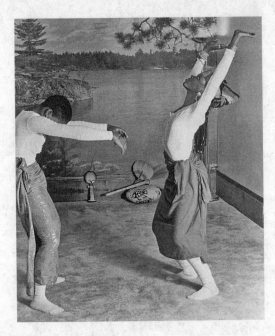

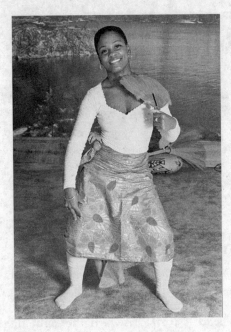

## 20. Praise the Creator/Creatress: Through Womb and Breasts

*Description of Movement:* Bend your knees. Inhale and contract arms, ribs, and abdomen, tucking head and chin into chest. Reverse by releasing and arching back as you exhale. Swing arms up and backward. Swing forward and backward as you repeat the contracting and releasing movement. Keep rhythm to drums as you contract and release your breasts, hips, and womb.

*Benefits:* Afrakan dance, as well as native dances of various other cultures, increases circulation, which cleanses and purifies the blood in the arms, breasts, back, stomach, and womb. It also increases circulation. So dance, Sacred Women, dance!

*Affirmation:* "I unite with the Spirit of the Creator/Creatress to heal my womb and set me free. I dance in the rhythm of divinity."

## 21. Planetary Motion: 360-Degree Hip Rotations

*Description of Movement:* Standing up, spread your legs apart and bend your knees. Place your hands on your hips and sway hips from right to left, then forward and back. Then swing hips all the way around in a 360-degree circle, first to the right, then to the left.

*Benefits:* Tightens womb, hips, and thighs as it increases circulation.

*Affirmation:* "As I dance, I rotate all pollution out of my womb as she travels the four directions and orbits the omniverse."

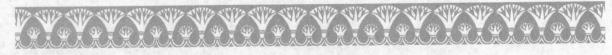

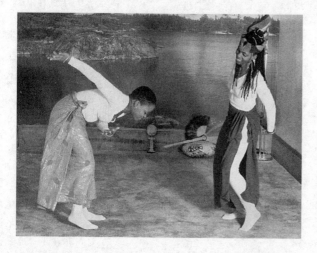

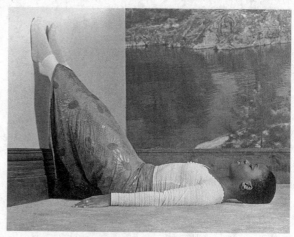

### 22. The Volcano Erupts: Pelvic Hip Vibrations

*Description of Movement:* Shake your hips as you move your body from side to side. Or lean forward as you lift your feet right, left, right, left, as your hips relax and vibrate to the rhythm of drums or other music you may be playing or making.

*Benefits:* Breaks down and releases dead cells, increases circulation, purifies your body while feeding your spirit.

*Affirmation:* "In jubilation I shake every past and present negative condition and circumstance out of my womb, my sacred nest."

### 23. The Pyramid Mountain Pose: 45-Degree Angle

*Description of Movement:* Place your feet against the wall with your legs at a forty-five-degree angle to allow your internal ocean to wash your womb clean, or lie down on a slant board with your legs at a forty-five -degree angle. Hold this position for three to ten minutes. While you have your legs up, do vaginal squeezes—tighten all muscles in the vaginal area, and hold for thirty counts, then release and rest for twenty counts. Squeeze again and hold for ten counts; release and rest.

*Benefits:* Relaxes the body as the inner water of the body flushes toxins out of legs, hips, and especially your sacred womb.

*Affirmation:* "I seek healing from the earth for the seat of my womb. The earth replenishes me."

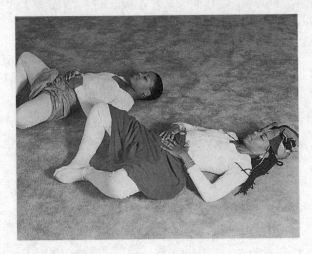

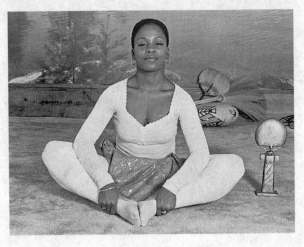

## 24. Rebirthing Pose: Womb Meditation for the Restoration of Peace in the Womb

*Description of Movement:* This is a repeat of #1. Lie flat on your back and draw your knees upward toward your hips. Place the soles of your feet together and open your thighs. Relax your back deep into the floor as your knees drop closer to the floor. Place palms gently and lovingly over your womb. Be sure to keep your elbows down. As you tune in to your breath, begin your womb meditation. Relax even more deeply as you meditate.

*Benefits:* Unblocks the tightness and stress within the pelvic area.

*Affirmation:* "I have come full circle. Now my womb is completely open and receptive to absolute wellness."

## 25. The Altar: Womb Pelvic Stretch

*Description of Movement:* To conclude your Dance of the Womb movements, return to womb affirmation and meditation with the Altar pose, #8. Sit up, back straight, shoulders down, neck long, chest lifted, feet together, thighs open, elbows resting on inner thighs. Now inhale with legs slightly open, then exhale as you press thighs open with your elbows. Do this until your legs are completely open and relaxed. Rock slowly from side to side, from hip to hip.

*Benefits:* Opens pelvic region, lubricates joints as it keeps you supple.

*Affirmation:* "I sit upon my inner throne and I affirm that the peace and harmony of my womb are my divine domain."

## A Free-Flowing Spirit

Not long ago, a sister came up to me and told me the following story.

*For some time my womb was in pain. I was experiencing all kinds of discomfort. I looked for help everywhere. Then one night in deep prayer, I stretched my soul and my arms up to the Creator/Creatress and woke up with a renewed attitude. I resolved to take my life seriously, and lovingly took my womb into my care and nurtured it as best as I could.*

*I did a sunbath and a womb dance. I vibrated my hips and shook out all of my years of madness. I took my womb into my care and I shaped her in the image of my Creator/Creatress.*

*I began to eat holistically, think high thoughts, exercise daily, pray continuously, meditate upon the coming of dawn by day, and by night I release malice out of my heart. I learned from my lessons. I forgave myself.*

*Now I am whole and my womb is whole and my spirit is free and flowing. I move my hips and my spirit in divine right rhythmic order, to flow with the Celestial Body that dwells inside of me.*

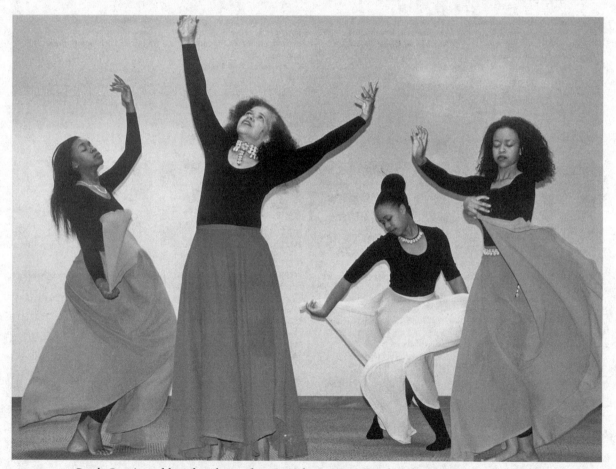

Starla Lewis and her daughters (l to r) Aisha La Star, Starla, Sherehe, Yamaisha Rozé, and Khaleedah Ishe founded CELL (Celebration of Everlasting Life and Love).

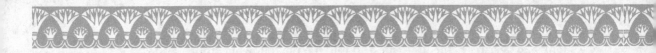

# THE DANCE OF THE WOMB CREED FOR SPIRIT REJUVENATION AND PURIFICATION

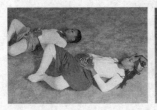

(1) Rebirthing Pose: I rebirth myself into existence through spirit, breath, sun, water, and roots . . .
*Key Vision: Womb Release*

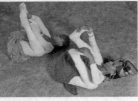

(2) Advanced Rebirth: The Great Mother dwells within me.
*Key Vision: Womb Expander*

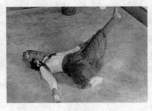

(3) The Lotus: I open up my lotus petals of Nefer Atum, expressing my inner beauty and harmony.
*Key Vision: Womb Opener*

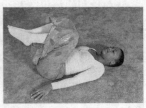

(4) The Womb Seat: Born out of my seat.
*Key Vision: Womb Balance*

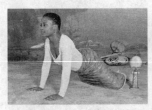

(10) The Waterfall: My womb is unlimited. She transforms into a soothing, cooling waterfall that allows waters to flush and baptize me, leaving my womb fresh like a lotus garden.
*Key Vision: Womb Cleanser*

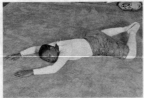

(11) The Offering: I surrender. I offer myself to the Great Mother Earth Ta-Urt to save me from womb catastrophe. Mama, take me in and keep me safe from harm and life's dangerous crossroads.
*Key Vision: Womb Rest*

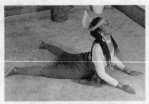

(12) Rennenet / The Cobra: I, the cobra, rise up the spine from the womb, the seat of Serpent Power of enlightening fire, to reach the heights to the all-knowing eye; opening myself up to Shai Destiny.
*Key Vision: Womb Stretch*

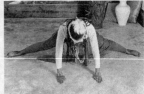

(13) Birth: I take on the challenge through *Meshkenet* of birthing myself again and releasing and learning from the pain of my lessons.
*Key Vision: Womb Stretch*

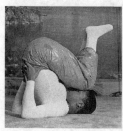

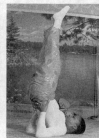

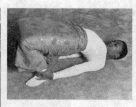

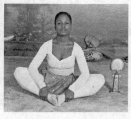

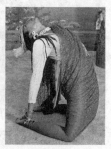

(5) Inner Reflection: I reflect my womb destiny. *Key Vision: Womb Lift*

(6) The Great Womb Purge: I ascend into the Mother Healer, the Great Womb Purge, allowing my ocean to wash and render my womb clean. *Key Vision: Womb Purger of Toxins*

(7) Bridge Over Troubled Water: I'm just like a bridge over troubled water. I'm clearing the tide of womb calamity. So I press on and on and on and up . . . *Key Vision: Womb Strengthener*

(8) The Altar: I go to the altar of peace and tranquility. *Key Vision: Womb Harmonizer*

(9) The Mountain: I climb this mountain to where my Womb Power maty be recharged and fulfilled. *Key Vision: Womb Stretch*

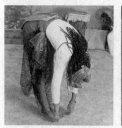

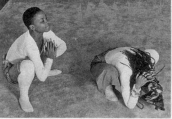

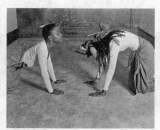

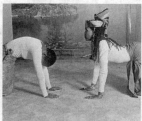

(14) Nut: Great Mother Nut of the Day and Night Sky of Illumination, I go into you. *Key Vision: Womb Release*

(15) The Seat of Mother Ast: And I come out filled with light, as only you can place me into the Seat of Ast, the Mother of Healing and nurturing. Upon this rock I sit in this seat and I shall not be moved. *Key Vision: Womb Realignment*

(16) Bes / The Cat: I am Bes, the Cat of Art and Creativity. I will create you a renewed Khat (womb) filled with energy. *Key Vision: Womb Energizer*

(17) Bes / The Cat: Come breathe through me. I will open you up to a softness and an inner grace that will set your soul free. *Key Vision: Womb Energizer*

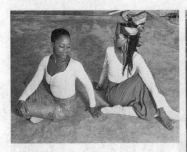

(18) The Moon: I am the Moon! Welcome home, sit down with me and glow. I rule the moon of your emotion. I live in the tide of your womb. Become one with me and I will give you sweet harmony.
*Key Vision: Womb Twisting Out Toxins*

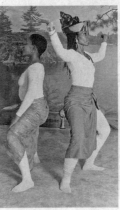

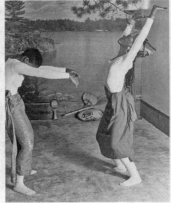

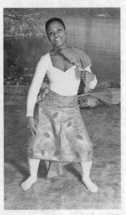

(19) Sun Ra: My womb is like Sun Ra—expansive, powerful, and radiant; and like the sun, my womb shines and shines and shines. She is free of all disease.
*Key Vision moves 19–22: All the active womb dances bring vitality and power to the physical and spiritual body of the womb, unleashing joy and gratitude*

(20) Praise the Creator/Creatress: I give praise to the Divine because my soul has a shine.
*Key Vision: Joy and Gratitude*

(21) Planetary Motion: I rotate my hips to the four directions—East, West, North, and South. Nut (Sky), Geb (Earth), Shu (Atmosphere), and Tefnut (Moisture). Womb, reaching every good and glorious part of me. Creating a new world, a higher calling, a pure humanity.
*Key Vision: Joy and Gratitude*

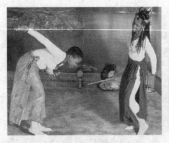

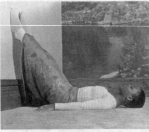

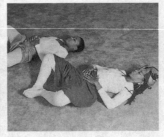

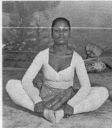

(22) The Volcano Erupts: Dancing the Dance of the Womb, causing Sekhmet (fire) flames to activate a global world healing through my womb's emancipation.
*Key Vision: Joy and Gratitude*

(23) The Pyramid: My dance helps me to join with my enlightened self as I rest in my ancestral pyramid of higher wisdom, causing me to have dominion over the heavens and the earth.
*Key Vision: Womb Flusher*

(24) Rebirthing Pose: After a long journey of womb wisdom in motion through the sacred Dance of the Womb, and after the sun of my womb has set, I return to yet another womb rebirth where my soul takes me to an inner womb reflection, and to the depths of my womb transformation.
*Key Vision: Womb Restabilizer*

(25) The Altar: As I sit at the light of my womb altar, I contemplate the Dance of the Womb, lifting me up like Hu (a sphinx), causing me to fly like Heru (a falcon). I give thanks for being pulled up and out of spiritual calamity and being gifted with complete womb peace and serenity.
*Key Vision: Womb Harmonizer*

# SACRED MOVEMENT: SEVEN-DAY TRANSFORMATIVE WORK

- *Perform the Dance of the Womb daily* (from the Dance of the Womb chart) for 20–45 minutes. If you have a friend or a mate, it's an added joy to perform this dance together.

- *Put your favorite music on and let the spirit move in you* as you dance to your sacred songs.

- *Study Sacred Movement,* such as Ari Ankh Ka/ Egyptian Yoga, or Afrakan, Brazilian, Haitian, Caribbean, or belly, jazz, or modern dance. These are my preferences, but don't be limited by them. Choose your own form of Sacred Movement.

- *Dance!* Dance can be performed before your altar, in your living room, throughout your house, or in Nature.

- *Expand your dance repertoire.* To make your Sacred Movement more elaborate, fun, and free-flowing, dance with bells, a drum, fans, scarves, or feathers. If you have a Het-Hru love blockage, dancing with bell waist beads helps to free your feminine energy. The sound of the bells as your hips gyrate forward and back and side to side inspires your womb to rotate in absolute ecstasy.

- *Dance with your eyes* as in Gateway 4: Sacred Beauty. This is a captivating and stimulating practice.

- *Dance together as a family* at least once a week, or as often as possible. Invite the whole family to dance together—mate, children, friends, mothers, fathers, grandparents, everybody. Sacred Movement will help to create a happy, free-flowing family.

- *After your dance take a warm salt bath* sprinkled with rose petals, and give thanks for the dance in your life.

- *Be careful not to dance on a full stomach* to avoid cramps.

- *Dance with what moves!* During your menses, you don't have to dance with the full body. You can stand or sit, and dance very gently with your arms, neck, and head, stretching your shoulders and rotating your ankles.

## My Sacred Movement End-of-the-Week Commitment:

I commit myself to establishing and continuing the wisdom of Bes and the power of Sacred Movement in all the areas of my life.

Signature: _____

Date: _____

# WOMAN RHYTHMS

*Gerianne Francis Scott*

*(Written for my mother, performed for my father)*

The Women of Dakar carry
Drumbeats in their hips
*da doom da doom*
Their breasts echo
Soft tom-tom rhythms
Their hands
sometimes staccato, sometimes still
on the way to market.
The Women of Dakar
wear many colors at one time
Embracing
All the magic power of a rainbow
as sisters of the sun
which glints off their smiles
and takes refuge in their ebony
    knowing eyes.
Gold wears the Women of Dakar to
    make itself look good.
The Women of Dakar
sauna on white-silver beaches,
allow Atlantic waters to caress
their feet and souls.
The Women of Dakar
anoint their liquid limbs with oils of
    coconut, peanut.
Pride is an ancient easiness
carved in their cheeks
woven into their braids.
The old Women and the tree
    monkeys watch carefully

as the Women of Dakar sing love
    noises that curl with village
    smoke
around cornstalks, peanut plants,
    and the men of Dakar.
Broad bowls of fish, fruits, fabric,
    flowers balanced on tall heads.
The Women of Dakar
know how to get the laundry clean
    without phosphate detergent.
The Women of Dakar.
And if the Women in Detroit,
    Brooklyn, Indianapolis,
    Memphis, Philadelphia,
Chicago, Watts,
Rio de Janeiro, Montreal, Atlanta,
    Portsmouth, San Juan,
Baltimore, Kingston, Georgetown,
    your town,
don't walk with music in them
    anymore
then something TERRIBLE has
    happened.
The Women of Dakar
carry music in their walk
to the market, to the Pier,
to the University, to the airport
And the children watch the women
and learn how to become
REGAL.

To receive the updated, expanded Womb Yoga Dance Teachings,
purchase Sacred Woman Womb Awaken in chapter 7 by Queen Afua.

# GATEWAY 4: SACRED BEAUTY

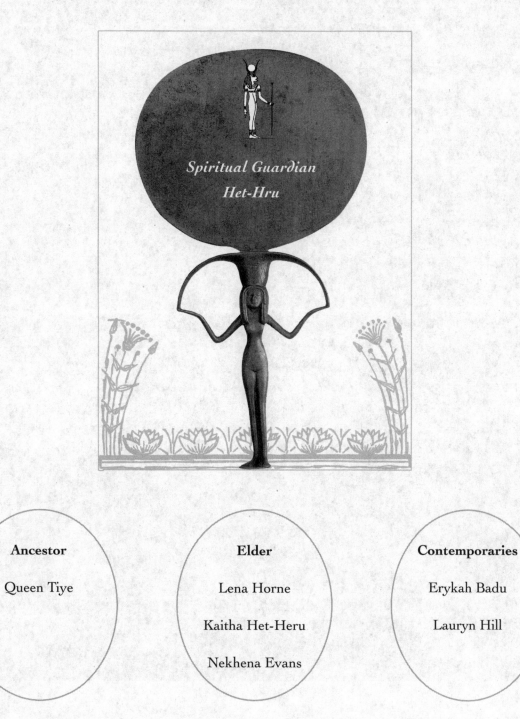

*Spiritual Guardian*
*Het-Hru*

**Ancestor**

Queen Tiye

**Elder**

Lena Horne

Kaitha Het-Heru

Nekhena Evans

**Contemporaries**

Erykah Badu

Lauryn Hill

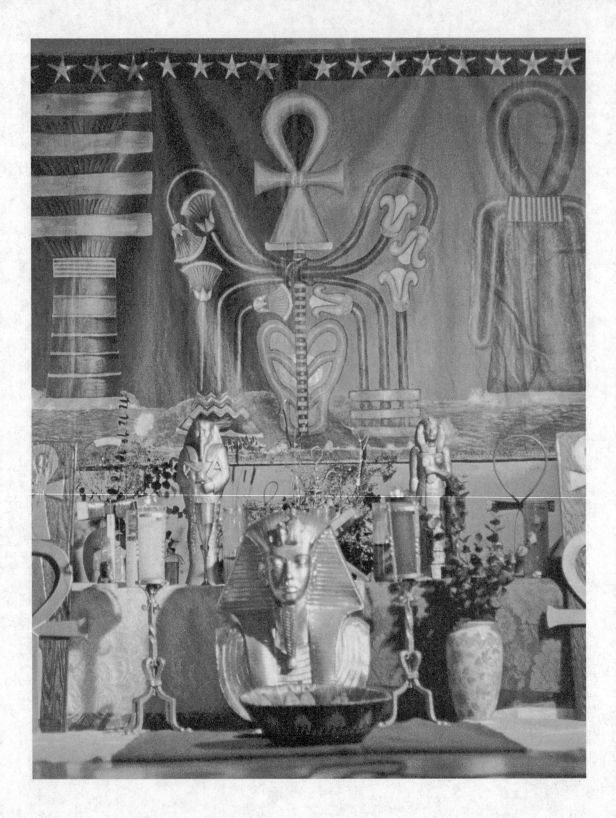

# SACRED BEAUTY ALTAR WORK
## Face Your Heart to the East—to the Rising Sun
*(Layout from top view)*

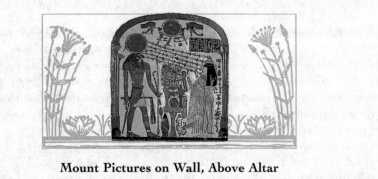

**Mount Pictures on Wall, Above Altar**

| | | | | |
|---|---|---|---|---|
| Picture of Spiritual Guardian | Picture of Ancestor | Picture of Sacred Self | Picture of Elder | Picture of Contemporary |

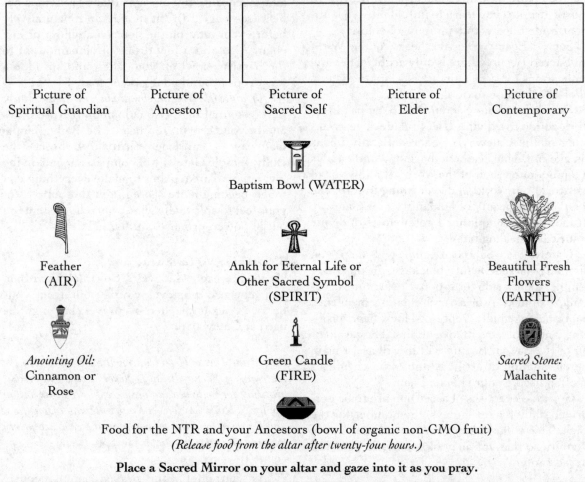

Baptism Bowl (WATER)

Feather (AIR)

Ankh for Eternal Life or Other Sacred Symbol (SPIRIT)

Beautiful Fresh Flowers (EARTH)

*Anointing Oil:* Cinnamon or Rose

Green Candle (FIRE)

*Sacred Stone:* Malachite

Food for the NTR and your Ancestors (bowl of organic non-GMO fruit)
*(Release food from the altar after twenty-four hours.)*

**Place a Sacred Mirror on your altar and gaze into it as you pray.**

Sacred tablecloth (green) and scarf to wear during prayer.
Sacred color cloth to lay before altar. Sacred instruments to be played as you pray.

# GATEWAY 4: SACRED BEAUTY DAILY SPIRITUAL OBSERVANCES

## Gateway Element: Earth

Sacred Beauty embraces the divine aesthetic of harmony within and without. It offers us a healthy alternative—the way of natural beauty to enhance our divine loveliness. Sacred Beauty brings harmony to every aspect of life through Khamitic etiquette, an ancient form of grace and beauty expressed through the Khamitic Nubian spiritual path. It will cosmically attune you to holistic dress as you learn to unfold into a beautiful attitude filled with a rainbow of colors.

Sacred Beauty rules the heart center. Without Sacred Beauty, there is only artificial beauty: applications for skin, hair, breasts, lips, and eyes, all of which cause toxic shock.

Developing your Sacred Beauty helps to create devotion to a divine, beautiful life. The awakening of the Gateway of Sacred Beauty opens the eye of divine aesthetic harmony and rids us of a mundane vision of the world. It allows us to transform our world and everything in it for the good and the beauty of humanity. This Gateway attunes us to the unlimited possibilities of divine beauty as a healing balm.

Gateway 4: Sacred Beauty will help you eliminate Sacred Beauty blockages in the Body Temple: boils, skin eruptions, deformities, eczema, baldness, psoriasis, circulation problems, emotional instability, repressed love, heart problems, and problems in love affairs. The awakening of the Sacred Beauty within will assist us in the elimination of artificial and toxic chemicals so often used on our skin and hair.

Spiritual exercises of ascension are to be performed daily for seven days, the number for the spirit. This will awaken your inner Gateways of Divinity so that you may blossom into your full sacred center.

## 1. The Spiritual Bath

Rose oil or cinnamon oil promotes love, forgiveness, compassion, and peace. Cinnamon oil helps to eliminate circulation problems, emotional instability, repressed love, and heart problems. (Avoid using it directly on your skin if your skin is sensitive.) When bathing, add 4 to 6 drops of cinnamon oil to the bathwater.

## 2. Your Altar

Set up your sacred altar on the first day of your entry into this Gateway. You may set up your altar according to your spiritual or religious beliefs (see page 18). Sit quietly and meditatively before your altar on the floor on a pillow, or in a chair. Also add a few drops of cinnamon oil to the baptism bowl on your altar, and sprinkle a few drops around your prayer space.

*Anoint with rose or cinnamon oil.* Select only pure essential oils. Use cinnamon or rose oil to anoint your crown, forehead (the Body Temple Gateway of supreme spirituality), heart (the Body Temple Gateway of compassion and divine love), womb area, palms to make everything you touch become more sacred, and the bottoms of your feet to spiritually align yourself for stepping out in power, promise, and faith.

## 3. Opening the Gateway

To invoke each Gateway's Spiritual Guardian, you may use whatever words pour from your heart. For example, here's a prayer that might be used at Gateway 4:

*Sacred and Divine Het-Hru, Spiritual Guardian of the Gateway of Sacred Beauty, please accept my deepest gratitude for your healing presence on my altar and in my life. Thank you for your guidance and inspiration, and for your love and blessings, and please accept my love and blessings in return.* Hetepu.

As you offer your prayer, simultaneously shake, ring, beat, or rattle a sacred instrument (sistrum bell, drum, shekere, or bells) to awaken the NTR that is indwelling.

### 4. Libation

Pour a libation for the Sacred Beauty Gateway from a special cup, or sprinkle water from a bowl onto the earth or a plant, as you call out this prayer of praise and adoration.

– *Pour a libation* as you say, *All praise and adoration to the Spiritual Guardian, Het-Hru, the Protector of Sacred Beauty.*
– *Pour a libation* as you say, *All praise and adoration to the Ancestor of Sacred Beauty, Queen Tiye.*
– *Pour a libation* as you say, *All praise and adoration to the Elders of Sacred Beauty, Lena Horne, Kaitha Het-Heru, and Nekhena Evans.*
– *Pour a libation* as you say, *All praise and adoration to my Divine Self and my Contemporary Divine Sisters, Erykah Badu and Lauryn Hill who honor Sacred Beauty.*

### 5. Sacred Woman Spirit Prayer

Ring a bell or play another sacred instrument at the beginning and end of this prayer. As you open your palms to the Sacred Spirit or gently place them over your heart, recite:

**Sacred Woman Spirit Prayer**

*Sacred Woman in the making,*
*Sacred Woman reawaken,*
*Sacred Spirit, hold me near.*
*Protect me from all harm and fear*
*beneath the stones of life.*
*Direct my steps in the right way as I journey*
*through this vision.*
*Sacred Spirit, surround me in your most absolute*
*perfect light.*
*Anoint me in your sacred purity, peace,*
*and divine insight.*
*Bless me, truly bless me, as I share*
*this Sacred Life.*
*Teach me, Sacred Spirit, to be in tune*
*with the Universe.*
*Teach me how to heal*
*with the inner and outer elements*
*of air, fire, water, and earth.*

### 6. Sacred Beauty Prayer

Shake bells, beat a sacred drum, or play another instrument at the beginning and ending of this prayer:

*Beloved Creator/Creatress, may my Body Temple become a sacred altar, clothed in an array of rainbow colors, reflecting the beauty and the boundless creativity of your light, so that my Body Temple may honor my beautiful spirit.*

*May divine beauty be anchored in my harmonious thoughts, and may my peaceful attitudes and consciousness be reflected in the sacredness of my dress. May I be a walking embodiment of the Beauty of the Creator/Creatress, so that others may be uplifted by the sacred beauty I emanate in all my ways.*

### 7. Chanting Hesi

Chant this *hesi* four times:

*Nuk Pu Ntrt Hmt* — I am a Sacred Woman.

### 8. Fire Breaths

Prepare for your Fire Breaths by slowly inhaling four times and exhaling four times. Then when you are totally at ease, begin your 500 Fire Breaths. Inhale deeply like a pump through your nose (mouth closed) as you expand the breath down into the abdomen, then back up to the chest. Completely exhale out through your nostrils from your abdomen as it contracts and the lungs release your breath completely. Repeat this breath rapidly in and out, in and out.

Allow each deep Fire Breath—rapidly inhaling and exhaling through your nostrils—to represent the opening of the thousand lotus petals of illumination and radiance to ultimately reach Nefer Atum—the ultimate Afrakan lotus station of Divinity.

### 9. Gateway 4: Sacred Beauty Meditation

Increase the length of time you spend in meditation every seven days. The longer you are in meditation, the deeper your inner peace will be, and the more solid your *ba* (spirit) will become.

The cleaner your Body Temple, the sooner it will be able to live permanently in the peace and inner balance of the meditative state.

As a Sacred Woman, I affirm that beauty is my divine inheritance; beauty is one of my sacred powers. I beam and radiate my inner Divinity, by adorning my outer Being with garments that befit my royal form.

Everything you wear reflects your inner consciousness, and that in turn has an effect on your soul. Experience this truth through the following meditation.

- Sit comfortably, close your eyes, and elevate your awareness to the blossoming lotus of your Divinity.
- Breathe in and out seven times, then visualize that you are in your home putting on a pair of red shorts with a black tank top and thick-soled sneakers.
- During your visualization, go outside and down the street in your mind's eye and see how you feel wearing these garments. Then observe how others react to your choice of clothing. Breathe in, breathe out. Let it flow.
- Go back home and put on tight blue jeans and an army surplus jacket with army boots. Now go outside and walk down the street in your mind's eye and see how you feel and observe how others view you. Breathe in and out.
- Go home and put on a short, tight skirt with a low-cut blouse and red high-heeled pumps. How do people respond, and how does what you are wearing affect you?
- Now see yourself in an expensive business suit, with jacket and skirt and silk blouse. Your hair is straightened and pulled back in a tight bun. You're wearing panty hose and high heels and carrying a briefcase. How do you feel about who you are? How do other people respond to you?
- Return home and put on a flowing dress that falls below your knees or down to your ankles. Put on dressy sandals or low-heeled shoes. Go outside. How do people around you respond? How do you feel?
- Return home and put on a grand buba and jewelry and accessories, with a flowing scarf. Does this outfit speak to you of balance, harmony, strength, softness, joy, high self-esteem, sensuality, grandeur? How do you visualize others responding to you?

Once you decide on what you want to project through this active meditation, then you will intuitively know what to wear and what garments you have outgrown. You will know what garments reflect your spiritual and mental growth, demonstrating how you think and feel about yourself.

Dress is also a code that speaks to the world about who you are. Choose your garments wisely, for they can close or open doors for you. The way in which you dress can even protect you in some cases. For example, when you dress in a culturally affirmative way and walk through a violent or aggressive neighborhood, see how much respect you'll receive. Dress creates an aura around you; through what you wear you can stir up positive or negative vibrations in your world. Your dress has the power to soothe a wild beast, revitalize low energy, bring serenity to a troubled soul, or just make you feel beautiful. It's amazin'!

Slowly open up your eyes and breathe in and out once again as you become one with the beauty that is dressed from your soul. Always remember your Sacred Beauty Meditation and that beauty is in the eyes of the beholder. So behold your beauty close to your heart, and your beauty will heal yourself and all others.

*Color Visualization.* Visualize the color of the Gateway: green for regeneration, fertility, and growth. As you perform your meditation, wear green and/or place a green cloth on your altar.

*Sacred Stone Meditation.* While in meditation, hold in your palm over your heart the sacred healing stone of Gateway 4: malachite—a green stone that aids in balancing and calming all those who come in contact with it. This stone energizes the fourth *arit* (chakra), which regulates the heart center, the seat of love and compassion. The tool of the Gate of Het-Hru is *khepera* (transformation), and Het-Hru's sacred instrument is the sistrum (a tambourinelike rattle). Play the sistrum as you do the transformative work of this Gateway to lift the vibration of Het-Hru from deep within you, so it shines through you and all around you.

### 10. Herbal Tonics

Drink aloe vera juice or tea. Remember, what's bitter to the taste is sweet to the spirit. Aloe vera creates a lovely disposition in women.

Aloe has been found in Khamitic tombs thousands of years old. It was used in abundance by our ancient Afrakan Ancestors to enhance beauty and health.

Taken internally, it is a powerful blood purifier and colon cleanser. Applied under the arms, it acts as a deodorant, and for internal cleansing it can be used as a powerful douche—all of which aids in our beautification, within and without.

Aloe vera gel is excellent for treating burns, scars, blemishes, sores, and wounds. It helps to remove dead skin and stimulates normal growth of cells. It also acts as a moisturizer for the skin, and is wonderful as a natural shampoo for the hair.

Drink your herb tea or tonic for seven days to receive the full benefits of tuning in to Gateway 4. Enjoy your herb tea in your favorite mug during or after spiritual writing.

*Preparation.* Use 1 tbsp. gel (scraped from inside the fresh leaves) to 1 cup of water. Boil water, turn off flame, pour water over gel, and stir. Drink before or after your morning bath or sacred shower. Drink with joy and peace as you breathe between sips and settle into easy contemplation and reflection.

### 11. Flower Essences

To deepen your experience of Gateway 4, choose from the following flower essences. Take 4 drops four times per day directly on or under the tongue, or add the same amount to a small glass of purified water and sip. For instructions on how to choose flower essences, see page 23.

- *Pomegranate:* Conflicting creative desires, especially in expression of the feminine part of self.
- *Iris:* Creative inspiration and artistic expression, especially from the higher realms.
- *Indian paintbrush:* Bringing vitality to creative expression, especially from earthly forces.
- *Pretty face:* Beauty that radiates from within; self-acceptance through understanding that true beauty is an attribute of the soul.
- *Pink monkeyflower:* Addresses issues of fear of exposure and rejection; hiding essential self from others.

### 12. Diet

Follow the Sacred Woman Transitional Dietary Practices presented for Gateways 4–6.

### 13. Sacred Beauty Journal Writing

This is best done after internal cleansing (enema) and/or meditation. When you are cleansed and centered, you can receive spiritual messages from the One Most High with grace. When you are in the spirit, messages travel down through your spirit mind, to your heart, into your hand, and onto the paper. (This is how I do all my writing.)

The best time to receive your spiritually inspired written work is after you have completed your altar work, between the hours of 4 A.M. and 6 A.M. Keep your journal and a very special pen by or on your altar to work with the power, force, and stillness at the coming of dawn, the hour of Nebt-Het.

Affirm your daily life. Write in your journal at this time thoughts, activities, experiences, and interactions that present themselves. You can also write down your visions, desires, dreams, and affirmations so that you will be able to draw on these resources when help and support are most needed.

*Consult Sesheta.* If you find that you are unable to contact your inner voice during your journal work, call Sesheta, the keeper and revealer of secrets (who is indwelling), to assist and speak through you.

### 14. Senab Freedom Shawl or Quilt

Choose a new piece of cloth that corresponds to the Gateway color (indicated in exercise 9 of your Daily Spiritual Observances or in Sacred Altar Work) to add to your Senab Freedom Shawl or Quilt. This cloth will serve as a mini-canvas to represent your experience in the Gateway you're working in.

Also, collect meaningful symbols that can be added to your shawl or quilt in appliqué or patchwork style. You can add stones, other natural objects, collectibles, family heirlooms, photographs that have been reprinted on fabric, or any other significant items that embody the essence of your experience. Give your imagination free rein and let your craftswoman spirit tell your story. For more information about the Senab Freedom Shawl or Quilt, see pages 122–125.

### 15. Sacred Tools

Four yards of cloth to practice wrapping and draping your Body Temple with simple beauty.

### 16. Sacred Reminder

Throughout the week, you are to observe closely the wisdom presented in Gateway 4: Sacred Beauty. For maximum results, live freely in tune with the various systems of wellness presented, and practice the Seven-Day Transformative Work at the end of the Gateway.

### Closing Sacred Words

*Mother/Father, help me to keep a beautiful. sacred Body Temple within and without, that I might live my life as a work of beauty in the world.*

# TRANSITIONAL DIETARY PRACTICES FOR GATEWAYS 4–6

Continue the same dietary practice that is presented in Gateways 1 to 3. The difference in dietary practices for Gateways 4 to 6 is that now you will eat 50 percent cooked (steamed), 50 percent raw (live/uncooked). Live enzymes are stored in live, uncooked foods.

## Before Breakfast

Kidney-Liver Flush (see page 72).

## Breakfast

Drink fruit juice and/or eat fruits one hour before or after other foods, for better digestion.

Freshly pressed fruit juices, 8 to 12 oz. (diluted with 8 to 12 oz. pure water), with Heal Thyself Green Life Formula I, 1 to 2 tbsp.

*Fruits:* Acid fruits: grapefruit, lemons, limes, oranges, tangerines. Subacid fruits: apples, pears, plums, cherries, berries, peaches. No bananas. Keep acid fruits together. Keep subacid fruits together. *Do not mix acid and subacid fruits together.*

Include live-food breakfast.

You may have cooked whole-wheat, dairy-free pancakes with maple syrup one to three times a week. Or rice, soy, sesame, or almond milk.

## Lunch

Freshly pressed vegetable juices, 8 to 12 oz. (diluted with 8 to 12 oz. of water), with Heal Thyself Green Life Formula I, 1 to 2 tbsp.

Large raw salad. No tomatoes, but include plenty of sprouts, such as alfalfa, mung bean, etc. Include any of the following: okra, kale, cauliflower, turnip greens, mustard greens, broccoli, seaweed in any form (i.e., kelp, hijiki, wakame, nori), to add to soups or salads.

*Proteins:* Choose one only:

- Sprouts soaked in water overnight
- Peas
- Lentils
- Beans
- Tofu
- Texturized vegetable protein (TVP)

If you are a flesh consumer in transition, prepare baked fish (no shellfish), soy chicken, or organic chicken one to three times a week. You can also choose from raw soaked nuts (almonds, filberts, walnuts, pecans; avoid cashews and peanuts) and seeds (sunflower, pumpkin).

*Starches:* Choose one of the whole grains, four to seven times a week. Soak light grains (tabouli, couscous) 10 minutes before eating; soak denser grains (bulgur, wheat, millet) 1–2 hours, or cover overnight.

During this transition period, you may also have cooked brown rice, baked potatoes, or whole-wheat and sprouted bread (dry toasted) or corn on the cob (lightly steamed or raw).

## Dinner

Repeat lunch. Increase freshly pressed/juiced vegetable juices to 12 to 16 oz. (diluted with pure water), with Heal Thyself Green Life Formula I, 1 to 2 tbsp. After the sun goes down, do not eat proteins or starches! Eat only live foods: salads, fruits and vegetables, steamed vegetables, vegetable soup/broth.

# DIETARY SUPPORTS

### Nutrients

Take three times a day with juice or some form of chlorophyll, such as one of the following:

- Powdered wheatgrass (1 tsp. to 1 tbsp.), or liquid, 1 to 2 oz., with distilled water.
- Powdered spirulina (1 tsp. to 1 tbsp.), or liquid, 1 to 2 oz., with distilled water.
- Powdered blue-green manna (1 tsp. to 1 tbsp.), or liquid, 1 to 2 oz., with distilled water.
- If stressed, take 25 to 50 mg of vitamin B complex, or you will have skin eruptions.
- For poor memory and poor circulation, take 1 tbsp. of granulated lecithin.
- For a debilitated immune system, also take 500 to 1,000 mg of vitamin C a day.

### Internal Cleansing

Take an enema seven nights straight, then three times a week throughout the weeks to follow. Herbal laxatives: 3 tablets of cascara sagrada *every other day*. Colonics: one to two during the twenty-one-day cleansing period.

### Physical Activity

Practice the abbreviated Dance of the Womb fifteen to thirty minutes daily, or the complete two-hour regimen, and do five hundred Fire Breaths daily.

### Rejuvenation Baths

Epsom salts, 1 to 4 lbs., or 1 lb. Dead Sea salt in your bath, seven nights straight. Time for soaking: fifteen to thirty minutes. Then shower off the salt. (Do not use bath salts if you have high blood pressure.)

### Heal Thyself Master Herbal Formula II

At bedtime daily, boil 5 to 6 cups of purified or distilled water, turn off the flame, and add 3 tsp. herbs. Steep overnight. Strain in the morning, and drink before 2 P.M. (See chapter 3, and see the product list in the appendix.)

### Queen Afua's Rejuvenating Clay Application

Optional, according to need. Follow instructions on pages 91–92. (See the product list in the appendix.)

### Other Nature Cures

Drink at least 2 to 3 quarts of distilled water daily. You may add the juice of 1 lemon or lime and/or a sacred stone or crystal to the water. (Do not swallow the crystal or stone.)

# FEMININITY
### by Hazelle Goodman

See I ain't got time for all them batting of the eyes
    and whispering in your ear
I'm just gon' tell you loud how I feel — You HEAR?!

## I WANT YOU AND THAT'S THAT!
I ain't got time to play hard to get 'cause all I may get
    is left back!

I can't waste no time with hushed tones and feathery
    steps cause you may just not get who I am
And when I come for my check you might act like you
    done forget
In which case I'm gone have to go upside yo head with
    my hard nonfeminine hand

See when I was young and trying to be sweet, life
    got together with some friends and beat the mess
    outta me

Then by the time my x husband broke my jaw — I
    jumped up and said, "Dammit, I ain't gon' be sweet
    no more!"

Walking around all sweet, battered and abused — Uh
    Uh, forget it!
I'm not gon' be on 60 Minutes or in the Daily News!

So that's when I got up and started fighting back
That's when I started to scream and talk loud in your
    offices and on your trains

I was gonna make sure you didn't never forget my
    name

That's why I took my femininity and put her in an ol'
    shoe box underneath my bed, next to where I hides
    my opportunity money.

But every time I go to gets me some cash for an oppor-
    tunity, I see my femininity sitting there all
dusty and sad looking at me, hoping I don't come to get
    her at last.

Asking for my sweet ol' femininity to come back to my
    heart.

Then I got still and noticed that my steps become
    lighter like I was running on air, and my tears
were honey sweet and a loving feeling filled the atmo-
    sphere.

My hard hands became soft and silky smooth, and I
    couldn't get my scream above a hushed kinda
    croon.

Then suddenly I realized my femininity was back,
    back inside of me.
I'm not scared no more about not being heard 'cause
    I've got all the strength I need in a soft word.

But let me tell you this, don' get smart and try to walk
    all over me and my femininity, 'cause we'll knot
    you gently upside yo head!

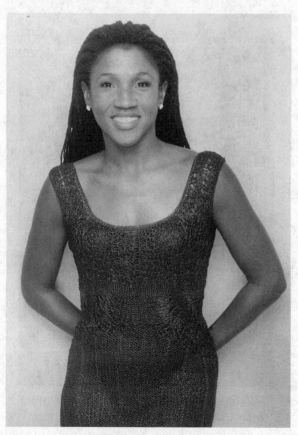

Actress and Writer Hazelle Goodman

# RECLAIMING OUR ANCIENT AFRAKAN BEAUTY

Thousands of years ago, Afrakan beauties were the most sought-after women there were. Foreigners went absolutely insane when they saw our Ancestors' sun-ripened, melanin-rich Nubian skin and honeydew hips. Afrakan women had the capacity to squat in a childbearing position and birth all the many colors of the world. Afrakan women were amazing!

Centuries later, we are wearing somebody else's garments. Where are the symbols of our natural beauty? Where are our adornments, our woven linens, our drapes, and our shawls, our turquoise and amethyst neckpieces, our silver and bronze bracelets, our lapis lazuli headpieces and anklets, our cowrie-shell waist beads, our gold and silver toe rings, our lotus flower earrings worn by our sisters Queen Tiye and Nefertari? When did we stop wearing quartz crystals and gems in purple, blue, white, green, bronze, and topaz? What happened to our sacred perfumed oils, lavender, sandalwood, and almond? Have we forgotten that black kohl protects our eyes and gives them mystery?

Here, take back your gray suits and trench coats, the garments you wear to "dress for success" and prosperity. We can no longer be hypnotized away from our true Afrakan self by commercials and marketing tricks.

## Reclaiming My Ancient Afrakan Beauty

*I now reclaim my sacred Afrakan beauty legacy that was designed to empower me!*

*I will express my own natural beauty and grace: from the ancient Afrakan lotus flower that sat on my crown and draped over my first eye to indicate my thoughts of divine perfection and illumination, to the crown I wore on my head to indicate high spiritual consciousness; from the headband swirling around my first eye to protect my higher mind and keep me in tune, and the circular earrings that link me to the infinite continuum of the cosmos, and my earrings of gold and silver, of faience and gems I see worn by my Ancestors carved on the walls of Abydos, Amarna, and Philae; to the floral colors that bathe me in rainbow radiance, and my formfitting and full-flowing wraps and robes.*

*I anoint myself with spiritual oils—with mandrake, frankincense and myrrh, sage, and cedar—to protect me from any harm and danger. I will do all these things and more to create harmonious vibrations around myself and my mate. I will lovingly do my part to restore the love and respect that by nature we have for each other. I will groom, calm, and dress my soul by playing and listening to the sounds of the Divine NTRU, with the sounds of harps, bells, strings, flutes, and drums—surrounded by the melodic voices of my ancestry that continue to live in me.*

*You ask where is my ancient Afrakan beauty? I am here, and thus it is here. I defend my right to be—here I stand!*

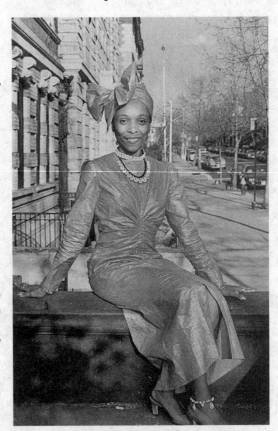

This cultural Sacred Dress that affirms natural beauty was designed by Ntr Tehuti's Touch.

## Call for a New Era of Afrakan Beauty
### by Kaitha Het-Heru

*The world is indebted to us for the benefits of civilization. They stole our arts and sciences from Afraka. Then why should we be ashamed of ourselves?*

— MARCUS GARVEY, HONORABLE ANCESTOR

Telling our story from an Afrakan perspective is important. It gives us the truth about ourselves. It is our way of looking into our past and remembering with the aid of images and writings found on temple walls, tombs, and monuments how we worked, played, dressed, and lived every day. Without our story, researched and written by us, we have no link to our past, no connection to our Ancestors.

Without our own identity, we are adrift in a sea of constantly changing images controlled by the image makers of the larger culture. We are left searching for self, being "in style" with whatever is the current fashion of the day. One day it's Jheri curls we maintain by wearing plastic shower caps in the streets; next day, it's blue or green contact lenses; next it's pants worn down below our behinds . . .

Beautiful Nubian Afrakan women existed before the beginning of recorded history. Their timeless beauty reflected their inner state of mind. Over five thousand years ago, in the ancient days of our Nubian Afrakan civilization in the land of Tawi (predynastic Egypt), the temples were schools of learning where the sacred arts of beautifying and ennobling the Body Temple were taught.

In the Temple of Het-Hru, dedicated to the sacred principles of divine love, beauty, nurturance, joy, music, and dance, young women were initiated by Wise Women called *abutu*, or Priestesses. They were taught the sacredness of the Great Divine Universal Mother, Mut Ast (renamed Isis by the Greeks). They learned that love and beauty are divine in essence and begin with inner harmony at the center of one's being that radiates out to the world. Beauty was not just cosmetic, only enhancing the appearance; it was also cosmological. True beauty involved knowing the spiritual, mental, and physical laws governing the universe. The young initiates learned that to be beautiful was to be in harmony with Nature.

We always saw ourselves as beautiful. Knowing that we were beautiful generated respect for our body as a sacred, divine gift to be honored and cared for. Beauty to Nubian Afrakan women meant taking the time to nurture the self. We knew that being beautiful meant taking charge of our thoughts and actions. The word for "beautiful" in our ancient Mtu NTR language is *nefer.*

We are descendants of beautiful royal Afrakan women. Queen Tiye (1415–1340 BCE) was a powerful Nubian Afrakan queen from the land of Kush. This great royal spouse of Amenhotep III was the mother of Pharaohs Akhenaten and Tutankhamen, and mother-in-law of Nefertiti, one of history's most classical beauties. Tiye reigned as Queen Consort and Queen Mother of Khamit for half a century. She had a great influence on arts and the fashions of the time in Khamit, from the changing of hairstyles—she adorned her head with short Nubian-style wigs instead of the long-haired wigs fashionable at the time—to the wearing of jewelry.

### Reclaiming Our Heritage

The consequences of more than three hundred years of transatlantic slavery, beginning in the early sixteenth century, and the continuing mental enslavement of our people today, have had devastating effects. Much of the knowledge of our story, our love of life, as well as the true meaning of being beautiful, was lost or suppressed. There was not much time for beauty, culture, or body care when you labored from dawn to dusk in the cotton fields.

Our rallying cry, "Black Is Beautiful," arose in the revolutionary 1960s. We began to wear our hair in a "natural" or "Afro." It was a visible statement of a shift in our consciousness. It was a time when we began to love ourselves and to reclaim our ancestral link to Afraka, our Motherland.

Sadly, the pride we felt in the '60s has become a far too distant memory. Today, most of us have been seduced by the mass media into a hypnotic trance. It is time for a new era of Afrakan Beauty Culture and *Love of Self*. The current fad of external youthful beauty being fed to us will fade with time. We must awaken from this soul sleep, which is orchestrated by the dominant media and advertisers who tell us what to wear, what to eat, and what to think to make us conform to their standard of beauty.

Such confusion causes us to emulate the Afrakan American models with blue eyes and blond hair we see on TV and in magazines. We are bearing witness to the lightening/whitening of ourselves. The messages we continually receive are that we are not, and will never be, good enough unless we Europeanize, homogenize, and pasteurize ourselves into their mold.

We must remember this: We are the Original Model. The Original Model was perfect; excellence was the pattern. "We have been created and come forth from the limbs of NTR, the One Most High," states our Holy Book, *Prt M Hru M Ghr, The Book of Coming Forth by Day from Night* (misnamed *The Egyptian Book of the Dead*). Let us stop patterning ourselves after mediocrity. The world is already filled with mediocre people.

The Sacred Het-Hruian principles of Divine Love and Beauty are a philosophy that each of us can put into practice in our daily lives. The tools needed to produce a new beauty culture based on this ancient Afrakan paradigm are: researching and studying our ancient Hapi (Nile) Valley High Culture, living in accordance with the Forty-Two Laws of Maat, prayer, meditation, maintaining an attitude of thankfulness, eating a balanced natural diet, proper exercise, daily grooming, and natural body care.

It is the knowledge of the beauty of our ancient Nubian Afrakan Hapi Valley High Culture, love and respect for ourselves, all beings, and Ta-Urt, the Great Earth Mother, that will assist us as a people in bringing forth the seed of a new world in which love, beauty, peace, and harmony will be restored within the Sacred Circle of Life.

*Sankofa!* (which means going back to fetch what is due to you). Go back and fetch it! Go within and get it! Our greatness, our beauty, our love, is within us, encoded in our genes. As we return to the realization of our Divinity and the first seed teachings that made us the greatest civilization the world has ever known, we will begin to have a different perspective of ourselves.

## The Melting Pot

I'm in total agreement with Het-Heru. From my point of view, our lost legacy is further compromised by the "melting-pot syndrome."

They say America is a melting pot. I've heard this most of my life. I was always concerned about that concept because I kept wondering whose pot we're all being melted down into. How willingly we jump into this pot headfirst and take on all the ingredients of the mix, which is predominantly from European cultures. So what happens to us as Afrakans? What happens to our particular gifts as a race? What happens? What has already happened!

We go to school and get our education and indoctrination. We give praise in the rituals of foreign religions. We wear other people's clothes, follow their customs and traditions. We oftentimes trade ourselves off to become the successful corporate professional. We break our fists trying to break through the glass ceiling. We become a part of the great melting pot.

We melt ourselves down to what? And we come out as who? Surely not ourselves. Do we melt out what makes us uniquely Afrakan, and become one of "the guys" or one of "the gals"? In this melting pot, most of my sister girlfriends and family have learned to press the kink out of their hair just to identify with the look of another woman's tribe. We're the only women on earth who consistently impose violence on our crown to take on the ideal of another tribe's beauty. Our kinks had to be melted down no matter what the cost.

Then came the 1960s to rescue our looks and our souls as sacred, strong, beautiful Afrakan women. As we dressed in our traditional clothing, we received the ritual healing of our self-image. Unfortunately, in the 1990s we've regressed, and we're back trying to melt into someone else's image of beauty, trying to melt into anybody's pot but our own. In the 1960s, African cultural schools came along to save our children's minds. We opened up independent businesses and hired our own people when no one else would. We were growing freer and more and more independent.

Then, in the early 1980s, drugs were poured into our communities by people in high places. We began working for the government and corporations. We had to dress for success, so our clothes and our natural hair just had to go. Our ways as natural Afrakans could not be accepted by this melting pot. To quality for employment, only a European look would do. Many of our people have had surgery to shape their once round Afrakan noses to pointed tips. Others have trimmed down their lips. Still others have bleached their dark skin to a lighter hue. We've taken on a more so-called acceptable look of the economically dominant race, who gained their "old money" from the hands of our forebears in slavery.

When we put in green, blue, and hazel contact lenses to cover our Afrakan brown eyes, do we melt down our intuitive nature, that part of us that functions from a high spiritual plane? Do we sacrifice what is most humane for what is most efficient? Our lives become less about how we feel as people, and more about what we think. Do we melt down all of our Afrakan traditions and customs, our way of being, our expressions of spirituality?

With this melting pot continuously boiling all the ingredients into one taste, where's the spice? It tastes bland to me. In the process of the makeover, I am posing as a stranger to myself. And what about the other cultures of people of color? Must we all wear suits and ties to participate in the American way of life? And whose excellence are we talking about in this great big melting pot? Surely not my own.

Thank you very much, but I'm not getting into your melting pot. I'll make my own soup with my own taste and freshness and richness, the soup that my ancient Afrakan mother prepared in the Nile Valley. Matter of fact, if you act right, you're welcome to come over to my pot and taste some of my simmered greens smothered in sage and other rich, secret tastes. I don't wanna be cooked down or toned down or blended into someone else's pot. Cooking from my own pot and spicing things up with my own taste, especially for me, is what I'm looking for.

My cultural diversity is what gives color to the human family.

## BEAUTY IS POWER

*Love and Beauty is within . . . what is within must manifest. The greater the awareness of the truth of our own Being, the greater your power.*
—KAITHA HET-HERU

As Het-Heru has said, "Don't judge a book by its cover." How many times have you heard that saying? However, you are judged by your cover—your dress. How you present yourself to the world tells a lot about you. It identifies you with a group, tells the world where you're from, who you are, and what you think of yourself. It signals others how you expect to be treated.

Sisters, as Nubian Afrakan women, you must set the standard of excellence in your demeanor and appearance. Wearing no panty hose or bra on the street and gyrating to monotonous music on national TV in skintight minidresses is not the image our children and our men need to see.

The simple, elegant lives of our classical dress shown on the temple walls from the Hapi Valley can provide inspiration and a new source of income for those of you seeking to become economically self-sufficient. European fashion designers have used our Nubian cultural dress to inspire their design collections for many years.

### You Are What You Wear

Increase your magnetism by energizing your natural beauty.

Whatever moved you to wear a garment, let it express your inner beauty. This is how we stay in tune with Nature's beautiful sky, green meadows, spring flowers, and mysterious ocean—all gifts of the elements of the Creator/Creatress.

Beauty in dress is a force that we as Afrakans traditionally combined with purpose. It is how we remain in keeping with the natural flow of beauty in womanform. Every wrap, drape, color, gemstone, headdress, or flower that was worn indicated your past history or present lifestyle and condition. Garments made a statement and had a purpose; this was the Afrakan way. Dress that was spiritually directed was worn for tribal ceremonies and rituals. Members of the same family often wore the same colors or made clothes from the same kind of cloth. Women wore particular drapes and jewelry to indicate their marital status.

The Ancients understood that what you place on your Body Temple is of great significance. This is why we must wear our clothes consciously. Clothes can ward off demons and summon the angels. Observe and keep a mental record of how your world is affected, and in turn how you are affected, by what you wear or what others wear.

## Cultural Sacred Dress

On one of my many trips to Washington, DC, to facilitate Wellness Seminars, I noticed that everyone traveling on the plane was wearing dark colors—black, brown, dark blue, and gray. I stood out, draped in my cultural colors of purple and white, with a small delicate feather in my hair representing Maat (harmony). Everyone kept smiling at me as though they wished they could have the same kind of freedom, to be different and to live a color-filled life.

Maybe one day all of us will begin to wear our culture and stop assimilating into one look and one way, trying to fit into another's limited view of who we are supposed to be. Reuben Amber, author of *Color Therapy*, puts it this way: "Life is color . . . colors must vibrate (within, on and around us) to keep harmonies balanced and rhythmically functioning."[1]

Wearing our various colors keeps us emotionally and mentally balanced, joyous and healthy, both as individuals and as part of the collective world. Color is what reminds us that we're unique expressions of life and not clones. When we are dominated by having to wear black, brown, and gray, it's a sign that we are dying. With the so-called European dress-for-success policy, we seem to be globally living through perpetual late autumn and winter with our dark colors.

It's time to declare the spring of the self. Behold the summer sun and let your colors glow and shine. Envision the beauty of Afrakans dressing in their color-filled tradition, Native Americans draped in their culture, Asians, Irish, East Indians, Brazilians, Norwegians, Inuit, and Middle Easterners all wearing our different, beautiful, colorful traditions. What an energy charge it would give our world.

What would happen if we all just broke out one day and said, "No more! I am what I am—colorful and unique. From now on I'm going to express myself and my cultural heritage through the colorful clothes I wear." All of us vibrating with the freedom to be—a rainbow of human colors. I believe this planet would vibrate on a higher level if we stood our cultural wellness ground, creating world harmony and respect.

## Dresses, Lappas, Wraps, Pants, Shawls

Cloth, textures, style, and colors speak to how I feel, what I think, my message, my peace, my alone time, my sacredness. When I wear my array of colorful velvet dresses, I feel mystical and chic. (It is appropriate that I am sometimes referred to as the Velvet Sword.) When I wear my shawl over my shoulder, I feel spiritually protected. When I wear my lappa (a traditional Afrakan skirt), I feel connected to my indigenous roots. When I wear a Grand Buba (a traditional Afrakan robe/dress), I feel royal. Wearing my yoga attire, I feel flexible and powerful. With my pink mountain climbing boots on, I feel like a force of nature. When I am wearing purple, I feel like Nebt-Het, the Lady of the House, the Healing Realm. Wearing my whites, I feel like fasting. When I wear beautiful lace cotton pants and a loose-fitting blouse, I feel strong in my loveliness.

Over the last twenty years, I've found that clothes speak to me like the Ancestors and help identify where I am in my life at that time of my life. Clothes, like food, like sunshine, air, and water, have become a part of my medicine. As I dress my body or an altar or a window or a table, the cloth, whether simple or elegant, becomes a beautiful dance that I use to encourage, to transform, to enlighten myself and all those I meet on my journey. My attire has opened doors, told my story, and ended chapters. The next time you get dressed, keep in mind what you want to accomplish. What you want to create will be enhanced by your choice of garment. Follow your heart and your intuition to wear what you are inspired to. Your dress, lappa, wrap, pants, shawl in combination with color, texture, and style can bring you a greater life of communication and therefore give you greater opportunities to deliver your message.

# CLASSICAL AFRAKAN NILE VALLEY WEAR

Our Sacred Nebt-Het/Ast (sister-to-sister) shawls, wraps, and drapes are blessed to evoke the Nile Valley spirit of our ancestors when worn in a state of meditation, protection, inner peace, and *smai tawi* (unity).

## The Lappa

Dress represents a people exactly the way food represents a people. For example, people get into Hatha Yoga for body conditioning and for mindful meditation. But it's not just Hatha Yoga, it's a practice that also reflects Indian culture. It may not be your culture, but you can dress within that cultural realm, you can eat within that cultural realm, you can recite Sanskrit prayers and chants and experience that same cultural realm.

The ancient dress of our Afrakan cultural base is the lappa. Lappas come in many designs and represent a wide range of cultural expression. So if you're committed to expressing your Afrakan woman-self, then it's important to take on the cultural dress that represents us as a people. The more you take on, the more you will feel like a Sacred Woman wherever you go in the world.

## Lap Your Lappa for Simple Elegance

Your lappa may be wrapped at the length of your ankles, your calves, or just below your knees.

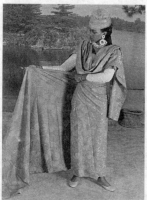

**Step 1.** Separate your legs a few feet apart as you wrap the cloth around you; this is so you have room to walk in your lappa. Next bring your legs together and continue to wrap your cloth around your hips.

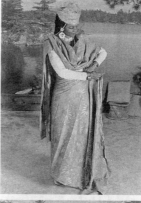

**Step 2.** When you bring the cloth around the second or third time, your legs are together.

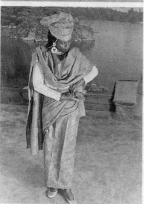

**Step 3.** Next, fold over the top end of your fabric to create a natural waistband. For reinforcement, add a belt or scarf at your waist or, better, attach a drawstring at each end of the lappa from the same cloth to go around your waist. Or feel secure and leave it as it is and go into your day with beauty and zest. Know that you're looking your Afrakan best!

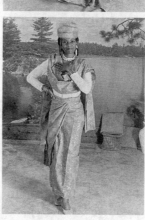

**Step 4.** You can drape one to two yards of cloth over your shoulders. Or create a *pedessa*, a protective sacred garment.

# Cosmic Dress

You can tune in to the universe through color. Coordinate your entire outfit or accessorize in the color of the day with a scarf, blouse, or head wrap. Initiates of the Shrine of Ptah organize their wardrobes to reflect the planetary influence through the color of the day. Let this way of Cosmic Dressing put your life in divine order.

| Day of Week | Ruling Heavenly Body | Color | NTRU (Divine Principle) | Function of Ancient Principles |
|---|---|---|---|---|
| Sunday | Sun | Orange | Hru | Will and determination |
| Monday | Moon | Blue | Ast | Divine mother or divine teacher |
| Tuesday | Mars | Red | Hru Khuti | Warrior |
| Wednesday | Mercury | Yellow | Tehuti | Wisdom, power of the word |
| Thursday | Jupiter | Purple | Ptah | Craftsperson, foundation, creativity |
| Friday | Venus | Green | Het-Hru | Nurturer, divine love |
| Saturday | Saturn | Red or pure indigo and black | Set | Grounding |

Families in Afraka show unity by the way they dress. You might see all members of the family—husband, wife, parents, children, co-wives—wearing the same cloth or color. So it should feel natural if you and your sister(s) desire to wear the same style or same color outfit at the same time—it's the Afrakan way! Maasai men and women show oneness by wearing the same styled orange cloth as a body wrap. And the Ashanti people are known the world over for their beautiful kente cloth.

## Sacred Beauty at Home

Your attire at home must be pleasing. You know how we dress sometimes—we slouch around in the worst garments that we own, things that are too tight, or falling off, or all worn out. We don't get dressed up for ourselves—we get dressed up for the world. When we're at home, we just throw stuff on.

So today, you're going to stop throwing things on. Keep a close watch on how your spirit feels when you begin to dress yourself in beauty. It's as simple as finding yourself some special fabric that's beautiful to you. Any kind of material is suitable. It could be cotton or silk. It takes just two yards of material to make a lappa. So you can't say, "Well, I don't have money for an outfit." Two yards of cloth at $10 a yard, and you can have a whole outfit. Your mate will love it, your children will think you've been recharged, and when you look in the mirror you'll feel good.

You'll come home, take off your war clothes, and wrap your lappa around you. You'll put your waist beads on, and now you're a Bush Woman, you're an Afrakan woman. You're feeling gorgeous. And then if you want to get really divine because someone is coming to visit, you can energize your womb to create a beautiful frame of mind.

Next, take those tired old gray slippers and throw them out. I know they feel so comfortable. My mother raised me wearing her tired robe. It wasn't until she got a little older that she started to honor her beauty.

There are different times when we wake up in our lives. This is one of them. It's your beauty wake-up time, because you deserve that kind of beauty within and all around you. The Body Temple is a sacred altar; we have to honor ourselves by dressing beautifully. It's the least we can do in our sacred space—our homes—and for ourselves as Sacred Women.

## Beauty for Your King

When a woman beautifies herself within and without, her mate is inspired and uplifted. He responds to her beauty the same way we all respond to a beautiful flower. There is nothing more appealing than looking at a beautiful flower, and women are Nature's flowers, just as men are Nature's trees. When a woman is beautiful before her man, she has the capacity to soften his temperament. He is inspired to become more flexible and gentle in his attitude toward life and toward her, his Queen, when he looks upon her beauty.

A word to the wise: Beauty within and without puts an end to conflicts and arguments of all kinds. When he sees our beauty, he becomes Divine; by contrast, anger, frustration, and pain dissolve beauty.

## Outerwear Expresses Inner Beauty

### Footwear

High-heeled shoes may be attractive to some, but generally they are a health hazard for a Sacred Woman. Constantly wearing high heels can cause lower back pain and/or pain in your spine because you are forced to tighten your lower back muscles when wearing high heels. It can also cause a tilted pelvis. For health and comfort, wear low pumps and be sure your shoes are wide enough; Afrakan women's feet are known to be slightly wider in general than those of other groups of people. Better still, wear attractive flat shoes.

Don't hesitate to wear assorted colors, the latest spring and summer wear, open-toed shoes, or sandals. Give your feet a chance to breathe and bathe them in sunlight, which is excellent for their health. Plastic shoes or sandals are a no-no. Plastic traps toxins that need to escape freely through the feet to help maintain the health of the rest of the body.

### Adornments

The sacred name for jewelry, according to Hru Ankh Ra Semahj, is *sas*. Some women don't wear any. Some wear a few pieces. Some wear it all! When you use jewelry, it should be for beauty and for a sacred purpose. For example, a crystal necklace is beautiful, and it also cleanses your energy field. A purple head wrap is decorative, and it also protects your crown from any negative vibrations in the atmosphere.

Accessorize with waist beads; silver, gold, brass, or crystal wrist and ankle bracelets; and neck jewelry made from gems, stones, or cowrie shells, as worn by the Nubian and Watusi women.

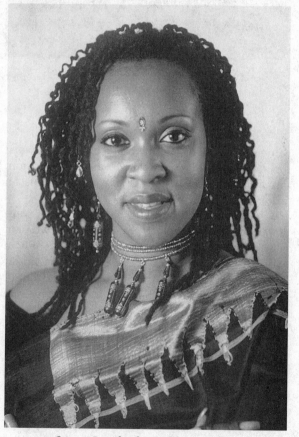

*Sas* or Jewelry by Nekhena Evans

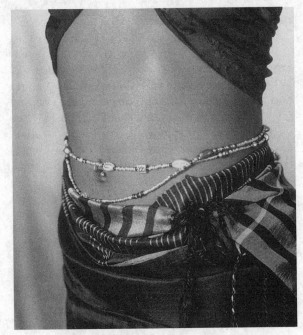

Waist beads are an adornment that
symbolize beauty and fertility.

## Waist Beads

Since antiquity Afrakan women have worn waist
beads around their hips to represent protection,
fertility, and the beauty of the womb. It is an
adornment of femininity.

Among the Saramaka, waist beads were
given to young women by older kinswomen.
They were used only for lovemaking; only a
woman's husband saw these beads. She might
even send her waist beads off with her husband,
as a symbol of her intended fidelity, when he
went far away to work over long periods. After
death, they must be laid in her coffin along with
the rest of the clothing required for a proper
burial.

I see waist beads as a form of femininity and
grace, a symbol of womanhood. As an Afrakan
dancer, I have worn waist beads when I danced,
as do many tribal women to this day. I also wear
rose quartz beads, which I never take off, that
were blessed and handed down from my mother.

A recurrent item of Afrakan female adornment was the cowrie shell girdle, "which was
worn slung low around the hips . . . and apparently had protective significance for that part of

a woman's body perhaps because the shell re-
sembles the outer female genitalia."[2]

During the time of the Crusades, European
women were forced by their men to wear locked
iron chastity belts. The departing Crusader kept
the key to represent his dominance and control
over the womb, and to be certain that his woman
did not get intimate with any other man while he
was away at war.

A growing number of women living in a
European-dominated culture, whether it be
Afrakan or European or other, have begun to
experience a renewed womb consciousness
symbolized by the freedom and beauty of waist
beads, and these women have healthy womb histories. At the same time, the majority of women
today still live a chastity-belt existence of womb
control and submission. These include women
whose wombs are constantly infused by medica-
tion to ease pain and to stop discharge; women
who have suffered clitoridectomy; women who
have been raped; and women who have had "unconscious" hysterectomies.

I say to these women: Remove your chastity
belts. It's never too late to heal the womb and to
psychologically, physically, and spiritually put
on your sacred waist beads of freedom as you
claim your sacred seat.

### Making Your Own Waist Beads

Cowrie shells represent fertility and creativity
and abundance, and this is what ancient women
wore as part of their waist bead attire. So if
you're making your own waist beads, bring
your beads and cowrie shells, and bring your
sacred thread—it may be purple or white. Everything you touch with conscious intention is
Divine.

While you're doing your meditation and your
prayers, string the shells onto your waist beads.
You may use four shells for foundation. You may
use seven for your spirit. You may string nine for
completion. You might also want to use beads of
rose quartz, which is for the heart. Be as creative
as you like. You can put other kinds of beads on
it and other sacred stones, such as amethyst for
healing. You can also add a clasp for getting
your waist beads on and off, but it isn't necessary.

# Headdress Beauty and Spiritual Protection

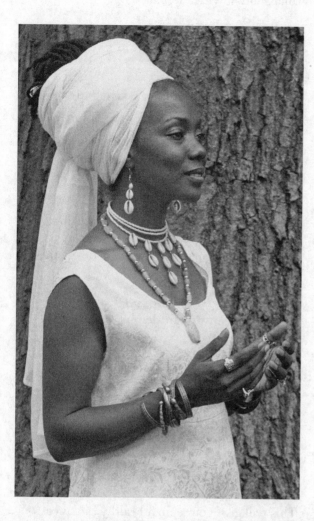

The name for the Nubian Afrakan Khamitic crowns Kaitha Het-Heru designs is *senu-Nu-sa*, which means "my hair is protected by Nu." Nu is the guardian of the primordial waters from which all life came forth.

The wrapped *senu-Nu-sa* headdress is fashioned from fabric and wrapped in two distinctly different styles.

The *senu-Nu-sa* crown band is designed to leave the top, or crown, of the head open to divine guidance.

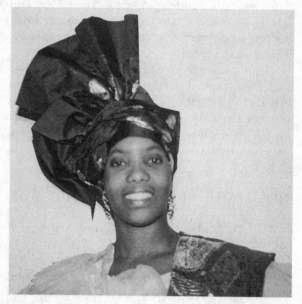

## How to Wrap Your Headdress

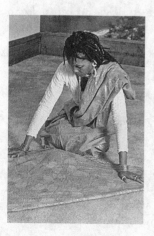 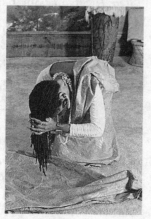 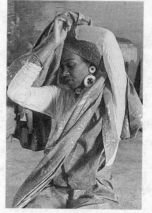 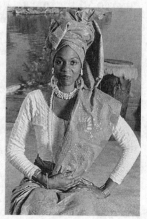

## Undergarments

Beautiful undergarments are as important as your outer garments. Wearing a foundation of beauty garments underneath your outer attire reminds you of your own inner beauty. As with outerwear, choose the appropriately colored undergarments to enhance your particular purpose while wearing them. For example, choose red for fire, energy, and power; choose blue for peace, gentleness, quiet, and spiritual empowerment throughout the day; choose green to intensify the rejuvenation of the womb.

Remember, your mate will also appreciate your beautiful undergarments. The color and fabrics you choose can increase passionate lovemaking or support your commitment to celibacy. The choice is yours.

Your garments should be porous and light so that your vaginal area and breasts are able to breathe. Use cotton, silk, or satin, for these fabrics aid circulation. Tight garments around the breast can cause discomfort or constriction, which in time can support the creation of cysts or tumors.

## BEAUTIFUL SKIN THE NATURAL WAY

### Methods of Internal Skin Care

- Drink 2 to 3 quarts of pure water every day.
- Take weekly enemas to keep your colon clean. Maintain two or three bowel movements daily.
- Eat okra for velvety skin.
- Eat greens and drink juices from live greens two or three times a day.
- Take 500 mg of vitamin C two or three times a day.
- Keep your blood pure—eat absolutely no dead flesh.

### Beautiful Skin Care—The Body Scrub

Once your skin has air-dried after your bath, try the following four-step system.

**Step 1:** Make a scrub of organic grits, cornmeal, and oats—¼ to ½ cup of each, mixed with 1 to 2 cups of distilled water. Add the juice of 1 lemon to the mixture. Scrub your body in a gentle circular motion with a loofah.

**Step 2:** Rinse off the scrub without soaping and take a sauna or steam bath to sweat out pores and increase circulation.

**Step 3:** Rinse first with hot water, and then with cold water.

**Step 4:** Massage your body with castor oil and/or olive oil and/or oil containing vitamin E for smooth, radiant, healthy skin. Or try the Edgar Cayce–inspired almond oil from the Home Health Products company.

This skin rejuvenation process should be done at least three times the first week you begin this beauty regimen. After that, do it once or twice a week for maintenance.

### Affirmation: The Sun Is Hidden in Your Face

My deeds, experiences, pain, peace, successes, and emotions are all recorded on my face. I now light the way through my life with a radiant, glowing face, pure in thought and pure in deed. My face expresses a life of good deeds and blessings, now and forever.

### A Natural Face-Lift in Seven Steps

This will give your skin a healthy radiance.

**Step 1:** Steam your face for five minutes. Lean over a bowl of freshly boiled water and cover your head with a towel that is big enough to surround the bowl. You can add dried flowers and herbs to the water, such as rosemary, chamomile, elder flowers, lavender, rose petals, lemon balm, and myrrh. If it gets too hot, give yourself a few seconds in the cooler air, then go back under the towel.

**Step 2:** Make a mixture of 1 tbsp. organic cornmeal, 2 tbsp. organic oats, and the juice of half a lime. Add enough hot water to create a paste, and allow it to sit for five minutes before using.

Apply the paste to your face and neck area, starting at the neck, massaging it on with an upward motion. Let the mask set for a few minutes after scrubbing. Then rinse off.

**Step 3:** Apply Queen Afua's Rejuvenating Clay (represents Asar, the Resurrected One) or use black mud from the Dead Sea or red clay, available in health food stores. Avoid the delicate skin around your eyes. Allow to dry for twenty to thirty minutes. Take this time to meditate and repeat the Clay Vow Affirmation (below).

**Step 4:** Rinse off gently, first with warm water, then with cool water.

**Step 5:** Lie down on a slant board or with your legs propped against the wall at a forty-five-degree angle. Relax and let your face air-dry.

**Step 6:** Apply fresh aloe vera gel, straight from the plant, or vitamin E oil to your face.

**Step 7:** Sunbathe in the rays of Ra for fifteen to thirty minutes. Do all sunbathing early in the morning or late in the afternoon—*never* in the full heat of the sun, from 11 A.M. to 3 P.M.

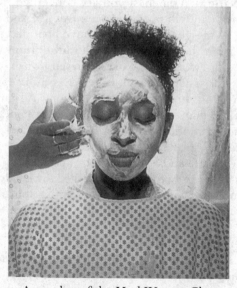

A member of the Mud Woman Clan enjoys the healing power of Queen Afua's Rejuvenating Clay.

### The Clay Vow Affirmation from the Mud Woman Clan

As a Mud Woman, a woman of the Earth and of the Divine Spirit, a devotee of the Clay Movement, I give thanks and honor to the Mother side of the Creator/Creatress. I offer this vow to the Great Earth Mother Ta-Urt who nourishes, nurtures, and heals us through the power of the land.

As a Mud Woman, a devotee of the Clay Clan, I vow to use clay daily and holistically to beautify my Body Temple. I vow to use the Earth as a source of drugless therapy to draw out all that ails me and to enhance my true, radiant beauty!

## NATURAL HAIR IS FREEDOM

Hair is a sensitive subject for most black women, but I want to discuss it as a part of our healing.

I was listening to Donnie Hathaway sing "Someday we'll all be free . . . ," and I began to sway to the rhythm, remembering the joyful days of my youth. I remembered raising my fist, testifying, "Power to the people!" when I was eighteen, fine and free. In those days we followed Bobby Seale, Huey P. Newton, Rap Brown, and of course, sister Angela Davis.

In the midst of the black cultural explosion I revolutionized my life by washing my hair and going naturally nappy. My mama thought I had lost my mind, but I was no longer ashamed of being me, no longer afraid of running from raindrops for fear of the "kink," no longer needing to imitate or adhere to the European woman's expression of beauty. Now I had my own classical look as a young Afrakan Queen. I wore my natural crown proudly. I washed centuries of slavery and self-hate out of my hair, and I finally loved me.

Then, in the 1970s, came the riots for our liberation in New York, Chicago, and Washington. The revolution for Afrakan American liberation had broken out everywhere, in the North and the South and throughout all of the colleges. We were waking up. Even James Brown was saying, "Say it loud, I'm Black and I'm proud."

I was attending Brooklyn College and about to take a trip to the Motherland with Doris Green, my Afrakan dance professor. That trip was canceled, but with faith and vision, I did manage to arrive in the Motherland at a later date.

I felt a revolution growing within me—I was moving from a dead state to a state of being fully alive. I was an Afrakan woman dressed in a long lappa and a headdress. I felt so majestic.

I remember that I was always listening for the drummers playing in Bedford-Stuyvesant Park. When the drumbeat started, I would stop everything and run toward that ancient Afrakan sound as my heart began to dance. My soul was set free as I stood face-to-face with my reality: that Afrakan drum and me.

The drum would bring forth my remembrance that I was not a "Negro," but an Afrakan woman, a sister Queen. Glory to the Creator/ Creatress, I was proud of this realization. Oh, yes, I was proud! Proud of all the things about me that this society had told me were all negative. I discovered within the revolution that I did love my dark skin and my round nose. I was proud of my big hips and broad feet and full lips.

Yet nothing topped the love and peace I experienced in claiming my natural Afrakan "kinks," my crowning glory, my powerful, magnetic, organic hair. I claimed then that I would never again let them take away from me my Afrakan hair. I would hold on tight and would not be swayed no matter what anyone did or said. No, I couldn't be tricked, for I was now convinced of my natural Afrakan beauty.

Since that time my hair has gone through the full range of natural hairstyles, and I loved each one, all the varieties and choices—from cornrows and Afro to braids and wraps. As much as I love and respect the Rastafarian way of living, I am not a divine Rasta. I am, however, a Natural Afrakan Woman living on Turtle Island, a Priestess of Ancient Earth Medicine, a Sacred Woman with Khamitic Nubian Ancestry. At this time my crown is filled with beautiful Nubian locks, growing from my head so grandly that they make a statement of who I am, a radiant Afrakan woman. No one outside of me can determine my beauty. They don't have the authority.

In the twenty-first century we must be totally in tune and fine-tuned as well. In these times of trouble and transition and spiritual power, my "antennas"—every hair on my head—are wired to pick up directions and instructions from the Creator/Creatress, the One Most High. I keep tuned in through these antennas. This level of communication with the Creator/Creatress can happen only when you are a Sacred Woman.

Afrakan Women everywhere, make a revolutionary statement of freedom and power. Put down that straightening comb that is brutalizing your spirit, your crown, your mind. Put down the lye—the lie—that represents the image of European beauty the larger culture has told us to seek. Their goal is to put you to sleep. We've been fooled, blinded in our view of our beauty. Can't you see? We must become instead natural Queens.

The moment you take back your natural lovely hair, a mental, spiritual healing, a deep love of self, will come over you. Be brave—do it now, before it's too late. Recapture your natural beauty, your crown, your high state. It's all right. Come on, wash out those foreign toxins and negative vibes. Set your hair free!

Natural Women, if you are concerned that a Negro man will not find you attractive and may stop loving you because you have liberated your hair from the straitjacket of cultural brainwashing, stop worrying. Love yourself, wash your hair, and style it beautifully as you "keep the faith" and hold on to the vision. A natural Afrakan man who loves himself, one who is on higher ground, is working his way toward you, beautiful Afrakan Queen.

My mate and I were on tour in Jackson, Tennessee, where we proudly received the key to the city for our work and service for the upliftment of our race. While in Tennessee, we gave a Rites of Passage Workshop to a group of brothers and sisters. As the training went on, I took the sisters to a separate area to talk of women's issues in a healing way.

I was speaking on self-love, and through love having the courage enough to embrace your natural hair, when all of a sudden a beautiful sister began to cry out.

She told us that after reading my first book, *Heal Thyself: For Health and Longevity*, she'd been inspired to become a vegetarian, and for three months now, she had been incorporating fasting and Natural Living into her lifestyle. As a result, she had gotten a new lease on life. She was healthier and stronger than she'd ever been, both spiritually and physically.

She went on to say, "As I became more natural I began to have the desire to claim my natural hair, for I know it would be in Divine Order. But I'm afraid that our Afrakan men won't find me attractive anymore."

All of us sisters—those of us with natural hair and those of us with straightened hair—began to pray as one. We all knew that sometimes acting consciously can be lonely, and that we needed to heal our vision of ourselves. We prayed that we as women would heal enough so that the Afrakan men we love would accept and cherish our natural beauty. We prayed for the healing of the consciousness of our Afrakan men. We prayed that, as with people in other races, Afrakan Americans and those born Afrakan who have bought into another woman's beauty trip would learn to recognize and appreciate their own natural beauty.

Sisters, stop passing around the straightening comb and hair relaxers. Throw them out with fast foods, flesh foods, and cow's-milk ice cream. It's time to release it and let it go!

### Special Notes on Hair Exposure

Muslim, Rasta, and other Sacred Women who keep their crowns covered regularly for spiritual or other purposes, please take heed! It is imperative that you expose your head to the air and to the sun's rays so that the natural elements can reach your hair follicles and your scalp can become nourished by the elements. Otherwise, your hair can dry out and become brittle, weak, and damaged over a period of time. This can also result in forgetfulness, depression, and headaches.

You need the sun's rays to bathe your scalp (your crown) because your hair is a living organism. It needs sun, air, and water to stay alive. The sun's rays feed your brain cells and open up your spiritual gateways. They also help you to think clearly and make more positive decisions about your life. So as you take sun/air baths, meditate on the Creator/Creatress. At least one hour a day—early in the morning or in the late afternoon—expose your crown to the beloved sun, our source of regeneration. While in your home, remove your headdress or wear a porous cotton headpiece. If you must wear a head covering, place a wrap over the head very lightly. Never wear a tight headdress.

The same advice applies to constant hat, wig, or scarf wearing. Let your hair breathe. Let it inhale and exhale. Hair is a living and breathing entity, your crown, your glory.

### Black Rose

Black Rose, an Afrakan Queen I know, was busy one day massaging her oils into my scalp as she locked my hair. She was also showing me her book of natural hairstyles from the 1970s. When she proceeded to show me a twelve-month calendar that highlighted various Afrakan beauty queens, a calendar in which she had designed the natural hair and Afrakan garments of each sister Queen, I was amazed!

I said, "So it was you and other Queens like you and Empress Akwéké who helped me and other sisters to embrace and love our own image of self. Our image as Afrakan women in America was beautiful because of Queens such as you!" I dropped to my knees, as one does before his/her Elder in Afrakan tradition, thanking her for holding on throughout the many years, for she has empowered Afrakan women, men, and children to celebrate our beauty in all its brilliant manifestation.

The title Black Rose, Goddess of African Culture, was bestowed on her by the *Evening Times*, the largest newspaper in Nigeria, West Afraka. It is a title she will cherish forever, for in our Afrakan tradition, when you are given a title, you do not put it in the closet. You live up to the honor bestowed on you and wear it with pride and dignity.

**Dedicated to My African Sisters by Black Rose, goddess of African culture for more than twenty-five years**

*This is the Interlude to the awakening of the beauty.*
*You are the Unbelievable Truth,*
*the Rebirth of Our Ancient Afrakan Beauty,*
*Radiantly flaunted with Pride.*
*Enchanting Afrakan Queens*
*and Beauteous Women of "Our Race"*
*are envied by all.*

Again, history repeats itself in the cycles of time. It compels us to regard ourselves as ascendants of African womanhood—not descendants, but ascendants, for we are ascending into our cultural magnificence. We are determined to adhere with unwavering devotion to ourselves and our race. African locks are not limited to one type, so be creative with your natural hair.

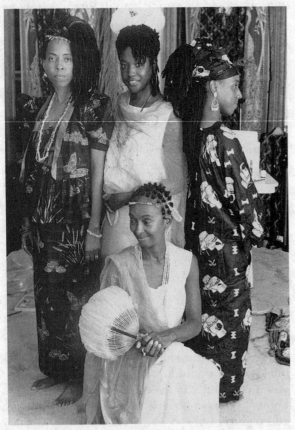

Beautiful Afrakan Locks

## Natural Care for Your Natural Hair

1. Wash hair with herbal soap, clay soap, or black soap.
2. Lightly dry hair, then apply Queen Afua's Rejuvenation Clay (see the product list in the appendix) to hair and scalp. Wrap head in a clean white towel for three to four hours or until the clay is dry. Then wash it out with warm water.
3. *Hair Conditioner I:* After you wash out the clay, rinse hair with the following homemade herbal rinse: 1 tsp. each of rosemary, thyme, horsetail, and sage, steeped overnight in 1 quart of boiled water. Leave mixture on hair for thirty minutes, then rinse out with warm water.
4. *Hair Conditioner II:* Use fresh aloe vera gel from the plant.
5. *Hair Oil Formula:* Combine equal parts of almond oil and olive oil. Add a few drops (25,000 IU) of vitamin E oil. After you wash and rinse, massage and dress your hair with oil. For a nice scent, add a few drops of essential rose or lavender oil to Hair Oil Formula.
6. After you oil your scalp, sit outside in the early morning or late afternoon for at least thirty minutes and allow the sun's rays to charge your crown.
7. As you sun yourself, speak positive affirmations about your hair and then meditate quietly. This activity will give you vision and inner wisdom.
8. As protective nutrients for the hair, take vitamin B complex, 50 mg, two or three times a day.

### What to Drink and Eat for a Full Head of Healthy Hair

Try this Chlorophyll Daily Herbal Tonic for the Hair. Make a tea of horsetail, oatstraw, alfalfa, and dandelion. Sip as a tea internally, and use externally as a hair rinse.

To make a green juice hair tonic to drink, juice 2 stalks celery, ½ cup of greens (broccoli, kale, brussels sprouts, etc.); add ½ to 1 cucumber.

## AIR BATH

In a private place, remove your clothes and allow the air to dance all over you.

Allow your pores to finally breathe. Allow yourself to take a look at yourself—don't turn away. Smile and admire yourself in all ways: big, small, fat, light, dark, thick, and thin. Look at how the Creator/Creatress made you so uniquely beautiful.

Go on and love what you see. Tell yourself: "I got a right to allow the air to dance all over me."

Once a week, or every day if you can manage it, take an air bath with yourself—and, if you so choose, with your mate. An hour or two will do. Most of our lives we constantly cover our bodies, so our skin ages quickly and develops all kinds of disease.

An air bath will add bounce, luster, and glow to your skin. In other words, the more your body can receive fresh air and particularly the rays of the sun, the more you'll have healthy skin. So throw off your clothes and don't be shy. Allow the air to be your divine lover as it dances all over you.

## ANCIENT BEAUTIFICATION OF THE EYES

Ancient Afrakan women had the most distinctively beautifully dressed eyes known to humankind. This was because the black kohl powder they painted around their eyes was not merely for cosmetic purposes but also for healing and spiritual purposes.

Ast (Isis), the Great Mother of humankind, was the first woman to wear "Egyptian eyes." The glyph for the eyes means "the Creator/Creatress, the Doer, the Maker." She set the example for all other Egyptian women to follow. Ast, with her kind husband Asar (Osiris), civilized Egypt (Khamit), teaching agriculture, medicine, and divine principles to those in the Nile Valley.

The healing purpose of kohl was to protect the eye from the intense rays of Ra, the Sun. But it was also to prevent the clustering of flies around the eyes and thus protect them from the disease and infection that is endemic in the Middle East. The spiritual symbolism of the black circle around the eye represents Nut (the Heavens), Het-Hru (divine love and beauty), and Ra (the power, energy, and light of the sun).

### The Eyes: Natural Eye Care

The eyes are indeed the windows to the soul. They must receive great care to prevent them from becoming weak.

### Eye Exercises

Exercises are very important in maintaining beautiful, healthy eyes.

1. Rotate the eyes to the right in a full circle four to twelve times. Rotate the eyes to the left in a full circle four to twelve times. Raise and lower the eyes twelve times. Relax and breathe deeply.
2. Now move the eyes on a diagonal. Look up to the right then down to the left. Do this slowly several times, then rapidly several times.
3. Close your eyes and cover them with cool, fresh cucumber slices. Meditate for five minutes. See peace and beauty with your inner eye as you care for your outer eyes.

### Clay Packs for Eyes

Make and use a gauze-wrapped clay pack over your eyes for a few moments once a week for rejuvenation. You can also apply a gauze clay pack for one to three hours, while you're napping, or until the clay dries. Shower off very gently with warm water; the skin around the eyes is very delicate.

While you apply the clay eye pack, meditate quietly and recite this Clay Prayer:

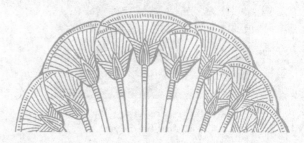

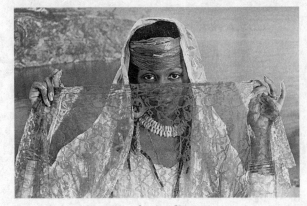

Exercise for Radiant Eyes

Another easy way to care for your eyes is to put a warm-water compress over them, using a white cotton washcloth or white flannel. Try a wheatgrass eye rinse, with ½ oz. of fresh wheatgrass diluted with 2 oz. of water.

Eyebright tea strengthens the eyes. Drink 1 to 2 cups daily until eyes are healthier, or 1 to 2 cups a few days during the week for maintenance. Use eyebright tea compresses over tired eyes as you meditate for ten to fifteen minutes.

Do this eye care work with your eyes until the whites are just that, white, and until there are no circles or crow's-feet under the eyes.

### The Dance of the Eyes

Adorned art thou, thy beauties are in my two eyes and they are shining rays upon my body.

Put a veil over your lower face, leaving your eyes exposed. Play some beautiful flute or string music and allow your eyes to come alive by "dancing" rhythmically to the music. Up, down, around—let the eyes dance freely. Speak through your eyes. Express joy, gladness, sadness, anger, peace, and ecstasy.

### Care for Your Hands and Nails

Cover hands and nails in clay one to three times a week and wrap in gauze overnight. Shower off in the morning. Then massage, one finger at a time, with castor oil or olive oil.

Exercise hands by stretching them, fanning the fingers outward and inward three times. Then open and close them rapidly three times. Shake several times and relax for beautiful hands.

Get a manicure weekly or biweekly, along with a pedicure.

### Dress Your Feet in the Spirit: Ancient Ceremony for Wearing Toe Rings

*Reti-A M Ptah*
*My feet are of Ptah.*

Ptah is the NTRU (Divine Principle) of foundation and stability. We tend to neglect our feet in this Western society. But our Ancestors were mindful of beauty and care from head to foot.

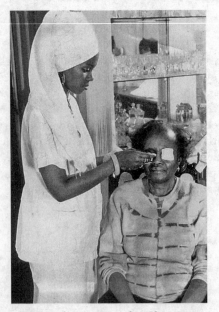

Natural eye care—the Clay Eye Pack for tired eyes

You will notice that if you are caring for your feet in a divine and sacred way, it indicates that you have already given full and proper love and attention to your entire Body Temple.

This ceremony can be part of a closing ceremony for your Rites of Passage, as each Sacred Woman's mentor blesses and washes her spiritual daughter's feet so that she will walk in power throughout the rest of her life. Or you can perform whenever you decide to honor your sacred feet by adorning them.

- Wash your feet with almond soap, clay soap, or black soap.
- Massage your feet gently with almond or olive oil. For self-healing, learn the skill of reflexology or zone therapy, which is a form of foot massage for healing the internal organs. The foot is a "road map" of the entire body, so daily massage of the feet will stimulate, relax, and energize your bloodstream, nerves, lungs, vision, sinus, mind, etc. It's all in the feet!
- Smudge your feet with desert sage.
- Anoint your feet with rose water, sandalwood balm, or any sweet oil that inspires you.
- As you put your toe ring(s) on, bless your feet:

    *My feet are of Ptah, solid and strong. I can walk through any challenge successfully and confidently.*

- If you are wearing a Maat Toe Ring, then say:

    *My feet are of Maat. I will walk in Maat, with truth, balance, and righteousness.*

- For the Lotus Toe Ring, say:

    *My feet are of Nefer Atum. I will walk in beauty, grace, and divinity.*

- For the Ankh Toe Ring, say:

    *My feet are of the Ankh. I will walk in full respect of life.*

- Place fresh rose petals around your feet and rest in quiet meditation as you absorb the divine spirit of beauty through and around your feet.

*Note:* This ceremony can be done with or without toe rings. The blessing of your feet and making them sacred is what is most important.

## Proper Body Temple Etiquette for Royal Women

Gentleness in conduct of every kind causes the wise to be praised. Do not make your mouth harsh or speak loudly with your tongue. For a loud voice does damage to members of the body just like an illness.[3]

- *Speaking Voice:* The speaking voice is like music to the soul. It should be clear, like a bell. Your voice sings a song of life, love, peace, power, energy, honesty. Your voice is the expression of your spirit. If your spirit is in tune, then your voice reflects the inner condition of the Body Temple. When you are in tune, you can pierce someone's heart with the sound of your voice. You can end a war with the texture of your voice. You can begin a healing ministry with the power of your voice.
- *Walking:* Without realizing it, the charm schools of today use Afrakan etiquette as a guide for the proper manner of walking, sitting, and standing. It began with our Ancestors. Stand tall, head straight, neck long, shoulders down as you walk with your feet parallel. Walking in a strong, straightforward way was shown on the temple walls of the first people. Perfection in stature was our way.
- *Sitting:* The ancient way of sitting was a pose of power: shoulders down, back straight, legs long, feet forward, hands placed quietly on your thighs. This type of sitting aligned you physically and spiritually.

Baba Ishangi once said, "Beauty is a spirit." So be certain to dress your spirit in the fashion of kindness, understanding, tolerance, patience, gentleness, and love, for then you will possess the true spirit of beauty.

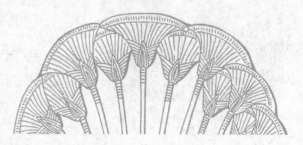

# THE CONTEMPORARY AFRAKAN WOMAN

I am honored to introduce to you a Divine Priestess of our Khamitic Nubian legacy. Her beauty has inspired Afrakan women everywhere to regain the magnificence of their ancient Afrakan beauty, physically and spiritually.

As Chief Priestess of Beautification, Snt-Urt Kaitha Het-Heru is keeper of the Shrine of Sekhmet/Ta-Urt/Het-Hru, and the author of *I Love My Beautiful Body Temple.* Here, we use her image and dress to show how our appearance can be deeply spiritual and inspire those around us as well as empower our own energies and beauty.

## Kaitha Het-Heru's Facial Adornments

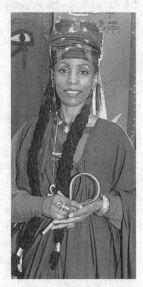

- Kohl outlines her eyes.
- Her nose ring is a design using the cow horn and lunar disk, the ancient symbol of Het-Hru (divine love and beauty).
- Her Sacred Circle hoop earrings represent the interconnection of all life.
- The *uja* covering over her first eye or pineal gland is Mtu NTR (a hieroglyph) for strength.
- Her Falcon of Heru earrings represent the inner light of Spirit.

## Her Clothing

- *Pedes-sa* means "protective wrap"; it is the ancient name for our Afrakan Nubian dress.
- Het-Heru's braided Nu-Locks are adorned with a wrapped *senu-Nu-sa* crown.
- In her hand is an Ankh. On her finger is an Ankh ring. *He sa,* her protective jewelry, was designed by Hru Ankh Ra Semahj in the Studio of Ptah.

## The Beauty of the Sacred Woman

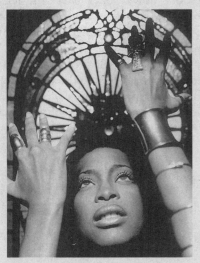

Erykah Badu

*As a Sacred Woman, I embody beauty, dignity, majesty, and grace.*

*We honor you, Het-Hru, for you embody absolute beauty, sensuousness, and grace, like that which came through Makeda, Queen of Sheba of the Nile Valley; like the beauty that Sarah Vaughan sang; like the beauty that moves through Judith Jamison when she dances and brings our souls with her to "wade in the water."*

*"The nature of creation is that it is always progressing toward beauty. Allah is beautiful, and Allah loves beauty," says the Qu'ran. "The nature of the body is to beautify itself; the nature of the mind is to have beautiful thoughts; the longing of the heart is for beautiful feeling."*

*The Sacred Woman is the most radiant and beautiful woman. She is the female manifestation of the Most High, and the Most High within her brings unmeasurable beauty. Everyone who looks upon this Sacred Woman is captivated by her divine beauty. It's yours to admire and enjoy, just like the natural beauty of rose petals and dew drops. Wherever a Sacred Woman journeys, she leaves the essence of beauty behind her.*

## SACRED BEAUTY: SEVEN-DAY TRANSFORMATIVE WORK

Before you start on the Gateway 4: Sacred Beauty Seven-Day Transformative Work, be sure that you have read the entire Gateway thoroughly first. Familiarize yourself with its contents and purpose before you undertake any of the work of this Gateway.

- *Think beautiful thoughts daily.* Meditate in Nature—in gardens, parks, or woods, or by a stream, river, lake, or ocean—one to three times during the seven days to enhance your inner beauty and healing. As you visit Nature in meditation, keep a journal of beautiful thoughts as affirmations come through to you. Use this Gateway in your journal to release all obstacles or disharmonies that separate you from your beauty. Once recorded, transform your negative thoughts into divine, beautiful possibilities and visions.
- *Create sacred attire for yourself.* Design special garments that add sacred beauty to every aspect of your wardrobe. Seek out help from designers, seamstresses, and sister queens who embody the sacred beauty that you seek. Choose the colors of the day to empower you (check the chart on pages 132–133).
- *Love and pamper your Body Temple daily,* not just on holidays and birthdays, because every day you live is a special occasion.
- *Give yourself a clay facial* every other day to keep skin radiant and weekly thereafter.
- *Give yourself a hair and scalp herbal or clay treatment* once a week to rejuvenate and cleanse hair and scalp.
- *Revitalize your original beauty.* Be brave—strive for natural hair or at least avoid putting chemicals in your hair if straightened. There are many natural hairstyles to choose from—investigate them. Adorn your hair with beautiful hairpins, shells, beads, crystals, etc.
- *Take an air bath* after your water bath or shower as often as possible.
- *Wear the Ast/Nebt-Het sacred shawl* to remind you of your sacred beautiful self when in morning prayer, or as spiritual protection when you go out into the world.
- *Create a beautiful healing song and/or dance a healing beauty dance* to the most inspiring music that mirrors your beauty back to you.
- *Make a Sacred Beauty collage* to define your vision of Sacred Beauty. What colors call their beauty out to you? What fabrics? What scents? What sounds? What locations?
- *Make a sacred collage filled with images of ancient Khamitic Egyptian beauty.* What adornments, hairstyles, and beauty habits come through to you from the Ancestors at this Gateway?
- *Design a Sacred Beauty natural hairstyle book.* Share your favorites in your Sacred Circle and allow your unique vision of beauty to be affirmed.

**My Sacred Beauty End-of-the-Week Commitment:**

I commit myself to establishing and continuing the wisdom of Het-Hru and the power of Sacred Beauty in all the areas of my life.

Signature: _____

Date: _____

## CHAPTER 10

# GATEWAY 5: SACRED SPACE

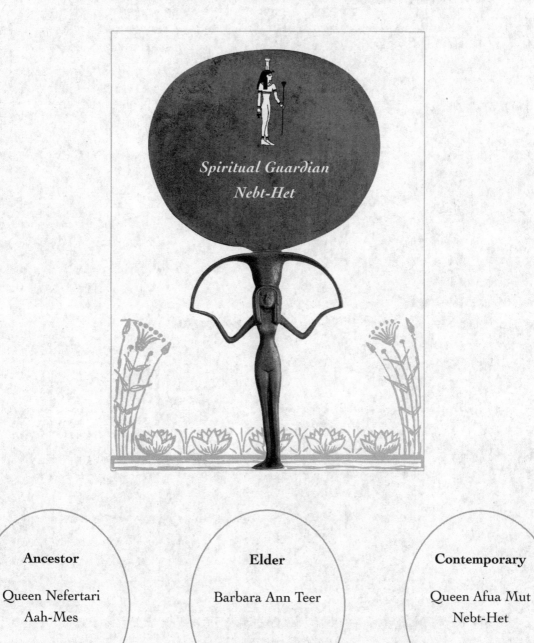

*Spiritual Guardian*

*Nebt-Het*

**Ancestor**

Queen Nefertari
Aah-Mes

**Elder**

Barbara Ann Teer

**Contemporary**

Queen Afua Mut
Nebt-Het

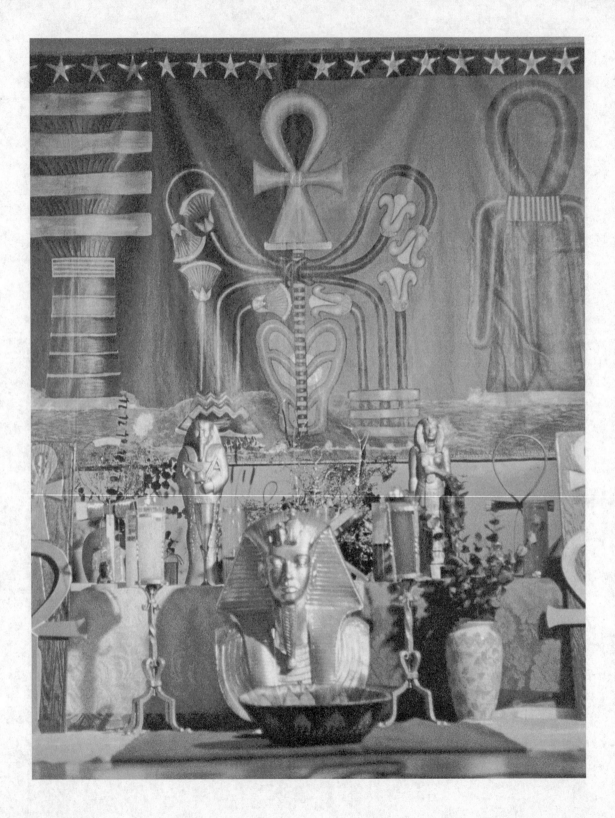

# SACRED SPACE ALTAR WORK
## Face Your Heart to the East—to the Rising Sun
*(Layout from top view)*

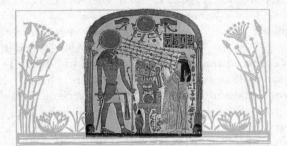

**Mount Pictures on Wall, Above Altar**

| | | | | |
|---|---|---|---|---|
| Picture of Spiritual Guardian | Picture of Ancestor | Picture of Sacred Self | Picture of Elder | Picture of Contemporary |

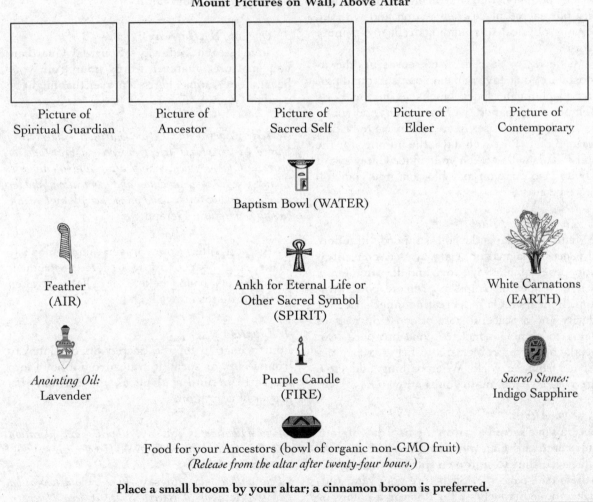

Baptism Bowl (WATER)

Feather (AIR)

Ankh for Eternal Life or Other Sacred Symbol (SPIRIT)

White Carnations (EARTH)

*Anointing Oil:* Lavender

Purple Candle (FIRE)

*Sacred Stones:* Indigo Sapphire

Food for your Ancestors (bowl of organic non-GMO fruit)
*(Release from the altar after twenty-four hours.)*

**Place a small broom by your altar; a cinnamon broom is preferred.**

Sacred tablecloth (purple) and scarf to wear during prayer.
Sacred color cloth to lay before altar. Sacred instruments to be played as you pray.

# GATEWAY 5: SACRED SPACE DAILY SPIRITUAL OBSERVANCES

## Gateway Element: Air

Sacred Space will clear out cluttered space, confusion, and loss. Sacred Space will assist you in bringing your home and work space into divine clean order that will create balance and harmony within and throughout your life. Nebt-Het, the Spiritual Guardian of Sacred Space, will bring peace, stability, and nurturing. She will purify our sacred place from within and without, for our physical surroundings reflect our inner world.

Gateway 5: Sacred Space represents the atmosphere, our environment, our surroundings. It will eliminate space blockages in the Body Temple: constipation, worms, toxicity, polyps.

Spiritual exercises of ascension are to be performed daily for seven days, the number for the spirit. This will awaken your inner Gateways of Divinity so that you may blossom into your full sacred center.

## 1. The Spiritual Bath

A bath with lavender oil supports intuition, aliveness, imagination, clairvoyance, concentration, peace of mind, wisdom, and devotion (*atum ra*). Lavender oil helps to promote concentration. It clears the mind, creating inner space for clarity and a peaceful state of consciousness. It helps to eliminate lack of concentration, fear, headaches, eye problems, and being overly detached from the world. When bathing, add 4 to 6 drops of lavender oil to your bathwater.

## 2. Your Altar

Set up your sacred altar on the first day of your entry into this Gateway. You may set up your altar according to your own spiritual or religious beliefs (see page 18). Sit before your altar quietly and meditatively on the floor on a pillow, or in a chair. Also add a few drops of lavender oil to your baptism bowl on your altar and sprinkle a few drops around your prayer space.

*Anoint with lavender oil.* Select only pure essential oils. Use lavender oil to anoint your crown, forehead (the Body Temple Gateway of supreme spirituality), heart (the Body Temple Gateway of compassion and divine love), womb area, palms to make everything you touch become more sacred, and the bottoms of your feet to spiritually align yourself for stepping out in power, promise, and faith.

## 3. Opening the Gateway

To invoke each Gateway's Spiritual Guardian, you may use whatever words pour from your heart. For example, here's a prayer that might be used at Gateway 5.

*Nebt-Het, Sacred and Divine Spiritual Guardian of Sacred Space, please accept my deepest gratitude for your healing presence on my altar and in my life. Thank you for your guidance and inspiration, and for your love and blessings, and please accept my love and blessings in return.* Hetepu.

As you offer your prayer, simultaneously shake, ring, beat, or rattle a sacred instrument (sistrum bell, drum, shekere, or bells) to awaken the NTR that is indwelling.

## 4. Libation

Pour a libation for the Sacred Space Gateway from a cup, or sprinkle water from a bowl into the earth or into a plant, as you call out this prayer of adoration.

- *Pour a libation* as you say, *All praise and adoration to the Spiritual Guardian, Nebt-Het, Protector of Sacred Space.*
- *Pour a libation* as you say, *All praise and adoration to the Ancestor of Sacred Space, Queen Nefertari Aah-Mes.*
- *Pour a libation* as you say, *All praise and adoration to the Elder of Sacred Space, Barbara Ann Teer.*

- Pour a libation as you say, *All praise and adoration to my Divine Self and my Contemporary Divine Sister, Queen Afua Mut Nebt-Het, who honors Sacred Space.*

## 5. Sacred Woman Spirit Prayer

Ring a bell or play another sacred instrument at the beginning and end of the prayer.

> *Sacred Spirit, hold me near,*
> *close to your bosom.*
> *Protect me from all harm and fear*
> *beneath the stones of life.*
> *Direct my steps in the right way as I journey*
> *through this vision.*
> *Sacred Spirit,*
> *surround me in your most absolute perfect light.*
> *Anoint me in your sacred purity, peace,*
> *and divine insight.*
> *Bless me, truly bless me, as I share*
> *this sacred life.*
> *Teach me, Sacred Spirit, to be in tune*
> *with the universe.*
> *Teach me how to heal*
> *with the inner and outer elements*
> *of air, fire, water, and earth.*

## 6. Sacred Space Prayer

Shake bells, beat a sacred drum, or play another instrument at the beginning and ending of the prayer.

*Divine Creator/Creatress, assist me in keeping my inner and outer space sacred and clean, whether the space is in my body, my home, my office, or at play. May all the space in me and around me be free of clutter, confusion, and dismay. May my environment be pure, open, and in divine order, as the sky, ocean, Sun, and Planet Earth were in its early days, when the world was clean and whole. May we respect Nature, our environment, and our space, and return to purity as it was in the beginning. May my space always emanate serenity so that you, Creator/Creatress, may dwell there. Today, I deem my space a sacred space.*

## 7. Chanting Hesi

Chant this *hesi* four times:

*Nuk Pu Ntrt Hmt*—I am a Sacred Woman.

## 8. Fire Breaths

Prepare for Fire Breathing by slowly inhaling four times and exhaling four times. Then, when totally at ease, begin your six hundred Fire Breaths. Inhale deeply like a pump through your nostrils (mouth closed) as you expand the breath down into the abdomen, then back up to the chest, and then exhale fully out as your abdomen contracts in and the lungs release your breath completely. Repeat this breath rapidly and release your breath completely in and out, in and out.

Allow each deep Fire Breath to represent the opening of the thousand lotus petals of illumination and radiance to reach Nefer Atum—the ultimate Afrakan lotus station of Divinity.

## 9. Gateway 5: Sacred Space Meditation

Increase the length of time you spend in meditation every seven days. The longer you are in meditation, the deeper your inner peace will be, and the more solid your *ba* (spirit) will become. The cleaner your Body Temple, the sooner it will be able to live permanently in the peace and inner balance of the meditative state.

- Sit on the Lotus Bed of Divinity, the very core of your sacred center. Breathe in Nebt-Het, the Guardian Lady of the Divine House on Earth, who comes from the Heavenly Realms.
- Fill your inner house with purple light as you become one with the light that is indwelling.
- Inhale, then breathe out of your Sacred Space internally and externally, as you envision confusion, disarray, and uncleanliness leaving through your breath. Repeat seven times.

*Color Visualization.* Visualize the color purple for spiritual liberation. As you perform your meditation wear purple, and/or place a purple cloth on the altar.

*Sacred Stone Meditation.* While in meditation, hold an indigo sapphire in your palm over your center. This is the Sacred Healing stone of this Gateway, and it helps to transform and raise the soul into the higher realms, making your inner space more peaceful and meditative.

## 10. Herbal Tonics

Drink gotu kola herbal tea. Parts used: seeds, nuts, and roots. Gotu kola is the "memory" herb. When used with cayenne, it stimulates blood circulation in the brain, helping to create a clearer and more efficient inner space, so that clarity will manifest externally.

Drink your herb tea for seven days to receive the full benefit of tuning you to Gateway 5. Enjoy your herb tea in your favorite mug during or after spiritual writing.

*Preparation.* Use one teabag to 1 cup of water. Boil 1 cup of water in a glass, clay, or stainless steel pot, turn off the flame, and add the teabag to steep before or after your morning bath or sacred shower. Strain the herbs from the water, then drink with joy and peace as you breathe between sips and settle into easy contemplation and reflection.

## 11. Flower Essences

To deepen your experience of Gateway 5, choose from the following flower essences. Take 4 drops four times per day directly on or under the tongue, or add the same amount to a small glass of purified water and sip. For instructions on how to choose flower essences, see page 23.

- *Indian paintbrush:* Addresses issue of scattered or disheveled quality in living environment.
- *Mountain pennyroyal:* To purify home or environment, especially when contaminated by negative energies.
- *Iris:* Helps address drab, dull, or ugly living environment; inattention to color and form.
- *Canyon dudleya:* Helps address the inability to identify with ordinary household tasks or daily living responsibilities.

- *Star tulip:* Allowing "home" to become a source of soul experience.
- *Sagebrush:* Purifying and simplifying one's lifestyle, especially when surroundings are congested and disorderly.
- *Shasta daisy:* Bringing parts of living environment into greater wholeness and relatedness; bringing harmony to chaotic or disorderly home.

## 12. Diet

Follow the Sacred Woman Transitional Dietary Practices presented for Gateways 4–6.

## 13. Sacred Space Journal Writing

This is best done after internal cleansing (enema) and/or meditation. When you are cleansed and centered, you can receive spiritual messages from the One Most High with grace. When you are in the spirit, messages travel down through your spirit mind, to your heart, into your hand, and onto the paper. (This is how I do all my writing.)

The best time to receive your spiritually inspired written work is after you have completed your altar work, between the hours of 4 A.M. and 6 A.M. Keep your very special pen and journal by or on your altar to work with the power, force, and stillness at the coming of dawn, the hour of Nebt-Het.

Affirm your daily life. Write in your journal at this time thoughts, activities, experiences, and interactions that occur to you. You can also write down your self-inspired hopes, visions, desires, and affirmations so that you will draw from them for help and support when in need.

*Consult Sesheta.* If you find that you are unable to contact your inner voice during your journal work, call Sesheta, the keeper and revealer of secrets (who is indwelling), to assist and speak through you.

## 14. Senab Freedom Shawl or Quilt

Choose a new piece of cloth that corresponds to the Gateway color (indicated in exercise 9 of your Daily Spiritual Observances or in Sacred Altar Work) to add to your Senab Freedom Shawl or Quilt. This cloth will serve as a mini-canvas to represent your experience in the Gateway you're working in.

Also, collect meaningful symbols that can be added to your shawl or quilt in appliqué or patchwork style. You can add stones, other natural objects, collectibles, family heirlooms, photographs that have been reprinted on fabric, or any other significant items that embody the essence of your experience. Give your imagination free rein and let your craftswoman spirit tell your story. For more information about the Senab Freedom Shawl or Quilt, see pages 122–125.

### 15. *Sacred Tools*

Cinnamon brooms—a small one to place by your altar and a large one to place by your front door. Portable cast-iron pot for burning sacred oils.

### 16. *Sacred Reminder*

Throughout the week, observe closely the wisdom presented for the Gateway you're in. For maximum results, live freely and harmonize with the various systems of wellness, and practice the Seven-Day Transformative Work at the end of the Gateway.

### *Closing Sacred Words*

*Mother/Father Creator/Creatress, help to purify me and keep my Sacred Space in divine order.*

---

## HOUSEKEEPING IS A HOLY EXPERIENCE

I've heard women say: "I'm just not good at keeping a house clean." "Being a housekeeper is not my thing." If you don't view your home as a sacred space, you may be experiencing some serious chaos in your life. Keeping your home clean and pure is not merely a physical act; it is a spiritual discipline that teaches you how to maintain divine order in your life. Your home, your living temple, directly reflects your spiritual condition and worldly state. So get out of the habit of just rushing out of your home for something so important or demanding that you had to leave dishes in the sink, clothes on the floor, the floor unswept, and papers everywhere. The purification of your home sets the tone of your day.

As a result of leaving your home in disarray, you are sure to meet confusion in the streets. So happily wash those dishes; joyfully hang up your clothes; place books on their proper shelves and important papers in a file and out of sight; peacefully make your bed. Know that all the good housekeeping that you are performing is actually prayer in motion.

Snt Tehuti's grandmother used to say, "Always prepare your clothes the night before, keep your hair, nails, and body clean and looking nice. Clean up the dishes in the sink, and have your clothes neatly pressed and clean. Make up your bed, and always make sure your home is in order before you leave the house." Your home is sacred, and it should be quiet, comforting, clean, and at peace.

### Transforming Your Home into a Temple

As a Sacred Woman, I endeavor to transform my domestic atmosphere into a paradise! My environment radiates my inner tranquility. The very walls of my sacred home engender the divine sanctity and safety of a womb. Whoever enters this temple shall be lifted to the heights.

## A pure, sacred home can:

- heal and create oneness within the family.
- dispel illness.
- balance emotions.
- create love between a man and woman.
- create peaceful, relaxed children.
- be a place of inspiration and motivation.
- act as a battery to charge you to be ready for the outside world.
- provide spiritual uplift and peace.

Each room in your temple has a different purpose and creates a different mood.

*Kitchen Healing Laboratory:* This space has creative fire and can provide peace through purification.

*Bathroom:* This is the hydrotherapy room.

*Living room:* This is the spiritual center, the prayer room, and the communal room. This room can create balance and harmony for members of the family as well as for visitors.

*Regeneration chamber:* This is a space allotted to create rejuvenation, energy, and love—usually the bedroom.

### Beautifying Your Palace

Make a commitment to your divine home in the following ways:

### Kitchen Healing Laboratory

- Use stainless steel or cast-iron pots and pans.
- Put an aloe vera plant in the kitchen—it's pretty and its gel is excellent for burns and dishpan hands.
- Use green healing colors in the tablecloths and curtains.
- Put fresh eucalyptus branches in vases.
- Purchase dark-colored jars to keep herbs fresh.
- Use beautiful long-stemmed glasses and pottery mugs.

*Suggested colors* are lime green for healing, some orange or yellow for vitality, and/or white for cleansing.

### Living Room

- Use low furniture and pillows. Sitting on the floor is healthy for your womb and increases the flow of earth energy within you.
- Decorate with plants and indoor trees.
- Put a silk cloth over the television.
- Have your prayer books readily available.
- Create an altar. (Do not use a mirror. Check the Gateway in which you're working for the appropriate candles to use. Also have present one to two glasses of fresh water to absorb all negative vibrations in the atmosphere, seen or unseen. Water also represents life. See each Gateway for other altar suggestions.)
- Display pictures of spiritual guides and/or Ancestors.
- Display pictures of yourself, your mate, and your family in poses of joy, spiritual heights, and inspiration.

*Suggested colors* are lavender or white for spirituality and the coming together of divine harmony and purity.

### Receiving Area
(for welcoming guests to your sacred home)

- Place a cactus plant there for protection. Cacti demand little care and have a reputation for high survival. According to Dr. John E. Moore, herbalist, cacti absorb lower energy forces.
- Place a runner rug to welcome people.

*Suggested colors* are white or eggshell to clear and open the way, or peach for vitality.

### Regeneration Chamber

- Use a brass headboard bed or a futon bed.
- Create an altar for private evening prayer.
- Have a glass lantern.
- Place plants in windows and use silk curtains.
- Have a love seat and small breakfast table for private natural drinks with your lover.
- Use pillows of various colors, especially purple.
- Use silk, satin, or cotton sheets for covers while making love.
- Have a throw rug on the floor.

- Have a fruit bowl filled with fresh fruits.
- Have a candle—blow out before retiring.
- Have a large bowl of water with a cover and fresh washcloths by the bed.

*Suggested colors* are blue for peace, lavender for spiritual oneness and better use and awareness of dreams, and some soft pink for pure love and sweetness.

### Hydrotherapy Room

- Have a footstool or squatting stool.
- Have a loofah brush.
- Use peppermint, clay, oatmeal, cucumber, and/or castor oil soap.
- Use potpourris to absorb odors.
- Have an enema bag and a douche bag.
- Have a plant in the window.
- Have green clay for morning facials.
- Have a Water Pik for dental hygiene.
- Have a handheld shower massager.
- Extra wonderful: Install a whirlpool bath.

*Suggested colors* are shades of blue to represent water, spirit, and peace. Also use white and/or lavender.

Cleansing spiritually and physically also applies to your work space. So apply these principles to your business area as well as your home space—this will put all the areas of your life in divine order.

## SPIRITUAL HOUSE CLEANSING

Air out your house year-round. Open the windows, even if it's for only a few moments during the cold-weather season.

1. Burn jasmine incense in the mornings for peace. Our ancestors used various sweet-smelling oils in every ritual, ceremony, offering, and celebration, as shown on the temple walls of Dendera in Upper Egypt, Kham in Luxor, and throughout the many sacred temples.
2. Wash your house down first with ammonia (to cleanse) and then with Florida water (to sweeten), then burn frankincense and myrrh incense for purification.
3. Use a pendulum to detect specific spots of imbalance. There are numerous books on how to dowse (read vibrations) with a pendulum, or you can study pendulum reading in workshops (see pages 274–276).
4. Smudge or smoke negative areas with white desert sage or sweet grass. Smudging and smoking were practiced both in ancient Khamit (Egypt) and on Turtle Island (America). Light desert sage leaves in a small pot with a handle, or use a sage smudge stick, and walk through the house with the pot or smudge stick as the leaves smoke. Leave windows open to provide an exit for negativity.
5. Clean and wash out drawers and closets. Baba Ishangi says that demons hide in the closets, so beware: Clean and cleanse those closets!
6. *Affirm:* "My home is as pure as it can be. It is clear of all negativity." As you cleanse your home, over and over, place sea salt in the corners of your home for additional cleansing. Purification rituals with salt were practiced by our ancient Ancestors (Priestesses) before performing rituals or ceremonies. This can be seen in the conception scene on the walls of the Temple of Edfu at Aswan.

### Sweeping Out Bad Vibes with Your Cinnamon Broom

When I was in Ghana, West Afraka, I watched women sweeping their earthen floors with a deep sense of purpose. Keeping the home clean always began with sweeping away physical dirt. But this activity also symbolizes getting rid of negative vibrations. For example, if someone negative comes into your home, pick up a clean broom and sweep out the low vibes after they leave. For deeper cleansing after traumatic events such as death or fire or violence, "sweep out" your Body Temple as well by eating green leafy vegetables and fresh fruits.

For protection once you have swept your home, place a braid of fresh garlic above or by your door. Keep a broom by the door for emergencies. When a negative person or experience departs, simply sweep the bad vibrations out of your sacred space.

If you can, use a cinnamon broom or sweet-scented broom to sweep in good vibrations and to send sweetness and kindness to the individual who has just departed the house. Use compassion when you sweep out and release negative vibrations.

To make a cinnamon broom, boil a large pot of water, turn off the flame, and add 2 tbsp. of powdered cinnamon. Place the pot on the floor on a trivet and place the broom in the water. Allow the broom to steep in the pot for four to eight hours. Remove the broom and shake off the excess water in a bathtub or outdoors. Let the broom dry in the sun if possible.

## RULES FOR THE DIVINE HOME

The following rules were written by Etta Dixon, Elder Mother of Purification, now sixty-five years young, for Etta's family members so that there would be peace within the home, making it a Healing Home. It indicates how serious it is for us to bring our homes into Divine Order.

Mother Dixon is a vegetarian, a faster, a mother of all who desired healing and claimed wellness. Her goal is to spread the word to the Elders that we are to prepare ourselves with clean living and a determined spirit to accomplish our true purpose in life.

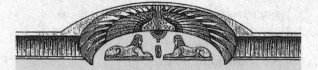

**Healing House Requirements**
*by Etta Dixon*
**(Mother of Purification)**

This is a Healing Place.
This is a Healing House,
you are here to heal.
No opposite-gender overnight
guests in the Healing House.
No oven on in the Healing
House during the summer months.
No profanity in the Healing House—it
impedes all of us from healing.
No playing loud, disruptive
music in the Healing House.
No one has to deal with STRESS!
Healing is the dealing!

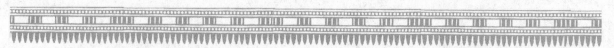

# SACRED SPACE: SEVEN-DAY TRANSFORMATIVE WORK

- *Honor your home with a new name.* Charge yourself to full strength in your own home space before emerging into the world each day, so that you can perform your life's purpose in a mighty way. Empower your home by giving it a power name. Choose the name carefully, for the name you use wields its own power. Charge your home with a name that has purpose and meaning to you. For example, you could refer to your home as a temple, palace, healing center, sacred ground, rejuvenation space, or some similar name. Be creative. Watch how your attitude toward your home changes after you name it. Use this technique to lift up your home and your life and to give you peace.

- *Perform a house purification and give your home a new spirit.* Rejuvenate, purify, and cleanse your home of any negative vibrations or demonic spirits. Wash your entire home with ½ cup of ammonia, 1 tbsp. sea salt, and a few drops of frankincense and myrrh oil added to a pail of clean water. From door to door, closet to drawer, inside and out, do an absolute wash with the cleaning solution as you pray for peace, love, and harmony within your temple, your sanctuary. A pure and restful spirit needs to be housed in a pure home. This should be done once a week until the vibrations in your home feel healed and balanced. Wherever you put your altar, no matter how small it may be, place white carnations on it to aid in drawing negativity out of the environment. A clean house allows you to live life more harmoni-

ously. After the cleansing ritual, rejuvenate your home with greenery such as aloe or cactus plants, which absorb negativity as they heal the environment. Or place white carnations in each room of your home for seven days. Then anoint your home and work space with sacred oils. Place a braid of garlic bulbs above your doorway for house protection.

After washing, clearing, smudging, prayer, and calling on the Divine to dwell within, carry your Maat feather to each corner of your space clockwise to seal in the Divine Order of peace, harmony, and cleanliness.

- *Perform an office purification.* Wash, cleanse, and purify your work space for clarity in your business affairs.

- *Commit several hours into both home and office cleansing over the next seven days,* according to the depths of cleansing needed. In your journal, record daily your state of mind, attitude, and transformation as you set things in order. Witness how what goes around comes around. By your claiming a sacred home, this transformation will show up in your outer life, so record your growth as you heal, energize, and clean your space.

- *Smudge your house with cedar, sage, or frankincense and myrrh* as you move about your home and work space in a clockwise direction before you begin your busy day. For the office, just one or two drops of sacred oil on a hot lightbulb will scent the entire environment and help reduce stress in your environment.

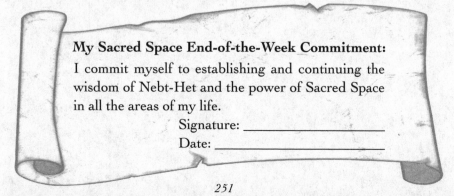

**My Sacred Space End-of-the-Week Commitment:**
I commit myself to establishing and continuing the wisdom of Nebt-Het and the power of Sacred Space in all the areas of my life.

Signature: _____

Date: _____

# CHAPTER 11
# GATEWAY 6: SACRED HEALING

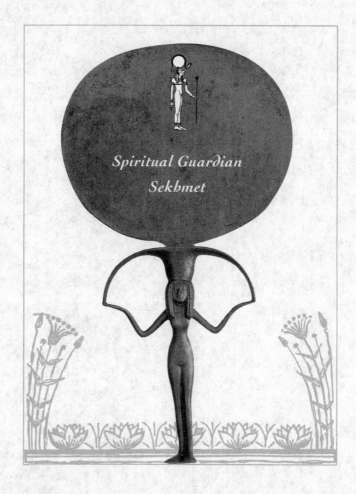

*Spiritual Guardian*
*Sekhmet*

| **Ancestor** | **Elder** | **Contemporary** |
|:---:|:---:|:---:|
| Ankh Hesen Pa Aten Ra | Berlina Baker | Dr. Sharon Oliver |
| Dr. Alvenia Fulton | | Earthlyn Marselean Manuel |

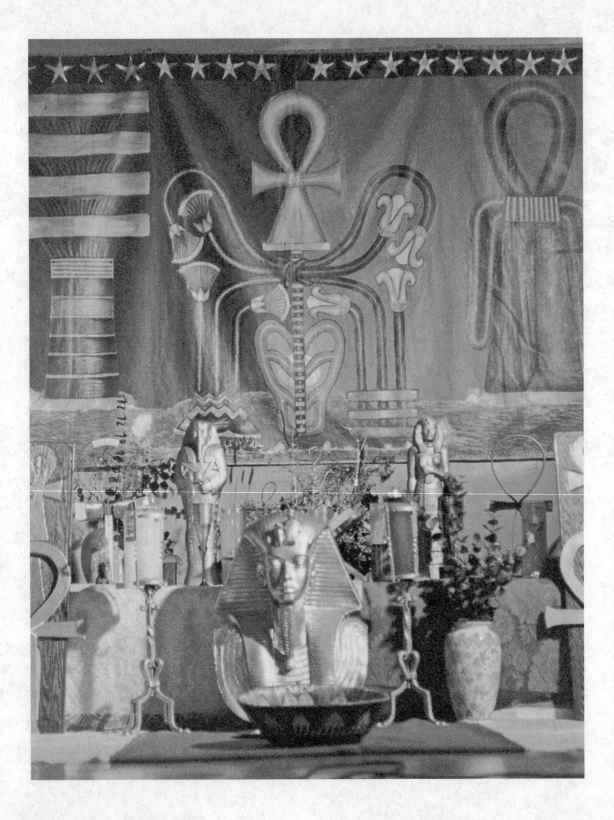

# SACRED HEALING ALTAR WORK
## Face Your Heart to the East—to the Rising Sun
### (Layout from top view)

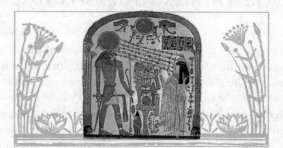

**Mount Pictures on Wall, Above Altar**

| Picture of Spiritual Guardian | Picture of Ancestor | Picture of Sacred Self | Picture of Elder | Picture of Contemporary |

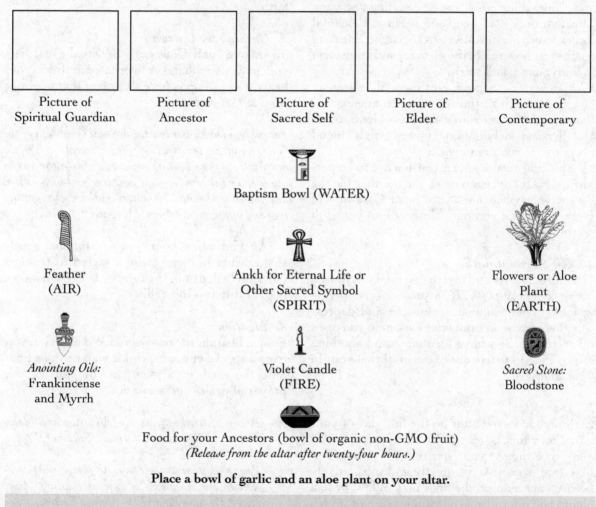

Baptism Bowl (WATER)

Feather
(AIR)

Ankh for Eternal Life or
Other Sacred Symbol
(SPIRIT)

Flowers or Aloe
Plant
(EARTH)

*Anointing Oils:*
Frankincense
and Myrrh

Violet Candle
(FIRE)

*Sacred Stone:*
Bloodstone

Food for your Ancestors (bowl of organic non-GMO fruit)
*(Release from the altar after twenty-four hours.)*

**Place a bowl of garlic and an aloe plant on your altar.**

Sacred tablecloth (red) and scarf to wear during prayer.
Sacred color cloth to lay before altar. Sacred instruments to be played as you pray.

# GATEWAY 6: SACRED HEALING DAILY SPIRITUAL OBSERVANCES

## Gateway Element: Fire

Sacred Healing helps you release the notion that someone other than yourself will heal you. Once you go through this Gateway, you will gain the confidence and the knowledge to Heal Thyself and your family in body, mind, and spirit.

The Sacred Healing Guardian Sekhmet calls us into the fires of transformation by activating and unleashing our innate healing powers. Through the use of hands-on healing, elemental forces, and the intuitive arts, Sacred Healing teaches us how to purify, elevate, and transform in body, mind, and spirit.

Gateway 6: Sacred Healing will eliminate blockages, such as those leading to anemia, inflammation, fatigue, circulatory problems, overall physical debilitation, fevers, high blood pressure, premature aging, and cancer.

Spiritual exercises of ascension are to be performed daily for seven days, the number for the Spirit. This will awaken your inner Gateways of Divinity so that you may blossom into your full sacred center.

## 1. The Spiritual Bath
Use frankincense and myrrh essential oils for the divine oneness of NTR inspiration and divine wisdom. They eliminate confusion and depression, help to balance out emotions, help you open up to others, and have a calming and soothing effect. Place 4 to 6 drops of either of these oils in your bathwater.

## 2. Your Altar
Set up your sacred altar on the first day of your entry into this Gateway. You may set up your altar according to your spiritual or religious beliefs (see page 18). Sit quietly and meditatively before your altar on the floor on a pillow, or in a chair. Add a few drops of frankincense or myrrh oil to your baptism bowl, and sprinkle a few drops around your prayer space.

*Anoint with frankincense and myrrh.* Select only pure essential oils. Use frankincense and myrrh to anoint your crown, forehead (the Body Temple Gateway of supreme spirituality), heart (the Body Temple Gateway of compassion and divine love), womb area, palms of your hands to make everything you touch become more sacred, and the bottoms of your feet to spiritually align yourself to step out in power, promise, and faith.

## 3. Opening the Gateway
To invoke each Gateway's Spiritual Guardian, you may use whatever words pour from your heart. For example, here's a prayer that might be used at Gateway 6:

*Sacred and Divine Sekhmet, Spiritual Guardian of the Gateway of Sacred Healing, please accept my deepest gratitude for your healing presence on my altar and in my life. Thank you for your guidance and inspiration, and for your love and blessings, and please accept my love and blessings in return. Hetepu.*

As you offer your prayer, simultaneously shake, ring, beat, or rattle a sacred instrument (sistrum bell, drum, shekere, or bells) to awaken the NTR that is indwelling.

## 4. Libation
Pour a libation for the Sacred Woman Gateway from a special cup, or sprinkle water from a bowl onto the earth or a plant, as you call out this prayer of praise and adoration.

— *Pour a libation* as you say, *All praise and adoration to the Spiritual Guardian, Sekhmet, Protector of Sacred Healing.*

— *Pour a libation* as you say, *All praise and adoration to the Ancestors of Sacred Healing, Ankh Hesen Pa Aten Ra and Dr. Alvenia Fulton.*

— *Pour a libation* as you say, *All praise and adoration to the Elder of Sacred Healing, Berlina Baker.*

— *Pour a libation* as you say, *All praise and adoration to my divine Self and my Contemporary Divine Sisters, Dr. Sharon Oliver and Earthlyn Marselean Manuel, who honor Sacred Healing.*

### 5. Sacred Woman Spirit Prayer

Ring a bell or play another sacred instrument at the beginning and end of this prayer. As you open your palms to the Sacred Spirit or gently place them over your heart, recite:

#### Sacred Woman Spirit Prayer

*Sacred Woman in the making,*
*Sacred Woman reawaken,*
*Sacred Spirit, hold me near.*
*Protect me from all harm and fear*
*beneath the stones of life.*
*Direct my steps in the right way as I journey*
*through this vision.*
*Sacred Spirit,*
*surround me in your most absolute perfect light.*
*Anoint me in your sacred purity, peace,*
*and divine insight.*
*Bless me, truly bless me, as I share*
*this Sacred Life.*
*Teach me, Sacred Spirit, to be in tune*
*with the universe.*
*Teach me how to heal*
*with the inner and outer elements*
*of air, fire, water, and earth.*

### 6. Sacred Healing Prayer

Shake bells, beat a sacred drum, or play another instrument at the beginning and ending of this prayer.

*Benevolent Sekhmet, help me to be in alignment with you, the Source of All Spiritual Healing. Help me to create a beautiful mind capable of opening to Spirit in every way. Strengthen me, renew me, baptize me in Spirit, that I may be free of the chains of earth. I am in need of spiritual healing. Grant me this, I pray.*

As I heal my spirit more and more every day, please allow me to become an instrument, a tool, to inspire sacred healing in every soul I meet that is seeking spiritual union with the Divine.

### 7. Chanting Hesi

Chant this *hesi* four times:

*Nuk Pu Ntrt Hmt*—I am a Sacred Woman.

### 8. Fire Breaths

Prepare for your Fire Breaths by slowly inhaling four times and exhaling four times. Then, when totally at ease, begin your seven hundred Fire Breaths. Inhale deeply like a pump through your nose (mouth closed) as you expand the breath down into the abdomen, then back up to the chest. Completely exhale out through your nostrils from your abdomen as it contracts and the lungs release your breath completely. Repeat this breath rapidly in and out, in and out.

Allow each deep Fire Breath to represent the opening of the thousand lotus petals of illumination and radiance, to reach Nefer Atum—the ultimate Afrakan lotus station of Divinity.

### 9. Gateway 6: Sacred Healing Meditation

Increase the length of time you spend in meditation every seven days. The longer you are in meditation, the deeper your inner peace will be, and the more solid your *ba* (spirit) will become. The cleaner your Body Temple, the sooner it will be able to live permanently in the peace and inner balance of the meditative state.

- Be brave. Sit still and be quiet. Relax deeply.
- Hold your bloodstone in your hand now and breathe in the healing fire of the Sacred Guardian Sekhmet. Visualize the violet flame as you breathe in through the entrance of your body, your feet.
- Continue to breathe in to a count of four all the way up into your crown, purging the impurities that are nesting and hiding within the Body Temple.
- Now ease your Body Temple with a cooling breath by exhaling. As you cool the body

down, blow out the sound of Shu, the guardian of the Air (the atmosphere), through your mouth or nose to the count of seven.

• Repeat seven times.

*Color Visualization.* Visualize the color of opalescent red fire for vitality, health, power (but avoid red or limit its use if you are hypersensitive). As you perform your meditation, wear vitalizing shades of red or violet, and place a corresponding cloth on your altar.

*Sacred Stone Meditation.* While in meditation, hold in your palm over the center of your body the Healing Stone, bloodstone.

Vibrational healing can be done by wearing and adorning your body with stones as a necklace, waist beads, or belt. You can place them under your pillow when you sleep, or at the four corners of your bed. You may also put your stone in your bathwater, as well as soak it in your drink, to fill your system with stone healing. Finally, you may let the stone sit in your clay to enhance the rejuvenation and cleansing energies of your clay applications.

## 10. Herbal Tonics
Drink ginger herbal tea. Part used: fresh root. Ginger helps to quicken the healing spirit in a woman, so that she is equipped to purge and heal others. Drink your herb tea or tonic for seven days to receive the full benefits of tuning in to Gateway 6. Enjoy your herb tea in your favorite mug during or after spiritual writing.

*Preparation.* One teabag to 1 cup of water. Boil water in a nonmetallic pot, turn off flame, pour water over teabag, and steep. Drink before or after your morning bath or sacred shower. Drink with joy and peace as you breathe between sips and settle into easy contemplation and reflection.

## 11. Flower Essences
To deepen your experience of Gateway 6, choose from the following flower essences. Take 4 drops four times per day directly on or under the tongue, or add the same amount to a small glass of purified water and sip. For instructions on how to choose flower essences, see page 23.

• *Self-heal:* Contacting true inner healing capacities; courage to ignite self-responsibility in the healing process, especially to encourage the belief that one can be healed.
• *Love lies bleeding:* To allow and understand intense and deep feelings of suffering.
• *Shasta daisy:* Ability to think holistically and to integrate different therapeutic approaches.
• *Pink yarrow:* Helps suppress hypersensitivity to the healing process or adverse reaction to the therapeutic process because feelings seem magnified.
• *Black-eyed Susan:* For any form of denial during the healing process.

## 12. Diet
Follow the Sacred Woman Transitional Dietary Practices presented for Gateways 4–6.

## 13. Sacred Healing Journal Writing
This is best done after internal cleansing (enema) and/or meditation. When you are cleansed and centered, you can receive spiritual messages from the One Most High with grace. When you are in the spirit, messages travel down through your spirit mind, to your heart, into your hand, and onto the paper. (This is how I do all my writing.)

The best time to receive your spiritually inspired written work is after you have completed your altar work, between the hours of 4 A.M. and 6 A.M. Keep your journal and a very special pen by or on your altar to work with the power, force, and stillness at the coming of dawn, the hour of Nebt-Het.

Affirm your daily life. Write in your journal at this time thoughts, activities, experiences, and interactions that present themselves. You can also write down your visions, desires, dreams, and affirmations so that you will be able to draw on these resources when help and support are most needed.

*Consult Sesheta.* If you find that you are unable to contact your inner voice during your journal work, call Sesheta, the keeper and revealer of secrets (who is indwelling), to assist and speak through you.

### 14. Senab Freedom Shawl or Quilt

Choose a new piece of cloth that corresponds to the Gateway color (indicated in exercise 9 of your Daily Spiritual Observances or in Sacred Altar Work) to add to your Senab Freedom Shawl or Quilt. This cloth will serve as a mini-canvas to represent your experience in the Gateway you're working in.

Also, collect meaningful symbols that can be added to your shawl or quilt in appliqué or patchwork style. You can add stones, other natural objects, collectibles, family heirlooms, photographs that have been reprinted on fabric, or any other significant items that embody the essence of your experience. Give your imagination free rein and let your craftswoman spirit tell your story. For more information about the Senab Freedom Shawl or Quilt, see pages 122–125.

### 15. Sacred Tools

Crystal pendulum and pendulum charts, oracles such as the Metu Neter Oracle, Sacred Woman's Prayer Cards, Black Angel Cards, Motherpeace Deck, or the Medicine Woman Tarot Deck.

### 16. Sacred Reminder

Throughout the week, you are to observe closely wisdom presented for the Gateway you're in. For maximum results, live freely in tune with the various systems of wellness presented and practice the Seven-Day Transformative Work at the end of the Gateway.

### Closing Sacred Words

*Mother/Father Divine, help me heal my Sacred Life.*

# SACRED WOMAN, HEAL THYSELF

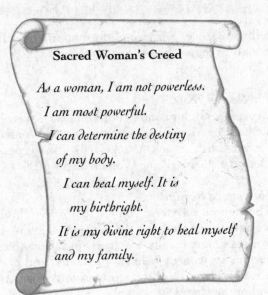

**Sacred Woman's Creed**

*As a woman, I am not powerless.*

*I am most powerful.*

*I can determine the destiny*

*of my body.*

*I can heal myself. It is*

*my birthright.*

*It is my divine right to heal myself*

*and my family.*

Reawaken your natural capacity to Heal Thyself from every affliction, for no disease is greater than you and your Divinity. Use this chapter to transform yourself into the woman you know you can be by working on your self-healing daily. The more you commit to self-healing, the more you understand that in order to experience true Divinity, you must become divine. Know that all matters of imbalance, disarray, or turmoil can be eradicated to the degree that we purify and honor our Body Temples, minds, and spirits.

## Sacred Medicine Women, Come Forth!

*These women of wisdom were respected by their people. These women could see beyond the obvious, predict the future, settle disputes, find lost property, and heal the sick.*[1]

In ancient Khamitic times there were—and are to the present day, in all parts of Afraka—Wise Women, Healers, and Priestesses.

Still you rise, Afrakan women of today, after all you've gone through for thousands of years. You, Medicine Women, Wise Women, Healers capable of all things, still you rise to go on and heal the Nation.

## Sacred Medicine Woman Affirmation

*As I fan myself from right to left while loosening my big dress, I proceed to squat and rotate my hips to the sacred four directions, so that I may bring balance to this incredible earth. I anoint and bless my womanness with frankincense and myrrh. I give praises that I can see the unseen and hear the unspoken.*

*Hear me now! I'm fully in the spirit, as natural as one can possibly be, for I don't travel anywhere without my herbs. I'm a believer in complete transformation as I move forward in my active meditation. Let it be known wherever I am in my life, I chant: "Ankh khepera, for life, transformation." And so it is, from the crown of my head, from my heart, and from the palms of my hands, I send out absolute healing to everyone I meet.*

## Channeling for Sacred Medicine Women from the Most High

All those in tune, the bell has rung. The changing of hands is taking place. Now the righteous are taking the lead. The pure of heart, the pure of Body Temple, are coming forth. Let it be you. The Most High said to me as I received in the spirit:

*I am gathering my obedient and faithful—gathering them up, training them in the spirit, sending them out to heal the sick, to heal the land.*

*Come forth, you Freedom Fighters, you Healers Divine. Come forth, you Harriet Tubmans and Sojourner Truths. Come forth, you Asatawas, righteous Warrior Queens. Come forth, Queen Nzinga and Queen Hatshepsut, too. Come forth, you Wise Women, Medicine Women, Ancient Women, Sacred Women, Sanctified and Holy Women. Mother Ast and Mother Mary come forth with the old ways, the first ways, the power and spirit knowledge of our great beginnings. Come forth, stand firm, and heal our dark Nubian race.*

*Demons and fallen angels have been cast out. The road is clear. The gates are open now as your aritu are opened due to the purity in your Body Temple.*

*Snap! The spell has been broken. You can go free, to heal the earth from sea to sea. I, the Most High, put the power right in your hands to heal the people and free the land. Don't you hesitate. Don't you wait. I am guiding you, so keep the faith.*

*Men tune in to the womb through you. Remember the Ancient Healing is coming through you, too. Be wise, be humble, be strong, be brave. Allow my healing to come through.*

*Ancient Women, Sacred Women, Medicine Women, Sanctified Women, Wise Women, remember the old ways from the Great Mother Spirit. Hear My call, the call to Divine Order, to the Ancient Ways of My Sacred Earth Medicine. Come forth; awaken to your natural self.*

*Remember the Medicine Women of thousands of years ago, the Original Women, sacred and divine. They are you, returning Ancestors with the initiative and knowledge from Me, the Great Mother Spirit, to heal every condition. I am the Great Mother Spirit, and I say to you that your tools are the old medicine, that I speak through the mud, the waters, all natural whole foods, the sacred herbs that grow from my rich soil.*

*Children of Light, Sacred Women Pure and Divine, come gather round here. The time is up, it's growing near. Stay in tune, go within. You'll find me there. Follow my lead; follow it now, for "I am that I am." My guidance will show you how to heal all those on the land.*

Thank you, Dr. Alvenia Fulton and Dick Gregory, original sources of inspiration for fasting and Natural Living. Thank you, Dr. Fulton, my Elder and mentor, for reminding me to make soup when strangers appear.

## Wife as Healer / Mother as Healer

There was a King Man named Kali whom I met at a Nubian spiritual gathering. He spoke of a back condition that had him in pain and flat out in bed. He spoke of Zebilah, his dear wife, giving him a healing by applying clay to his back. After three applications he was pain-free, able to move once again.

I asked him, "Are you aware that your wife is an ancient Medicine Woman?" He replied, "Yes, I know. Had it not been for my wife, Zebilah, my enemies would have destroyed me." This let me know that Zebilah has been there, patiently and lovingly healing her man, for many a day.

It's a fact that the most visible healers have been men—from Imhotep to Afrakan American surgeon Dr. Ben Carson. But isn't it the woman who maintains the health of the family? Day-to-day healing comes right from the home. If the woman stays in her natural state, then sickness and disease can be prevented through the grace of the Creator/Creatress. Natural healing in the home through each and every healthy meal prevents the need to seek outside cures because you have not gone against the flow of Divine Natural Laws.

### Affirmation: Inner and Outer Harmony

*As a Sacred Woman, I am the Original Healer. I call upon my brothers and sisters, the elements—air, fire, water, and earth—to heal physically, mentally, and spiritually, for I am the great-granddaughter of Mother Nature herself!*

## Healers Are Coming Through

Women, stir that pot. Let the spirit move in you. Heal your mother, your father, your children, your friends, and your coworkers, too—even the strangers the Divine places in your path— because you've got the power in your hands. All women are healers, so go and do your work.

Medicine Women have insurmountable, unwavering power, and when it is unleashed it can raise the dead. Medicine women heal with herbs, mud, food, air, water, and spirit. When men create unnatural laws that tell women they cannot heal themselves and their families and their loved ones, it is a spiritual travesty. It is a crime that will be judged and sentenced upon departure from this earth.

Don't try to suppress a Healer coming through. If you do, you'd better look over your shoulder, for disharmony is on its way to you. What form will it take? Only the spirit knows. But there is no need to invite disease to your door. So please sit down, so the Healer can heal you.

The Healer's work has been ordained from birth, from the Creator/Creatress who rules the heavens and the earth. Let it not be told that you stood in the way of human salvation, for Grandmother Earth will get upset, causing a volcanic eruption or hurricanes if necessary. So, whatever you do, don't stand in the way of a Healer coming through.

Sacred Woman, when you take a stand as a Healer and you heal yourself, you know you have the power and authority to heal every condition and circumstance in your life. Women, Sacred and Divine, when you complete this initiation process, you begin to activate your true healing self. Healer! Yes, you are. Healer! Your life will be glorified and you will know how to be divine!

### Meditation from an Unknown Healer

*I thank Thee for rain in its season, for gentle winds, and merciful clouds, for heat and cold, all adapted by Thy love to meeting human comfort and Nature's needs. For all of these Thou hast appointed a time so that the beauty and productiveness of Thy creation may increase. Let nothing hinder the harmony of the whole, but let man and Nature work together to restore the perfection of Thy kingdom on Earth.*

*I now speak peace and harmony to the elements, that all Nature may receive directly from Thy hands and fulfill its purpose of beauty and productiveness, in the name and through the power of the One who said to the waves and winds: "Peace. Be still," and received instant recognition and obedience. I speak to all Thy creation: "Let harmony and peace reign supreme in you, that it may be so in the elements."*

I've carried this meditation for over thirteen years now. These words are anointed in my heart. Unknown Healer, may peace reign supreme in you, whoever and wherever you may be, for you have been a blessing to me and to those who read your inspired words. May your life be sweet and filled with blessings.

## ACCESSING THE HEALING SPIRIT THROUGH THE BREATH

We're now going to explore several approaches to healing yourself and others. We will begin with the breath, the source of Spirit in our Body Temples. Then we will move on to healing with the hands, with water, with sacred stones, and healing through inspiration.

Elders and wise people know that it's necessary to get beyond their busy schedule for a moment to sit, be still, close their eyes, and go within for meditation. Do as the wise ones do: Open up in prayer, and then allow your mind and body to relax in total stillness. After ten or fifteen minutes of stillness and peacefulness, ask your questions. Then listen with your inner ear for the answers.

If you are still not able to immediately access your answers, try these techniques:

- Drink a pint of warm water with the juice of one lemon.
- Perform one to three hundred Fire Breaths and/or twenty-five deep, deep inhalations and exhalations to relax your body.
- Now tune into Spirit once again and become an open channel for guidance.

Our Elders knew the importance of doing our inner work. As they rocked in their rocking chairs, they pondered on the how, who, and why of the puzzling issues of life, and they listened for answers from deep within. You can rest assured that as our Elders rocked to and fro, the answers would flow.

Our grandmothers and grandfathers knew how to listen and receive in the Spirit. My grandmother would be so self-assured about what she heard that she'd tell me: "Child, don't you worry, don't you fear. Listen up. Don't you hear?" They were so perfectly in tune, living and rocking and humming in the Spirit, that they could guide us and support us each and every step of the way.

Thank you, beloved Elders, for showing us the natural way of tuning in to the Holy Spirit.

### Breath and Spirit Are One

To do your inner work and to be fully alive, breath must be supreme, for the Creator/Creatress and the breath are one. If you have breathing problems and blockages, you have spiritual problems and blockages. Mend the breath and you heal the spirit. Increase your breathing capacity and you increase the quality of your life.

Breath is life; without breath there is death. All your activity should include attention to the breath. Your food must contain breath, so your foods must be of the highest quality—live, organic whole grains, uncooked fruits and vegetables, fresh juices and herbs full of live enzymes. Cooked food, fast foods, and all flesh foods lack breath. These foods put the Body Temple into a deathlike state.

There must also be breathing space in all your relationships. They should have free-flowing light and air and room for true communication; otherwise toxic associations can lead you to a premature death. Your home must be clean and pure, with oxygen flowing through to support your life force.

Inhale and exhale deeply when conducting all your affairs and in all your circumstances. In this way you will be filled with breath, with life. The breath must flow smoothly between the inhalation and the exhalation. Your breath is crucial. The more conscious you become of your breath, the more you feel the presence of the Creator/Creatress dwelling within you. So before, during, and after meditation and prayer, keep your breath deep, quiet, and even.

If you notice that your breath becomes shallow and uneven when you're around certain people, it may be due to a lack of communication between them and you. Or it may be due to their inner negativity, or your own. It is best to discontinue your association with them until you are fully empowered with a lifestyle that supports the free flow of oxygen to your spirit despite the negativity around you. Once your breath/life is strong, you will be able to balance out your interactions with all and every association, for breath is life and peace.

*An Herbal Tonic for the Lungs:* For cleansing and developing strong, balanced lungs, boil 3 cups of water, turn off the flame, then add 1 tsp. mullein leaves, 1 tsp. eucalyptus leaves, and 1 tsp. of freshly juiced or grated gingerroot. Instead of sugar or honey, use the water of soaked dates or raisins to sweeten this tea, or drink it in its pure form.

## Two Daily Meditations: Using the Breath for Renewal

When your cup is brimming with life's challenges, confusion, and pain, it's time to do an emptying meditation so you won't accumulate any additional spiritual, mental, and emotional toxins. To clear yourself, you will perform these meditations for seven to twenty-one sunrises and sunsets. The meditations also work as prevention against spiritual toxins and offer mountains of peace, especially when you need sacred centering the most.

### Emptying Meditation

- Before you begin, drink 1 pint of pure water, and smudge your sacred space with sage or jasmine to clear the atmosphere.
- Inhale slowly while counting backward from ten to zero. As you hold your breath for ten counts, pray to let any circumstance or individual ready to be released appear in your mind's eye. Then, as you exhale, count from ten to zero. Breathe out and release from your Holy Temple whatever circumstances—persons, thoughts, or actions—you need to let go of. As you move closer to zero, you will be releasing the toxic situations that block your blessings, and your cup will become empty.
- To enhance this meditation, hold a clear quartz crystal in your hand for clarity, or lie down and place a crystal over your sixth *arit* (chakra), on your forehead between your eyes. Now allow your mind and body to just float. Anchor your emptying work naturally by seeing yourself in the ocean being baptized and feeling clean. Or see yourself on a high mountain, breathing in the rarefied air. Or just be as you sit on a field of grass with the sun pouring energy and light into your Body Temple.
- After you are done, drink 18 oz. or more of pure water and give thanks.

This emptying meditation will keep you ageless. To become more cosmically energized, perform this meditation for three or four days after the night of the new moon. You may also want to fast for two to four hours on the new moon.

## Filling Up or Rejuvenation Meditation

- Fill up your Body Temple with love and light and supreme peace as you slowly inhale and exhale from deep within while counting slowly from zero to ten.
- On each inhalation and exhalation, sense the positive energy building within you. See yourself becoming stronger and more potent. See each breath of life filling you with love, peace, joy, and abundance.
- With each breath, affirm that your condition, circumstances, feelings, and relationships are all being healed.

Do these emptying and filling up meditations daily, and whenever you're inspired to do so. To enhance their effect:

- You may hold clear quartz crystals in the palm of each hand while performing these meditations.
- Throughout the day give thanks and praise for your purification and rejuvenation.
- Drink 4 to 12 oz. of some form of chlorophyll (green drink)—for example, water or juice mixed with spirulina or wheatgrass, or alfalfa and dandelion herb tea, or Heal Thyself Green Life Formula I, or a freshly juiced mixture of broccoli, kale, and parsley.
- Anoint your seven energy centers or *aritu* with essential oils.

## THESE ARE HEALING HANDS

The One Creator/Creatress transmits love through our hands for spiritual healing, if we are willing to be a living vessel of the glory and grace of the Creator/Creatress.

How many people have you healed with these hands without even realizing it? Every time you served a troubled friend a cup of herb tea, or stroked your child's head when she was sad, or opened the door to someone in need and gestured for them to come in, you extended healing, encouragement, and peace with your hands.

Honor all the love that you've given out all these years through your hands. Now take those hands and wrap them around yourself; hold on real tight. Receive the love and care that you are in need of through your own healing hands. Pour the love on thick. Embrace yourself deeply. Then when you've received enough, open your hands back to the world so your hands may extend that all-powerful love to others, for your healing hands are a gift from on high.

As a Sacred Woman, whatever or whomever you touch is charged with healing. When you tuck a baby into bed, the baby receives wellness and sleeps deeply. When you rub an Elder's feet, he or she then walks with less pain. When you prepare a crying sister-friend a bowl of soup, she dries her tears and takes a new look at her life. When you sweep your home with your hands wrapped around a cinnamon broom, blessings begin to flow. When you serve your family natural foods filled with love, profound healing takes place—all because you have healing hands, blessed and cleansed by the Creator/Creatress.

The laying on of hands opens you to the laying on of High Spirit from one soul to another. It opens you to the laying on of heart, of compassion. And it opens you to the laying on of healing words so that when you speak, the sound, the tone of your voice, and the words that you utter create wellness in those you meet.

### Prayer for Laying on of Hands

Open your palms facing upward and call upon the Lord, NTR, Mother/Father God, Jehovah, Allah, Olodumare, Krishna—the Creator/Creatress is one.

*Divine Creator/Creatress, living and breathing in me, I empty myself of all negativity. I open my mind, my soul, my heart, and my hands to you. Please fill my hands with your divine power and light. Charge and guide my hands so that I may follow and do your will, so that I may be your instrument of healing, so that I may be your instrument of peace. Do with me what you will. With hands blessed and pure, Creator/Creatress, I give thanks and praise to you.*

Laying on of hands, the first form of energy work, was clearly depicted on the temple walls in Khamit, by Ast and Nebt-Het. They are shown resurrecting Asar the King on what appears to be an ancient massage table. Ast is sending healing energy through Asar's feet through her hands, posed in a Kes (a pose of praise).

Nebt-Het is simultaneously standing by Asar's head (crown), as she is sending the healing Life force of breath through Asar with the Maat feather.

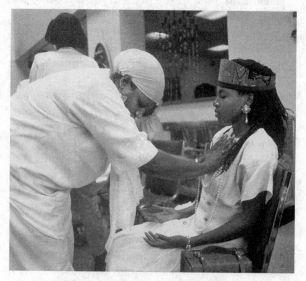

These hands are Healing Hands.

## LAYING ON OF HANDS

### How to Do Hands-on Energy Work

1. Smudge your work area.
2. Drink 8 oz. of pure water.
3. Do a spiritual wash for yourself and the person who will be receiving the laying on of hands. With a small bowl of hyssop water, very lightly wash down the face, throat, arms, hands, legs, and feet.
4. Anoint your chakras and the recipient's chakras with essential oil of frankincense and myrrh or lotus.

- Wash your hands thoroughly with black Afrakan soap or clay soap (from the health food store) and with pure water or with hyssop, which you make as an herbal tea.
- Call for the presence of the Source of All Healing, the Most Divine, who is indwelling, for the highest good of the person who has re-quested the laying on of hands energy work. (Never do hands-on work, not even at a distance, with anyone who has not given you their permission.)
- Make certain your own protective energy field is in place. To do this, center and quiet yourself, and visualize yourself completely surrounded by pure white or golden light. Always remember to establish your protective field before doing any energy work.
- Now breathe deeply seven times. Breathe in light and healing energy, and exhale all blockages, confusion, or doubt that will interfere with the flow.
- Ask that Sekhmet Ra light this work through you. Call on Ast and Nebt-Het to work through you with the laying on of hands skills that they used to resurrect Asar, the king, so the Nubian race would continue.
- Continue your breathing, but now focus your awareness on the *aritu* (chakras) in the palms of your hands. Rub your hands briskly together, as the healing breath of Nebt-Het breathes life into your hands.
- You can test for the presence of the healing energy by turning your palms toward each other about six inches apart, and very gently and very slowly attempting to bring your hands together. You should feel some resistance, as though you were holding an invisible ball between your hands.

If you don't feel the energy, center and quiet yourself again, and repeat the breathing.

- Before you begin to work—on yourself or someone else—offer a prayer to the Divine One, using your own words, or perhaps this example:

*Divine Sekhmet, allow me to be a clear instrument of your healing energies. I open myself up so that your sacred healing may flow through me to assist in easing the pain and suffering of _____ [person receiving hands-on work]. May this work assist in reawakening his/her abilities to heal himself/herself. Tua NTR (Thanks to the Divinity).*

- The first step in working with someone is to do a body scan, using your palm chakras as the "eyes" to read their energy field. Have them lie down and breathe quietly while you are doing your preparatory work, so they are calm and ready when you begin.

Hold your palms about three inches or so over the body of the person you are working on—you can begin at the feet or at the head, whichever area calls to you first. Very slowly move your hands along their body, getting a sense of their energy.

Stop whenever you come upon an unusual feeling—a cold spot, a hot spot, or an empty spot, an area where you sense there is an intense energy blockage or hole.

Keep in mind where the unusual imbalances exist, and continue your scan, until you have covered the person's entire body.

- When the scan is complete, you can discuss the areas where you felt problems existed, or you can simply return to these spots one at a time and work on them for a few minutes.

- Focus the heat of your hands on a problem area. Some people like to move the energy clockwise with their hands over the spot, then pull up, push out, or draw out pain and negative energy, returning it to Nut, the Heavenly Mother, or into Ta-Urt, the earth, for purification. Each time you do this, shake your hands vigorously several times to remove the energy being discarded.

When you feel a release, a letting go, a sigh, or a deep breath from the person, your work on that spot is complete. You will sense that the energy balance has been restored or that the work is sufficient for now.

Don't overactivate any one spot; you can return to it later if necessary. Remember, energy work is powerful, and you don't want to tire out the person you're working on or yourself.

Repeat this process for the major problem areas you encountered in the scan. Never work longer than forty-five minutes to an hour.

- If images arise in your mind, or the person you're working on tells you that they're seeing a scene of some sort in their mind, talk about it. This may be a hidden memory of a trauma from this life, or perhaps a past life that's coming to the surface to be released. The body remembers major injuries, even from life to life. But when the memory comes to consciousness,

it can be released, along with the pain and difficulty it has caused.

For example, a person may have suffered from a stiff shoulder that has ached for years and years with no relief. But when they discover that in a past life someone ran them through the shoulder with a lance or sword and they died from this wound, this recall can release the pain in the present life once and for all.

- As the session is ending, call upon the Divine to fill this person with a sense of Maat, harmony, *hotep*, and Nefer Atum (illumination). Say this out loud. And do a final scan, putting the white light of protection around the person, and tell them that you are doing this.

- Let the person lie quietly for a minute or two, then have him or her rise slowly and gently and sit in a chair for a few minutes, sipping the glass of water with the juice of half a lemon that you have prepared, or even better, wheatgrass and/or juice made from any fresh green vegetables.

- You might want to caution the person that energy work essentially speeds up the body's own self-healing abilities, and it will fast-forward through the healing process. So they may feel a bit worse for the next two or three days, comparable to the experience of a cleansing crisis when you purify your diet. But after that they should start to feel truly energized and renewed.

- Suggest that the person might want to take healing baths, drink cleansing herbal teas, and eat a light, meatless diet for the next few days to enhance the effect of the energy work.

- While the person is sipping, shake your hands out one more time, and wash them thoroughly with salt water, and/or rinse with hyssop water.

- Drink at least 8 oz. of purified water with the juice of ½ lemon or drink a glass of juice made from any fresh green vegetables. This restores the balance of electrolytes in your system, which may get depleted when you do energy work of any sort.

- Check your own energy field to make sure all is well. If you have time, take an Epsom salts bath with a few drops of frankincense and myrrh essential oil. And thank the Source of

All Healing for the assistance and guidance you received.

## CHANNELING THE GATEWAYS

We all have the capacity to receive the Divine. Through conscious channeling work we allow ourselves to become vessels for the spiritual Guardians. If we have been adequately cleansed in body, mind, and spirit and are pure in our intentions, our request for guidance is granted. And the Spiritual Guardians funnel information, guidance, and healing to us, from the *heavenly realm to the earthly realm.*

If you are blocked and you need answers to questions, then open a channel into the appropriate Gateway. To channel is to allow light to come through you. Before you begin, offer the following prayer:

### Prayer for Divine Guidance, Protection, and Purification

*Mut (Mother), Atef (Father) Divine, who are indwelling, I ask that you open the way for me to receive a healing. I pray that the secrets of my heart be revealed to me. Oh, Mut Ammit, spare me from your jaws, which consume the hearts of the unjust. I pray that you guide my every movement, protect and purify my heart and my breath as I seek the wisdom of Tehuti. I pray that Maat will honor me with her wings of truth, that I may dwell in the lotus heart of Nefer Atum for all eternity.*

### Preparation and Protection Work for Channeling

- Purify the space and all those who are to take part in the channeling first by smudging the space with frankincense and myrrh or sage.
- Smudge the participants in the channeling session.
- Purify yourself by drinking bitters. Bitters detoxify evil thoughts, which come from evil spirits. Drink a glass of bitter herbal tea (i.e., goldenseal, ¼ teaspoon to 8–16 oz. of water; or add juice of 1 or 2 limes to 8–16 oz. of water; or aloe vera, ¼ teaspoon to 8–16 oz. of warm water). Avoid goldenseal during pregnancy.
- Prepare the Nefer Atum lotus bath formula: Combine 1 quart of distilled water or rainwater, 3 or 4 drops of frankincense and myrrh essential oil, 2 drops of lotus essential oil, and and 2 tbsp. hyssop essential oil.
- Give yourself or the seeker of truth a Maat spiritual bath for purification, sweetness, and protection. Pour the Nefer Atum lotus bath formula in a calabash or a glass bowl, which you hold in both hands as you pray. You need a heavy bath for heavy concerns.
- Soak in a tub of water with 2 to 4 lbs. of Epsom salts or 1 to 2 lbs. of Dead Sea salt for thirty minutes. Rinse, then pour the Nefer Atum lotus bath over you.

### To Channel

- Lie down on your back or sit in a chair, close your eyes, then begin to call your Guardian. The Guardians that you call upon are all indwelling divine aspects that you can tap into whenever needed.
- Begin breathing full body breaths, slowly inhaling on the count of four and exhaling on the count of eight. Do this several times, until you are completely relaxed and centered.
- Now chant the name of the Guardian who rules or represents your quest several times until you are one with the indwelling spirit of the Gateway.
- Visit the Holy of Holies by going into your heart center. Visualize yourself standing before the Gateway that symbolizes the truth you seek.
- Open up the Gateway with your mind. Go deep inside. You are now facing the Altar of your Ab (heart), the altar of your quest where you are seeking guidance.
- Place your request upon your altar. Breathe, release your fears, apprehensions, and judgments, and listen with your innermost ear for the answers. Just listen, let go, and relax, and you will hear Maat (truth). If you feel a little blocked in gaining the answers, then repeat the breathing until you feel relaxed.

If you still cannot hear the answers you seek, then call on Sesheta, the Keeper of Secrets, to reveal what you wish to know. Make your connection by repeating her name or by speaking to Sesheta from within. Say: "Sesheta, divine inner guidance, I ask that you reveal the secrets of my heart to me that I may heal."

## Advanced Initiates

Determine which Gateway you need assistance from. Call inwardly for the Guardian of that Gateway as you face the altar of your Ab. For example, call for Maat to speak through you if you have a Maat issue of finding out the truth. Or call for Ast to speak through you if your question is about relationships. The Guardians of the Gateway will speak through you according to your need. They will speak through your mind or your mouth on your behalf as they bestow answers to your questions from within.

## Departing from the Channel

Once you have received your answer, you are ready to return from your innermost journey to the Holy of Holies.

- Begin to inhale and exhale deeply and fully. With each breath say, *"Tua NTR, Tua Maat,"* Thank you, Divine, thank you for truth and balance. *"Tua Tehuti,"* Thank you for divine wisdom.
- Give thanks to the Guardian of the Gateway where you received guidance. Or you may simply and always say, *"Tua NTR,"* which covers all the indwelling aspects of the Divine.
- Now that you have returned to the more material world, stretch your body with gratitude, for the journey is now complete.

Sacred Woman, the level and depth of your channeling depends on your ability to be in a state of divine detachment. In this state you are unafraid of knowing truth, for the truth will set you free. Only through Maat (truth) can you experience *khepera* (transformation) leading to Sekhmet (healing).

## If You Need to Unblock Your Healing Powers

When you need your healing power to come through, say:

> O, Afrakan Spirit of Yemaya,
> bring forth my khepera [transformation].

If for any reason you are unable to send out healing, then cleanse, meditate, and pray. There's a part of you that needs to purge deep within. Examine yourself for anger and depression. Are you using the evil eye on anyone, or holding on to vengeful thinking?* Are you putting yourself down? Are you blocking your sister's good? Are you putting dead or processed foods in your mouth, drinking from depression, smoking from habit, eating flesh because you say, "This is how Mama raised me"? Are you being impatient with children, cursing your husband, or eating or sleeping to suppress emptiness? All of these things block our ability to heal ourselves—and others.

If you desire to change your attitude, thoughts, and actions, then repeat the following daily or as often as needed:

> *I have destroyed my defects. I have made an end of my wickedness. I have annihilated the faults that belong to me. I myself am pure. I am mighty.*[2]

* *Warning!* The evil eye can be used only in matters of life and death, for if the force behind it is strong enough, it can destroy an unrighteous enemy who is genuinely threatening your life or the life of your family.

# Who Says You Can't Be Your Own Doctor?
## by Kwasausya Khepera

*I was attracted to healing because of a picture of my mother that stayed in my mind. She was young and fine, around nineteen years old, standing in a playground. I wondered how she, my aunts, and grandmother had come to change so drastically. At what point did disease set in? Where did the high blood pressure, diabetes, and obesity get their start? I'd had fragile health in my earlier years, and I knew that I could also wind up sick. But I believed that through Natural Living I could break the cycle—beginning with me.*

*My grandma, Geraldine Burgess, died afflicted by many diseases. Although she took laxatives regularly, used vegetable salt, and ate plenty of raw grated carrots and salad, her feet still burst open from diabetes—perhaps because she also liked corn bread, hog maws, chitterlings, and steak. Sometimes she was bedridden or in the hospital, miserable and in pain.*

*When I learned that my great-grandmother Mackey was heavy into herbs and nature cures, I was surprised. She passed at ninety very peacefully, without pain, and without a wrinkle on her face. They said she died because she never went to the doctor. But it seemed to me that she lived as long as she did because she took her health and healing into her own hands.*

*Just as the medical doctor has diagnostic tools and medicine, you also have your medicine bags and healing tools: herbs, wheatgrass, enema bag, natural live and raw foods, freshly pressed fruit and vegetable juices.*

*Vegetable sprouts contain large amounts of easily digestible protein, and when your fruits and vegetables are taken raw, their enzymes, vitamins, and minerals are intact and work like medicine for your Body Temple. However, in addition to consuming lots of raw foods, we also take nutrients. This is because much of our food is grown in soil that is devitalized, and deficient soil produces foods that lack complete nutrients and minerals. Much damage is done to the soil by chemical fertilizers that are toxic to us as well.*

*Taking baths with ingredients from the elements—air, fire, water, and earth—is also crucial, as the body is made up of the elements. Exercise is important because only activity will burn fat and toxins, contrary to the popular notion that diet pills can burn fat while you sleep.*

*With the health care crisis and skyrocketing medical costs, it's in our best interests to know how to "Heal Thyself." Vegetarian food is the safest "fast food" (raw or steamed in mere minutes), and it is not*

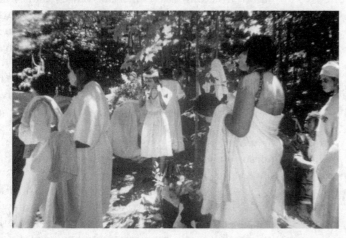

*expensive when you stick to the basics and begin preparing all your own food in your own Kitchen Healing Laboratory.*

*Like a good doctor, it is important to be well read, well informed, and aware of your health options. More importantly, it is necessary to reorient our people to the mind-set that disease is not normal and you should not grow debilitated, be sick, and wither away as you age. The opposite is true: The quality of the total sum of our lives can be improved and enhanced.*

## HEALING WITH WATER

Healing with water is one of the most powerful transformational methods. It puts us in the flow of the spirit and energy of the earth, whose surface is two-thirds water. Doing meditations and self-healing in the shower, baths, pools, ponds, rivers, and the ocean—all of it is restoring, cleansing, and purifying. We ourselves are 60 percent water, and being in the flow renews us inside and out.

### Baba's Spiritual Healing Bath: To Purify the Body Temple, Release, and Renew

In the summer of 1984, Baba Ishangi, a Yoruba Priest, Afrakan historian, and vegetarian for over thirty years, prepared a Spiritual Bath formula for me that helped me clear my path, cast out fear and negativity, and open the way to many blessings in my life.

Baba Ishangi, along with the entire Ishangi family, was honored at the United Nations for excellence in the teaching and the spreading of Afrakan culture and dance. This extraordinary family has gained worldwide acclaim.

This is how Baba told me to take a Spiritual Bath:

1. First, prepare a quart of spiritual wash.

- Use rainwater or purified water (temperature of the wash should be cold or room temperature).
- Add approximately 1 tbsp. of raw honey to water for sweetness.
- Cinnamon is optional.
- Add one handful of hyssop leaves.

2. Cover mirrors in the bathroom.
3. Burn frankincense and myrrh to purify your condition, and add cinnamon to sweeten your situation.
4. Get on your knees in the tub and scrub yourself with black Afrakan soap, or coconut or clay soap. Use warm water or room-temperature water with a sponge or washcloth as you wash downward and pray.
5. Sing spiritual songs that apply to your condition.

6. Now pour a bowl (or gourd) of spiritual wash over your head and let the wash run down your entire Body Temple.
7. Repeat this anywhere from three to seven times until your inner voice reveals that you have completed your task. I usually did three washings in one sitting. It could go up to as many as seven if there was a major spiritual blockage or problem.
8. Baba told me that when I was finished I should apply pure white clay or powder over my body to represent the High Holy Spirit within me and upon me. I then went to my altar to pray and to receive further spiritual guidance.

Baba recommended that the Spiritual Bath should be taken at the following times:

- At the New Moon, and at the beginning of new projects, in order to energize them
- At the Full Moon, to subdue or stabilize one's energy; also to bring forth an idea, concept, or situation
- Before, during, and after a cleansing fast; before traveling; before marriage; before and on one's birthday, and during one's birthday month; before and after birthing a baby
- To purify oneself from adversity
- If one is experiencing any physical, spiritual, mental, or financial blockages

I've been blessed to have assisted Baba Ishangi in countless Spiritual Baths that were given at the Heal Thyself Center in my early years as a vessel of healing. After he performed the baths, he would give the person a very clear and concise spiritual reading. I recall that Baba would fast during his readings to stay in the spirit even though his readings would last five, six, even eight hours. He would drink only an herbal brew with blackstrap molasses in it. Then he would pray, sing spiritual songs, and read the person's past, present, and future as he sat in this pure state.

I will never forget my own first Spiritual Bath. It was a soul-stirring cleansing that will live with me a lifetime. Since then, spiritual bathing by the ocean or in my home has been a part of my evolution on the Path of Purification. It is earth-changing for me.

# HEALING WITH SACRED STONES

Since antiquity, people have revered the healing properties of the bones of the earth, our mother. Deep within her heart, in her dark and secret places, she creates minerals and gems of astonishing beauty and color and healing properties. We need only hold her wondrous bounty in our hands to feel their inner power and energy. We need only listen to their slow earth heartbeat to learn what parts of the body and spirit they have an affinity for.

The following sacred stones—semiprecious stones and gems—were worn by our ancient Nile Valley ancestors to energize, empower, and purify the seven *aritu* (energy centers). Not only were these precious stones beautiful and captivating to the eye, they also contained healing power that maintained the wellness of the Body Temple. These stones were worn thousands of years ago and are still available to us today to use as talismans for spiritual protection; as necklaces, earrings, pendants; as stones for healing rituals; as a part of body work when doing massage, auric cleansing, or water healing; as room activators; and as calmers.

The Khamitic people worked closely with the system of *aritu*—subtle energy centers in the body, also known as chakras. Each *arit* corresponds to a particular stone that our Ancestors wore as sacred jewelry. These various stones aided in opening up the seven energy centers.

*Arit 1—Hematite* is a steel-gray to iron-black form of iron oxide. This stone stimulates, unblocks, and heals conditions that relate to the first *arit*—the energy center that grounds us on earth and regulates the base chakra, and our basic survival energies. Hematite is highly effective when placed at the base of the spine or by the buttocks.

*Arit 2—Amber* is a tree resin that often contains fossilized forms of flowers or insects. It ranges in color from orange to dark brown. Amber is connected to the electromagnetic energies of the etheric body. This stone represents the second *arit*, the sacral energy center that regulates the sexual and reproductive system. Amber is also said to stabilize the spleen, heart, and base of the spine.

*Arit 3—Carnelian* is a reddish opaque stone. It helps to regulate the intake of food, as well as assimilation and circulation. It helps the digestive system properly filter. It gives you the ability to handle and break down challenges that come into your life. This gem represents the third *arit*, the solar plexus, the energy center that regulates the digestive system gateway.

*Arit 4—Jade* is a green stone ranging from light to deep shades that generates Divine love. It aids in promoting altruism and unconditional love by aligning the subtle bodies. It serves as a balancing and calming energy to all those who come in contact with it. This stone represents the fourth *arit*, the energy center that controls the heart, the seat of love and compassion.

*Arit 5—Turquoise* is a blue-green stone that gives us wisdom and brings good fortune. It can absorb negative feelings and vibrations and sends healing to the wearer. This gem represents the fifth *arit*, the energy center that regulates the throat, which aids in intelligent creativity and divine communication, so the sacred words from On High can come through.

*Arit 6—Lapis lazuli* is a deep blue stone that stimulates both love and beauty, and helps to illuminate the mind. Lapis lazuli builds a sense of unity in man and woman. This stone is known to have healing, curative, and purifying properties. Its high vibratory spiritual color opens our capacity for inner seeing, prophetic visions, and clairvoyance. This stone represents the sixth *arit*, the energy center in the forehead, between the brows, the first eye that activates the high spiritual mind.

*Arit 7—Amethyst quartz* dispels anger, rage, fear, and anxiety. It aids in eliminating pain and cleansing the Body Temple. Amethyst purifies the lower nature so that you can reach Asar higher consciousness. This gem represents the seventh *arit*, the energy center that regulates the crown of the head—the gateway of the highest spiritual knowledge and union with the Divine.

## INTUITIVE HEALING

Now that you have done so much healing work on yourself and your life—with diet, exercise, baths, herbal preparations, prayer, altar work, meditation, journaling—you have truly begun to open up your inner channels of communication with the Highest Source. You have probably begun to experience flashes of intuition or inner "knowing." What this means is that you're opening to your gifts of clairvoyance and prophecy.

This could not have happened until you journeyed through the preceding Gateways, because you would not have been clear enough to receive accurate answers to your questions. Also, by doing your inner healing work on a steady basis, you have developed a powerful sense of self-responsibility and compassion for others.

The most important thing is to use these awakening gifts to express respect and gratitude for the Source. The world is made up of both light and dark, and it is our job as Sacred Women to maintain the balance between these opposing forces within ourselves and in our lives.

Our Ancestors knew that our spirits face tremendous challenges on a daily basis—from our inner forces of temptation and negativity to outer attacks both subtle and overt. This is why we have the presence and protection of Maat—truth, clarity, and balance—and this is why our hearts are weighed against the feather of Maat every day, to make us consciously aware of when we are out of balance, for only then can we make the proper changes in ourselves.

We all have our times of weakness and doubt, Sacred Woman! But we have tools for recovering from these states. We have the love and protection of all the Spiritual Guardians we have met as we moved through the Gateways. We have the love and protection of Maat. And above all, we have the protection of NTR, the Highest Source of Love. We only need to ask for their help and protection.

It's as simple as that. And as hard as that. Because the Universal Law says, "To get help, you must ask for help." We must be responsible to ourselves—to see where we are, to know when to ask for help. There is no room for ego in a Sacred Woman. We must recognize and honor our true needs. That's when we need to do an inner cleansing, to fast, meditate, pray, take a sacred bath, write in our journal, or go out into Nature. We must ask for help, and we must know, deeply in our heart of hearts, that help is instantly there.

### Consulting Time-Tested Oracles

I read life. I read life's symbols by observing by how the feather falls at my feet to remind me to step in balance, or I read why a person who has asthma is my devoted client, which is a reminder to me to take better care of my lungs. For almost ten years, I lived as a hermit in order to channel the works of Sacred Woman.

I have been personally reading cards to help me raise my children and to learn to see with my first eye. Now it's time for me to open up and reach out, so I have developed the Sacred Woman's Prayer Cards to help you work with the Sacred Guardians of each Gateway. I have channeled and developed these cards for the spiritual support of Sacred Woman initiates and devotees to the Light of Truth. (See the product list in the appendix.)

Sen-Urt Kaitha Het-Heru, the Priestess of the Gate of Het-Hru, designed a divine personal set of oracle cards inspired from our ancient Khamitic legacy to assist her in her spiritual reading with clients and divinations. She points out that in ancient times temple Priestesses were carefully trained to perform this service.

To prepare your Sacred Woman Divination Cards for use, first prepare your deck by smudging it with sage for purification. Next, to maintain your deck's high vibratory level, select a silk cloth to keep your deck wrapped in when you're not using it.

You don't always have to do a whole complex reading. You can choose one card for daily meditation, guidance, and journal work. To do this:

• Shuffle the deck five times, then spread the cards facedown on a flat surface.

- Close your eyes and move your right hand over the deck until you feel energy coming into your hand from one card.
- Open your eyes, choose that card, and turn it over to see which sacred principle has come to guide you for the day. You might want to dialogue with it in your journal to see what it has to tell you, or to ask it questions.

### The Sacred Woman Spread

If you would like to do a reading for yourself, or someone else, try this spread.

- Shuffle the cards five times, then hold them to your heart as you silently ask the question uppermost in your mind at the moment. If you're reading for someone else, have them hold the cards and ask the question.
- Cut the deck into three piles in a horizontal row, facedown. Again, if you're reading for someone else, have them do this.
- Now turn up the top card on each pile. You can consult your book for the message on the Sacred Woman's cards and listen from within for the intuitive messages they are sending you. If the spread is for yourself, read it as gently and compassionately as you would for someone else.
- If you would like additional information and background to clarify the answer, you may turn up another card in each pile; place it below the pile. If you would like more information on where you're going or processes you're going through, you may turn up one additional card in each pile; place it above the pile.

If you do the full reading, you will have drawn nine cards, one for each of the Sacred Gateways. But if the information is clear from the first three cards, there is no need to go further.

Remember, the Sacred Woman Prayer Cards will answer the deepest question of your heart, the one you are truly asking. So if the reading doesn't seem to answer the question you originally asked, go deeper into yourself and into the images, and see if the answer you received was the one you truly needed to help you grow and evolve.

You can also try these other divination decks.

- Shoké Cards: The Black Angels, by Earthlyn Marselean Manuel, bring you heavenly, melanin-enriched guidance on a daily basis. Pull one card a day for meditation, protection, and joyous companionship.
- I often use the Mother Peace Deck, from Vicki Nobel and Jonathan Tenney, myself.
- Another deck that might interest you if you feel strongly pulled to Nature and to Native American ways is the Medicine Cards of Jamie Sams and David Carson, both of whom are well-respected and powerful Medicine People. The animal oracles in this deck are beautiful and wise and bring their healing medicine to you straight from Mother Earth.

### Numerology

Another tool for learning to access the intuitive realms of signs and portents is the science of numbers. Numerology is an ancient modality, often attributed to the Greek master mathematician Pythagoras. Recorded history confirms that Pythagoras spent many years of study in ancient Egypt before he established his college and philosophy of numbers.

The science of numerology is brilliantly explained in Lloyd Strayhorn's *Numbers and You*. This informative guidebook will be particularly useful as you investigate the meaning of the key numbers in your life—your name, your birth date (and those of your loved ones), your address, and your phone number—that will lead to harmony and prosperity.

Strayhorn's national bestseller is packed with useful information and easy-to-follow instructions about the power of numbers.

### The Pendulum

The more that we are able to purify our Body Temple, the more sensitive we become to subtle energies. Working with a pendulum teaches us how to sense or tune in to the subtle energy fields that surround us. The pendulum serves as a powerful bridge between the conscious and unconscious mind.

Learning to use a pendulum can teach us how to access and trust our intuition, while bypassing the judgments and distortions of the conscious mind. The pendulum works by allowing invisible energetic signals to be converted into visible movement through the response of the pendulum.

Most Sacred Women are pendulum workers. Use of the pendulum is an ancient technique based on dowsing, in which sensitive people were able to use a forked stick to find the ley lines, or earth energy meridians, to find the proper sites for buildings and towns, or to find sources of underground water. Today we tend to use a pendulum instead of a forked stick, because in our rushed modern world, we're faced with having to make instant decisions and consult our guidance on a moment's notice.

All you need is a small weight on a chain or string or ribbon that will swing freely. Many people like to use a crystal pendant on a chain, a dangly earring, even house keys in an emergency—any weighted object suspended from a 3- to 6-inch string or chain will do. If you're using something on a fairly long chain, wrap the chain around your forefinger so that only 2 or 3 inches remain—you don't need a wide movement to get an accurate answer.

- Hold the chain or string lightly between the thumb and forefinger of your right hand (for incoming information and energy). Hold your hand still; trust the pendulum to move all by itself.
- Now take three deep breaths, relax, and put yourself into a light meditative state.
- Call upon the Divine Light that is indwelling for guidance to give you clear, truthful answers to your questions.

### Tuning Your Pendulum

The first time you use your pendulum, hold it in your hands and ask for the light of Sekhmet to bless your sacred tool. Begin by asking it which direction means yes, which no. If the pendulum moves in a clockwise motion, it means yes. If the pendulum moves in a counterclockwise circle, it

means no. Another indicator of yes and no answers with the pendulum is when it moves in a vertical direction (yes) and a horizontal direction (no). Remember, always allow the pendulum to come to its point of stillness, hanging straight and motionless, in between questions. If the pendulum stands still when you ask the question, it means the question is void—there is no energy surrounding this issue. If you are not clear, the pendulum will jump from the right to the left, then back and forth, almost all at once.

If you don't get very much movement, that's okay. The pendulum will move more precisely with practice and as you simply relax into the process of using it. Like all good things, it just takes time.

As with all oracles, don't keep asking all the time, or every day. Give life a chance to happen.

The quieter, more detached, and less emotionally involved in the answer you are, the more accurate your reading will be. Try not to use the pendulum in a state of panic or high emotional distress. If the situation is critical, sit quietly and meditate until you regain your center. Then, call out from within the One Creator/Creatress for your highest guidance and try the pendulum.

### Spiritual Guardian Pendulum Reading Chart

You can use the pendulum to ask which Spiritual Guardian or source of guidance to consult each day.

### ELEVEN GATEWAYS PENDULUM READING

As you enter each Gateway, you will take a pendulum reading once a week to receive an overall assessment of your condition. As you hold the pendulum over each Gateway of the Pendulum Reading Log, ask, "What is the condition of . . . ?"

For example, do a reading of Gateway 8: Ast. If the pendulum swings counterclockwise (adverse), it means you are having challenges with your Sacred Union. If the pendulum does not move, then the reading is void and it means your Sacred Union is chronically shut down. If you get a neutral swing, then the Sacred Union can

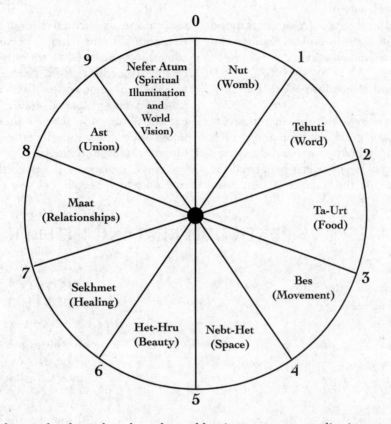

# SPIRITUAL GUARDIAN PENDULUM CHART

0

9 — Nefer Atum (Spiritual Illumination and World Vision)

1 — Nut (Womb)

Ast (Union)

Tehuti (Word)

8

2

Maat (Relationships)

Ta-Urt (Food)

7

3

Sekhmet (Healing)

Bes (Movement)

Het-Hru (Beauty)

Nebt-Het (Space)

6

4

5

To use this chart, take three deep breaths and begin to access a meditative state. Then take your pendulum in your right hand, hold it over the dot on the center of the chart, and ask which Guardian you should seek out for guidance and advice at this time. Wait quietly, with your mind empty, and allow the pendulum to find the path to the appropriate Guardian. Then you can do journal work or dialogue with the NTRU that has come to you.

be better but it's holding its own. If the pendulum swings very positively, in a clockwise direction, it means your Sacred Union is very charged and positive.

Rate your pendulum readings as indicated on the Pendulum Reading Interpretations (below). Observe your progress as well as your blocked areas as you grow into and maintain your Sacred Woman Wellness Lifestyle. Watch as your readings go from void to adverse to neutral to positive. If you fall off your seat of Sacred Woman Principles, you'll watch the situation worsen as you decline in wellness. Your healing is in your own hands.

## Pendulum Body Reading

You can scan your entire body with your pendulum and read every body part. As you travel over your body with the pendulum, begin with your head. Ask if your mind and spirit are clear. Move on to your eyes, ears, sinuses, throat, breasts, lungs, internal organs, womb, legs, arms, and back. If the pendulum swing is positive, the body member you are reading is healthy and there is good circulation and wellness. If the swing is less positive, this body member needs some care and attention to return to balance.

You can also hold your pendulum over an

anatomy chart and use it to indicate the degree of energy and light that your body contains and where any blockages may be.

Always remember that you are never trapped by what appears in a reading. The reading can change according to how you live.

### Additional Pendulum Work

The pendulum is a very useful tool for discovering which foods are good for you and which foods are not. Simply hold your pendulum over the food item and ask whether it is beneficial for your Body Temple. If the answer is yes, then you're free to eat it. If the answer is no, there's another item to cross off your grocery list.

If the answer is neutral, then do a little research on this particular food; see what is positive about it and what is negative. Perhaps it's something you need to eat only once in a while, or for a specific reason. For example, leeks are very helpful in your diet if you're going through a bout of high blood pressure. But you should eat them for only a very short time, because taken for a longer period they can lower your blood pressure too much.

You can also use the pendulum for information on which herbal teas you need at a particu-

## ELEVEN GATEWAYS PENDULUM READING INTERPRETATIONS

| PENDULUM READING | CODE | ROAD TO TEMPLE (BODY) BALANCE |
|---|---|---|
| Void (motionless) | V | Entrance of the Temple (a far cry from the Temple Gates). Wellness shutdown. |
| Adverse (counterclockwise swing) | A | At the gate of the Temple (this also applies if organ related to element has been damaged or removed). Partially blocked. |
| Neutral (horizontal line / back-and-forth swing) | N | Inside the corridors (Inner Circle). Midway to wellness level. |
| Positive (clockwise swing) | P | Throughout the Temple (Upper Room). Wellness level. |
| Positive + | P+ | Reach the Nebt-Het Purification Bowl (roof) within the Upper Room. Advanced wellness. |

# THE ELEVEN GATEWAYS PENDULUM READING LOG

| GATE | WEEK 1 | WEEK 2 | WEEK 3 | WEEK 4 | WEEK 5 | WEEK 6 | WEEK 7 | WEEK 8 | WEEK 9 |
|---|---|---|---|---|---|---|---|---|---|
| 0. Nut (Womb) | | | | | | | | | |
| 1. Tehuti (Word) | | | | | | | | | |
| 2. Ta-Urt (Food) | | | | | | | | | |
| 3. Bes (Movement) | | | | | | | | | |
| 4. Het-Hru (Beauty) | | | | | | | | | |
| 5. Nebt-Het (Space) | | | | | | | | | |
| 6. Sekhmet (Healing) | | | | | | | | | |
| 7. Maat (Relationships) | | | | | | | | | |
| 8. Ast (Sacred Union) | | | | | | | | | |
| 9. Nefer Atum (Sacred Lotus Initiation) | | | | | | | | | |
| 10. Seshat (Time) | | | | | | | | | |
| 11. Meskenet (Work) | | | | | | | | | |

lar time, which essential oils, which flower essences, and which dietary supplements you need to take. You can even check which dosage is correct for you. For example, your dialogue with the pendulum might go as follows: "Should I have one tablespoon of this formula?" No. "Should I have less?" No. "Should I have more?" Yes. "Should I have two tablespoons?" No. "Three tablespoons?" Yes. "Should I take it at night?" No. "In the morning?" Yes.

Be creative in the uses you find for your pendulum.

The more detached you are about the pendulum, the stronger and clearer and more accurate your readings will be. You actually are a pendulum yourself. If you are clean, clear, open, and tuned in, you can read directly from your spirit. Your inner voice speaks the truth. Listen!

## Prayer

Another important part of your spiritual work as a Priestess-in-Training is to create your own prayers. Prayers that come fresh from your soul, using the words of your heart, are nearly always more effective than even the most beautiful prayers you may have read in a holy book or find in *Sacred Woman*. Your own prayers are filled with "inspiration"—the inbreathing of spirit.

Instead of always asking for something, try filling your prayers with praise and gratitude for all the things that are going right in your life, in the lives of your loved ones, and in the world. Even at the darkest moments, fill your prayers with light and love and blessings, for another Universal Law is that what you send out is returned to you a hundredfold.

So be brave. Trust yourself, trust Spirit moving through you—whisper your prayers, speak your prayers out loud, sing your prayers, dance your prayers. Trust that you will be heard.

## Dream Work

My ancient Afrakan Ancestors used dreams and fasting to discover truths about themselves and others. Your dreams are filled with information and insights, healing and inspiration. All you need to do is learn to retrieve them, record them,

work with them, even program them as you would a computer—our minds are the software, and dreams are the spreadsheets of our lives.

None of these things is difficult to do:

• You can use your Sacred Woman Journal to record your dreams, or you can use a special Dream Journal and pen kept right by your bed so it's easy to reach when you first wake up.

• The Sacred Woman Wellness Diet is ideal for remembering dreams, since drugs, alcohol, or eating heavy or sugary foods before bedtime disturbs sleep and interferes with dream recall.

• You can program your dreams, which is called "incubating," to find the solution to a question or problem, or to receive a healing or a creative inspiration. In as few words as possible, state your intention; for example, "Dreams, please show me how to solve my problems with my boss." Or, "Dreams, please bring me a healing tonight." Repeat this to yourself like a mantra at least three times just as you're falling asleep. Be patient and give your dreaming mind at least three nights to come up with a response. It responds to repetition.

• When you wake up, try not to move for a few minutes while you rerun the dream in your mind. Reach down to the side of the bed, pick up your Dream Journal and pen, and write down what you remember. The more you write, the more you usually remember. But even if it's a scrap of an image or a few words, write it down.

• Date your dream. Give it a brief title and write a very brief description of it, like a movie review. When you review your Dream Journal in a few months, you'll use these descriptions to find the information you want to review, for dreams often make more sense to you over time.

• There are many ways to work with dreams, but the one that will probably be easiest and most familiar to you is simply to dialogue with the person, place, or thing in the dream that is the most mysterious, scary, or puzzling to you. Ask this element to tell you why it appeared in your dream and what it means to your life now.

• Dialoguing with frightening images, people, or

situations is an excellent way to get rid of nightmares, for it allows you to work your way through to your healing.

- You don't need to do dream work with every dream—only the most important ones, and especially the ones you have incubated. And your dream work doesn't have to be done first thing in the morning. Just get your dream down, and save a few pages to do your dream work when you have time and a meditative space to work in.
- Ask your dream for a gift. Be prepared to offer one in return if asked.
- Take the wisdom of your dream with you into your day.

Sweet Dreams!

## FOUR SACRED WOMAN HEALING MEDICINE BAGS

Sacred Medicine Women, Bush Women, and Wise Women of power and grace, spread the word—let's heal our race. The time has come for you to step forward to do the work of the Creator/Creatress. Your Sacred Medicine Bag will grow and transform just as you do. Like an old-fashioned doctor's black bag, the Sacred Woman's Medicine Bags contain the earth and spirit medicine necessary to help heal what ails you and your loved ones. Just remember, for good medicine always let Spirit guide you.

Create a special bag or buy a beautiful ready-made bag that has your spirit in it. Use this bag only to carry your ju-ju tools and to help keep your energy balanced as well as the energy of those who are in need of assistance. With your Sacred Woman Master Healing Medicine Bag, you will be ready for whatever comes up in your life travels.

In my Medicine Bag I also carry my Sacred Spirit Watcher Doll. She sits in the center of the bag as a gift from Sister Queen Sirus, a loving Lotus Blossom and Sacred Artist from Los Angeles, California. I travel with this sacred image to use when I set up my altar for Sacred Woman Initiation Training.

One afternoon while teaching a Sacred Women's Training, I asked all the women to pull out their Sacred Medicine Bags, which 90 per-

cent of them had. Each Sacred Woman spoke about what was contained in her Medicine Bag and why. One corporate sister's Medicine Bag stood out because of its simplicity. It contained only a pendulum and a sacred stone—a crystal clear quartz.

It was really important for us to see the range of Medicine Bags carried by different women. It sparked the idea that we each use different Sacred Medicine Bags for different situations. And this led me to share the contents of the following four medicine bags. As a rule of thumb, always use your intuition to guide you to the right bag and its contents. Trust your divine self. Again, create the medicine bag that fits your needs as you draw from the Master Medicine Bag to empower you.

### Sacred Woman's Master Healing Bag

Include all the items listed below so that you will be ready for most any situation.

1. Goldenseal—extract or capsules. Blood Cleanser—20 to 40 drops to 8 oz. of water and juice of 1 lemon twice a day, or 2 to 4 capsules three times a day.
2. Cascara sagrada—tablets or capsules. Laxative—2 to 3 tablets or 2 to 3 capsules at night with water.

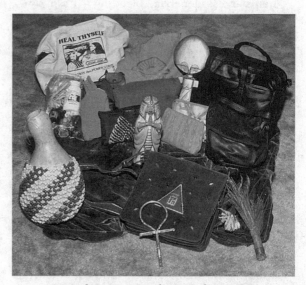

Sacred Woman Healing Medicine Bag

3. Aloe vera gel. Blood cleanser and laxative—2 tbsp. of pure gel scraped from inside of leaf (or an unadulterated brand made directly from the plant from the health food store) mixed with juice of 1 lemon or lime in 8 oz. of water.

4. Cayenne. ¼ tsp. of powdered cayenne increases circulation.

5. Organic apple cider vinegar—breaks up mucus. 2 to 3 tbsp. in 8 oz. water, or add 4 tbsp. to enema bag to flush out congestion and mucus.

6. Heal Thyself Green Life Formula I—rejuvenator. 1 to 2 tbsp. to 8 oz. of freshly pressed vegetable or fruit juice.

7. Clear quartz crystal—for clarity, mentally or spiritually. Carry with you in your hand or pocket, or wear as a necklace or talisman in small drawstring bag. Remember to purify your crystal daily.

8. Heal Thyself Colon Ease—3 tbsp. in 8 oz. warm water and juice of 1 lime, or 2 tsp. of olive oil or castor oil.

9. Kyolic—liquid garlic extract—for respiratory system/high blood pressure. 12 drops a day with distilled water or with Kidney-Liver Flush.

10. Shepherd's purse—extract. Stops bleeding—10 drops to 8 oz. of water.

11. Cinnamon. Brings forth a sweet disposition, helps arrest menstrual bleeding—1 tsp. powdered cinnamon or as a loose tea or one or two teabags to 1 to 2 cups of warm water. Steep for 30 minutes and drink.

12. Desert or white sage leaves. For spiritual cleansing of self, home, altar, and clothes. Burn sage in a seashell or ceramic dish and smudge. If possible, always keep a window open when performing this kind of purification. Use Weleda Sage deodorant spray for instant smudging in spaces where you cannot perform a traditional smudging.

13. Frankincense and myrrh. For spiritual cleansing. Anoint self with oil or add a few drops of oil to a pot of boiling water to cleanse self and environment.

14. Valerian—extract. 10 drops to 1 to 2 cups of water. Calms and quiets. Good for nervous conditions and sleeplessness.

15. Kava kava—extract or capsules. Relieves stress, has a natural tranquilizing effect. The famous South Pacific herb has been used for centuries—20 to 40 drops in a small glass of water two to four times a day or up to 100 mg in capsule form three times a day.

16. Queen Afua's Rejuvenating Clay. Relieves aches and pains. Make a gauze-covered clay pack for best results. For deep rejuvenation, leave on a few hours or overnight until dry.

17. White willow bark—extract. Relieves pain and headaches—10 to 15 drops one to three times a day.

18. Heal Thyself Breath of Spring (or equal parts eucalyptus and peppermint oil). Good for respiratory system, hay fever—1 to 3 drops under tongue and drink with water with a few drops of lemon juice squeezed into it. Or boil a few drops in a pot of water to ease your breathing.

19. Bach Flower Rescue Remedy Cream. For abrasions, burns, bruises, and skin discomfort.

20. Salt and honey. For drawing out poisons and adding sweetness. (Recommended by Iyanla Vanzant, an Honorary Professor of Heal Thyself, a loving and caring friend and best-selling author.)

21. Candle to light the way.

22. Lemon to eliminate congestion.

23. Crystal pendulum. A sacred instrument to do energetic readings.

24. Crystals, such as clear quartz, amethyst, the Mother of Healers, or rose quartz.

25. Cowrie shells to promote womb wellness and to summon the voice of the womb.

26. Oracle or spiritual reading cards (see Intuitive Healing, page 272).

27. Bach Flower Rescue Remedy—a composite, five-remedy flower essence. For emergencies and high stress.

28. Feather to bring balance to any situation.

29. Favorite prayer. Laminate on cards.

30. Several favorite spiritual music tapes.

31. Small sacred image or sculpture.

32. Silk scarf to make an instant altar.

*Note:* Extracts of herbs must be nonalcoholic and taken with liquid as tea. (Try brands such as Liquid Farmacy or Nature's Answer.) Follow directions on bottle.

## Sacred Spirit Medicine Bag

1. Sage (leaf or essential oil).
2. Stones or gems for all seven *aritu* (chakras).
3. Frankincense and myrrh (rocks or essential oil) for emotional and spiritual balancing. (See the master Gateway chart on pages 130–135 for appropriate oils.)
4. Small ceramic or metal incense burner, and charcoal to burn the incense.
5. Small feather (optional) for Maat meditation.
6. Purification prayer to balance out the heart, emotions, and traumas, to soothe and bring harmony.
7. Small bell or tuning fork to harmonize energetic imbalances.
8. Sacred Healing Prayers (either transcribed into small book or photocopied and laminated).

## Nine-to-Five Healing Medicine Bag for Work

1. Small crystal (choose from the master Gateway chart on pages 130–135).
2. Seven chakra crystals and surgical tape to place stones on appropriate chakra according to the needs of the day.
3. Rejuvenation herbal extracts—dandelion, alfalfa, gotu kola (brain food for power and drawing in positive vibrations), kava kava, and Siberian ginseng; 10 to 20 drops in a glass of water as needed.
4. Sekhmet healing prayer.
5. Protection prayer.
6. Frankincense and myrrh essential oil for protection.
7. Bach Flower Essence Rescue Remedy, 2 to 4 drops on the tongue or mixed in a small amount of water, and Rescue Remedy Cream.
8. FES (Flower Essence Society) Yarrow Root Essence to protect aura from radiation from computers, televisions, microwave ovens, etc. Use 2 to 4 drops under the tongue or mix in a small amount of water.

## Traveling Healing Medicine Bag

1. Herbal laxative (cascara sagrada tablets). 2 to 3 tablets or 2 to 3 capsules at night with water.
2. Enema bag.
3. Kyolic garlic extract (liquid form), 12 drops a day with distilled water.
4. B complex tablets or capsules—nerve strengthener. For relief of stress, take 25 to 50 mg twice a day.
5. Wheatgrass or spirulina powder. Take 1 tsp. to 1 tbsp. one to three times a day in juice or water for energy, memory, and rejuvenation.
6. Ester vitamin C, 500 mg capsules or powder. Strengthens immune system. Take twice a day with meals.
7. Echinacea and/or echinacea and goldenseal extract for infections, fevers, compromised immune system. Take ¼ tsp. or 10 to 20 drops in 8 oz. warm water.
8. Juice of 1 to 2 lemons. Take with warm water to keep the body cleansed.
9. Aloe vera gel. Breaks addictions; good laxative and blood cleanser. Use 2 tablespoons gel to juice of 1 lemon in glass of water.
10. Pendulum to read the energy of a person, place, or situation. (See Intuitive Healing on page 272.)
11. White leaf sage with small seashell for burning, or Weleda sage deodorant spray. Lavender oil for bath or anointing.
12. Divination cards for spiritual readings.
13. Favorite prayers.
14. Favorite spiritual music tapes.

## TWO HEALING CEREMONIES

### Releasing Baggage That Causes Disease

If release work is to be done within a group or healing circle, smudge the space, yourself, and everyone else in your healing circle with sage or frankincense and myrrh. Then pray together with palms open, saying in unison:

*Divine Creator/Creatress, help us right now to let go of all that is not You, all that is not truth. Allow Your light of love to flow through each and every one of us on this, Your holy day.* Tu, ashé.

- One or two sisters should then come up to the altar that has been sweetly arranged with flowers, candles, and crystals to release all their past hurts.
- Have them place their hands inside a wooden bowl filled with purified water, crystals, and hyssop and sage oils or leaves. You may use the Nebt-Het purification bowl on the altar.
- Pray hard, and as you dip into the holy water, let go of all conditions, attitudes, and diseases that have blocked you from your blessings. Let the Spirit move you to reveal your new self to you when you are done.
- As a strong affirmation to seal each release within the water work, say: *"Tua, ashé." Tu* is a Khamitic word meaning "yes," and *ashé* is the Yoruba word for "yes."
- While your hands and heart are still in the purification bowl, someone chosen in the circle should ring a bell or chime for each person or condition you call out to be released, until you are free of all burdens.
- Once the ritual is completed say, *"Tua NTR,"* meaning "Thanks be to the Creator/Creatress." Or say, "Give thanks and praise."
- Then the presiding Priestess will anoint everyone's crown chakra of high wisdom, heart chakra of love, or throat chakra of expression, or bless all seven chakras or *aritu* (spiritual centers) with sweet-scented essential oil such as rose or jasmine, so that all may go in peace.

Remember, the cleaner your lifestyle, the easier it is to release and let go of all negativity, blockages, and end-of-cycle experiences.

### Healing Your Past

- Bless and purify your sacred space and everyone within the gathered circle.
- Each woman, Sister, or Queen writes down on plain paper with a pencil whomever and whatever she wants to be released—everywhere she holds resentment, jealousy, or anger. This allows her to finally let go and be free of the negativity that surrounds the experience, person, or thing.
- Start a fire in the center of the circle in a cast-iron pot using charcoal and frankincense and myrrh or white leaf sage to purify the situations or individuals to be released. As the fire gets strong enough, each sister, one by one (or if a large group, in twos or fours), places her letting-go paper in the pot.
- After each sister releases her pain on paper into the fire, all the sisters support these releases by playing instruments or singing in celebration.
- Each sister who is experiencing release dances around the full circle of women in celebration of her letting go.
- When she returns to the circle and sits down, the music stops. The Priestess or leader or Elder places the feather symbolizing Maat on her heart as a reminder of inner harmony.
- The Elder says, "May your heart remain weightless and as light as a feather eternally."
- The circle continues until everyone has completed the ritual. Then everyone rises, plays their instruments, and dances together in the joy and release of letting go of past hurts and wounds.
- Once the celebration has come to a resting place, make a final closing circle to offer a prayer of thankfulness to the Creator/Creatress and the Sacred Women within the healing circle.

## VIOLENCE UPON A RACE: HEALING THE COLLECTIVE

Afrakan women and men were stolen from their people and sold into slavery in Europe, the West Indies, and in the Americas. They were subjected to the worst kind of violence that one people on the face of the earth has ever perpetrated upon another—to be enslaved and controlled and abused and raped.

We as a people still carry the scars of slavery; these tarnish all our relationships and activities in one way or another. Soul-deep hurt has been passed down from one generation to the next, from mother to daughter, from father to son, from husband to wife.

My hurts are endless. My Afrakan family was ripped from me. My man was lynched before my eyes. My baby was cut out of my belly. I drowned my sweet innocent babies to save them from the brutality of slavery. When my children were of age they were sent away to another plantation never to see me, their mama, again. I cannot express how deep my wounds are, how much they bleed.

Light-skinned and dark-skinned women were placed at odds—one thinking she's better than the other; one feeling she's less valuable because she compares her kinky hair with another sister's straight hair. Full hips and small hips are at odds; round noses and pointed noses are at odds; big behinds and flat behinds are at odds. So here we are today, a product of the violence committed upon our race. Our race has been poisoned by European inhumanity. My land, language, dance, song, traditions, and dreams were taken from me. My people, the old ways, and the wise ways were taken from me.

Today, we Afrakan people must call to our Ancestors to move through us as we liberate, wash, cleanse, and pray the violence and grief away. We must call on the Most High for a renewed body, a renewed mind, and a renewed, revitalized spirit. We must release the pain, the hurt, the anger, and the rage because it keeps drawing us back to even more violence, which is reflected back to us in our closest relationships.

We must go through our Sacred Woman Initiation, lying on the bosoms of Elder womenfolk so that our souls may be nurtured and washed clean. We must celebrate who and what we are as we, the Afrakan race, begin to recall ourselves as great, unbending, strong, enduring, creative people, unlike any other. We must heal our grief and rage. We must recover ourselves and heal our past to have a future worthy of all that we are!

### Violence and the Sacred Woman

*As a Sacred Woman, I can never accept abuse by man, woman, child, or nation, for I represent the active presence and power of the Almighty Creator/Creatress.*

As a Sacred Woman you have the power to stop violence and injury. Hold up your hand of purity and peace and speak out. Say, "I've got the power because I am a Sacred Woman!"

When you experience violence, it often indicates that your toxic inner elements are drawing violence to you. Stop the violence within. Bring your elements into harmony by loving and caring for self.

I was able to stop my own violence because I've got the power and the power of the Creator/Creatress within me. Through the years I have had the opportunity to work through my own healing by changing my relationships, replacing violence with peacefulness. Relationships with my mate, my ex-husband, my mother, my children, and my kin and friends have improved. I've watched many, many women who have come to me for guidance eliminate violence from their lives.

I bear witness that the peace that we now experience is a direct reflection of our own internal healing and purification. The level and intensity with which we cleanse and rejuvenate ourselves indicates the level to which violence will no longer be a part of our times.

When you take healing baths, don't simply wash your skin and pores. Take the opportunity to wash blemishes out of your soul as well. Let peace flow like water as it warms your heart, your mind, your body, your spirit. Affirm:

*I release the anger that is within me and draw out the peace that dwells within me—the peace that is buried under the anger.*

### Violence Begets Violence: Let Peace Flow

Ingesting violence-inducing foods such as animal flesh, fast foods, dead or processed nonfoods, sweets, alcohol, drugs, and cigarettes ultimately creates disease in our Body Temple. As a result, we find ourselves having to take medications and poisonous chemicals to suppress the diseases we developed by eating violent foods. Often such a diet forces us to cut away a deteriorated organ, to tear away a uterus, to slice off a woman's breast, or to irradiate lungs, bones, or a cancerous throat. We have to transfuse blood. We lose our minds. All this is due to self-inflicted toxic, violent foods (actually nonfoods).

Consumption of violent foods causes us to fall into a zombielike state and live out our lives as sleeping giants. Violent nonfoods create a demonic state internally and externally that draws in demonic circumstances and/or people who mean us no good.

On the other hand, when we eat and drink pure foods, heavenly foods, organic fruits and vegetables, and pure water, violence of all kinds will flee from us. When we fast and pray, we draw blessings to us and we begin to live in a more heavenly state, for heaven is within a pure Body Temple. There is much untapped power within our Body Temples.

No matter what has happened in your life up to this moment, accept peace in your life right here and now. Meditate on this Peace Prayer.

---

### A Peace Prayer

*I am a sacred being. I epitomize and personify peace. There is peace within my soul. I live a life of peace. I think thoughts of peace. I eat the foods of peace. I pray a peace-filled prayer. There is power in peace and peace in power. Not a moment passes that I don't meditate on peace. I am supremely peaceful, so I draw all peace unto me. I'm full of peace. Peace is my refuge, for peace is my divine friend, light, love, and protection. Peace is my refuge and strength.*

---

As you meditate on these words of peace, smudge your Body Temple with desert sage smoke from head to toe to deepen your peaceful ways. Smudge your home with sage for the sake of peace (if no one around is opposed). The herb sage grows in our Afrakan Motherland. It was used thousands of years ago in ancient Khamit. The Native American people of Turtle Island also widely use wild sage in many of their sacred ceremonies.

Come to work early, before staff or coworkers have arrived, and smudge your work environment with herbs of peace such as sage, cedar, and sweetgrass. In silent meditation, put a handful of sage in a pot of water and boil it. Put a drop of sage oil or cinnamon oil in a pot of water. Drop a dash of sacred oil onto an aromatherapy lightbulb ring.

This brings forth sweet dispositions in body, mind, and spirit. No one will know what you've done, but everyone around you will be more considerate, patient, and peaceful as you raise the positive vibrations of the area in which you work.

## From Violence to Peacefulness Through the Foods We Eat

Food is our fuel. What and how we eat determine the effectiveness of our lives. There are natural-food alternatives, so we don't have to feel deprived. We can simply make better choices.

### Symptoms from Eating a Violent Toxic Diet

- Women verbally abusive to men
- Men physically abusive to women
- Stressed-out parents unable to talk to children, using blows instead
- Gossiping
- Inability to let go of resentment, depression, and worry
- Abusive, animalistic, or uncontrollable sexuality

The following formulas and activities will help you eliminate violence from your life. This includes violence from your mate, boss, parents, children, and even girlfriends. Most times when we think of violence, we think only of male-on-female violence. When we are abused, put down, or taken advantage of, or when we experience violence, we may receive it from various directions—even from our sisters, children, mates, or friends.

## The End of Violence: The Peace and Love Diet Fast and Pray—Cleanse and Purify

Let's work for a full three-month season with these principles:

- **Diet.** Eat beans, peas, tofu, soy meats, live and organic vegetables, fresh and unsprayed fruits. The diet must consist of 60 to 75 percent raw foods and 25 to 40 percent steamed foods for inner balance and rejuvenation of thoughts, attitudes, feelings, and overall wellness. Foods such as wheatgrass, spirulina, turnip greens, mustard greens, kale, and celery are best taken in the forms of live juices or steamed lightly. Consume these two to three times a day.

- **Bath.** To your bath add 2 to 4 lbs. Epsom salts, a few drops of lavender essential oil, and an infusion of chamomile (3 tsp. herbs steeped overnight in 1 quart boiled water). Stay in tub one to two hours. Begin by doing this bath seven nights straight, then three times a week. Burn a small pink candle and give yourself a self-massage from head to toe in the bath. Embrace your body and say:

*I've got the power to heal myself. I've got the power to stop my violence. I depend on myself, I support me, I allow only the best for me. I eat only the best, most peaceful, nonviolent foods.*

Woman, let it be known that you are a Healer of your life, and that anyone and anything that crosses your path is due for a healing. When you heal everyone who comes near you, you heal their violence. Nothing stops violence like purity and inner peace—not guns, not the strap, not punches.

Joy is a choice; hold on to it. Whatever happens, don't give up your joy. If someone is angry or hostile toward you, learn and study what they're expressing. Allow yourself to grow from it. But all the while, very quietly, hold on to your joy, your sanity, and peace.

Inner peace draws external peace to you in the end, as inner love of self draws external love. Inner happiness manifests as bliss externally. Hold on to your peace. Peace is a precious gift from the Most High to those who are obedient to the Natural Laws.

## HEAL A WOMAN, HEAL A NATION

I'd like to share with you a powerful work by Lady Prema, author of *My Soul Speaks*. It has encouraged and uplifted a multitude of women, and I am sure it will do the same for you, Sacred Woman Healer, as you become a nurturing source in our Nation Building.

### Heal a Woman, Heal a Nation
### by Lady Prema

*Celestial Channel of our human birth*
*Wholesome womb of creation*
*Devoted daughter to divinity.*
*Heal a woman. Heal a nation.*

*Envisioned in her radiant form*
*Exalted, she'll rise supreme*
*Rebirthed to her innocence*
*True love will be redeemed.*
*Sacred spirit for peace on earth*
*Virtuous vessels of inspiration*
*Earthy essence of femininity*
*Heal a woman. Heal a nation.*

*She dances to her own rhythm*
*Sings with all in harmony*
*Shares with all what she can give them*
*Through her love she sets us free*
*Glorified through her inner grace*
*Liberated through purification*
*Nurturer of humanity.*
*Heal a woman. Heal a nation.*

*Engaged to her eternal mate*
*She serves through charity*
*Bestowing her gifts on everyone.*
*Let her live, let her love, let her be*
*Mother of civilization.*
*Heal a woman. Heal a nation.*

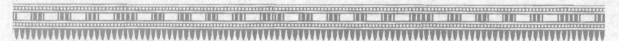

# SACRED HEALING: SEVEN-DAY TRANSFORMATIVE WORK

- *Continue to keep your Sacred Journal Writing alive.* Consult Sesheta and Sekhmet to reveal what most needs to be healed in your life.
- *Talk to the Most Divine throughout your journey;* open your heart and speak your soul. Become one of mind with the Divine, one of voice, one of action. This is the time to allow total crystal-line clarity to move through your spirit mind, into your heart, through your hands, and into your journal, so you may reflect on what your soul speaks through the harmony of Maat.
- *Renew your commitment to your Sacred Woman Transitional Dietary Practices.*
- *Encourage one to four friends, family members, or co-workers* who are willing to follow the Heal Thy-self plan to join you on the road to wellness.
- *Record your Sacred Healing Circle's results.*
- *Empower your partners in healing by supporting their achievements,* no matter how small, until they are able to come into complete balance. Remember, everyone around you reflects where you are in your own wellness cycle.
- *Consult a licensed holistic medical professional,* such as a naturopathic physician or holistic medical doctor or Chinese medicine practitioner, for a thorough examination to establish a baseline for your physical health.
- *Take on healing as a way of life.* Apply Nature cures and Natural Living and fasting tech-niques offered in *Sacred Woman.*
- *Continue to maintain your wellness program without fail.* Meditate and live in a state of absolute wellness daily as you allow the Healer within to come through.
- *Receive a colonic every fourteen to twenty-eight days;* take enemas one to three times a week; get a massage treatment once a week (exchange massages with friends or family, or get it done professionally) to benefit your lymphatic and circulatory systems. Relax and energize through the power of sacred touch.
- *Sweat (steam or sauna) daily, or as often as possible,* to flush out years of accumulated toxins.
- *Create your Sacred Woman Medicine Bag.* Sew it yourself and let it reflect your own spirit medi-cine.
- *Place a bowl of garlic and an aloe plant on your altar,* both of which are ancient Khamitic sources of healing.
- *Grow medicinal plants* in your backyard or on your windowsill.
- *Get a pendulum and learn how to read energy levels* in yourself, foods, herbs, and so on, so that you can track your level of wellness. (See Intuitive Healing on page 272.)
- *Perform a Sacred Woman Prayer Card Reading.*
- *Practice the "End of Violence—Peace and Love Diet" for one full season.*
- *Practice Laying On of Hands* with those in need of healing energy.
- *Pray for the end of racism* and its toxic effects on Afrakan people and all the people of our planet.

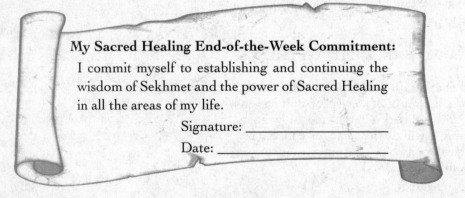

**My Sacred Healing End-of-the-Week Commitment:**
I commit myself to establishing and continuing the wisdom of Sekhmet and the power of Sacred Healing in all the areas of my life.

Signature: _____

Date: _____

## CHAPTER 12

# GATEWAY 7: SACRED RELATIONSHIPS

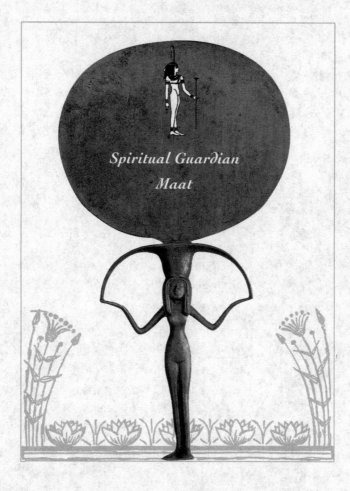

*Spiritual Guardian*

*Maat*

**Ancestors**

Sojourner Truth

Sarah and
Elizabeth Delany

**Elder**

Queen Nzinga
Ratabisha Heru

**Contemporaries**

Oprah Winfrey

Iyanla Vanzant

Lady Prema

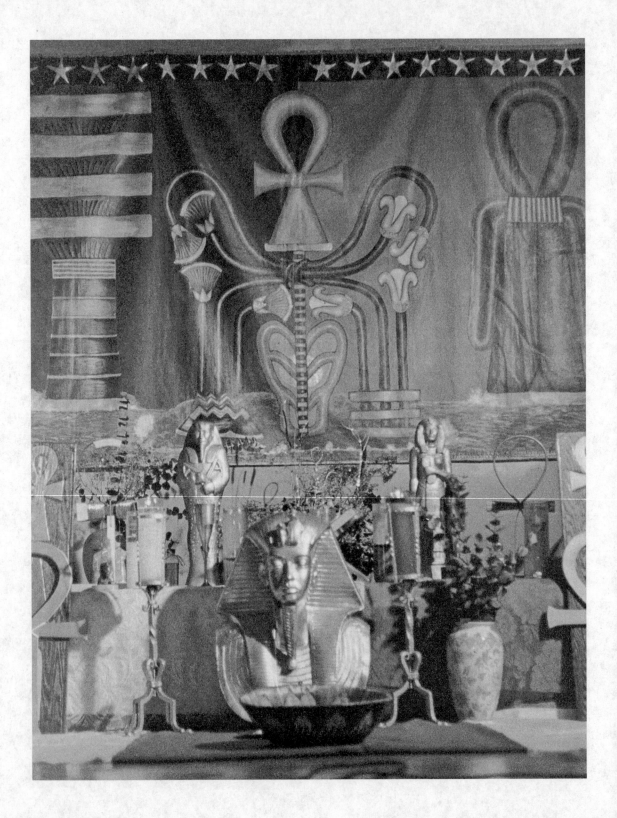

# SACRED RELATIONSHIPS ALTAR WORK
## Face Your Heart to the East—to the Rising Sun
*(Layout from top view)*

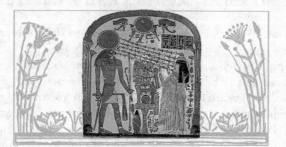

**Mount Pictures on Wall, Above Altar**

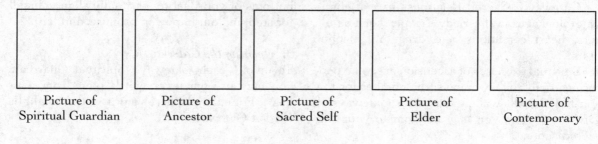

| Picture of Spiritual Guardian | Picture of Ancestor | Picture of Sacred Self | Picture of Elder | Picture of Contemporary |

Baptism Bowl (WATER)

| Feather (AIR) | Scale of Maat with Heart and Feather (SPIRIT) | Fresh Flowers or Flowering Plant (EARTH) |

| *Anointing Oils:* Lavender, Ylang-Ylang | White or Rose Candle (FIRE) | *Sacred Stone:* Rose Quartz, Pink Tourmaline |

Food for your Ancestors (bowl of organic non-GMO fruit)
*(Release from the altar after twenty-four hours.)*

**Place on your altar a diagram of your blood and extended family tree.**

Sacred tablecloth (rose) and scarf to wear during prayer.
Sacred color cloth to lay before altar. Sacred instruments to be played as you pray.

# GATEWAY 7: SACRED RELATIONSHIPS DAILY SPIRITUAL OBSERVANCES

## Gateway Element: Air

Sacred Relationships eliminate toxic, dysfunctional, and disjointed relationships that destroy one's life. Sacred Relationships create cleansed, honest, and harmonious relationships that energize one's life. Fulfilling, healthy relationships are the result of establishing Sacred Relationships.

Gateway 7: Sacred Relationships will eliminate blockages in the Body Temple, such as ulcers, heart conditions, and drug and alcohol abuse.

Spiritual exercises of ascension are to be performed daily for seven days, the number for the spirit. This will awaken your inner Gateways of Divinity so that you may blossom to your full sacred center.

## 1. The Spiritual Bath

Place 4 to 6 drops of lavender or ylang-ylang oil in your bathwater. Lavender oil acts as a sedative for the nervous system. It also acts as an anti-inflammatory and heart tonic. It is very effective in treating burns, wounds, and sores. It promotes concentration, peace of mind, wisdom, and devotion (Atum Ra). It will eliminate mood swings, restlessness, fear, headaches, and eye problems. Ylang-ylang treats anger, rage, and nervous depression. Ylang-ylang is a very potent scent and should be applied sparingly.

Sprinkle a few drops on a tissue or handkerchief and place by your pillow to inhale while sleeping; this helps to promote emotional balance due to stress, worry, impatience, and shock.

## 2. Your Altar

Set up your sacred altar on the first day of your entry into this Gateway. You may set up your altar according to your spiritual or religious beliefs (see page 18). Sit before your altar quietly and meditatively on the floor on a pillow, or in a chair. Add a few drops of any of lavender or ylang-ylang oil to your baptism bowl on your altar, and sprinkle a few drops around your prayer space.

*Anoint with lavender or ylang-ylang oil.* Select only pure essential oils. Use lavender or ylang-ylang oil to anoint your crown, forehead (the Body Temple Gateway of supreme spirituality), heart (the Body Temple Gateway of compassion and divine love), womb area, palms to make everything you touch become more sacred, and the bottoms of your feet to spiritually align yourself for stepping out in power, promise, and faith.

## 3. Opening the Gateway

To invoke each Gateway's Spiritual Guardian, you may use whatever words pour from your heart. For example, here's a prayer that might be used at Gateway 7:

*Sacred and Divine Maat, Spiritual Guardian of the Gateway of Sacred Relationships, please accept my deepest gratitude for your healing presence on my altar and in my life. Thank you for your guidance and inspiration, and for your love and blessings, and please accept my love and blessings in return.* Hetepu.

As you offer your prayer, simultaneously shake, ring, beat, or rattle a sacred instrument (sistrum bell, drum, shekere, or bells) to awaken the NTR that is indwelling.

## 4. Libation

Pour a libation for the Sacred Relationship Gateway from a cup, or sprinkle water from a bowl onto the earth or a plant, as you call out this prayer of praise and adoration.

— *Pour a libation* as you say, *All praise and adoration to the Spiritual Guardian, Maat, the Protector of Sacred Relationships.*
— *Pour a libation* as you say, *All praise and adoration to the Ancestors of Sacred Relationships, Sojourner Truth and the Delany Sisters — Sarah and Elizabeth.*
— *Pour a libation* as you say, *All praise and adora-*

tion to the Elder of Sacred Relationships, Queen Nzinga Ratabisha Heru.

— *Pour a libation* as you say, *All praise and adoration to my Divine Self and my Contemporary Divine Sisters, Oprah Winfrey, Iyanla Vanzant, and Lady Prema, who honor Sacred Relationships.*

## 5. *Sacred Woman Spirit Prayer*

Ring a bell or play another sacred instrument at the beginning and end of this prayer. As you open your palms to the Sacred Spirit or gently place them over your heart, recite:

### Sacred Woman Spirit Prayer

*Sacred Woman in the making,*
*Sacred Woman reawaken,*
*Sacred Spirit, hold me near.*
*Protect me from all harm and fear*
*beneath the stones of life.*
*Direct my steps in the right way as I journey*
*through this vision.*
*Sacred Spirit,*
*surround me in your most absolute*
*perfect light.*
*Anoint me in your sacred purity, peace,*
*and divine insight.*
*Bless me, truly bless me, as I share*
*this Sacred Life.*
*Teach me, Sacred Spirit, to be in tune*
*with the universe.*
*Teach me how to heal*
*with the inner and outer elements*
*of air, fire, water, and earth.*

## 6. *Sacred Relationship Prayer*

Shake bells, beat sacred drum, or play another instrument at the beginning and ending of this prayer.

*Divine Creator/Creatress, I stand in need of Sacred Relationships. I pray for Sacred Relationships in my life. First, may I create a Sacred Relationship with you, Creator/Creatress, and with my parents, children, sisters, brothers, friends, associates, coworkers, teachers, and students, with Nature, and with all my other relations. Divine Creator/Creatress, help me to attract and establish harmonious, wholesome, and healthy relationships. Help me to unblock and release old hurt feelings, resentments, and hostility that are trapped within my Body Temple. Help me to have the vision and the strength to learn from all my relationships, as they are all my reflection, each and every one. If by chance my relationships do not change, may I remain unfazed and on point. May I be the one to create new links of change and transformation for my Ancestors, my descendants, and myself, for all healing really begins within me. I affirm that each one of my relationships has value and in some way has forced or helped me to grow into a more sacred relationship with my self. As I reflect on the true purpose and sacredness of relationships, I give thanks to the Divine in me and the Divine in all others.*

## 7. *Chanting* Hesi

Chant this *hesi* four times:

*Nuk Pu Ntrt Hmt*—I am a Sacred Woman.

## 8. *Fire Breaths*

Prepare your Fire Breaths by slowly inhaling four times and exhaling four times. Then, when you are totally at ease, begin your eight hundred Fire Breaths. Inhale deeply like a pump through your nose (mouth closed) as you expand the breath down into the abdomen, then back up to the chest. Completely exhale out through your nostrils from your abdomen as it contracts and the lungs release your breath completely. Repeat this breath rapidly in and out, in and out.

Allow each deep Fire Breath to represent the opening of the thousand lotus petals of illumination and radiance, ultimately reaching Nefer Atum—the ultimate Afrakan Lotus station of Divinity.

## 9. *Gateway 7: Sacred Relationship Meditation*

Increase the length of time you spend in meditation every seven days. The longer you are in meditation, the deeper your inner peace will be, and the more solid your *ba* (spirit) will become. The cleaner your Body Temple, the sooner it will be able to live permanently in the peace and inner balance of the meditative state.

- Hold your rose quartz stone inside your palm. Visualize yourself sitting in the blue and green heart of the lotus blossom, unfazed by the adversity of the world, living and breathing in a balanced, beautiful centered breath of ease and grace.
- Breathe in your heart center, visualizing Mother Ast protecting, nurturing, and loving you with each breath. Breathe, purge, and flush out from the heart of the lotus, from the arms of Het-Hru, from the bosom of Ast, your mother, all anguish, all mistrust, hurt, pain, fear, and resentment that have poisoned your relationships. Flush these out of your heart of compassion and love. Then breathe five hundred Fire Breaths into your heart until it becomes light as a feather.
- When you are calm and have completed your breath work, place your palms over your healed heart and repeat these soothing words our Ancestors said before us:

*My heart, my mother*
*Ab-a en mut-a*
*My heart, my mother*
*Ab-a en mut-a*[1]

Most of us have embraced the Father aspect of the Most High for inner balance and harmony of your womanself. Now sit in your seat, the heart of the Lotus, within the arms of the Mother and revitalize this most primary relationship. Rest easy and breathe fully. Vow never to forsake your Holy Mother again.

*Color Visualization.* Visualize the color of the Gateway you are in—blue, for communication and inner peace. As you perform your meditation, wear white or blue, and/or place blue cloth on your altar.

*Sacred Stone Meditation.* While in meditation, hold a rose quartz or pink tourmaline stone in your palms over your heart. It is the Sacred Healing Stone of the Gateway and helps to illuminate the heart. The opaque light of these deep pink stones stimulates both love and beauty. These stones are known to have healing, curative, and purifying properties. They unblock the heart area, allowing compassion and understanding so that the sacred healing from upon high can come through. These stones represent the fourth *arit* (chakra), or energy center, at the heart, which activates Divine Love.

### 10. Herbal Tonics

Drink chamomile herbal tea. Parts used: flowers and leaves. Chamomile tea helps to heal all relationships that the mother / Sacred Woman births. Use for seven days to receive the full benefit of tuning you to Gateway 7. Drink your herb tea in your favorite mug during or after spiritual writing.

*Preparation.* One teabag to 1 cup of water. Boil water in a nonmetallic pot, turn off flame, and add tea to steep. Drink before or after your morning bath or sacred shower. Drink with joy and peace as you breathe between sips and settle into easy contemplation and reflection.

### 11. Flower Essences

To deepen your experience of Gateway 7, choose from the following flower essences. Take 4 drops four times per day directly on or under the tongue, or add the same amount to a small glass of purified water and sip. For instructions on how to choose flower essences, see page 23.

- *Calendula:* Communication, receptivity, listening to others; heals argumentative tendencies.
- *Fawn lily:* To develop intimate and warm contact with others.
- *Mallow:* Ease in developing friendships, warmth, and trust; greater social warmth; ability to sustain soulful relationships with others, especially friendship.
- *Violet:* Helps address inability to share one's essential self in a group situation, fear of losing one's identity if too close to others.
- *Pink yarrow:* Helps address oversensitivity to others, lack of emotional boundaries.
- *Forget-me-not:* Perceiving deeper karmic bonds within relationships; ability to acknowledge spiritual destiny and intent of relationship.

- *Poison oak:* Helps address difficulty in yielding or showing a soft side, fear of vulnerability, creating barriers; displaying hostility.

## 12. Diet

Follow Sacred Woman Transitional Dietary Practices presented for Gateways 7 and 8.

## 13. Sacred Relationship Journal Writing

This is best done after internal cleansing (enema) and/or meditation. When you are cleansed and centered, you can receive spiritual messages from the One Most High with grace. When you are in the spirit, messages travel down through your spirit mind, to your heart, into your hand, and onto the paper. (This is how I do all my writing.)

The best time to receive your spiritually inspired written work is after you have completed your altar work, between the hours of 4 A.M. and 6 A.M. Keep your journal and a very special pen by or on your altar to work with the power, force, and stillness at the coming of dawn, the hour of Nebt-Het.

Affirm your daily life. Write in your journal at this time thoughts, activities, experiences, and interactions that present themselves. You can also write down your visions, desires, dreams, and affirmations so that you will be able to draw on these resources when help and support are most needed.

*Consult Sesheta.* If you find that you are unable to contact your inner voice during your journal work, call Sesheta, the keeper and revealer of secrets (who is indwelling), to assist and speak through you.

## 14. Senab Freedom Shawl or Quilt

Choose a new piece of cloth that corresponds to the Gateway color (indicated in exercise 9 of your Daily Spiritual Observances or in Sacred Altar Work) to add to your Senab Freedom Shawl or Quilt. This cloth will serve as a mini-canvas to represent your experience in the Gateway you're working in.

Also, collect meaningful symbols that can be added to your shawl or quilt in appliqué or patchwork style. You can add stones, other natural objects, collectibles, family heirlooms, photographs that have been reprinted on fabric, or any other significant items that embody the essence of your experience. Give your imagination free rein and let your craftswoman spirit tell your story. For more information about the Senab Freedom Shawl or Quilt, see pages 122–125.

## 15. Sacred Tools

A beautiful white ostrich feather to be your Maat feather. A sacred scale for weighing your heart and your Maat feather. Beautiful feathers to create a feather fan for purifying the atmosphere when you seek to harmonize your relationships.

## 16. Sacred Reminder

Throughout the week, you are to observe closely the wisdom presented in Gateway 7: Sacred Relationships. For maximum results, live freely in tune with the various systems of wellness presented and practice the Seven-Day Transformative Work at the end of the Gateway.

## Closing Sacred Words

*Mother/Father Divine, help me to heal and honor my significant relationships and to transform them into Sacred Relationships.*

# TRANSITIONAL DIETARY PRACTICES FOR GATEWAYS 7 AND 8

Continue the same dietary practices presented in Gateways 4 to 6. The only difference in Gateways 7 and 8 is that now you will eat 60 to 75 percent raw (live/uncooked) and 25 to 40 percent cooked (steamed) food.

### Before Breakfast

Kidney-Liver Flush (see page 72).

### Breakfast

Drink fruit juice and/or eat fruits one hour before or after other foods, for better digestion.

Freshly pressed fruit juices, 8 to 12 oz. (diluted with 8 to 12 oz. pure water), with Heal Thyself Green Life Formula I, 1 to 2 tbsp.

*Fruits:* Acid fruits: grapefruit, lemons, limes, oranges, tangerines. Subacid fruits: apples, pears, plums, cherries, berries, peaches. No bananas. *Do not mix acid and subacid fruits together.*

### Lunch

Freshly pressed vegetable juices, 8 to 12 oz. (diluted with 8 to 12 oz. pure water), with Heal Thyself Green Life Formula I, 1 to 2 tbsp.

Large raw salad. No tomatoes, but include plenty of sprouts, such as alfalfa, mung bean, etc. Include any or all of the following: okra, kale, cauliflower, turnip greens, mustard greens, broccoli, seaweed in any form (i.e., kelp, hijiki, wakame, nori), to add to soups or salads.
*Proteins:* Choose one only:

- Sprouts soaked in water overnight (alfalfa sprouts, mung bean sprouts, sunflower sprouts).
- If you are a flesh consumer in transition, prepare baked fish (no shellfish), soy chicken, or organic chicken one to three times a week.
- 2 to 4 oz. raw soaked nuts (almonds, filberts, walnuts, pecans, Brazil nuts); avoid cashews and peanuts.

- Seeds (sunflower, pumpkin).
*Starches:* Choose one of the whole grains or starches. Soak in water with herbal seasonings and vegetables for 10 minutes. No cooking needed.

- Tabouli
- Bulgur wheat
- Couscous

### Dinner

Repeat lunch. Increase freshly pressed/juiced vegetable juices to 12 to 16 oz. (diluted with pure water), with Heal Thyself Green Life Formula I, 1 to 2 tbsp. After the sun goes down, do not eat proteins or starches! Eat only live foods: salads, fruits, and vegetables.

## DIETARY SUPPORTS

### Additional Nutrients and Herbs

- Heal Take Green Life Formula 1—Heal Thyself Super Nutritional Formula (see the product list in the appendix) contains all the vitamins and minerals the Body Temple needs. Take three times a day with juice or take some form of chlorophyll, such as powdered wheatgrass (1 tsp. to 1 tbsp.) or liquid, 1 to 2 oz., with distilled water; powdered spirulina (1 tsp. to 1 tbsp.) or liquid, 1 to 2 oz., with distilled water; powdered blue-green manna (1 tsp to 1 tbsp.) or liquid, 1 to 2 oz., with distilled water.
- If stressed, take 25 to 50 mg of vitamin B complex or you will have skin eruptions. Vitamin B complex also strengthens the nervous system and rejuvenates skin and hair.
- For poor memory and poor circulation, take 1 tbsp. of granulated lecithin.
- Take 500 to 1,000 mg of vitamin C daily, to build the immune system and fight colds and infections. Ester C is easier on the digestive system.

- Heal Thyself Breath of Spring (optional), 3 drops twice a day with warm water, particularly during hay fever season. (See the product list in the appendix.)
- 1 tbsp. lecithin. This brain food helps to clear out the arteries for increased circulation.

## Internal Cleansing

Take an enema seven nights straight, then three times a week throughout the weeks to follow. Herbal laxatives: 3 tablets of cascara sagrada *every other day*. Colonics: 1 to 3 during the twenty-one-day cleansing period.

## Physical Activity

Practice the abbreviated Dance of the Womb fifteen to thirty minutes daily, or the complete two-hour regimen (see Gateway 3: Sacred Movement), and do four hundred Fire Breaths daily.

## Meditation

Meditate five to fifteen minutes daily.

## Rejuvenation Baths

Epsom salts, 1 to 4 lbs., or 1 lb. Dead Sea salt in your bath, seven nights straight. Time for soaking: fifteen to thirty minutes. Then shower off the salt. (Do not use bath salts if you have high blood pressure.)

## Heal Thyself Master Herbal Formula II

At bedtime daily, boil 5 to 6 cups of purified or distilled water, turn off the flame, and add 3 tsp. herbs. Steep overnight. Strain in the morning, and drink before 2 P.M. (See chapter 3, and see the product list in the appendix.)

## Queen Afua's Rejuvenating Clay Application

Optional, according to need. Follow instructions on pages 91–92. (See the product list in the appendix.)

## Other Nature Cures

Drink at least 2 to 3 quarts of distilled water daily.

---

# SACRED RELATIONSHIPS

Relationships are the arms and legs of the womb, the extensions of a woman's "inner space."

In order for a woman's womb to be at peace, she needs to be at peace in all of her relationships—those with people, with food, with Nature, and, of course, with herself.

Review each of your significant relationships in your own way and allow each one to become your teacher. Empty your heart of all resentment and become receptive to the lessons that each relationship brings to you. Surrender to the love that each and every lesson offers so that you will not hold on to pain. Undigested pain or grief or anger held in your body grows into illness.

Relationships have the potential to provide both joy and sorrow. Unfortunately, there can be many sources of relationship pain. Perhaps the most tragic is the hurt and disappointment caused by intimate relationships with family members or friends, someone known and trusted. Emotional or energetic harm or violation from a person you thought you could trust to love and respect you creates deep resentment, anger, or rage that requires committed healing work.

Too often we retreat from dysfunctional relationships or deny the true depths of the problems in an effort to soothe our wounds. Yet we must take self-responsibility now and begin to try to understand the lessons of our relationships. Relationship wounds must be healed or their repressed energies will solidify on the spiritual, emotional, and physical levels.

*Affirm now, and from now on:*

*My womb is my sacred nest in which I hold all my relationships. No one will enter into the womb of my mind, the womb of my heart, or the womb of my womb unless they are at their best; pure and clean. Join me, all my relations, in my Natural Living lifestyle. Join me in my peace of mind, in my state of divine bliss. My womb speaks peace to all my relations and so my relationships speak peace to my womb. I bless all my relationships.*

## My Mother, My Heart . . .

The relationship we daughters have with our mothers is primal. It is the first and most potent connection we have with anyone. It began by living inside our mother's body for nine months before emerging into the world. She was our first caretaker and nurturer.

Even if we've had a difficult relationship with our mother from the very beginning, we still have an irreplaceable bond. Thus mothers and daughters have shared life energy from the Creator/Creatress. We've shared things that we share with no one else.

And whether we think so or not, no matter what human shortcomings our mother may possess, she does love us—in her own way. And we love her, sometimes in spite of ourselves—in our way. And when our mothers pass over, we discover that there is an empty place in our hearts and our lives that no one else can fill.

The ancient Afrakan Priests and Priestesses of Khamit prayed to the Great Mother:

*Ab-a en mut-a. Ab-a en mut-a. Ab-a en mut-a.*
*My heart, my mother. My heart, my mother. My heart, my mother.*

Reading these words, I opened up my sacred first eye right above my brow where my melaninized nectar pours forth to allow me to receive from the Spirit. I asked the meaning of "My mother, my heart," and this is what I was given in my moments of prayer:

*Within your heart is your Sacred Mother. There she sweetly sits and holds council; there she handles all matters of your heart center. Come to Holy Mother in prayer for the healing of hurt feelings and emotional disharmony in all your relationships. Come to Holy Mother for soothing, for comfort. Come for heart wounds and scars that are ready for healing.*

## A Healing Meditation of the Heart

- Lie down on your back and focus on the Great Mother spirit center, the Ast (Isis) center.
- Choose one of the following Heart-Healing Symbols to use during your meditation:

  — *Rose quartz crystal or pink tourmaline.* May be used in your heart-healing meditation.
  — *The scarab.* Represents the heart space transformation. It is a tool our Ancestors used to guide us into a renewed heart place, and thus a renewed life.
  — *The feather.* Represents the balancing and lightening of your heart from the sorrows of the world. As you call forth the Great Mother and breathe, rest the feather or the scarab over your Ab center to help magnify peace within your heart.

**Rose Quartz Meditation**

- First rest a rose quartz crystal over your heart center to cleanse heart blockages. Keep it there as you relax. Breathe slowly and deeply and repeat, "My mother, my heart."
- When your intuition has spoken and the cleansing has taken place, remove the rose quartz. Then place a clear quartz crystal over your heart center to energize and magnify the love that is in you by nature.
- When you are filled with a deep sense of love all through your Body Temple, then slowly get up, as you breathe deeper still, and go about your day. Carry the love that has been activated and generated to all your relations, for they all are merely reflections of the level of

love that you give to and receive from your Holy Mother.

## Scarab or White Feather Meditation

- Place a scarab or a white feather over your heart center and breathe deeply and slowly as you recite over and over again: "My mother, my heart."
- As your harmony and sensitivity deepen, continue to breathe into the Great Mother Spirit center until you finally reach a trancelike state. In this state you might find yourself weeping. Just let it flow, for these are your tears of bitter or sweet release. Let it be so. Know that the Great Mother Spirit has connected to and touched the depths of your heart and freed your soul.
- Perform this simple heart-healing meditation, particularly during your initiation in the Gateway of Sacred Relationships over a seven-day period, or whenever you're in need of it.
- If your heart is heavy, acknowledge and call upon your Spirit Mother and she will cradle you in her bosom, illuminate you, lighten you, and fill your heart with love, joy, and unending compassion. She does this to help you move through this earthly realm with greater ease and sublime sweet assurance.

### A Love Message on Behalf of Our Earthly Mothers

If you are carrying resentment for your earthly mother, release your burden; cleanse your heart in your meditation. Open up and just thank your mother no matter what. Hug her body and kiss her hands in the flesh, or if she sits among the Ancestors, embrace her spirit sweetly and offer her a spiritual gift—for your mother did the best she could with what she had to work with. Forgive her, and your blessings will flow like a waterfall.

## SACRED MOTHERHOOD

As far back as I could remember, I felt in my soul that mothering was an all-important work, and I wanted very much to become one. I waited most of my life to finally become a mother. Well, it did happen. I birthed and mothered three children, nurtured and mothered a few husbands, and many friends and clients, and other people's children.

But of all the nurturing work that I've ever done in my life, birthing and mothering my children was by far the most supreme experience of mothering. To mold a being from inside your womb, to share your body with a soul that feeds from your person until he or she arrives on this earth, is a mighty miracle.

As a mother giving birth, you are given the opportunity to be an active part of Creation, to experience the volcanolike eruption of the earth within you as you crack open into your power. When you are in that birth space, that sacred place, you ride on a sacred wave with each birthing contraction. How brave you are as you transcend pain and use it as an opportunity to usher in new life.

As you give birth to yourself through your child, you will witness your own and your mate's combined love prayer.

Motherhood will make you over if you allow it to. It will create muscle—spiritually, mentally, emotionally, and, yes, even physically. Mothering will keep you in counsel with the Creator/Creatress from moment to moment, so that you will be properly and wisely guided. Motherhood, if you don't fight it, run from it, or rebel against it, will teach you how to master your very life. Mothering will show you the way to unconditional, all-embracing love. It will teach you how to absolutely put your trust in the Creator/Creatress. To receive the position of motherhood is truly honorable work. This station can help you to evolve to your highest of highs.

However, if you are not supported by a loving husband, the children's father, or blood or extended family, the task can break you down. Even when you have full support for your mothering, you may still find this the most challenging transformational work you've ever undertaken. Motherhood is a test of faith, love, and strength. Motherhood forces some and aids others to blossom into their absolute womanness.

And yet the birthing of a baby is not a requirement for developing the art and science of mothering. To mother means to master the art of the nurturing spirit. Mothering calls you to order. It demands that you move beyond being weak, impatient, quick to anger. Mothering calls on you to speak and act from your spiritual center, which may supply you with the answers for all your questions and concerns on mothering. Mothering is the ultimate healing work.

Mother Earth teaches us, through the Creator/Creatress, how to be good mothers. For Mother Earth loves her children one and all, she feeds us from her waters and land, she gives us her pure air. Mother Earth supports us in peace as we rest on her fields, grass, and trees so that we can feel secure. Mother Earth takes care of us, and this allows us to continue to care for our children everywhere.

In the act of mothering there are moments when our children and the conditions surrounding them may be harsh and unyielding. You may from time to time feel unappreciated, and reciprocity may not be in the air. A tear drops, the pain of motherhood pulls at your heart. Sometimes the lessons of motherhood come from child to mother. That's when you need to hold on with all your might to the Supreme Mother. She is there eternally, to nurture you, heal you, and lighten your heart.

To be a mother is to be in a supreme position of power, peace, and strength. Sometimes motherhood feels so good and comforting, it's like eating corn bread, barbecued soy chicken, and meatless collard greens with a jar of honey lemonade at a family reunion in Grandmother's backyard on a hot summer day. Motherhood — yum. I'm full.

## Mother to Daughter

Mothers, take time to teach your daughters, whose wombs have not yet been touched by the world. Show them, by your example, what is and is not to be. Follow your intuition and your knowledge. Guide them about how to respect their sacred wombs. Anoint and bless your daughter's womb, heart, and mind every new moon, or at the onset of her menses. Teach her

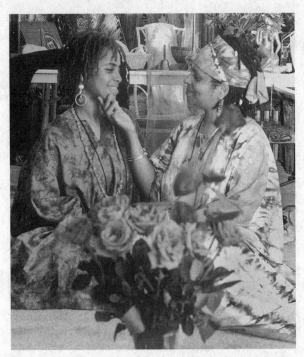

A Village of Mothers and Daughters

how to care for her sacred, holy womb through the teachings of Natural Law. Whisper in her ear at night, like the old folks did. Tell her, "Your womb is sacred, for you are sacred."

Tell your daughter that she is beautiful. Tell her she is like a crystal, a pearl, or another precious gem. Tell her that she is as lovely as roses and orchids. Your beloved daughter is to be appreciated as one of the flowers of Mother Earth.

Let your daughter know that she is worthy of all of the love and blessings of the Creator/Creatress. Hug her often, kiss her crown, rock her when possible so she will know you as her foundation, her solid ground.

Talk to her and tell her what's in your heart. Listen to her closely. Let nothing be so big or small that she cannot talk to you.

Keep her heart sweet by exposing her to the beauty of the world. Keep her mindful of the world and its adversity in order to help her develop her highest compassionate and intellectual level.

Let her know her womb is an extension of her mind. Adorn her mind with lots of love, so her life will be sublime.

## A Village of Sister-Mothers

At a workshop where we'd been talking about mother-daughter relationships, Sharon came up to me and told me that at the age of twelve, her daughter, Lajuana, had come to the conclusion that Sharon had certain gaps in her mothering abilities. This isn't unusual around this sensitive age, but instead of attacking or fighting with her mother all the time, Lajuana tried what she later called her "village of sister-mothers" approach.

Lajuana approached four of her mother's closest friends, each of whom had a special gift—at least in Lajuana's eyes—that represented an aspect of her education as a young woman that she felt she couldn't get from her mother. She picked a mother who ran her own store, for practical in-the-real-world advice; she asked another mother, a designer and the most elegant and alluring woman in the village, for advice on clothes and hair and makeup—and boys. She picked a healer mother for spiritual advice, and a fourth mother, who was a high-school teacher, for advice about coping with all the stresses of school, getting into college, and dealing with the new challenges there. She also figured she could go to them for advice on how to deal with her mom, since they knew Sharon so well.

Lajuana then approached each sister-mother individually and asked if she'd be willing to be part of her village of sister-mothers circle. They were all flattered and genuinely pleased to support Lajuana in this way. It's one thing to become a godmother because the parents of the child ask you at the naming ceremony. But when the young woman herself asks you when she's older and more aware, it is a very special gift—especially to women who may not have their own biological children. Honorary sister-mothers are valued for who they are and the special gifts they have to offer.

Each potential sister-mother checked out this new relationship proposal with Sharon, who was surprised but delighted. She thought this was a brilliant thing for her daughter to do—and it would take a lot of pressure off them both. This was how the Sister-Mother Circle was born. Lajuana felt free to consult with any of her sister-mothers when she had a problem in their area of expertise. Before long, it dawned on both Sharon and Lajuana that their relationship had improved as well.

The Sister-Mother Circle still exists today, even though Lajuana is in her late twenties, married, and a new mother. Essentially what Lajuana created for herself was the old Afrakan tradition of extended family. She created her own village to help raise her, and now she's extending that wisdom to the raising of her own child.

There's no reason why we can't create a Sister-Mother Circle for ourselves, no matter how old we may be or whether our mothers are alive or no longer with us. We all need all the good mothering we can get. So think about who you might choose for your own Godmother Circle, and invite them in. And also think about suggesting to your daughter, the next time she criticizes you for your inadequacies, that she might want to create a Sister-Mother Circle for herself. Who knows, you may end up being in someone else's Sister-Mother Circle, and the circles of love and caring and mothering will keep expanding like the ripples from a stone thrown in a pond.

## Mother to Son

My son, SupaNova S.L.O.M. "Daoud," helped me to organize the contents of this book, and just as I was about to release it, he said, "Ma, you speak about all forms of relationships in your book, but what about me, your son? We really have such a great relationship. Why not write on mothers to sons?" After thinking about it for some time, here is what I have to say.

Being the mother of sons as well as daughters is so fulfilling, and also at times quite overwhelming and demanding. But whatever else motherhood may be for me, it contains many divine lessons, and I embrace them willingly. For example, a son at times may try to be a father and tell his mother what to do. When this happens to me, I just stand up on the kitchen table and shout: "Wait a minute! I'm the mother here, and I run this ship."

Dynamic, spontaneous mothering can bring so many marvelous happenings out of you. Stay

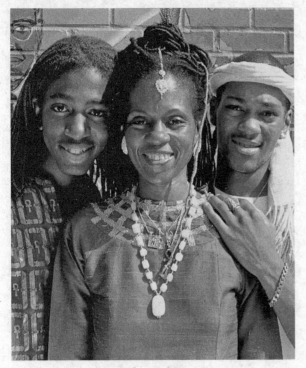

Queen Afua and Her Sons

in tune and witness how the Creator/Creatress will work through you.

My children's father and I separated many moons ago. As a mother, I was required not only to give the normal ratio of love and compassion that a mother gives, but I found myself having to pull out the father in me and be this firm, strong-armed person. Many times I felt like I was simply not enough. But as the years went on and the tears fell, I stayed prayerful and continued to purify, and I was shown the way.

The Creator/Creatress guides me and teaches me how to raise my sons to become whole human beings in a disjointed world. To make my life a little easier and my sons more balanced, I make sure they have access to many wonderful men who will assist them in their growth process. These men include physical and spiritual uncles, an attentive and caring stepfather, mentors, and friends.

Through their most formative years (grades one to eight), I sent the boys to Afrakan cultural schools that served vegetarian meals to enhance their living a clean, natural life. These schools also helped them strengthen and maintain a strong, positive self-image of who they are and where they came from. They were taught not a heritage of slavery, but rather a heritage of Maat (righteousness), dignity, intelligence, strength, and prosperity.

I was on a journey, all of their young lives, to encircle them with a rich sense of self-awareness, love, support, and high thinking. For example, my youngest child was sent to Endosha Martial Arts and Cultural School for discipline and for the character-building influences of powerful, upright men.

Both my sons went through their Rites of Passage just by coming into contact with the positive, influential male role models in the community. Together, they took the Shrine of Ptah Wat-Heru African Nile Valley Rites of Passage Training for a solid base in Afrakan spirituality and self-knowledge. Their birth father gave them a spiritual bath and words of wisdom as they took their final step into manhood.

As a result, my sons are growing up to be strong leaders and mentors for other young males. They are sensitive, loving, strong, intelligent, vegetarian visionaries. We talk a great deal, my sons and I, about our individual and collective aspirations, inner feelings, hopes, and dreams. Ours is truly a blessed relationship.

For those women who have been able to maintain a healthy marriage—which helps in raising healthy children—all power! For those like myself who become divorced or single parents, you must expand yourselves to be wiser and more loving. Hug harder, talk more, play with great vigor, love deeply, and let loose all your creativity. It's what I had to do to be both a mother and a father to my sons.

For the love of my boys I would go through fire. And I did on many occasions, with all of the early challenges that came with raising my sons into young men. When he was seventeen I had to send my elder son, SupaNova, to his father's people in South Carolina for a year, to get him off the streets of New York and save his life. I took myself and my younger son, Ali, to St. Thomas, Virgin Islands, to live and attend school for six months, to help him tap back into his soul. I traveled up and down the highways of life as I followed the healing voice of the Creator/

Creatress for help. Oh, yes, I was driven to stretch myself wide open to rise in the Spirit so that my sons would grow into whole men.

The Afrakan mind-set is that traditionally our children inherit what and who we are as part of their legacy. I affirm this to be true, for one day my younger son was assisting his grandmother in producing some of our Heal Thyself products in our Kitchen Healing Laboratory when he looked up at me and said, "Ma, besides becoming a medical doctor and helping to deliver babies, when I grow up I'm going to help manage our family business, the Heal Thyself Center, to help your work to grow." And then he went back to work.

My elder son, at nineteen, said to me when I was feeling down and bewildered over my life's work, "Don't worry, Ma, I'll represent you. I'll enforce your teachings. You see, I'm a Warrior of the Creator/Creatress, so I must hold up the banner of 'Liberation through purification.' I can represent you well because I'm a chlorophyllion [one who eats and drinks mostly green vegetables]." He then leaned forward and kissed my forehead, which warmed my heart.

When your reflections, in the form of your children, turn their hands and hearts back to you, their mother, when they are led to support, heal, and uplift you . . . my, my, my. Words fail to convey the gratitude that a mother has for the world of Divinity expressing itself through her children.

Many a time my mama would say that it would not be easy raising boys, and she was right. But Lord, it has been good for my soul. I can only offer endless thanks and praise for being the mother of these two precious sons of mine!

### Thank You, Mama, for Loving Me

Mama is so rich in her ways, she loves life by living effortlessly. She's like a beautiful meditation. Mama has cultivated me with as much care as one would cultivate a beautiful rose garden.

Thank you to my mother, Ida Robinson, who has been a wonderful example of the total personification of "Peace; be still." No matter how intense life got to be, or how turbulent the roller

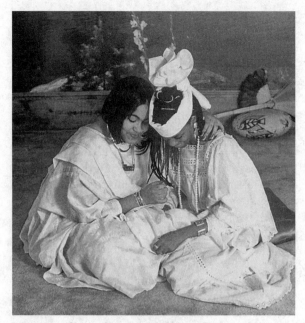

Queen Afua and Her Daughter, Princess Sherease

coaster of living became, you were always like the dove sitting peacefully, undisturbed by the confusion or the challenges of life's ups and downs.

Thank you, Mama, for showing me what peace looks like. Thank you, Mama, for the graceful way you walked, the regal way you sat, the gentle way you laughed, and the soft way you spoke. What an exquisite image you gave me about the beauty there is in being a woman.

Thank you, Mama, for supporting my entire life—my children, my work, my associations, my mate, my whole being. The work that I was destined to do could not have happened without you.

Thank you, Mama, for keeping me on the stoop, in the house, and out of trouble as a young girl. It paid off later on as you and the old folks knew it would.

To my Ancestor "Big Mama" Ford, thank you for birthing Mama Ida, and for pressing into my young memory the beauty and necessity of strength in an Afrakan woman. Thank you, Big Mama, for raising my nine aunts and four uncles with Grandfather Ford so very well and so very upright. But especially thank you for giving me my mama. She is so rich in her ways. My mama's beauty and beautiful way surpass the beauty of the lotus, if that could be. My mama, she's supreme. She *is* a beautiful meditation.

To my precious daughter, Sherease, who's as pretty as can be, you have drawn me closer and closer to the Most High. I thank you. Thank you, daughter, for teaching me who I am at the core of my being. Thank you, daughter, for walking with me so I may garden you properly. I'm sincerely grateful that the Most High Creator/Creatress chose me to be your mother. With all of our ups and downs and the hard times, and oh so challenging times and sweet quiet times together, it's been good.

Our union has made me a mother of a daughter, and that's an extra-special reflection to learn and grow from, for in you I see clearly my own trials, my victories, my madness, my fears, my beauty, and my hope of lotuslike reflection coming through from me to you.

I promise to walk with you all the days of your life, even when I become an Ancestor. Worry not; I will be there for you. My love for you is steady; it has no mood swings.

Mothers, fathers, and extended family especially, love, pamper, and nurture your daughters deeply so that they will grow up accustomed to being treated well. Teach the women in your family to expect and receive the best treatment from the men in their lives through you. Good treatment should be the norm, not the exception. Encourage the family to love its women. In this way their self-esteem will be heightened, and they will not attract men who abuse women but instead find men to love, respect, and cherish women.

To our daughters, from mothers everywhere: There is a silver cord that runs from me to you. If you don't know what to do or where to go, just pull on the cord and I will send you what you need to help you. Seen or unseen, you can be sure I'll always be there for you, and if not me in person all the time, I'll send an extension of me — your grandmother, or your auntie.

May we all continue to be positive examples for our daughters and sisters everywhere.

### We Have Many Mothers

A sister newly on the Path of Purification was talking with me about her troubles with her mother. She said, "My relationship with my mother has never been good, and it hurts me because I keep going back and trying. I keep trying to bring my mother healing information, and she won't accept it. I had a big fight with her this week, so I think that's what triggered a binge of emotional eating."

Our first and most important relationship is with our mothers. And no matter how old we get or whether they're still on this planet or not, that relationship continues to affect us deeply.

What changes over the years is how we come to view them. With deep inner work and purification we can move from rage and noncommunication to compassion and acceptance.

But in the meantime, we don't have to do without the mothering each one of us needs, whatever our age. We all have different mothers in the world. In your meditations, tap into all the mothers in your life. We have a mother who brings us into the world. She's the gatekeeper who got us here, and so we give gratitude and thanks. We may not be able to get all we need from her, though. You know the principle that it takes a village to raise a child. And we're constantly being raised by others as we grow up. So that means we have a number of mothers. Give praise for them all. The Creator/Creatress is your mother. She doesn't leave this void. We're constantly getting what we need. We just need to open up our eyes and see.

There may be a woman at your job who keeps supporting you and assisting you and giving you advice. For example, my accountant has been my mother for the last two weeks. She's helping me acquire the building that we're in. She says, "I don't know what it is that has me calling up and checking and investigating for you and doing all this work and making all these doors open." But I know. It's because I am her true child. And I know she has wisdom that I don't have, and I submit to that. A girlfriend may mother you sometime.

So don't feel like you're empty. Feel glad about your birth mother. As a matter of fact, you may be the mother for your mother sometimes. And give her what she can't give herself, even if it's simply a good thought. You know how we can be in the same room and send thoughts to each other that knock us out? You say, "I wonder how come I'm feeling so bad." It's because you're in a room full of thoughts that have not been lifting up your spirit. So try sitting with your mother and thinking, "I love you, Mom. I thank you for the strength you've shown me." Know it's on not the physical plane but the spiritual one that you're connecting. And know that she's giving you the best mothering she has in her. If you can show her that gratitude, your daughters and your daughter's daughters will give you the same energy back.

### Healing Our Mothers and Ourselves

"My mother hurts to this day," a client told me. "Twenty years later she's in grief, because when she came with her children, her mother said, 'You can't bring those children here; you better go back to your husband.' But he abused her, so she had to go to a shelter."

That's why I say, if your mother ever opens up the door and lets you in, you can just kiss her feet in gratitude, because gratitude builds. If you just keep saying "Thank you, thank you, thank you," it creates light, and your mother will heal. This is her chance. You are her love energy.

### A Final Healing

A sister in one of my workshops said, "I had to write my mother a letter and tell her that I refused to be Cinderella anymore, and she said fine. And a friend of hers called me up and said, 'Listen, I've seen your relationship with your mother. Go about your life. If she ever needs you, I'll call you.' So for two years I was free.

"And when I got that telephone call that she needed me, I went to her. She was amazed that I would nurse her. I would nurse anyone. As a matter of fact, I told her that, and it broke up our relationship again. But that's what she did for me. She made me a person who would help anyone. Watching her die, I saw that she came to realize what she had created. She saw what she'd helped me become. She had a wonderful passing, but I can't say I don't have a sense of freedom with her gone.

"Now I see that our mothers come to terms with all this by watching how we're living our life, by how we transform, and how we make peace with ourselves. That's when your mother will come into your energy field. Right now she may be refusing to even acknowledge you—like 'You don't exist, you're not my daughter.' And you're constantly trying to live up to this image that she has in her mind of you. But you have to understand that you have to transform, you have to be at peace with yourself, and be patient. In time, your mom will come to learn who you are and what she has helped bring about."

## COMING TOGETHER SISTER-TO-SISTER

A sister once told me, "My grandmother said to me, 'Don't take anything from women.'"

We got scared of one another because of competition for men and scarce survival resources. As a result, we've tried to hurt one another and keep one another down.

But now we're going to begin to open up and look at one another and hug one another, and know that it's going to be okay. And when we do our inner work, life reflects who we are now. When we're out in the world, what we see is our own reflection.

When we take our loving bath and take time to do our affirmations while we're commuting from home to work, we're incorporating wellness into our whole life. So keep your lemon water by your desk. Have your Maat feather in your medicine bag, and pull it out at high noon when you feel really stressed out. Then it will be easy when you're with another sister because she'll be reflecting what you've done for yourself. Trust the womb in her as well.

### Sister-to-Sister Growing into Woman-to-Woman

As sisters, Queen Esther and I spoke the same language, shared the same visions, raised our children together. We sat around the table and talked—and sometimes our sessions seemed to go on for days. We became spiritual blood sisters. My sister was so young but yet so very wise. Her joy of living inspired me to see life in a more beautiful way, in a more ecstatic way. She added to my fire.

Queen Esther is a cultural activist, extraordinary Afrakan mother of two, entrepreneur, businesswoman, and dancer of pure grace. She is a lovely woman indeed, who above all has a love for her people that is profound and supreme. As sisters, we sat back-to-back with inquisitions of the heart, the mind, and the spirit. And, oh! how the answers did flow from me to her and through her to me. We made a pact that when we were old and still vibrant at a hundred years of age and beyond, we would come together and witness. We would share and remember our story of living.

Together, we explored our spiritual lives. We made a home in the Native American Sweat Lodge and received our sacred feathers. I was her support on a reservation in the Black Hills of South Dakota. Her father, Mr. Hunter (may he rest in peace), was part of the Blackfoot Indian people. His blood running through her Afrakan body allowed Queen Esther to be one of the first Afrakan women to dance in the sacred Sun Dance—a tradition that has been in place for thousands of years.

Every year, in the month of August, the tribes come together to pray for deliverance and for the earth, our mother and father spirit, the rock people, the two-legged and four-legged creatures, and the winged people. They came together to dance, fast, and sweat for liberation. They pray for the freedom of political prisoners in American jails.

During slavery many Afrakans fled to the Native Americans for refuge, and they were able to live together because of their common traditions, views, and rituals of family, sharing, and moral values. Both groups respect Nature, and both believe in the Sacred Feather. The Eagle of the Natives of Turtle Island and the Nubians' Sacred Falcon were birds that represented our spiritual ascension. From this coming together emerged such people as Mr. Hunter, part Blackfoot, part Afrakan.

Chief Crow Dog was a "bad" dude, which in Harlem means powerful in a positive way. He was also empowered and in tune as one of the leaders of the Sioux Nation. He honored and gave permission for my sister, Queen Esther, to

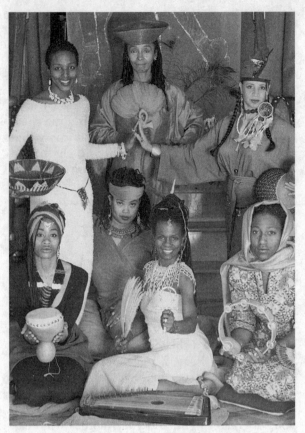

Maat Kheru: The Sacred Voices

dance in a Sun Dance of South Dakota's Black Hills. So did Marenzo—a sweat lodge leader, artist, and friend from Chicago.

Together with over 150 people who came out to be Sun Dancers and supporters, we pitched a tent on the reservation. We washed in a nearby lake when we rose at sunrise, and fasted (or ate "air sandwiches," as Queen Esther called it). The morning was filled with drums that woke us at five in the morning to begin the purification ritual, which went on for four days. Esther would dress in traditional Native American garb: feathers, shawls, and wraps. She would do a morning sweat, then dance for eight hours in the sun and the rain. I supported her and Marenzo during this sacred time.

Each night during the four-day dance, my sister and I sat on the Great Mother (Mut) in the sweat lodge, heated with twenty to forty hot rocks. One of the most amazing sweats was when we shared the lodge with some Native American women from Alaska. They were spiritually solid. We sweated out our old pains, unresolved anger, unfulfilled dreams, and disappointments. We sweated for hours, strengthened by the power of our people, until a freedom call rang out from deep within: "Freedom is at hand. Resurrection of a nation is coming forth."

As we grew into woman-to-woman, we sweated out negativity, old baggage that we picked up as we journeyed through life. At times we forgot to study and we let the unlearned lessons accumulate. We forgot to put down the excess baggage. But when we caught ourselves starting to dry up like raisins in the sun, we talked together, prayed together, meditated together, and rocked the pain away. We called on freedom, strength, love, power, forgiveness, and peace for ourselves, our blood families, and our extended families.

You will always be with me, my sister-woman Queen Esther, even if we are miles apart. Thanks to the Creator/Creatress, I know how to call you up without a phone.

My deep friendship with Queen Esther is a powerful example of a wonderful sister-to-sister relationship. It's great to have a soul connection with a generous, loving woman who's working on herself. But it's a whole other thing to have a relationship with a woman who's working with you! A relationship stagnates when the other person is capable only of offering negativity to you.

Why is it some women are able to claim the mantle of Sacred Woman while others proudly claim the mantle of Bitch? They can control and terrorize us for ages, but as we begin to work on ourselves we discover that in reality Bitches are wounded women in need of deep healing.

## OVERCOMING THE BROKEN

I have been observing Millennials, particularly those in the hip-hop family. (Generally, Millennials are recognized as those who entered adulthood at the turn of the twenty-first century.) In many song lyrics and in conversations, men sadly refer to girlfriends, mates, and wives as ". . . my bitch." The women respond, "I'm his bitch." Men and women who speak this phrase demonstrate a misguided usage of a term not of endearment—even if it's intended in that way—as well as an acceptance that one person can own another. Use of the B-word in lyrics and conversations is loud evidence of a culture gone mad. In this case, the "B" could correctly stand for "broken."

To detox from the name-calling and related negativity, I suggest you examine the B-word in its present use. Further, I suggest working to heal from the deadly, misguided effects of using this word. Supporting campaigns to radiate away from a "broken," toxic frequency to a positive, healed frequency would be fitting for a Sacred Woman and all her relations.

Encouraging news! Woman are beginning to speak up and out against the B-word, recognizing it as a form of verbal abuse. In the name of love and in order to heal, it is high time that women and men make the shift to overcome the strife, the struggle, and the pain of accepting and living with being seen and spoken to in a derogatory way.

As the Women, the Healers, we elevate ourselves to our true holistic nature. For as the Women rise, so do the men. Our men will begin to see and call us properly: Queen, Beloved, Precious, Beautiful, Lovely, Sacred, and so on. When all use the name Blessed, all will become blessed.

### How to Heal "the Bitch"

*What happens to a people when they are stolen away from their home, then endlessly used and abused by another group of people for personal, diabolical gain? What happens to the generations of women of such a tribe who are continuously raped for hundreds of years by their oppressors for pleasure and profit? What happens to a once-whole, beautiful Afrakan woman who was forced to bear the babies conceived under such defiling circumstances?*

One of the negative things that can happen to women under such circumstances is Bitch Possession. The Bitch is an unrealized woman, encased in pain and filled with fear. She's a woman who feels trapped by life, surrounded by and absorbed in her own waste. The Bitch is a negative (evil) entity or spirit that possesses the Body Temple of a woman who has already been filled with rage, hate, envy, and despair. The Bitch can possess any woman from any race or status. The Bitch is on the opposite pole from the Sacred Woman, and ultimately she will strangle and destroy the one who is possessed by her.

This piece is a response to some of what this society has rendered to my people and so to me. I have no choice but to share this message, because Bitch Possession in others has hurt me throughout the years. She has given me the blues, made me feel bad about myself, made me feel used. Sisters with Bitch Possession brought me to tears, leaving me feeling attacked and hopelessly in despair. I'd shut down so tight no one could get through because I was runnin' scared of her and intimidated. Even my children would tell me, "Mama, people mistake your kindness for weakness." SupaNova, my son, would say, "Mama, you got to get stronger. You gotta speak out and defend yourself."

Over the years, my own healing has helped me to see that the Bitch is a sick state in a woman,

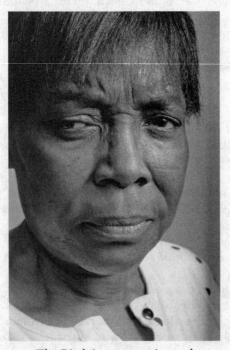

The Bitch is a woman in need
of healing.

and she needs psychospiritual and physical healing and purging. This understanding has allowed my fears of her to turn into compassion. It has allowed me to take the stance of a healer, pulling on my Ancestors for strength and clarity.

One early morning I was in my tub in a bath with eight pounds of salt, trying to heal from a Bitch encounter. I sat there, staring at the wall, while tears began rolling down my face. I cried out, "That's evil! Why is she so evil?" Then I started running an inner tape, going back to when I was seven, of built-up hurts from my sisters. Finally, after pondering, I said aloud, "That's a Bitch!"

My husband was in shock, for I'm known for not cursing. There was silence in the bathroom, and then my husband said, "It's time for you to write about your feelings before it kills your spirit."

I was in a trance as the tears kept silently flowing down my face, over my breasts, and into the water. Then I looked down at the water and saw that I was surrounded by a bath of tears. I was spellbound, locked in space, despondent.

That was a painful day, and to make things worse, it moved by in slow motion. I cried all day long. I cried to my mother, asking her why we women are so often this way. "What's wrong with us?" I cried to my friend Prema. I cried as I walked in the streets.

Finally, at the end of the day I began to write. I transformed my tears into these pages so that some healing could take place in my people who are suffering greatly from a postslavery conditioning that has gone as deep as our DNA—a conditioner that keeps us hurting one another, as woman to woman.

The *Random House College Dictionary* defines Bitch as "(1) a female dog; (2) a lewd woman meaning obscene, indecent, low, vulgar. Slang: a malicious woman (motivated by viciousness); an unpleasant, selfish woman, anything difficult or unpleasant. Characteristics of a Bitch, spiteful. Malevolent, which is also a characteristic of a Bitch. Wishing evil to another or others sharing ill will, ill disposed, vindictive, evil, harmful, injurious."

Why would I talk about the maliciousness and vindictiveness of the Bitch in *Sacred Woman*?

Because the Bitch has always been a part of my evolution as far back as I can remember, and I'm certain she's been a part of yours. She's shown up in the form of friends, associates, family members, coworkers, and even healers throughout my life. I was raised to be a "Brownstone Princess," and some people have called me "Miss Goody Two-Shoes." I was not raised to be a Bitch, and as a result, I was not given the tools or the skills to identify, recognize, cope with, work through, handle, or heal the scars the Bitch leaves behind. I had to go at it alone and learn as I went along, for no one was able to break down for me how to live with the Bitch—not in my blood family, in my extended family, or in the society at large.

From where I am now in my life I recognize that there are Chamomile Women—the calm and gentle type; Aloe Vera Women, who are direct but helpful; Cayenne and Ginger Women, who are quick, hot, and intense; and Clay Women, who are down-to-earth realists who thrive off Nature, grass, and trees. And, of course, there's the Bitch. Yet all women have the potential to be Lotus Women—spiritually enlightened, gracious, beautiful, compassionate, and whole.

Sometimes a Bitch develops in a woman who is running scared that she's not enough—not good enough, not strong enough, not powerful enough, not woman enough. When a woman gets more pressure than she can handle, she sometimes gets possessed by the Bitch. A first-class Bitch develops in a woman who's forced to live under tight conditions with limited space and limited resources and limited finances, with little or no support from a black man who has experienced his own set of unresolved issues—sexual abuse, rape, and mutilation. The Bitch is the result of a well-cultivated negative environment. The Bitch is a survivalist. She will take you down before she's taken out, because it's all about the survival of herself, her children, or her man at whatever cost. Problem is, she needs to watch out, for the Bitch in her will take her out, too, while she's in the process of doing her thing.

I speak here of the Bitch because through systematically adapting the Sacred Woman Principles she can indeed be healed. All women have the potential to be the Bitch to ourselves, to sister-friends, and to our men who are afraid to confront a woman with a Bitch possession. Therefore they end up fleeing to women from other cultures, who don't have the psychological baggage that the history of slavery in this country has passed down through our Afrakan genes. The black man runs to other women for refuge, turning their backs on us black women, because they say we're acting Bitchy. Bitchiness is becoming our reputation. We hear it from the lips of many of our men. They complain of our sometimes overbearing, dominating spirit—always seemingly fighting for survival. Come on, sister, if it's you I'm speaking to and you're tired of getting the old relationship blues, try to lighten up.

### 1. Part-Time Bitch Possession

There are part-time Bitches who emerge occasionally when the need arises. They appear to be a normal kind of woman much of the time, and may even show genuine kindness. Their sword is not active full-time. But if you catch them on the wrong day, you will get sliced and diced at the drop of a dime. And when they're done, it's business as usual.

### 2. Full-Time Bitch Possession

Some women are full-time Bitches—evil all the time, even when they're calmly smiling right at you. The wheels of deception are constantly turning toward evil doings. She stirs her pot with her sly words, her poisonous thoughts, and the proverbial "evil eye," which is in full effect. She steadily releases venom into the atmosphere, leaving a stench that infects passersby, for her mission in life is to destroy the very core and essence of life. Beware if you are her chosen victim, for when she strikes, your only way out is to strengthen yourself by raising your vibratory level through fasting and prayer.

### 3. The Sweet Bitch Possession

Please, let us not forget the sweet Bitch who manipulates you through apparent kindness. She's the one who will hug and embrace you, appear to be supportive of you, and utter gentle tones toward you as she moves with an easy glide. After being with her you'll probably feel ecstatic about an exchange, a project, or a promise. And then about a block later, a day later, a borough or a city away, a month or year later, you'll realize that you've been had. That something was stolen that you once had, and you have suddenly and drastically been made aware that the Bitch took your mind, your confidence, your money, your time, your gift, or your secret with a smile and left you bloody and wounded. The Bitch may be skillfully subtle at times and at others overtly ruthless, cutthroat, and deadly.

All the various types of Bitches are the strongest and their toxic symptoms most venomous during the full-moon period and during the time of their menses. Evilness rules within them especially during this period.

Some confuse Sekhmet, the fierce lion-headed Khamite female Spiritual Guardian, with the Bitch. But Sekhmet fights to destroy evil. She is not a Bitch. Sekhmet is a healer who won't take anything off anybody, be it a person, a warped society, or an institution. Sekhmet is motivated by Maat, or justice, whereas the Bitch feeds off a consistent diet of greed, lust, fear, anguish, selfishness, control, envy, bitterness, confusion, and deception.

The Bitch was greatly cultivated during slavery. She is a by-product of the mass rape of one people by another. She, the black woman, was the bed warmer, the property of the European slave owner. At the same time she was the servant of the European woman, herself notorious for using Bitch tactics when striving to control a black woman as a prisoner of slavery. This once-beautiful, highly spiritual Afrakan Priestess, Elder, Mother, Queen, Princess, and Herbalist, was brought to these shores violently. Then, through whips and chains, she was forced to submit to continuous rapes from the slave owners, from her man, or from any field hand by the slaveholder's command, resulting in impregnations for human profit. So like a cow in a herd, she brought forth as many babies as she was able for the profit of the wicked plantation system of slavery.

The head of a slave woman's captive family was the slave master. He had the upper hand. He was law. He, like welfare, was the provider of her room and board—a shack to live in, slop to eat, and rags for clothes for herself and her babies. The stolen woman's man or spiritual husband could be lynched, sold away, or forced to impregnate other women to provide more potential laborers. Plantation life had to grow, and this economic strengthening was created by the number of heads (slaves) put to work.

Forget about family ties. A little girl growing up without a daddy was our norm on these shores, and it created the postslavery conditioning that led to dysfunctional families and female heads of families. Those fatherless little girls grew up to be angry women who became possessed by the Bitch. (Now, ain't that a bitch?)

A Bitch attitude often comes out of an incest experience, yet another leftover from plantation life to make more slaves on a mass level, by any means. The criminal slave owners would force impregnation not just from a man and woman of age and from different families, but by any means available—mother and son, or father and daughter, or uncle and niece. So today incest runs rampant in our race. The disease spread and survived through the generations.

Black women are on the defensive from centuries of continuous crimes committed on their wombs, and so they have been left with dysfunctional lives—a perfect breeding ground for the Bitch. How can she help but be angry and evil and mad? The venom has passed down from one generation to the next through the eating of flesh, of pork, beef, chicken, and from sugar, drugs, and alcohol. All of this ensures ongoing Bitchiness.

Most of us womenfolk are fighting for our lives. The endless battle destroys some of us. But some women build out of misery. Some become freedom fighters. Some become cultural activists. Others become healers. Yet all of these women are postslavery prisoners of a hideous crime perpetrated by one group on another. This terrible legacy causes a number of overt reactions, and innumerable suppressed reactions.

Some women have become docile and debilitated. Some have become modern-day house Negroes, obedient prisoners. Some have demonstrated a lack of self-love so powerful that their self-hate ends up mutilating their Afrakan beauty. They bleach their dark skin to a lighter, so-called whiter tone. Others commit to surgically trimming down the broadness of their noses, surgically decreasing the size of their lips, or placing lenses of blue, green, or hazel over their beautiful brown eyes.

After the smoke cleared from the 1960s, when we all got a surge of Black Pride and natural hair, we then started getting equal opportunity and corporate jobs. This led most black women to revert right back to our slave training. We started relaxing our hair again—"Cause, girl, if you want the look, you better straighten out those kinks." Other women took on some of the other debilitating characteristics of postslavery conditioning and turned their unresolved anger, rage, bitterness, and hate in on themselves. These are the women who act out the Bitch. This residue of pain has been passed down from mother to daughter, causing generational spiritual genocide. We black women have been left wounded, with attitudes that won't quit.

These same attitudes result in systematic injustices being done to Afrakan people. It just never stops. Drugs were poured into our communities, keeping us weak. So we're angry. The AIDS virus was injected into the veins of our community, rendering the black women among the highest percentage of AIDS carriers in the world.

So black women are outraged. We receive the greatest number of hysterectomies of all women in the United States. Over 50 percent of black women in this country are single parents, because so many of our men keep walking, leaving their children behind to be raised by the mother. Our sons are filling up the jails. Our men are forsaking us for women from other races.

This is what we need to say: "Black men, don't leave us. Help us to repair ourselves. But at the same time don't be no toxic man and lie and cheat, because it's bound to make us real mad and have us act outside of ourselves."

It even appears that there aren't enough men to go around for all my sisters in need of a good man. So we claw at one another for just a taste of the chocolate, fighting for his time, his love, his arms, the security of having a man. And this really makes us Bitchy toward one another. We know things are getting really bad when we hear this out of our daughters' mouths. Queen B (meaning Bitch) rules in the Hip-Hop Nation. That's a hard-core reflection of how low we've sunk, when our girl children call themselves Bitches, or when our men say with pride, "That's my Bitch."

The Bitch gains massive support in the media, which only promotes the demise of Afrakan women, and of all women. Soap operas are based on the principle of the Bitch. Hollywood glorifies and presents a high profile of the Bitch. Only a sick society promotes and makes profit off women's pain and ignorance. A society is only as high as the status of its women, and if the women are degraded and doomed, so are the men.

Since we're sisters from the same family, let me help you come out of your lower state, this critical deformity, before we completely self-destruct and explode.

### Fourteen Steps for Purging the Bitch and Returning to the Lotus Clan of Sacred Womanhood

These fourteen steps will help you break the Bitch cycle to free yourself and to prevent the ways of the Bitch from being passed down to your daughters. Follow these fourteen steps closely for at least one season, but it's best to adhere to them through four full seasons to purge yourself of the Bitch. If you have a tendency to be dominating, harsh, judgmental, and sharp-tongued, with much attitude, acting as an occasional or a full-blown/full-time Bitch, this anti-Bitch lifestyle regimen will help you make a turn for the better and transform yourself into a Lotus of Nefer Atum.

1. Confess out loud or to another sister/brother or just yourself that you have been behaving like a Bitch, and that you are willing to release the Bitch in you.
2. Fast on green vegetable juice, fresh fruit juices, water, herbal blood purifiers, and herbal extract calmatives, such as valerian root, kava kava root, hops, or passiflora, during your menses and around the time of every

full moon. Take 10 to 20 drops in a small glass of water. It is at these times in particular that the Bitch can act up the most and cause absolute havoc.

3. To maintain Bitch blood, you have to eat a great deal of meat. The blood and flesh of an animal feeds the Bitch. Other foods that strengthen Bitch possession are sugar, fast foods, junk foods, and fried foods. For a healing change, take on a natural vegetarian lifestyle. As a protein source, consume beans, peas, soy meats (TVP), and raw soaked nuts and seeds. Limit your starch intake to small amounts of whole grains. Consume large amounts of fresh raw or lightly steamed vegetables. Be sure to drink 12 to 16 oz. of green vegetable juice daily, which will help you maintain a state of balance and harmony.

4. Drink a tonic daily of 2 cloves of mashed garlic with the juice of 1 lemon in 8 to 12 oz. of water. Also drink at least a quart of purified water daily.

5. Please stop wearing all that black, gray, dark blue, and especially red until you are well. Wear white and pastel colors to lighten up your spirit and to help you open to your higher spiritual Gateways (chakras or *aritu*).

6. Clean up your Karma/*Shai*. Make a list of all those to whom you've been Bitchy, and as you cleanse, write them or call them in person, one by one. Reach out and ask for forgiveness; offer them a supportive act to balance out your wrongdoing, and/or help someone else who is in need.

7. Say thank you more often for any large or small good deed done on your behalf.

8. Practice smiling from your heart regularly as you send out healings from your heart center.

9. Over seven consecutive days take seven baths with 2 lbs. of sea salt each time to draw the demon out. Take a white candle into your Hydrotherapy Chamber and meditate on its flame to clear your spiritual body. Or use a green candle to heal your heart center from the pain and conditions that created the Bitch qualities.

10. Practice the Maat Feather Meditation (pages 312–313) for forgiveness and to lighten up your heart.

11. Cleanse your colon of old toxic waste with three enemas a week over a twelve-week period.

12. Travel through and begin to incorporate the wisdom of the various Gateways of the Sacred Woman into your life.

13. Go on a talk fast for one to eight hours a day. Anoint yourself with frankincense and myrrh or eucalyptus oil before you begin your talk fast each day. Also before you begin, place the Maat feather by your lips so that your words and attitude will lighten up. This way you will begin to train your mouth to speak from a place of Maat.

14. Accept and affirm your sacred calling, which will return you to your original state. Allow your higher self to emerge and rescue you from the Bitch state. Allow the beautiful lotus in you to open and blossom in the sun!

We womenfolk can overcome the Bitch attitude, break the Bitch cycle, and come out of our possession as we make a conscious effort to put down the Bitch sword and pick up the Maat feather of truth and right, balance and purity. As we embrace our ancient Afrakan spiritual aspects of Divinity, which meet us at every Gateway of *Sacred Woman*, we will progressively rise out of the Bitch state. The Creatress didn't make any of her daughters to be Bitches. We are born out of the likeness and image of our Creatress into a divine being—a beautiful reflection of spirit.

## If You Have Been Attacked by a Woman Possessed by the Bitch

If you are a Lotus, Chamomile, or Aloe Woman and you have been attacked by a woman possessed by the Bitch, then you too must raise your vibration by following the fourteen steps as well, so that you will attract higher relationships from your sisters.

Keep in mind that the Bitch may even be the reflection of yourself, of your weakness. Or maybe she's been sent to bring out your assertiveness, your strength. Even a woman acting like a Bitch can teach you some valuable lessons.

If you are a Lotus Woman who has been at-

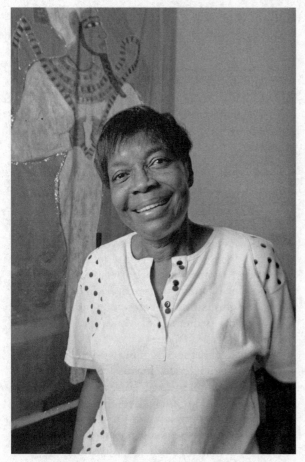

The Transformed Lotus Woman

## Journal Work: Sister-to-Sister Dialogue I— You're My Sister and I Forgive You

One of the best ways to promote sister-to-sister healing is to do a journal dialogue between your sister-friend and yourself. You might start by asking if she is willing to speak with you from her Highest Self.

Then write about how you feel about your relationship. Try not to be accusing, shaming, or blaming; remember there are no victims here, just relationships in need of purification. Write honestly about how the challenges in your relationship make you feel. Then let her speak, and keep going from there. You may be quite surprised about what happens between you by the end of your dialogue.

Your relationship with your sister-friend may not change as a result of this dialogue, because consciously she's unaware of it. The transformation will come through you. The healing will come through your new insights and understanding about your friend and your relationship—your behavior toward her will change. And in time, because all things change when we do, your friend's behavior will slowly begin to change toward you—for the better.

**Sister I** (the abused but forgiving and evolved sister): "Your words hurt. Why must you be so harsh and judgmental?"

**Sister II** (the sister filled with fear and anger, but seeking to cleanse her soul by pleading forgiveness): "I was just trying to protect you and keep you from hurting yourself again. I'm sorry. Maybe I could have done it another way, maybe taken a gentler approach."

**Sister I:** "It's all right. I forgive you, for you're my sister."

**Sister II:** "I always admired you and put you up on a pedestal. Then jealousy stepped in and I took a wrong turn. Please, won't you forgive me?"

**Sister I:** "It's all right. I forgive you, for you're my sister."

tacked by the Bitch, don't run. Have no fear. Turn on the flashlight. Let her know that you know what she's doing, and present her with the alternative of walking in righteousness so that both of you can be winners. Create a sister-to-sister support group, or a womb-healing circle. Purify and fast together.

In reality, no one wants to be a Bitch. The one acting out in her unnatural state is actually suffering from unbearable mental, emotional, and spiritual pain. She's calling out for help. Won't you give a sister your hand? For as the two seemingly opposed women come together and strive to be sisters, the highest degree of healing can be exchanged.

Let's just stop calling ourselves Bitches. Instead, let's start calling ourselves hurt women, wounded women, women in need of healing.

**Sister II:** "You got all of Mama's attention, I just hated you for it."

**Sister I:** "But you were the one who was always so together, my sister. I was always so undone, and Mama just knew. So it only seemed that she cared more for me than you."

**Sister II:** "Forgive me for my bad attitude, for in truth I always loved you. Through the years you always watched over me. Sister! Could you help me to be a better sister-friend and not bring harm to you, and me, by my words, thoughts, and deeds?"

**Sister I:** "Of course, my sister. I'll always be there for you, 'cause Mama wouldn't have it any other way. After all, we are sisters, born from the same womb."

### Journal Work: Sister-to-Sister Dialogue II—Sister, Don't Fret, 'Cause You Got It, Too

Sometimes sisters are envious of one another, and that toxic state makes us out of sorts. But when each of us reflects deeply enough into our own golden treasure chest, we will see that each sister-woman has been well endowed with blessings that fit her life path, her destiny. So sisters, don't you fret, 'cause you got it that way, too.

Vanessa is all depressed about what she thinks she does not have in life. To compound things, she feels her sister-girlfriend Ruby is blessed to a greater degree than herself. So she writes a dialogue with Ruby in her Sacred Womb Journal to get all those feelings up and out.

**Vanessa:** "Sister-girlfriend Ruby, you're more beautiful than me."

**Ruby:** "According to whose image of beauty?"

**Vanessa:** "You were educated better than me."

**Ruby:** "But, Vanessa, you're the one with street smarts and survival skills."

**Vanessa:** "You have more material goods than I."

**Ruby:** "But, sister, you're the one who's truly rich, 'cause you're always spirit-filled."

**Vanessa:** "You've always had a good man."

**Ruby:** "But, sister, you were always the one more contented with self. Vanessa, don't concern yourself with the way I've been blessed, 'cause if you reflect, you'll see you got it that way, too, all in your own way."

## THE MAAT FEATHER MEDITATION: BALANCING THE HEART

Maat is the cosmic order that permeates all creation. It represents truth, righteousness, balance, order, law, reciprocity, propriety, and sobriety. The ancient Khamites based spirituality, government, relationships, professions—their entire lives—on the principles of Maat, represented by the feather.

The heart in the Khamitic system is seen as the seat of intelligence. It was weighed with the feather of Maat on the scale, one against the other, as shown in the judgment scenes on the walls of many Egyptian temples.

The Khamites believed that if your heart became burdened through life's lessons, then the scale would be out of balance, opening the way to illness and plague. But if your heart maintained balance with the feather on the scale, then you would be in harmony with life, for your heart would be equal to the lightness of NTR, the One Most High. Then you would be free of disease in body, mind, and spirit. Our Ancestors believed that the heart is the Gateway to our higher self. They recommended that we check our hearts daily to be sure that we maintain this high spiritual state of Maat consciousness, for it is through Maat that we will experience heaven on earth. It is through Maat that every yoke that oppresses will be broken.

Place in your left hand a clear quartz crystal and visualize the white light. In your right hand hold the feather of Maat. Now begin.

If your heart is heavy due to accumulations of life's challenges, it will create depression, cancer, heart attacks, strokes, premature death, or a life full of anxiety, stress, and pressure. To keep the heart center clear and clean and filled with beauty, light, and vitality, neither an individual nor a community may continue to harbor past painful experiences. You must accept that every lesson is a blessing, and that every experience you receive has given you deeper insight.

In order to keep the heart as light as a feather and in a balanced state, we must remain in an active state of meditation so that Spirit may continue to reveal to us the divine plan of all circumstances. A light heart is reflected in one's peaceful state of body, mind, and spirit. Those who are in a state of Maat experience contentment, compassion, wisdom, and the constant inner freedom to manifest their life's purpose. Once in this divine state, one tends not to waver, regardless of the mood swings of other people or conditions. A Maat person is spiritually empowered with the ancient Afrakan spirit of Truth, Justice, Righteousness, and Absolute Harmony.

- Sit quietly for a few moments and connect to your heart center.
- Breathe into the heart and out again, very slowly and quietly. Do this seven times, for seven is the number for the Spirit. Every time you inhale, see the image of your heart as light as the feather.
- With each exhalation, release from the heart center, in degrees or all at once, emotions of anger, depression, disappointment.
- With each inhalation, breathe into the heart peace, joy, compassion, balance, and serenity.

This Maat meditation should become part of you all of the days of your life so that you will be disease-free. When the heart center—the Het-Hru center of Divine Love—is light and in balance, then you can experience Hru the Falcon, the Christ consciousness, the inner freedom that takes flight above the denser spirit of Seth—pain, challenge, disharmony.

### Maat Affirmation

*I live on Maat. I satisfy myself with the righteousness of my heart. On the walls of the pyramids the heart and the feather were weighed against each other to indicate that the heart must never become heavy. It must always be in balance, be as light as the feather. According to how I live, my heart will be weighed and judged daily. Whatever I carry in my heart will be revealed in my life. So I will guard my heart (my life) with much love and care and no burdens will weigh upon it.*

# SACRED RELATIONSHIP: SEVEN-DAY TRANSFORMATIVE WORK

The most important relationship on earth is your relationship with self. The extent to which you heal yourself is the extent to which you will be able to heal all your relationships.

I'm sure you have already improved—stay on the road, it gets better! Focus not so much on the outer world; as your inner environment is healed, the world around you will improve. Self-communication, love, unity, and compassion for your sacred self aids you in establishing a sacred relationship with all others. This week enjoy all of your relationships!

- *List all your relationships.* Explore the current state of these relationships and what you need to do to bring about Divine Order in each one. Keep praying about and purifying these relationships to understand the lesson that each relationship has brought into your life.
- *Practice forgiveness of self and others* as you do your daily altar work, so that you spiritually cleanse your heart and all your conditions.
- *Process old hurts from unhealed relationships,* by placing photographs of those who need forgiveness on your altar and chanting, "Love holds no grievances. What's past is past."
- *Perform seven-day prayer work for Sacred Relationships.* Place a photo of your mother and father on your altar in a beautiful frame. Write a love letter to your parents, expressing all the gratitude that you have for the relationship that birthed you.

  Even if right now you don't feel the emotions expressed by the words, writing this letter will begin to heal your heart, for once you come to grips with the foundational relationship in your life—that with your parents—then all other relationships will prosper and give you *hotep.*

- *Consciously release old relationship patterns through purification rites, journal work, prayer work, and affirmations.* Don't be erratic and jump into new relationships without ridding yourself of old toxic habits that drew in your previous toxic unions.
- *Within the next seven days, write a thank-you letter to all those in your life with whom you are or have been in Sacred Relationships.* Thank each individual for the special riches they bring to your life and place these letters on your altar. Infuse them with more love and gratitude each day, and when you complete this Gateway, put these love offerings in the mail. If the person has died or has vanished out of your life, then burn the letter with a little sage to begin to release the vibratory pain of your past.
- *Send love, light, and forgiveness to those you're sending letters to, or who are on your relationship list* during your morning meditation and prayers.
- *Ast is about nurturing the self—yourself—first.* Self-worth/self-love must be in place within you in order to establish any Divine Relationship. It's not about your relationship with him or her; it's about your relationship with self! Once you tend to this relationship, then all others will reflect your personal wellness and wholeness. As you do your journal work, ask yourself what it would take to establish a healthy relationship with self.

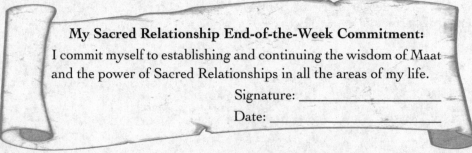

**My Sacred Relationship End-of-the-Week Commitment:**

I commit myself to establishing and continuing the wisdom of Maat and the power of Sacred Relationships in all the areas of my life.

Signature: _____

Date: _____

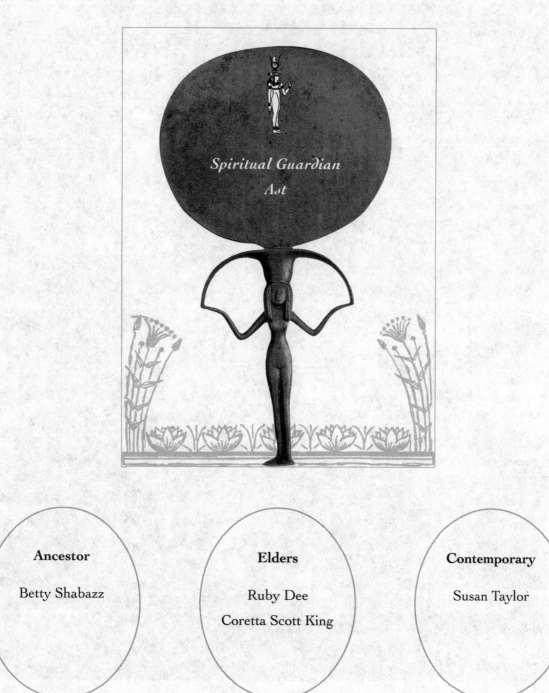

## CHAPTER 13

# GATEWAY 8: SACRED UNION

*Spiritual Guardian*

*Ast*

**Ancestor**

Betty Shabazz

**Elders**

Ruby Dee

Coretta Scott King

**Contemporary**

Susan Taylor

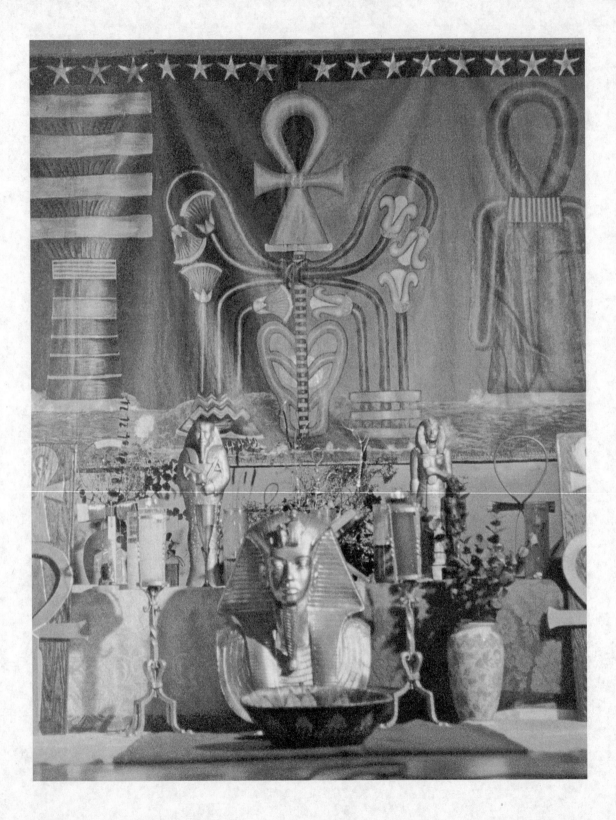

# SACRED UNION ALTAR WORK
## Face Your Heart to the East—to the Rising Sun
### (Layout from top view)

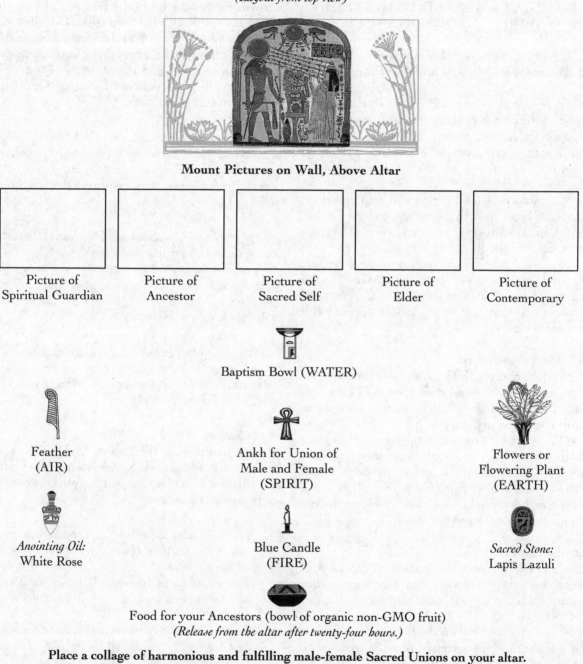

**Mount Pictures on Wall, Above Altar**

Picture of
Spiritual Guardian

Picture of
Ancestor

Picture of
Sacred Self

Picture of
Elder

Picture of
Contemporary

Baptism Bowl (WATER)

Feather
(AIR)

Ankh for Union of
Male and Female
(SPIRIT)

Flowers or
Flowering Plant
(EARTH)

*Anointing Oil:*
White Rose

Blue Candle
(FIRE)

*Sacred Stone:*
Lapis Lazuli

Food for your Ancestors (bowl of organic non-GMO fruit)
*(Release from the altar after twenty-four hours.)*

**Place a collage of harmonious and fulfilling male-female Sacred Unions on your altar.**

Sacred tablecloth (blue) and scarf to wear during prayer.
Sacred color cloth to lay before altar. Sacred instruments to be played as you pray.

## GATEWAY 8: SACRED UNION DAILY SPIRITUAL OBSERVANCES

### Gateway Elements:
### Water/Moon/Female and Fire/Sun/Male

Sacred Union eliminates toxic, dysfunctional relationships that destroy life, and creates and supports cleansed, honest, and harmonious relationships that energize one's life. Fulfilling, healthy relationships are the result of establishing Sacred Union.

Gateway 8: Sacred Union will help you eliminate all blockages that prevent Sacred Union: heart conditions, drug and/or alcohol abuse, ulcers, fear, anger.

Spiritual exercises of ascension are to be performed daily for seven days, the number for the spirit. This will awaken your inner Gateways of Divinity so that you may blossom to your full sacred center.

### 1. The Spiritual Bath
Use white rose oil. White rose oil is for the crystal/crown—for the divine oneness of NTR inspiration and wisdom. It eliminates separation, confusion, and depression.

Place 4 to 6 drops of white rose oil in your bathwater. This helps to promote emotional balance and relieve stress, anxiety, worry, impatience, and shock. Sprinkle a few drops on a tissue or handkerchief and place by your pillow to inhale while sleeping.

### 2. Your Altar
Set up your sacred altar on the first day of your entry into this Gateway. You may set up your altar according to your own spiritual or religious beliefs (see page 18). Sit before your altar quietly and meditatively on the floor on a pillow, or in a chair. Add a few drops of white rose oil to your baptism bowl on your altar, and sprinkle a few drops around your prayer space.

*Anoint with white rose oil.* Select only pure essential oils. Use white rose oil to anoint your crown, forehead (the Body Temple Gateway of supreme spirituality), heart (the Body Temple Gateway of compassion and divine love), womb area, palms to make everything you touch become more sacred, and the bottoms of your feet to spiritually align yourself for stepping out in power, promise, and faith.

### 3. Opening the Gateway
To invoke each Gateway's Spiritual Guardian, you may use whatever words pour from your heart. For example, here's a prayer that might be used at Gateway 8:

*Sacred and Divine Ast, Spiritual Guardian of the Gateway of Sacred Union, please accept my deepest gratitude for your healing presence on my altar and in my life. Thank you for your guidance and inspiration, and for your love and blessings, and please accept my love and blessings in return.* Hetepu.

As you offer your prayer, simultaneously shake, ring, beat, or rattle a sacred instrument (sistrum bell, drum, shekere, or bells) to awaken the NTR that is indwelling.

### 4. Libation
Pour a libation for the Sacred Union Gateway from a cup, or sprinkle water from a bowl onto the earth or on a plant, as you call out this prayer of praise and adoration.

— *Pour a libation* as you say, *All praise and adoration to the Spiritual Guardian, Ast, the Protector of Sacred Union.*
— *Pour a libation* as you say, *All praise and adoration to the Ancestor of Sacred Union, Betty Shabazz.*
— *Pour a libation* as you say, *All praise and adoration to the Elders of Sacred Union, Ruby Dee and Coretta Scott King.*
— *Pour a libation* as you say, *All praise and adoration to my Divine Self and my Contemporary Divine Sister, Susan Taylor.*

### 5. Sacred Woman Spirit Prayer

Ring a bell or play another sacred instrument at the beginning and end of the prayer. As you open your palms to the Sacred Spirit or gently place them over your heart, recite:

**Sacred Woman Spirit Prayer**

*Sacred Woman in the making,*
*Sacred Woman reawaken,*
*Sacred Spirit, hold me near.*
*Protect me from all harm and fear*
*beneath the stones of life.*
*Direct my steps in the right way as I journey*
*through this vision.*
*Sacred Spirit,*
*surround me in your most absolute*
*perfect light.*
*Anoint me in your Sacred purity, peace,*
*and divine insight.*
*Bless me, truly bless me, as I share*
*this Sacred Life.*
*Teach me, Sacred Spirit, to be in tune*
*with the Universe.*
*Teach me how to heal*
*with the inner and outer elements*
*of air, fire, water, and earth.*

### 6. Sacred Union Prayer

Shake bells, beat a sacred drum, or play another instrument at the beginning and ending of this prayer.

*Divine Creator/Creatress, I stand in need of Sacred Union. I pray for a Sacred Union with my self, with you, Creator/Creatress, and with my mate. Divine Creator/Creatress, help me to attract and establish harmonious, healthy relationships, and joyous oneness with my life partner. Help me to identify and release old hurt feelings, resentments, and hostilities that are trapped within my Body Temple. Help me to have the vision, strength, and courage to learn from all my past and present relationships, as they are all reflections of my own consciousness, each and every one.*

*If by chance my intimate relationships do not change, may I remain undaunted and fearless. May I be the one*

*to become the first link of change and transformation in my life, for all healing really begins within me. I affirm that each one of my intimate relationships, past or present, has value and has in some way prepared me to grow into a more conscious Sacred Union with my self. As I reflect on the true purpose of Sacred Union, I give thanks to the divine masculine and feminine in me and the divine masculine and feminine that unite to create Sacred Union—the life force from which all creation flows within us.*

### 7. Chanting Hesi

Chant this *hesi* four times:

*Nuk Pu Ntrt Hmt*—I am a Sacred Woman.

### 8. Fire Breaths

Prepare for your Fire Breathing by slowly inhaling four times and exhaling four times. Then, when you are totally at ease, begin your nine hundred Fire Breaths. Inhale deeply like a pump through your nose (mouth closed) as you expand the breath down into the abdomen, then back up into the chest. Completely exhale out through your nostrils from your abdomen as it contracts and the lungs release your breath completely. Repeat the Fire Breath rapidly in and out, in and out.

Allow each deep Fire Breath to represent the opening of the thousand lotus petals of illumination and radiance, to reach Nefer Atum—the ultimate Afrakan lotus station of Divinity.

### 9. Gateway 8: Sacred Union Meditation

Increase the length of time you spend in meditation every seven days. The longer you remain in meditation, the deeper your inner peace will be, and the more solid your *ba* (spirit) will become. The cleaner your Body Temple, the sooner it will be able to live permanently in the peace and inner balance of the meditative state.

• Hold your sacred stone for Gateway 8 inside your palm. Visualize yourself sitting in the blue-and-white heart of the lotus blossom, unfazed by the adversity of the world, living and breathing in a balanced, beautiful centered breath of ease and grace.

- Breathe into your heart center. With each breath, visualize Mother Ast as she protects, nurtures, and loves you.
- Breathe, purge, and flush out from the heart of the lotus, from the arms of Het-Hru, from the blossom of Ast, your mother, all anguish, all mistrust, hurt, pain, fear, and resentment. Flush these forces out of your heart and allow it to fill with compassion and love.
- Visualize yourself and your mate standing together in a sphere of pure white light, hearts cleared of all pain and grief and anger, feeling a deep upwelling of love and joy and compassion for each other.
- Now, place your palms over your healed heart and say:

*Sacred Mother Ast*
*Bless us*
*And bless our union.*

*Color Visualization.* Visualize the color of the Gateway you are in—blue for inner peace. As you perform your meditation, wear white or blue, and/or place blue cloth on your altar.

*Sacred Stone Meditation.* While in meditation hold a lapis lazuli stone in your palms, over your heart. It is the sacred healing stone of the Gateway and helps to illuminate the mind. The light of this deep royal blue stone stimulates both love and beauty. Lapis lazuli builds a sense of unity in man and woman. This stone is known to have healing, curative, and purifying properties. It unblocks the throat area, allowing free expression, so that the sacred words from On High can come through. This stone represents the sixth *arit,* or energy center, which is between the brows. It is the chakra that activates high spiritual mind.

## 10. Herbal Tonics
Drink lemon balm tea. Parts used: flowers and leaves. Lemon balm soothes the troubled mind

and heart and thus opens a channel for communication and dispels moodiness. Drink your herb tea or tonic for seven days to receive the full benefit of tuning you to Gateway 8. Enjoy your herb tea in your favorite mug during or after spiritual writing.

*Preparation.* One teabag to 1 cup of water. Boil water in a nonmetallic pot, turn off flame, and add tea to steep before or after your morning bath or sacred shower. Strain herbs from water. Drink with joy and peace as you breathe between sips and settle into easy contemplation and reflection.

## 11. Flower Essences
To deepen your experience of Gateway 8, choose from the following flower essences. Take 4 drops four times per day directly on or under the tongue, or add the same amount to a small glass of purified water and sip. For instructions on how to choose flower essences, see page 23.

- *Evening primrose:* Addresses inability to form committed relationships, afflicted relationships due to feelings of abandonment and rejection in childhood.
- *Chamomile:* Calming emotional trauma or hypersensitivity in relationships.
- *Forget-me-not:* Perceiving deeper karmic bonds within relationships; ability to acknowledge spiritual destiny and intent of relationship.
- *Sticky monkeyflower:* Addresses issues of intimacy and sexuality; overcoming fear of intimacy.
- *Snapdragon:* Addresses improper expression of emotions through verbal aggression and hostility.
- *Penstemon:* Strength and perseverance despite difficulties in relationships.

## 12. Diet
Follow Sacred Woman Transitional Dietary Practices presented for Gateways 7 and 8.

## 13. Sacred Union Journal Writing
This is best done after internal cleansing (enema) and/or meditation. When you are cleansed and

centered, you can receive spiritual messages from the One Most High with grace. When you are in the spirit, messages travel down through your spirit mind, to your heart, into your hand, and onto the paper. (This is how I do all my writing.)

The best time to receive your spiritually inspired written work is after you have completed your altar work, between the hours of 4 A.M. and 6 A.M. Keep your journal and a very special pen by or on your altar to work with the power, force, and stillness at the coming of dawn, the hour of Nebt-Het.

Affirm your daily life. Write in your journal at this time thoughts, activities, experiences, and interactions that present themselves. You can also write down your visions, desires, dreams, and affirmations so that you will be able to draw on these resources when help and support are most needed.

*Consult Sesheta.* If you find that you are unable to contact your inner voice during your journal work, call Sesheta, the keeper and revealer of secrets (who is indwelling), to assist and speak through you.

### 14. Senab Freedom Shawl or Quilt

Choose a new piece of cloth that corresponds to the Gateway color (indicated in exercise 9 of your Daily Spiritual Observances or in Sacred Altar Work) to add to your Senab Freedom Shawl or Quilt. This cloth will serve as a mini-canvas to represent your experience in the Gateway you're working in.

Also, collect meaningful symbols that can be added to your shawl or quilt in appliqué or patchwork style. You can add stones, other natural objects, collectibles, family heirlooms, photographs that have been reprinted on fabric, or any other significant items that embody the essence of your experience. Give your imagination free rein and let your craftswoman spirit tell your story. For more information about the Senab Freedom Shawl or Quilt, see pages 122–125.

### 15. Sacred Tools

- A special Sacred Union Ankh to symbolize the union of masculine and feminine to place on your altar.
- Your own special Sacred Union Dialogue Journal for recording, molding, and shaping the desires of your heart or dialoguing with your mate (see Seven-Day Transformative Work).
- Finding or discovering "His Pleasures"— objects or experiences that expand your mate's consciousness because they offer him special satisfaction or joy. Now explore your own pleasures and share them with your mate.

Throughout the week, you are to observe closely the wisdom presented for the Gateway you're in. For maximum results, live freely in tune with the various systems of wellness presented and practice the Seven-Day Transformative Work at the end of the Gateway.

### Closing Sacred Words

*Mother/Father, help me to heal all disunity within myself. Help me to heal all discord in my intimate unions past and present and to transform them into Sacred Unions.*

# SACRED UNIONS

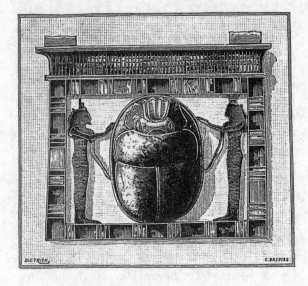

## With the Creator/Creatress

The union of the Creator/Creatress and ourselves is the most critical union, for all that we are begins with the Great One. In order to be inside the Creator/Creatress, to be fully aware of the presence of the Creator/Creatress within us, and to be guided by the Most High, we must first love ourselves as the Creator/Creatress loves us. When we truly love ourselves, we become one with the Divine. It is then that the Creator/Creatress can enter our house, and all of our unions will be blessed.

## With Self

We all have at least three or more active aspects or personalities within ourselves. Each of these personalities develops in divine time to aid our growth and development. To be effective, these various parts of ourselves must come into harmonious union and work together in concert for the greater good. For example, one self protects us, another self inspires us, a third is brilliant, and yet another is sensual. The male and the female parts of us must come together with love. These complementary aspects must unite into one team—one entity with the strength necessary to ultimately give us all that we need as we journey through life. Meditation and fasting will help us learn to honor our own Sacred Union within.

## With Our Mate

Once the two forces of male and female come together in complete harmony, heaven and earth become one. The wellness of the earth is determined by the union of these two opposite forces. When earthquakes, tidal waves, and hurricanes manifest, it is a direct result of lack of harmony between the masculine and feminine energies on the planet.

We must be committed to the Creator/Creatress and our planet, and begin the process of healing ourselves. We must develop harmony first within ourselves, balancing our own inner masculine and feminine forces. We must strive to become sacred, divine mates to our selves and others, learning to live in perfect union.

## The Union of Two Becoming One

Man is not the head of the house, nor is the woman the head of the house. It is the one with the knowledge, wisdom, and understanding in a particular matter that guides or leads the union to the shores of Maat (balance). In this way we use the wisdom of the union of two becoming one, representing the One Most High Creator/Creatress in a wise way.

Intimate relationships or divine unions are the arms and legs of the womb, the extensions of a woman's "inner space."

In order for a woman's womb to be at peace, she needs to be at peace in all of her intimate relationships—her relationships with all things that she consumes at a physical or energetic level and that become a part of her. Whether the intimate exchange is breathing air into her body or putting food into her mouth, all of a woman's intimate relationships are rooted in her relationship with her self.

So reflect on your unions in your own way and allow each to become your teacher. Empty yourself of resentment and become receptive to the lessons that your intimate relationships bring. Surrender to the wisdom that each and every union offers to your spirit so that you will not hold on to pain. Undigested or unprocessed pain held in the womb grows into tumors.

Intimate relationships have the potential to provide pain or joy. Unfortunately, there can be many sources of pain. Perhaps the most tragic is the hurt and disappointment caused by a negative or unbalanced masculine energy in our lives, that of a father, brother, uncle, mate, lover, or friend—someone known and trusted. Violation—physical, energetic, or emotional—from a person you thought you could trust to love and respect you creates deep hurt and resentment that requires committed healing work.

Too often we flee to a new relationship in an effort to soothe our wounds before we have begun to recognize them, much less heal them. This is an unfair burden to carry to your new mate and lover and puts undue stress on a new relationship. Pain must be released or it will solidify into permanent blockages on the spiritual, emotional, and physical levels.

## NO MORE LOVERS, IF YOU PLEASE

*There's a whole lot of women*
*who are hooked on a bad man*
*with a good orgasm.*

A Sacred Woman must have a committed lover within her mate, husband, or husband-to-be. For the salvation of her soul, she must strive to avoid men who are merely "hit-and-run" lovers who will violate her womb spirit and leave her high and dry. She cannot afford to be involved with someone who does not intend to go deeply, to make a commitment. She does not need a lover who is oh-so-sweet for a moment, only to have those moments turn into hours, days, even years of feeling insecure, resentful, angry, depressed, lonely, empty, and abused.

An uncommitted relationship can create these feelings in a woman, and even in a man. A woman who permits and encourages a man to deal with her predominantly on a sexual basis is setting herself up for emotional and spiritual danger. She can find herself on a collision course with pain. She can become needy, desperate, or hostile. For absolute healthy love to flow and be a healing experience, there must be commitment.

For a woman to really open up, she must be absolutely at peace with her soul, for when she trusts her man enough, she will not hold back on her love. A woman's love is like a deep vault. When she is confident in her man's love, and if love comes from the heights, she will not merely open up her thighs for sex; she will open her sacred vault to reveal the treasures of her Sacred Womanhood. In a committed union there will be many blissful gateways of ecstasy, joy, and peace. Yes, peace. When a woman truly experiences a loving union with a man, she will have no need to hold back for fear of being hurt. She will bless the union with her full self. For a woman to be at one with her mate she needs to know that her man is going to be there for her without excuses, without stories, without lies.

Women, you must first see and establish your worth, your value, your richness, your beauty, your power within yourself in order for the man to have a passion to commit to you, body, mind, and spirit. You tell me, "Oh, but he looks so good!" And to this I reply, "No more lovers, if you please!" For those of you who are not striving to go beyond, for those of you who do not intend to find and to become a divine mate, I can only say, sister, beware, for the lover you share your bed with is no different from the food you put into your mouth.

With the man presently in your life, or soon to be, strive not to have a hamburger-on-white-bread lover, or a frozen-food marriage. Keep your Body Temple clean and pure, so you will attract a sea-moss-and-sprouts man, a watercress-and-dandelion mate, a wheatgrass-and-mustard-greens-and-kale husband who is just like you, strong and pure. Watch your food intake and your thoughts, attitudes, and feelings, for what you embrace externally reflects your inner environment. So, women, take responsibility to model the level of union you seek. And by all means, while in waiting, stay away from any foods or herbs that stimulate the libido.

Be patient and cleanse, and your king will come. He will be compelled to drop rose petals at your feet, anoint and kiss them, for he feels so complete. He knows that to be in the presence of his divine mate, you, is a gift from the Most High, and that he has been waiting for you all his life. He too has longed for a divine union, and now you can both grow together in absolute Divinity. Purify, women, and rise into your sacredness, for there is no need to settle for less. Purify, rise up, and attract the best.

Queens, Sacred Women, sisters, when you have an itch, don't scratch it by finding just any man to go to bed with. The soul of a woman cries out every time she gets screwed as opposed to loved. His job, beautiful car, and being "fine" are not enough for you to give him even just a little. It won't do. Be patient and trust, for the right man for you is on the way. Keep the faith and look ahead. Stay in tune, remember your divine self. Place your consciousness within the Royal Court of Maat, the place of righteousness. Transfer your sexual energy to creative activity—take dance classes, learn to play an instrument, take voice lessons, write poetry, fast, and pray. Prepare yourself for your divine mate.

For the continuation of a race, the salvation of our people, and the enrichment of our nation, we women must stop having lovers who have no intention of being husbands. We must love ourselves, respect our wombs, and protect our souls from all harm, danger, or sickness, so that we will finally experience wholeness as women who are loved properly and sweetly. Reflect on our Ancestors. Watch the Elders, and witness how they made love work. Learn the lessons of Sacred Union. Observe the patience, the commitment, and the quality of the wise ones' love. Allow their vision to mold you, to support you as you embrace higher degrees of love, in tune with your inner self.

Keep echoing the following affirmation when you think you are getting weak, because you deserve so much more. Close your eyes, go within, and decree:

*No more lovers, if you please.*
*No more lovers, if you please.*
*I am preparing for Sacred Union*
*and I will accept nothing less.*

## A WARNING FROM THE WOMB

A sister called me from Atlanta, Georgia. Weeping on the phone, she said, "I just finished having my eleventh abortion!" I was silent for a moment as I caught my breath. Then we began to talk back and forth as she quietly processed her profound pain over the phone. "All my pregnancies were from the same man," she went on.

Do you think this sister was loving herself, or that she knew how to love and care for her overburdened womb? Do you think for a moment her "lover," her "boyfriend," was loving her or even knew how to love himself?

This sister needed to reestablish and evaluate the divine value of self, and of the many lives who were created through her womb and who were returned back to the Divine Source of All Things. This beloved sister was in bondage to low self-esteem. She needed desperately to take a long fast from intimate relationships and to lift up, love, purify, and heal as she opened herself to an intimate, caring union with her divine self.

Sisters in stress, stand back and witness who has deposited what in your sacred womb, your life. Chant: "No more lovers, if you please."

This is a loving but serious warning for those sisters who want to stop the pain and dry the tears of regret. Be celibate and wait for your true King Man, for a serious love candidate, so you don't find yourself in an abortion clinic in a strange state or, if you decide to bear an unwanted baby, find yourself alone raising sons and daughters without fathers, and so playing out the hard role of a single parent.

Please wake up before it's too late, for you, as a woman of light, can put a stop to this madness immediately. Stand up for your true sacred identity. To attract a divine high relationship and have a life of peace and serenity, you must begin by taking all the time required to deeply love and heal yourself before taking on any mate.

I say to my sisters who may be addicted to a man or men in general and take all kinds of physical, emotional, and spiritual abuse: Stop desperately looking for love outside yourself, for you are in need of help and detoxification. Commit yourself to the many self-healing principles of the Sacred Woman. Seek and connect to highly charged positive Elders as spiritual mentors for at least 365 days or more. Learn the lessons of self-love. Then, with grace from the Divine Creator/Creatress, you will be in a more centered, loving place, which will make it possible for you to bring a sacred male reflection into your space. When the time comes for the union of the two, the Creator/Creatress will speak through you, by way of a dream, or a vision, or simply through your sister-friend, or your Elder.

Don't make the mistake of getting yourself into yet another fix because you're feeling hot and need a little sex to tide you over. Slow down, cool off; drink cucumber and parsley juice. To receive complete love healing and attract a good man, don't rush into anything until you have been seriously renewed.

If you, Sacred Woman in the making, find yourself in a situation such as I have shared, know that you are not alone, that many women before you have shared similar life challenges. So, divine sister Queen, I humbly offer you this advice to help you liberate yourself from the drama.

### A Period of Celibacy:
### A Time to Return to Self

Be at peace; don't panic. A period of celibacy can be a wonderful time in your life. It can rejuvenate you when you have exhausted all of your mental, emotional, and spiritual energy reserves. For example, when you keep trying to start a relationship with a mate but it just never seems to work out, maybe it's time to consciously pull in your energy and recharge your battery mentally, physically, and spiritually by giving yourself a rest from sex.

When you become sexually active again, you will be making love with a man who is not just a random date, but someone who is to be your husband, your sacred mate. As you follow the Sacred Woman lifestyle, this will happen for and to you without fail. You will not have to settle for just any man. Your soul mate is being prepared for you as we speak. Go do your work so you can receive what you seek.

This time go about things a little differently. Have someone speak on your behalf. If a man that you might be receptive to is interested in you and you in him, then have your mentor, or

an Elder of your family, and one or two members of his family sit down together with the prospective brother and have a meeting of intentions. You will speak through your mentor, and he will speak through his. Anywhere between two to four people other than yourselves can be present to witness this meeting.

After this talking and observation, if the Elders see that this could be a good coming together, then gifts should be offered from the brother to the sister. This should happen before he even begins to date this Sacred Woman. The intention of dating is for a period of observation before a possible marriage can be considered.

Sacred Women are royal women, so your life must be handled in a sacred and divine way. The man that seeks you out and captures your heart must treat you as the very special woman that you are, since you, Sacred Woman, have taken the time to beautify, harmonize, and heal yourself to uplift your vibration to a high degree. Before you reach this place, you have to take the time to return to self, so it is your right and your destiny to be granted a proper mate.

### My Self-Love Letter

This love letter will strengthen, reinforce, and remind you of the love that you have for yourself. By reading your love letter daily, weekly, or monthly, according to your need, you will strengthen and reinforce the love you have for you. As your love grows and you are the recipient of the gift of love, you may be inspired to write other love letters. Just go with the flow.

Dear Spirit Most High, Whatever happened to me in my life up to now—it's okay.

I know that you can turn what now seems bad into good. Show me that what happened was a lesson, and that I don't need to love myself any less for it.

On this day I am writing a love letter to myself and I will observe the boundless blessings that this presents to me.

Date: _____

Beloved: _____

(your name)

## Journal Dialogue: "In Him I Saw Me"

Dear Journal:

I'm so unhappy . . . I'm content . . . I'm so confused . . . My mind is clear. I'm unfulfilled . . . I have what I need. Back and forth, up and down, my mood swings like a pendulum . . . I meet me wherever I go. I went to my lover and what did I see? In him I saw me. What a sight. I'm hurting. Oh, no, I feel good.

In him I saw me, so I abused him . . . but I love him, or so I thought. In him I saw me. I was bored . . . tired . . . uninterested . . . lonely . . . I thought he loved me . . . only . . .

In him I saw me. I scratched out his eyes. We fought day and night in word . . . and deed.

Out of my confusion, pain, discontent, I call on the Most Mighty Mother-Father-Creator/Creatress who dwells within me. I call for divine healing.

Time passes . . . Seasons change. I am healing. We're cleansing . . . In him I see me . . . I love, adore, and cherish him. I love me . . . at last. I can really be because in him I found me . . . In me I found me . . .

### Heart Release Visualization

The following Heart Visualization is a perfect womb and heart alignment that teaches us how to stay rooted in our sacred seat.

Sitting on the floor, in your seat of power, close your eyes and inhale deeply, just to tune in. Exhale. Now inhale again and breathe into your womb. Come into the womb with a breath. Then bring it to your heart—the womb of your heart and the womb of your mind.

#### Releasing Pain and Hurt

When you exhale, you purge the womb of all adverse thoughts that block you, and the fears lurking in your mind about what happened to your womb in the past. Focus on what's happening to it now.

#### Releasing Hurtful Relationships

Inhale, and release from the mind and heart any hurt feelings, any residue of toxicity from rela-tionships that has settled into your heart center. Release it now. Breathe it out.

Inhale and open up your womb. Exhale and purge all heaviness and toxicity. Now take a deep inhalation all the way from the heart up to the crown of your sacred mind, your sacred seat, and release it down and out. Exhale.

Breathe in deeply, eyes still closed, and just keep breathing, at your own pace. Breathe into your womb as you heal yourself. As you heal your womb, you heal your atmosphere, you heal your relationships with your daughters, with your sons, with your mates, with your mothers, with your Ancestors. We've been car-rying the entire world of our Ancestors with us.

### Breathing in Divine Help

Within us we also carry all the divine Afrakan angels. They manifest through our wombs as we connect to Mother Nut. She will help energize us and release us, for she is the heavenly body of stars that dwells within us.

### Men Are Seeking a Divine Mate, Too, *by Ellis Liddell*

Men are looking for someone to be close to their soul, what many people call a soul mate. It is quite interesting that as children we simply look for companionship and warm, caring friendship. From age sixty-five until we die we look for the same thing. But somehow from twelve to sixty-four we're on this roller coaster we call relation-ships. Why do we go through all this pain and upset? It's because no one teaches us how to be adult women or men. This is something we're forced to learn through trial and error.

As a result of this process, some of us develop better relationship skills than others. We com-municate with one another better. Some people have the ability to get along with anyone, mak-ing everybody feel a sense of value and self-worth, causing a rise in their self-esteem. But more important, such people lift others' sense of spiritual value by acknowledging the God pres-ence in us all.

Men are actually very committal by nature. They are slow to form new friendships or rela-

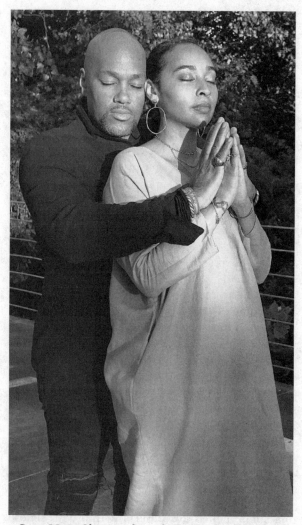

Supa Nova Slom, author of *Man Heal*, and La Lah Delia, author of *Vibrate Higher Daily*. A Sacred couple.

tionships, and as they grow older they will have fewer male friends. They usually replace their male friends with female ones. I also observed this pattern in some of my close women friends. They seem to develop closer female friendships after they have found a mate.

Men are looking for four basic things in a divine mate: affection, friendship, communication, and, most important, a deep spiritual connection.

*Affection:* On the affection side, men want it outwardly and inwardly. They want to know they are loved, and that the love their mate has for them is not a jealous love, or a "you do for me, I do for you" love.

*Friendship:* Men want to be able to talk to their mate about anything and everything, and know that she will be there for them.

*Communication:* Men want verbal and nonverbal communication to a point where both sense each other's need and thoughts—to a point where their thoughts are one.

*Spiritual connection:* Men want a mate with whom they can fast, walk hand in hand, and be able to connect even when there are thousands of people around or when they're a thousand miles apart.

### Het-Hru (Venus) Day Love Ritual: Visualizing Your Mate-to-Be

Do your spiritual love rituals on Friday, which is Venus Day.

- Do a twenty-four-hour fast on fruits and/or fresh fruit juices, and red fruits—cranberry, grapes, plums, blackberries, apples, berries, and cherries—to draw out spiritual sweetness.
- Drink nutmeg or cinnamon tea.
- Wear soft pink and/or white garments or a scarf.
- Wear a rose quartz necklace, earrings, and, of course, your rose quartz waist beads.
- Love bath: In 1 gallon of rainwater or distilled water, blend 12 oz. rose water, 1 bottle Florida water, 1 tsp. cinnamon, and 1 tsp. raw honey. Let sit overnight. Pour it into your bathwater in the early morning.
- Rise to meditate during the holy hours of 4 A.M. to 6 A.M. as you visualize your mate coming into your life. Repeat this affirmation: "Only sweetness comes from my lips on this Holy Day."
- Put a pink cloth and a vase of fresh roses on your altar. Burn jasmine, rose, or cinnamon incense in the morning or evening.

- Create your ideal mate on this day by using active visualization. Have faith in yourself and the power of the Divine Spirit to provide you with the sacred mate you deserve.
- Finally, dedicating this love ritual to yourself will draw love to you on every level of life—from mother to daughter, father to daughter, sister to sister, man to woman, love of work, love of self. If you do the love work, love will permeate everyone and everything around you.

## COURTING, SLOW AND STEADY

It is Afrakan tradition to maintain the sanctity, protection, and support of healthy unions, and to avoid the adverse results of women taking on partners without the full support of the family.

I think we need to reclaim this ancient tradition in our lives today in an appropriate way. My husband tells this story quite often:

"For five years, my father traveled fifty miles from San Pedro de Macoris to La Romana in Santo Domingo to court my mother. And upon his weekly visit my parents-to-be would sit under the observation of ten or more members of her family—Elders, sisters, brothers, all in the living room.

"Then, five years later, my father was given permission to wed this beautiful, sacred princess, Amancia Georges De Guerrero, the woman of his heart. All that time he'd had to prove his love and commitment to his beloved through the test of time and patience. It was intense, but a precedent was set.

"From the time of the courtship to marriage up to his transition from this earth, Father Georges had a deep respect, love, and appreciation for this divine Sacred Woman, his wife."

### The Elders Advise: Check His Background

We sat around the kitchen table drinking herb tonic and fresh juices. An hour later, I served a vegetarian dinner fit for my Elders. "Check his background," said the Elders, speaking from their collective 121 years of wisdom and life experience. They talked to my spiritual sister all night long, giving her advice in a wholesome,

profound way—the advice she needed to hear to avoid those after-the-wedding blues.

Don't be too quick to say "I do," they told her. Check his background, his people, and his people's people before you take him on. Observe him; see what he feels about the women in his life, past and present. Observe his actions with his mother, his sisters, or even your sister-friends.

"He might be your client, not necessarily your husband," said one of the Elders. "Don't confuse the two."

The Elders went on to ask a number of very important questions and to give clear advice. Consider the following questions:

- Does he resent women, or love and respect them?
- Check the records. Has he ever been abusive to women through physical or verbal means?
- Is incest interwoven into his family history, his genes?
- Find out about his previous relationships with the women in his life, especially his mother. Does he have an active relationship with his mother? This will give you an idea of how you will be treated once the doors are shut and the union settles in.

Remember, check him out closely before you take on a relationship. And while you're checking him out, check yourself, too. Are you carrying some tucked-away hurts within you? These have got to be healed first, otherwise you'll act out the real you—the hidden and hurting you—in your marriage. If needed, get help. Commit to cleansing yourself on the inner planes. Above all, do not rush into a union due to fear of being alone, or the mistaken belief that "this is my last chance." Come into the union with your whole self intact, knowing that what you give you're supposed to get back. Reciprocity is part of the divine order.

When your standards rise, there are certain things you will no longer stand for.

Don't check things out against your ego alone. Invite your spirit to sit in as well. Also ask your mentors and/or Elders, your honorable and balanced friends, and your extended family to assist you in this observation process.

Always keep in mind that in the end you can only attract a reflection of some part of you. So be sure to go within and clean up your negative thoughts, attitudes, habits, and patterns. Your observations and reflections need to be like a crystal or a diamond—brilliantly clear. Your future joy depends on it.

You might want to present the following Guide to Courting a Sacred Woman to your possible husband-to-be. His response will tell you a great deal about your potential for Sacred Union.

## Guide to Courting a Sacred Woman

"I am a Sacred Woman. Don't just pluck me out of my family. It is not done that way traditionally. I have been specially trained and groomed for this role in life. Bring me gifts of flowers, precious oils, jewels, and sacred cloth. Speak words of sweetness, and play me music of heavenly sounds. Handle me with loving care, just as you would a dove.

"I sit on my lotus throne surrounded by my blood and extended family, by my spiritual teachers, and by my mentors and Elders. Come through them and ask for me. In their wisdom and concern they will study you and observe me to see if we are to be together."

## LOVE PROGRESS REPORT

What follows are two Love Progress Reports—one for you and one for your mate. Fill them out during your active meditation. Use this report to witness your own inner growth as reflected in your past and present choices of a mate. Remember, there are no mistakes—everything happens for a reason. That's how we learn and grow within the confines of this earthly plane.

Chart your growth with a light and open heart, unafraid of your reflections and observations. You may discover that your growth has progressively reached higher levels of consciousness (awareness of self). Or you may find yourself in the depths of hell. Both states reveal to you lessons and insights about who you are, where you came from, and where you're going. Don't hold on to pain and get stuck. Be open and

objective as you record the few or many men, past and present, in your life. Use the various teachings from your choices of mates as a way to move toward positive change, transformation, growth, and development.

Before you begin charting yourself, take a very hot salt bath or herbal bath as you drink a glass of warm lemon water—the juice of 1 lemon to 8 oz. of purified water. This simple process will help liquefy you and put you in the right mood for self-reflection and healing work. This work is best done between the hours of 4 and 6 A.M., so that you will be spiritually guided as you unfold from a deep sacred place.

Once you have completed your report, think about what you've told yourself. Observe and learn from your life patterns. See how you and your past experiences and present attitudes have created all your love conditions.

Once you have examined yourself, you can begin to purify by taking on the lifestyle of a Sacred Woman. Start breaking up those unhealthy patterns; uproot and purge out any poisonous state. Face up to the part of you that's holding you back from your joy, that has locked up your love and squeezed the life out of your happiness.

Fight for your sacredness. Discover who you are, so that any inner imbalances you may have carried from one life to the next, and from one year to the next, will drain away. Release that spiritual cancer once and for all. That is not the real you. Let those emotional toxins ooze out of you. When the healing has taken place, you will be left whole and healthy and ready for your Sacred Union.

Check your Love Progress Report; you should be reaching for a complete union with yourself so that when you look outside of yourself you will see bliss and oneness showing up in your divine mate. If it is meant to be, even a dead union will come alive when you begin to purify.

A word to the wise: Fast, fast, and fast again, until he arrives. Rest assured, he will arrive. Also know that he will reflect the true you—the one who is divine and pure in every day—because within you there he is, and the one who lives within is the true you.

## Love Progress Report for Women

Serve this Love Progress Report to your prospective mate to evaluate his previous condition, which may very well lead up to his present state. This chart, when honestly completed, will give both you and your mate clarity. It offers pictures of what is happening individually and collectively in your union. As a result, it reveals ways to build a healthier union.

## PREVIOUS AND PRESENT HISTORY

| Relationship Status | Dates of Union | State of Consciousness | Dietary State | Feelings | Reflection | Purpose | Lessons |
|---|---|---|---|---|---|---|---|
| Indicate relationship status (mate, husband, intimate friend); write appropriate title next to birth name. | Dates of union (beginning and end). | Indicate your emotional, mental, and physical state during this union. | What was your food and drink intake during this period? | What did you feel for him? What did he feel for you? How would you treat each other? | If you could, would you go back and pick up the pieces? Yes? No? Why? | What was the divine purpose of this union? | What lessons, challenges, blessings did you receive from the union? Have you released this relationship? Why or why not? |

These questions will help you to identify and filter out some poisonous ideas, concepts, and conditions that have influenced your thoughts and attitudes in relationships.

### Reflections

- How do you feel about yourself right now?
- How do you feel about men—your father, brother(s), son(s), uncle(s), male friends, male coworkers?
- How do you feel about women—your mother, sister(s), daughter(s), aunt(s), female friends, female coworkers?

After going on a seven- to twenty-one-day fast, write about your mate in detail. Do you mirror your own needs and expectations in a mate? If so, then everything is in place. If not, then get busy. Raise your vibrations up to the level of the mate that you're calling forth.

According to our ancient Nile Valley Ancestors, the perfect union with self, mate, or Creator/Creatress was termed *smai tawi* (union of the double regions)—that is, masculine and feminine, or left and right brain, heaven (Nut) and earth (Geb).

## Love Progress Report for Men

Serve this "Love Progress Report" to your prospective mate to evaluate her previous condition, which may very well lead up to her present state. This chart when honestly completed will give both you and your mate clarity. It offers pictures of what is happening individually and collectively in your union. As a result, it reveals ways to build a healthier union.

## PREVIOUS AND PRESENT HISTORY

| Relationship Status | Dates of Union | State of Consciousness | Dietary State | Feelings | Reflection | Purpose | Lessons |
|---|---|---|---|---|---|---|---|
| Indicate relationship status (mate, husband, intimate friend); write appropriate title next to birth name. | Dates of union (beginning and end). | Indicate your emotional, mental, and physical state during this union. | What was your food and drink intake during this period? | What did you feel for him? What did he feel for you? How would you treat each other? | If you could, would you go back and pick up the pieces? Yes? No? Why? | What was the divine purpose of this union? | What lessons, challenges, blessings did you receive from the union? Have you released this relationship? Why or why not? |

These questions will help you to identify and filter out some poisonous ideas, concepts, and conditions that have influenced your thoughts and attitudes in relationships.

### Reflections

- How do you feel about yourself right now?
- How do you feel about women—your mother, sister(s), daughter(s), aunt(s), female friends, female coworkers?
- How do you feel about men—your father, brother(s), son(s), uncle(s), male friends, male coworkers?

After going on a seven- to twenty-one-day fast, write about your mate in detail. Do you mirror your own needs and expectations in a mate? If so, then everything is in place. If not, then get busy. Raise your vibrations up to the level of the mate that you're calling forth.

According to our ancient Nile Valley Ancestors, the perfect union with self, mate, or Creator/Creatress was termed *smai tawi* (union of the double regions)—that is, masculine and feminine, or left and right brain, heaven (Nut) and earth (Geb).

## GRANDMOTHER'S BASIC FOUR

One day when I was spending a winter in St. Thomas, Virgin Islands, on top of Old Mountain Road inside of Scott Free, I was looking out the window at the ocean, feeling bewildered by so many women complaining about their relationships. Then all of a sudden, my grandmother's spirit came through me and left me this message about Grandmother's Basic Four for keeping your man in the home:

"Honey, stop crying. Come here, sit down, and dry your tears. Listen, I'm an old woman, been married some forty-odd years, and during those years I have learned some basic lessons on how to keep a man coming home. I'm going to make it plain. Once you get your man—be it through beauty, intelligence, strength, purity, or all of the above—and you have wedded, use my wisdom for keeping your husband coming home and away from strayin'.

"One: Be sure to feed your husband wholesome meals made with your own hands and from your own pots.

"Two: Be mindful to keep looking attractive. Keep yourself well groomed, especially the feet. 'Cause when a woman is losin' her man, you can usually tell by the way she treats her feet.

"Three: Do not forget to keep the house clean and in order—either with your hands or with a trusted spiritual housekeeper.

"Four: Be loving to your man out of bed and in the bed. Give him good southern or island or Afrakan lovin'. It's all the same—good. Furthermore, don't go to bed or fall asleep with bad words between you and your man. Work it out before the sleep sets in."

"But Grandmother," I asked, "what about me?"

"What about you, honey? In order to truly love a man and keep him loving you, you must love yourself! Child, I've said enough. I'm an old woman and I'm going to go and get my rest now. Bless you, honey. It's gonna be all right. Just you never forget Grandmother's Basic Four."

## WHEN A SACRED WOMAN WEDS

At a Women's Rites of Passage Workshop a few years ago, I spoke about traditional Afrakan ways of healing through marriage, how problems between a husband and wife were solved in Afraka and also how a marriage was formed. I told them how the village, or family, would arrange a marriage, and how there was third-party intervention, too, by Elders and family members, in both arranging and maintaining the marriage.

Afterward a young woman came up and told me how surprised she was to hear that she had instinctively been using these traditional ways in her life. She said, "When my husband and I planned to marry, we had a lot of problems to work out. I spoke about my worries to my cousin. My husband also spoke to her of his concerns. She was able to convey our thoughts, feelings, and worries to each other without strife. She was able to make both of us understand the other's point of view without causing further problems. We were then able to come together in marriage.

"Later on down the line, my husband and I came to another crossroad. The paths we chose to follow this time could have destroyed our marriage. At this time there was another third-party intervention. I spoke to a dear Elder about my concerns and feelings. She was able to bring those things to my husband's attention in a non-threatening way while I listened in. He relayed to her his thoughts and feelings as well. When all was said and done, I felt closer to my husband than I had ever felt before, and I found a way to love him for his truly divine self."

### Before the Wedding:
### Create a Spiritual Balance

As we find our balance, our reflections will be healed. You see, there are no bad people. There are only unbalanced beings, who, no matter how much they search and experiment, find their relationships usually end in fear, frustration, and pain. Balance within a relationship must begin first with personal balance within each partner.

Pray daily that you and the mate that you draw to you will share the same goals and aspirations; that you are both traveling on the same road, so that together you will be going in the same direction. Study each other, take your time, and be guided in the Spirit. As women become more attuned, negative interactions, old hurts, experiences, and conditions drop from our being, flee from our souls, so new possibilities can unfold.

Do some form of water healing. For example, take a daily salt or herbal bath. If you live near the sea and if the weather permits, take a weekly ocean bath. Also drink a quart of purified water every day. Using water daily, inside and out, will bring about balance, harmony, peace, and inner wisdom. Also, fast for seven to twenty-one days. Once you have cleansed, you will be in harmony with your mate or your mate-to-be.

There are certain foods to avoid, foods that bring discord to the union. Eating meat makes both women and men overly aggressive, sexist, short-tempered, hard to get along with, and in an overall state of imbalance.

Meditate on this affirmation:

*I am a balanced being. Both my male and female selves are functioning in harmony within me. I love and am tapped into my strong, firm, expressive male qualities. I love and am tapped into my gentle, patient, creative, nurturing female qualities. I will say this daily until I have fully merged the two aspects of me in total harmony.*

You will know when you have merged the two within and accomplished the ultimate harmony because you will have excellent communication, love, and peace with your loved one and all the men in your life.

As a woman, you represent heaven, the great Mother Nut. Your man represents earth, Geb. Together, when in harmony, you strive for a divine balance between heaven and earth. The only way to experience this natural supreme state between man and woman is to first heal yourself from deep within.

## Seven Steps to a Healthy Relationship

Once your union is sanctified, follow these seven steps to maintain balance, clarity, and ever-flowing love and understanding. Trust in the Most High for guidance in all your relationships. In this way, when it is time, you will be able to give fully and beautifully, like Nefer Atum, the lotus within you, and forgive that you might be forgiven, love that you might be loved, send out compassion that you might receive it in return.

1. Purify the mind, body, and spirit. Be a light, an example, so that your mate and others you know may be inspired to grow.
2. Respect and support the natural diversity in yourself, in your mate, and in your blood and extended family. It's the variety of life that makes a garden beautiful.
3. Think before you speak. Your words can build or destroy.
4. Stay detached. Free your heart of malice, anger, and vengeful ways. Detox your heart so love will flow like a healing balm between you and your mate—and others.
5. Remember the lessons you've learned. Strive to use your relationship lessons as a guide toward maintaining a healthy union.
6. Strive to be a source of divine love, nurturing, and compassion.
7. Step onward. Pray for strength and divine direction as you both make decisions on transforming and building your lasting relationship.

## Before the Wedding: Create a Practical Maintenance Plan

In traditional societies, the husband was a provider for his wife and children. As a result, he received absolute respect from his woman and children. A man built a home for his woman, provided her with jewelry, cloth and/or sewing supplies, cows and domestic animals, a source of light—vegetable oil or animal fats—and canoes or whatever was needed for transportation. If he was a farmer, he tilled the land. Otherwise he hunted or herded.

The woman, on the other hand, foraged for wild foods and herbs and fuel for cooking and heating. She prepared and served her husband meals. In some cases, she worked the land that he prepared, in order to bring to the table vegetables, grains, and fruits. In other cases, she tilled as well. She often helped to build the house and kept it clean, and she wove and sewed most of their clothing.

The couple lived within a supportive family

compound that aided in providing everyone within the family or community what they needed for survival. The family had no choice but to live within their means, unlike today, where we live a charge-card existence that can create debt and anxiety, which produce stress in the union. Think about it!

However the two of you plan to handle your finances and family responsibilities in this day and age, the business talk must be taken care of before you say "I do." Be honest. Establish open communication, and trust that your union can handle truth on this very important issue. This will aid in securing the future of your marriage.

Below I suggest several different ways to approach the practical matters of running a home together. Be creative, but make certain you both have a clear idea of what you're going to do, and that you both wholeheartedly agree. You might even want to write it down, sign it, and date it. You can amend your plan as circumstances change, but always communicate clearly with each other and come to a loving agreement.

## Maintain Balance and Unity in the Home

### One Way
Men take financial care of the home, such as the rent or mortgage (leases or deeds should be in both names), and the following:

Electricity bill
Gas bill
Food bill
Phone bill
Attire for family members
Medical expenses
Insurance
Transportation
School expenses
Part of the child care

They may or may not share in the costs of vacations and evenings out.

Women should take care of:
Keeping the home pure and clean
Laundry

Preparing natural, unprocessed food in the Kitchen Healing Laboratory
Being the husband's personal healer, from baths to massages, clay packs, live juices, and herbal tonics
Most of the child care

### Another Way: One-Pot Afrakan Concept
Both the man and the woman put their money into one account or pot, and the couple maps out a budget that covers all expenses, including vacations, evenings out, gifts, clothing, and so on. They care for each other equally in the Kitchen Laboratory, Hydrotherapy Room, and Regeneration Chamber, and in caring for their children.

### Yet Another Way
Sit down and have meetings until you work out your maintenance plan. Be clear, open, and honest with each other, for sooner or later the truth of the matter will come out. If it's later, then be prepared for some misgivings and hurt feelings. Stand up for yourself, but also for the union. It can be worked out if your union is to be.

Whatever your maintenance plan is for marriage, it must be established up front so that you can best serve each other in a balanced, real way. Put your cards on the table, breathe deeply, drink plenty of pure water, and pray.

Remember: Whatever you decide, work it out before you say "I do."

## WEDDING BANDS

When the moment comes to consecrate your Sacred Union, let even the wedding bands you choose be reflective of your reclaiming your ancient and divine high culture. If you are in doubt about which signs and symbols to choose, look to the oldest Afrakan source possible—the Nile Valley.

The Studio of Ptah in New York City provides such wedding bands (see Harriette Cole's Afrakan American wedding book, *Jumping the Broom*). The Master Craftsman Sen-Ur Hru Ankh Ra Semahj, who designs such rings, is also a Khamitic High Priest. As a Nubian Minister who performs wedding ceremonies to invoke the

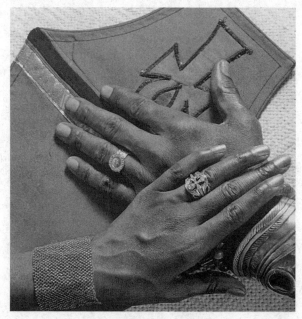

Sacred Wedding Bands

highest and most sacred traditions of the Kham-ite Legacy, Sen-Ur Semahj says, "As an Afrakan Priest, before I consent to perform a cultural ceremony or union, I counsel the couple to cleanse, fast, and purify their Body Temples. In this way they will create a perfect union—Smai Tawi."

## LOVING AND SERVING YOUR MATE

### Sacred Love Essence:
### Purifying the Sperm

Women, be wise when you enter a Sacred Union, for when we make love with our man, we become all of who and what he is. We women drink his essence into our womb, the entrance to our entire inner world. If he is troubled and in pain, or full of liquor or flesh or mind-altering substances, we become all of who he is through his sacred fluids. So be wise and heal your man, not only for his sake, but especially for your own. The healing work—the love, the joy, the fruits, the vegetables, the peace—that you bathe him in is what you will ultimately receive through your womb as his essence moves into your inner world. Inspire, encourage, and nurture your man. Help him cleanse the sickness and disease from his sperm, so that it becomes a source of health and wellness. Do not forsake the union,

for what you give your mate you receive back from him. Be patient and persistent.

If your man is out of balance, then when you're in the act of making love, your womb becomes filled with gases, toxins, and fluids that come from flesh, grease, devitalized starches, and so on. If your mate is not already on the path to wellness, then gently, lovingly, expose him to the new way. Pamper him. Share with him the information necessary to help him make his transition into sacredness.

Dr. Yosef Ben Johannan, a well-known Afrakan historian, said, "Heaven is between a Black Woman's thighs." If that's the case, then in order to enter into heaven, our men must first be purified. No flesh, no liquor, no drugs, no dead foods, and no dead thoughts may enter the sacred portals of my womb.

*Note:* In this day and age of extreme toxicity, for safe sex men must wear a condom to make love. But the moment of truth arrives when you desire to conceive a child. Then it's off with the condom. This is when you gotta "come" clean.

### Sacred Woman, Regenerate Your Mate
### in Twenty-One Days

After you, as a Sacred Woman, purify yourself, you are in place to give guidance to your mate. The better you feel, the more you have a desire to share. The next step is to begin taking your man through a twenty-one-day cleansing and rejuvenation regimen for wellness in body, mind, and spirit.

In order for a man to become healthy, with a clean, clear prostate, he must first get rid of that large stomach area. A colon wellness program is good for starters. Have your man use the Heal Thyself 7-Day/7-Step Colon Wellness Kit (see the product list in the appendix). He will feel more vibrant, more energetic, and younger as a result.

By the time you finish loving up your man over the next twenty-one days, he will be like a fireball of light. His love and respect for you will have come forth in a big way, for you acted as his healer, lover, and tender supporter. As you lift him up in the spirit of love, he will do the same and more for you.

During these twenty-one days, abstain from sexual intercourse to conserve power. But do not abstain from lovemaking. Lovemaking is about caring through holding, touching, kissing, and snuggling up—the physical contact that is needed to strengthen love. During these twenty-one days of preparation, love energy is building, healing, and empowering itself.

Activate this lovemaking on the new moon for new beginnings and a new union. If you come together on a full moon, the orgasm of love and beauty might put you out for a week, so be mindful of your level of heightened sensitivity!

## Meditation: Love Me, My King, Please Love Me Good

*Your sperm has to be organic for me, made from pure foods and pure thoughts so graciously.*
*For I rely on the Most High that dwells in you to feed me pure light, so true, so true.*
*Your sacred nectar when injected into me reaches my heart, my blood, my brain, and my veins.*
*I am Earth Mother, and Nut, Cosmic Queen. I need nectar that has been charged supreme with the green life of kale, sprouts, beets, and turnip greens.*
*No flesh, no grease to enter me.*
*No milk, no cheese to rest in me.*
*No mental poison, greed, or pain.*
*Just love, my darling, should remain.*
*In my palace of beauty, my corridors of bliss, shower your waters of power and purity; for I ingest what you give me and give it back effortlessly.*
*When sperm is pure and charged with light, each cell, each nerve shall then ignite.*
*As cycles come, and come, and come, I feed you my sweet nectar of melons and berries, pears and plums.*
*Pure male nectar leaves me tumor free—if I also take good care of me.*
*Love me, my beloved King, love me good, so I can be who I am, the Divine Earth Mother, and Nut, Cosmic Queen.*

### Heal a Man / Heal a Woman

A divine sister came to me with a tumor the size of a grapefruit, but there was nothing in her diet that would create that. She'd been a vegetarian for twenty years. She didn't eat any dairy or ice cream. She laughs a lot and is very creative. So I asked, "What is the state of your mate?"

She said, "He's so wonderful. But he eats everything."

"Do you wear protection?" I asked.

"No," she said. "We've been together for some years. I don't even want to talk about what he eats. But he eats steak. He eats fried chicken. He has a little beer on occasion."

What her man is doing is injecting the essence of his meals into her womb. He's helping to grow her tumor. We don't grow a tumor by ourselves, but we do participate in allowing it to grow. So what this sister must do is to take her womb knowledge and share it with her man—however she does it. She can pamper him into healing. She can give him juices such as fresh apple and pear juices, because the sweetness actually makes men want to heal in the goodness. And she can prepare healing baths for him and introduce him to some of the food alternatives.

She can work with him that way if she so chooses—or he can wear protection. But if he's consuming those foods, he might be imposing his aura on her even if he wears protection. She might stink of his aura.

If you're very sensitive, you're vulnerable to the vibes of someone close to you. When they hug you, you can feel the pain that comes from all those chickens or cows that were slaughtered to feed him. Forget about cows grazing in the grass. They're not doing it anymore. They're being shot up with hormones and antibiotics until they're all very sick. And we ingest that.

Even if we cleanse ourselves, our mates are going to poison us if they're not doing any cleansing. And if they cleanse and we don't, when they go into our wombs they will develop tumors and cysts and discharges, along with some rage and anger. So we're all responsible for each other.

### Carry Me on Wings of Air Ritual

Women, every now and again when you and your mate are in bed, particularly during the full moon, you should climb up on your King Man's back, sink your body into his, sink your trust into his, sink your beauty into his, sink your needs into his. You will come up more balanced, in tune, and powerful. He will know after this ritual that the bond of love and your pure love for him will bring all of his strength forth.

Size does not matter; your man's test has got to be that he can take the weight of your love. He will and must come forth and carry you on wings of air. As you breathe in, he breathes out, with the harmony of his breath (life). His back will melt and you will mold yourself into his being. This process harmonizes heaven and earth within and without. Breathe until there is complete stillness and complete oneness. This love ritual will help you avoid fights and enhance love and truth within your union. Whenever your union is disturbed, climb up on his back. As you both humble yourselves, fly on wings of air and invite a profound peace to come upon you both.

To further the love ritual, do the following:

1. Drink 8 to 16 oz. fresh apple or pear juice for gentle detoxification to create a sweet spirit.
2. Take a bath together in total silence (a talk fast). Massage his back, then have him massage your back, using olive or almond oil. Massage up the sides of the spine and neck to increase inner peace and soothe the nerves.

## THE SACRED MAN: A BROTHER-TO-BROTHER RESPONSE TO "NO MORE LOVERS" by Hru Ankh Ra Semahj

Beloved brothers, prepare yourselves to deal with a new order. The chant "No more lovers, if you please" is ringing throughout the Nubian nation. Sisters are tired of being receptacles for brothers who just want to masturbate into warm flesh.

Our women are heeding the Heal Thyself call: "Liberation through purification." They refuse to be held captive by keepers of toxic sperm. You cannot possibly be a lover of your mate if you have no intention of matching her cleansing for cleansing, healing for healing.

Brother King Man, we are going to have to seriously examine our ideas about a loving relationship. Can we be lovers without commitment,

without assuming responsibility for the living results of our loving?

Where did we learn to be lovers? Have we become cloned amateurs of scenes in Hollywood movies? This would appear to be the case. To correct this we must *sankofa* (go back and get) the ancient paradigm of our Nubian Ancestors.

Their word for "love" was/is *amer* or *mr* (the origin of *amour*?). It was spelled with ⌇, a plow, or ⊐⊏, a canal.

The plow, a male symbol, is a tool used for cultivation of the soil. Tilling the soil was and still is the most natural thing for a farmer to do. Cultivation of the soil by plowing, sowing, and harvesting is the beginning of culture. Our ancient Nubian existence was based upon *amer/mr*. The canal, a female symbol, channeled the flow of precious water to irrigate the thirsting fields.

A relationship is based upon sowing positive seeds to ensure a positive harvest. A relationship requires the proper channeling of emotions in order to be successful.

### Twelve-Point Action Plan for Men with Sacred Women in Their Lives

Men, how do you respond when your partner embarks on the Sacred Woman pathway, and you suddenly discover there is this illuminating brilliant light, joy, supreme strength, wellness, security, and serenity emanating from the woman in your life? She's different—she's better. Your life through her is changing around you—it's good, but it can be a little overwhelming. What do you do? How do you cope with this beautiful but challenging reflection?

There's no way out—it's time for you to empower yourself by becoming a Sacred Man. To help you through this process, I offer you twelve points of action for meeting your Sacred Woman face-to-face and heart-to-heart.

1. Purify your Body Temple. Meditate, fast, pray, and eat sacred foods—fresh fruits and vegetables, herbs, and purified water. Take salt or herbal baths. Use the book *Heal Thyself* by Queen Afua as your definitive how-to guide for reclaiming and maintaining your new healing self, your Nubian being.

2. Reclaim your ancestral heritage. Study your history—particularly the Nubian legacy of Asar and Hru. Identify your purpose for being.

3. Start really talking with your mate. We've overdone the "strong silent type" thing. The human ear is a feminine instrument. Harsh sounds and coarse speech are a no-no. Never, never even think of striking your woman. Walk away if necessary.

4. Dress and adorn yourself with the grace and dignity of designs based upon Afrakan culture. Stop being clones of European men. Remember, the suit and tie may be the perfect infiltration garments for moving up in the world of corporate sharks, but on your time off don the elegant, kingly robes of your Afrakan culture. Bring color to your community. Our children need color—enough of that blue-jean drabness!

5. Practice sexual hygiene to the max. Funk is good in music, but sexual funk is a turnoff. Remember, a Sacred Man does not eat dead flesh. It is these foods that cause unpleasant odors in the private parts of men and women. Your woman's vagina is the entrance of the "holy of holies." Enter this gateway to paradise with a clean mind, heart, and organ.

6. Exercise. Do your crunches. A potbelly has no place on the body of a Sacred Man. A potbelly is a storehouse of pollution and putrefaction—it will ruin your prostate gland and contribute to toxic sperm.

7. Set up your own altar of sacredness. Place upon it your Sacred Woman's picture and those of your children. Speak to them from your heart in spirit. Trust the ears of the invisible. Don't fail to invoke the feminine aspect of the Divine. Afrakan culture teaches us of a Mother/Father Creator/Creatress.

8. Treat each of the children of your union with the same respect and *mr* (love). Our relationships are being torn apart by men who molest their daughters and stepdaughters. This is a sure way to ruin a woman for life. She will carry the scars into adult life, and it will affect the way she deals with her future husband. Don't contribute to this tragic and vicious cycle.

9. Establish your mentors. Sit with the Elder men, learn from their wisdom—and from their errors. Do pass on to them in a respectful way the lessons you've learned in sacredness. Heal the relationship with your own mother. Remember your mother's and her mother's birthdays.

10. Discover, nurture, and relate to the woman within you. Until you do this, you will never be able to nurture and relate to the woman outside you who is your mate. Keep a journal and try dialoguing with your inner feminine energy. Feel her in action when you bring your mate gifts and flowers, and when you touch your mate's hair as you pass her chair. Little things mean a lot.

11. Most of all, trust your Sacred Woman. She is the most trustworthy of all women because she cannot just be laid. She does not sleep around; no man can touch her unless he is cleansed. So there is no need to be afraid or jealous if she is friendly with other men in her life. She does not mix essences.

    Because she has a natural live-food lifestyle, she is not hot all the time. A Sacred Woman will help you to save your seed. She is not oversexed because she has restored her natural balance. Match her as you support your dual resurrection as a couple of pure light and healing.

12. When your mate sees fit to accept her natural hair and stops using the hot comb and chemicals that have been killing her hair, don't be turned off. Let's end the schizoid behavior. Rejoice, for you no longer have split loyalties. She has taken back her natural crown. Give thanks and praise.

# SPEECH OF THE SEED
## by Hru Ankh Ra Semahj

**To Those Struggling.**
"B. boys" rhymin' inner city rap
curse not our women,
their wombs don't attack.
They're our sisters, our mothers,
NOT "bitches," NOT "hoes."
In their precious bodies
our nation grows.
They are the Queens of Nubian
    resurrection.
So check this out
a new direction
respect your first home—
the womb of your mama:
Bring women no insults, no curses, no
    trauma
no acid sperm
no seed hooked on crack
no forty-ounce highs
no dead foods, no violence, no anger, no
    pain.
The ANCIENTS are watching
as our lives we reclaim.

**To the Sisters.**
Oh, how you dance, WOMB!
You dance
I salute you.
Let us celebrate the joy of a freedom
    reclaimed.
You, WOMB,
first nest of the egg of creation
Khamitic, Black, source of all human life.
You, WOMB,
stir my Seed to dance with your egg
in your primordial waters of Nun.
Oh, how you dance, WOMB,
with living SEED.

**To the Brothers.**
Man your life stations!
Let us cleanse our seed—
No negative thoughts
No toxic foods
No adverse actions!
Dance, SEED, dance in the living
    WOMB.
The kind of seeds we sow
can make or break our rising nation.
No seed comes forth unless it
    lifts our station
and brings glory and healing to
    ALL our relations.
Speak, SEED, Speak!
Deliver to us the saviors of our race.
Living seeds need living food.
Herbs to make sperm-seeds stern
    and strong
in the Womb of Heaven
where we Dance,
living SEED in a living WOMB.

This is the New Order.
This is the New Day.
Be cleansed. Be purified.
It's the only way.
Let's dance! Let's celebrate!

## Advice to Husbands from the Elders of Khamit

"If you are wise and seek to make your household stable, love your wife fully and righteously. Give her food, clothes, and oil for her body, and make her happy as long as you live. For she is of great value to you, her husband. Be not brutal to her. Kindness and consideration will influence her better than force. Pay attention to what she wishes, aims at, and regards highly. Then she will remain with you. Open your arms to her, call her and show her your love."[1]

## Affirmation: From a Sacred Woman to Her King Man

*As a Sacred Woman, I am ever striving to resurrect and exalt the divinity of my mate and counterpart. I recognize that my inner balance must manifest externally in my relationship with my man if the true potential of the Higher Self is to be made known to me.*

*Love is like water, and you are like a plant. Are you thirsty? Then I will let my love flow like the river upon you.*

*Come and receive this love. Let me pour it all over you ever so gently as I watch us grow.*

*I must not be thirsty, for I can love you only when my own source is full.*

*The extent to which I radiate and contain love is the extent to which I draw love from you. With you, King Man, I share in love fiercely, knowing you'll give it right back to me.*

*I can forgive you only when I forgive me. I can nurture you only when I first nurture myself.*

*By loving myself unconditionally, I have the capacity to love you the same way. Ever since I've healed naturally into a Sacred Woman I've grown so vast and so potent, so fierce and so powerful, that I can lift you up and put you back together again. I can do for you what Ast (the Great Mother) and Nebt-Het (the Lady of the House) did for Asar (the Resurrection) in ancient times in Khamit so that the nation could continue to be.*

*Yes, I, a Sacred Woman, have the capacity to love, heal, and support you, King Man—in more than a thousand ways. It's something I do naturally.*

## REAWAKEN YOUR MAN'S *DJED,* HIS ORGAN OF REGENERATION

*When a man's rod has failed, the woman is supposed to go out and pull the leaves off the vines from the fields and make a tea. And, brother, his standing rod should be ready and hot in a couple of days.*

—DR. JOHN E. MOORE, ELDER AND MASTER HERBALIST

The penis or *djed*—the Khamitic term for both "penis" and "stability"—is an extension of a man's entire body. Once you inspire your man to eat natural, unprocessed foods, his whole body will reawaken. A flesh diet, cigarette smoking, alcohol, and drugs of any kind are the quickest way to destroy the organic long life of your man's penis.

The same toxic blood, due to wrong eating, that flows through his heart and lungs flows into his penis as well, and so he is weak, limp, and unable to get an erection. He is sexually congested and impotent. Diligently help your man detoxify to cleanse and rejuvenate all the systems of his body. The state of your man's *djed* is a direct reflection of how he's living his life. Reverse this process of death by adopting a Natural Living lifestyle.

Women more easily take to a Natural Living lifestyle for body, mind, and spirit wellness because they are eager to heal themselves. Most men, I've found, are not inclined to change old habits to improve their health. Brother Bey, a well-known Natural Living practitioner and owner of the Health and Happiness Institute in Washington, DC, says, "Most men are not going to change their diet or improve their health unless it is for their sexual powers and virility."

That's sad, but so be it. That's why I'm approaching the issue of detoxing our men through the body organ that matters the most to them—the *djed*. Once your man is convinced that his sexual performance can be improved through a taste of good healthy living and the many blessings that it brings, he will be encouraged to go deeper into the natural lifestyle.

Awaken your King Man into Natural Living, for this is just the beginning. Self-healing must take place by any means necessary to prevent cancer of the prostate. According to the American Cancer Society:

*Black Americans have the highest prostate cancer rate in the world. Over the past 25 years, the incidence in black men has doubled. The rate of prostate cancer is about 37 percent higher in African American men than in whites, and they are more likely to develop the illness at an earlier age. More than 6,000 black men die each year from prostate cancer, a rate that is rising—a shocking reminder that . . . black men are particularly at high risk of tumors of a gland that most black men know little about. Unfortunately, prostate cancer treatment does, in some cases, cause loss of bladder control and impotence (the inability to obtain an erection). . . . The good news, however, is that most men regain full bladder control within several weeks or months of the operation. Operations performed at advanced medical centers frequently bypass crucial sexual areas, making it possible for men to regain their potency. . . . Men can now give themselves erections with injections or opt for prosthesis or implanted pumps.*[2]

It's best, wisest, and easiest for men to just live naturally. The following directions, if heeded, can create a robust, healthy man.

### For a Healthy Prostate

- Have your Sacred Man drink an herbal tonic: Combine saw palmetto, dandelion, alfalfa, burdock. Use 3 tsp. of each herb to 3 cups of boiled water and steep overnight.
- Give him green vegetable juices twice a day.
- Eliminate dead foods from your diets.
- Your man must do squats daily to open his center. He must also drain and rejuvenate his whole body by putting his legs up at a forty-five-degree angle or, for the advanced man, by performing a shoulder stand or headstand.
- Abstain from physical lovemaking for at least three weeks. But be very loving toward each other to build up deep inner power and strength.
- During abstinence, direct sexual energies to activities such as bike riding, speed walking, Afrakan dancing, or swimming.
- When lovemaking is permitted again, anoint

yourself and your mate with essence of honeysuckle or sandalwood, or use patchouli to fully awaken his mental *djed*.

- The ideal goal for the Sacred Man is to experience internal ejaculation at the point of climax. This means retaining his seed (sperm) and redirecting his sacred fluids to his crown *arit* (chakra). This is accomplished through breathing and meditation, and can only be achieved through much practice and discipline. The benefits reaped include, first of all, natural birth control. It also strengthens the man, giving him longevity, and helps prevent premature graying of the hair.
- For superior wellness of the *djed*: If your man is advanced in his cleansing, or would like to be, then it is best to prepare with Natural Living for seven to twenty-one days, then proceed to a twenty-one-day Nutritional Fasting program with two vegetable juices, one fruit juice (all fresh), herb teas, and at least 2 to 3 quarts of purified water daily. Before bed, take an enema *or* herbal laxatives for the twenty-one days of fasting as needed. Investigate other Nature Cures that will aid in eliminating impotency, cancer of the prostate, and infertility.
- He should go on a meatless diet (or with as little meat as possible). For optimal wellness, use meat substitutes such as beans, peas, lentils, nuts, and seeds. If you still feel the need to eat flesh, eat steamed fish (no shellfish) not more than twice a week.
- Give him green supplements, 1 to 2 tbsp. three times a day: spirulina, wheatgrass, or Heal Thyself Green Life Formula I with fresh juices.
- Have him drink unsweetened cranberry juice. Combine 8 oz. juice with 8 oz. water.
- Mix beet juice with all the other green vegetable juices you're giving him, half and half. (Omit if he has high blood pressure.)
- Aloe vera drink: Scrape 3 tbsp. of fresh aloe vera gel from the plant and blend it with 8 oz. plain purified water; you can also add the juice of 1 lime.
- Gently massage your man's *djed* for five to ten minutes, massaging upward toward the heart to improve circulation.
- Commit to a weekly one- to two-day juice fast—two vegetable juices and one fresh fruit

juice daily, as well as the herbal tonic with male health-improving herbs (see the recipe in the first entry on this list), and a quart of purified water.

- Have him drink organic apple cider vinegar — 3 tbsp. in 4 to 8 oz. warm water, one or two times a day. To break up congestion throughout the body, have him drink this before bedtime. Tell him not to become frightened if a lot of mucus drains out the next morning. It really is a wonderful cleanser.
- Air-bathe the penis. A sun bath in the early morning or late afternoon is superior for re-generation of the *djed*.

*Note:* To begin to see results, follow these steps for a minimum of three weeks.

## Setting Up an Altar for the Spiritual Awakening of the *Djed*

Awakened men, or Sacred Women, set up an altar space on behalf of your own or your mate's sexual and spiritual regeneration in your Regeneration Chamber (bedroom). In the center of the altar you may place a hand-sized *tekhen*. The *tekhen* is the symbol of the Afrakan man's penis, and it represents regeneration and power.

*Tekhens* were created in the Nile Valley in ancient Khamit. Foreigners came to our land and stole them.

To rebuild your man's *djed*, once the *tekhen* is set up, place flowers around it and rub sweet oils on it, such as rose, jasmine, and particularly musk (a man's oil). Also on the altar, light a white candle for balance between your two spirits, and light a red candle for physical oneness and power. Place a bowl of water on the altar and a bowl of saw palmetto berries — an herb for the healing and rejuvenation of the *djed*. Place a picture of your mate on the altar. Write out your prayer for him in pencil on plain paper, then place the prayer request under the white candle or under the *tekhen*.

Encourage your mate to eat, drink, and think pure as he empties out all his hostility and rage into his sacred salt and herb baths. In this way he will once again become powerful and virile, and be able to bring forth strong, spiritual, loving offspring.

## The Myth of Ast (Isis) and Asar (Osiris)

In the myth of Ast and Asar, the jealous Seth slew his brother, Asar, dismembered the body into fourteen pieces, and cast them into the Nile. When Ast discovered this treacherous deed, she was overwhelmed with grief. Determined to res-urrect her beloved husband and bear a Sacred Child, Ast and her sister, Nebt-Het (Nephthys), searched the river until they had found and reas-sembled all the body parts but one. The *djed* of Asar had been consumed by a huge fish.

Ast created a new penis of gold and cedar-wood for her beloved. Then she began to dance around the body — dancing and singing and chanting prayers and magical incantations, faster and faster and more and more passionately, until her arms became vast wings. Ast hovered over Asar and breathed life back into his body. As his *djed* rose, Ast made sacred love to her beloved one last time and became impregnated with his seed. She conceived the Sacred Child Heru (Horus), the beautiful hawk-headed God of Light.

For years after the birth of Heru, Ast and Nebt-Het traveled the dusty roads of Egypt, teaching the arts of weaving, agriculture, and healing, and establishing temples for the worship of Asar. In the sacred precinct of each temple, Ast caused the *djed* of Asar to be created as a *tekhen* and placed it upon the altar as a symbol of regeneration and rebirth. This is the legendary origin of the worship of the sacred *djed*, and why we place the *tekhen* on the altar of a Sacred Man.

## HOLISTIC LOVEMAKING IS ALL ABOUT CREATION

Holistic Lovemaking comes to us from ancient Khamit, when Ast conceived the Sacred Child Heru (Horus) by regenerating the *djed* of her Beloved Asar.

The Sacred Woman of today uses her Kitchen Healing Laboratory to restore herself and her mate, re-creating the spiritual gold inherent in his organ of regeneration. This consciousness creates and enhances dynamic, holistic lovemaking.

In turn, holistic lovemaking creates a healthy future, for the Sacred Children of this union come into the world in a state of peace, harmony, and balance. So many of our children now are violent and angry. We must check the state we are in before and during conception so that we bring no more diseased and imbalanced children into the world.

My work and research on Holistic Lovemaking was inspired by three important issues:

1. I found it important for us to balance every part of ourselves in order to live to the fullest.
2. Future generations are at stake.
3. Too often TV and films present intercourse as violent and negative, and not as lovemaking at all. Holistic Lovemaking is the answer for total fulfillment and for peace between a man and a woman. Holistic Loving represents the restoration of the New Man and the New Woman.

• Holistic Lovemaking can lead to the creation of a divine baby. But it can also lead to the creation of love, peace, an idea, or a whole new world.
• Holistic Lovemaking brings a harmonious oneness within the union. It is an embrace of body, mind, spirit, and beauty.
• This level of lovemaking cannot be experienced if you don't have a committed union.

That level of trust and love allows you to be open, to express and exchange, to love freely and unhampered.
• An unhealthy union brings about false ideas and false reflections. A healthy union is able to create spiritual oneness, inner peace, joy, and rejuvenation.
• There are also certain love positions, along with breathing techniques, that can heal the body from disease. Read *Sexual Secrets: The Alchemy of Ecstasy*, by Nik Douglas and Penny Slinger.[3]
• Holistic lovers unblock energy, tension, and stress. In preparation for the full love embrace, the couple should take a salt and herbal bath, massage each other, and drink rejuvenating herbal tonics as well as live vegetable or fruit juices in order to be in the proper loving, meditative state. This way you don't come to the love exchange with devitalized fluids and body tensions only to release stress and anxiety into and through your partner.
• In Holistic Loving, one's orgasm is not localized. It works freely and intensely throughout the body. If you cleanse through a healthy diet, exercise, and prayer, you will experience a total-body orgasm that will be felt in your back, neck, head, and face. All parts of you will receive this positive, love-healing exchange.

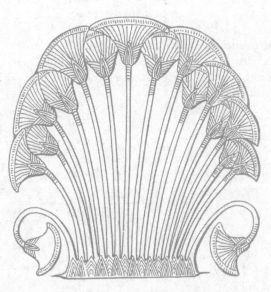

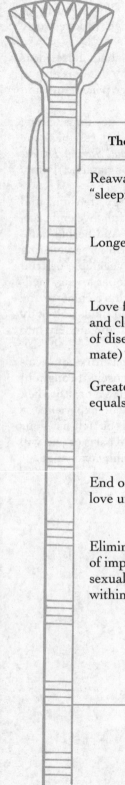

# HEAL THYSELF HOLISTIC LOVEMAKING

Holistic Lovemaking can be established only if you live a holistic lifestyle.

| The Results for Her | Holistic Tools | The Results for Him |
| --- | --- | --- |
| Reawakening of the "sleeping *shetet*" or vagina | 1. Live-food diet—fruits, vegetables, whole grains, protein<br>2. Herbs, natural hygiene | Reawakening "tired *bennenum*" or penis |
| Longevity / eternal youth | 3. Live juices—fruit and vegetables | Creates a profound spiritual balance and deep love within union |
| Love fluids are rejuvenated and cleansed (prevention of disease between you and mate) | 4. Clay work<br>5. Water work—internal cleansing and sacred baths | Enhanced creativity and energy level during lovemaking |
| Greater sensitivity, which equals greater orgasm | 6. Exercise, movement, massage<br>7. Spiritual work/prayer, meditation, and affirmation | Brings about respect and reverence for mate |
| End of violence within the love union | 8. Life mission clear and in harmony (Maat)<br>9. Self-love activity | Holistic loving reduces or eliminates low self-esteem |
| Elimination or prevention of impotency and other sexually related imbalances within men or women | 10. Breath work (air)<br>11. Cultural healing and balance (know thyself) | Seeing the body as a Divine Temple of love and beauty<br><br>If channeled, holistic lovemaking opens the sixth and seventh chakras (*aritu*)—the spiritual gateway to the Body Temple. |

## THE NEXT GENERATION—
## AN END TO VIOLENCE ON EARTH

Holistic lovemaking creates healthy parenting and a healthy future. Babies that are born of parents who make love under these conditions have a greater opportunity to be disease-free in body, mind, and spirit.

### Sacred Woman Exercises to Stimulate Delightful Divine Loving with Your Sacred Mate

- Squats
- Shoulder stands
- Resting with legs at a forty-five-degree angle (or on a slant board)
- Fire Breaths (rapid breathing), 100 to 500 breaths
- The Cat asana in Hatha Yoga
- Afrakan Dancing
- Belly Dancing
- Tightening and releasing vaginal muscles with tantric egg ten to fifteen minutes per day

### Sexual Orgasm Intensified for Regeneration with Your Soul Mate

The way to a true orgasm that is pure bliss comes from a pure diet. Mind-altering herbs alone create only temporary bliss.

### Herbs with Aphrodisiac Qualities

(Herbs and/or foods should be taken daily seven days prior to intercourse.)

- *Damiana.* Damiana and saw palmetto berries are very effective for improving and strengthening the male reproductive organs and for nerves. Avoid large doses and excessive use.
- *Passionflower* is an old island favorite.
- *Spearmint or peppermint* are cures for frigidity in both sexes.
- *Echinacea* stimulates sexual activity and has an-algesic as well as immune-stimulating properties.
- *Pure vanilla extract.* Stay away from vanilla if you are trying to be celibate; it's famous for its aphrodisiac properties.

### Fire Foods to Stimulate Passion in Your Soul Mate

Cayenne
Ginger
Red apples
Cherries
Beets
Strawberries
Raspberries
Red or purple grapes
Watermelon
Garlic

### How to Dress for the Rejuvenation Chamber (Bedroom)

- Waist beads (like traditional Afrakan women)
- Ankle bracelets
- Neck bracelets
- Manicure and pedicure, clear or colored polish
- Silk wraparound garment
- Dimmed lights (place a silk scarf over lamp)
- Drop of rose water or essential oil on lightbulb ring
- Incense

## MORE WAYS TO KEEP YOUR UNION BEAUTIFUL AND LOVING

Sacred Women, don't just assume a man knows what you want; teach him gently. Demonstrate or guide him to what your needs are. Usually a man needs and wants you to show him. It's easier on the union if he's not always required to read your mind or to know your feelings.

- Pamper him, serve him, and massage him.
- Encourage him to do the same for you by giving him gifts of flowers, fruit, candles, and books for consciousness raising.
- Allow your mate to advise you on how this helps to encourage his manhood and his leadership qualities—even if it's not always needed.
- Always keep yourself beautiful in body and in spirit.
- Keep developing your separate gifts as a unique person to ensure growth and excitement in the union.

- Have as many meals together as possible. Eat only natural, wholesome foods.
- Travel together. Take mini-trips together, even if it's once a week for a simple walk in the park.
- Go out together somewhere that's very special to you both, one to four times a month.
- Take evening walks together. Sit on the porch at night. Lie on the grass together during the day.
- Keep in shape. Exercise vigorously together whenever possible.
- Dress to impress each other.
- Be sure to dress beautifully around the house and in bed—never allow yourself to fall into a rut because you now have each other.
- Speak words of love and appreciation often to keep the fires burning within your Sacred Union.
- Speak words of sweetness and use honeyed tones of endearment to him.
- Get away from that television! Constant TV viewing is the quickest way to eat away at the beauty and creativity of your union.
- Don't argue. Always discuss issues in tones of peace so you can both remain clear enough to work out any and every challenge.
- Women, please be wary of the bobbing of your head, the hand on the hip, the pointing finger, the arched back. Instead of this behavior, which is both unnecessary and the opposite of sacred, breathe deeply several times. Be prayerful. Be confident that you can calmly talk it out, 'cause you got the power!
- The quickest way to end a war and begin the love dance is to perform the Talking It Out Ritual (see below).

Sacred Man, now that you feel empowered, show your mate that you care:

- Give her a clay facial.
- Run her an herbal-seaweed bath.
- Massage her from head to toe.
- Give her fresh juice and fruits in bed Saturday or Sunday morning.
- Read poetry to her; dance for her. Have fun.
- Take her to an interesting place a few times a month to keep the fires of interest and passion burning.

- Men—real men, balanced men, Sacred Men—under no circumstances ever lay their hands in a negative or destructive manner on their woman! Never! A loving touch is most effective in helping to resolve conflict.

This book is not for women only. If a man is aware of this knowledge, he becomes sought after, for he knows how to care for and love a woman. All women desire a man who is caring, sensitive, and loving. When a man shares with and serves his mate, he balances out and serves feminine energy in a powerful way.

If, after much time and care (you determine how much), he is unable to serve you as you serve him, then he is simply not the mate for you. Rethink your life, purify, and try again. Know that with every round of cleansing you go higher and higher on the Path of Purification. If you have children together, try not to separate; instead do a twenty-one-day fast and see what miracles fasting will bring.

## TALKING IT OUT RITUAL

If you and your mate must discuss concerns, first take a silent bath together in 2 to 4 lbs. of Epsom salts or 1 lb. Dead Sea salts in hot water. Add a few drops of rose water or pink rose petals and bubble bath in the bathwater. Soak for twenty minutes, and then pour more hot water into the tub and over your heads, faces, and backs before speaking.

When your bath is done, you will find that all is well as you emerge from the tub. Now take a warm shower together and gently come out of the tub. Gently towel-dry each other.

The next step is to massage each other's feet. It's important that the one receiving the massage is sitting up in a chair and the masseur/masseuse is sitting on a low stool. Masseur or masseuse, place a towel in your lap and then massage your mate's feet, one at a time, with natural earth oils, such as olive or almond oil; or simply lie flat in the bed to receive your foot massage.

This entire ritual is done in silence. Allow your eyes, hands, and heart to speak for you. This is a sacred dance between man and woman, which increases your level of sanity, love, and bliss.

If your mate is not advanced sufficiently due to anger or resentment or fear, then you be the one to set him or her free and give love effortlessly. Watch and see—in due time there will be reciprocity.

For advanced couples of this divine way, here is a ritual that is done occasionally, when you need help from the Heavenly Mediator:

Dress your King. Dress your Queen. Humble yourself to each other from head to toe, from brushing the hair to oiling the skin, from putting undergarments on to wrapping her skirt, buttoning his shirt, putting on socks, and pulling up stockings in total love and care. This absolute service will stop all internal wars.

Now if you need to speak, your words will be spoken in pure harmony.

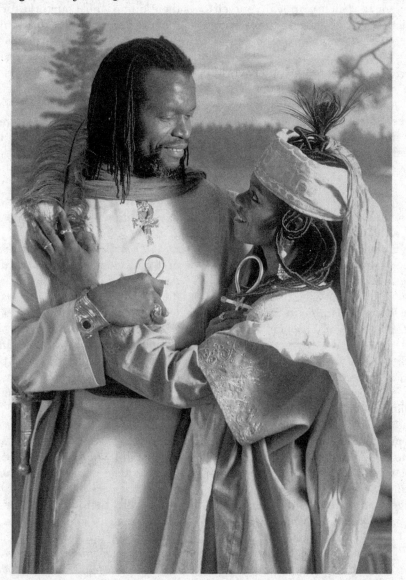

Sen-Ur Hru Ankh Ra Semahj Se Ptah, historical advisor of
Sacred Woman text, and Queen Afua, author of *Sacred Woman*

## SACRED UNION: SEVEN-DAY TRANSFORMATIVE WORK

The most important relationship on earth is your relationship with your inner self and the inner marriage between your masculine and feminine energies. The extent to which you heal yourself and come to union within is the extent to which you will be able to heal all your external relationships.

As you learn to focus less on the outer world and enter your inner environment, the world around you will improve. Establishing a strong foundation of love, honor, and compassion for all aspects of your inner sacred self will also help you establish a strong intimate relationship with your life partner.

- *Extend your use of the Love Progress Report* charts in Sacred Union and extend it to include, evaluate, and heal all your relationships that need strengthening, change, or release.
- *Write down the ten most important qualities you want to manifest in intimate relationships* in order to create union and a life of divine right order. Examine your past four intimate unions and reflect on the presence or absence of these qualities.
- *Identify four sacred unions from your past that need spiritual purification.* As you do your altar work, place symbols of these unions on your altar and practice the art of forgiveness of self and others so that you spiritually cleanse your heart and all disharmonious conditions. If you are not yet ready to forgive, still place the symbols of these intimate relationships on your altar and let Asar and Ast begin to soften your feelings of resentment, judgment, and anger.
- *Don't be erratic and jump into new relationships without cleansing* out the old toxic habits that created your previous poisonous unions. Perform purification rites, and activate them regularly through fasting, eating natural foods, taking enemas and colonics and spiritual baths, journal work, prayer work, affirmations, and purification of your environment at home and work.

- *Perform seven-day prayer/altar work for Sacred Union.* Place an image of the mother/father or an inspiring loving couple on your altar in a beautiful frame.

Write the Creator/Creatress and your parents a love letter about your understanding of their union and your gratitude for the union that created your life. Read this out loud every new moon. Explore the nature of your parents' union honestly. What was positive in their intimate relationship? What was negative? What needs to be purified? What needs to be healed? What energetic inheritance have you carried from their union into your intimate relationships? Even if you don't feel the words at the time, once you come to grips with the foundational relationship in your life—that of your parents—the letter will heal your heart. By healing the roots of this union, all other unions in your life will be healed and will prosper and give you *hotep.*
- *List all your past intimate relationships,* from your first childhood crush forward to the present. As you list each relationship, identify the core themes of the union. For example: "This is what I brought to the relationship . . . This is what my partner brought . . . This is what we created together . . ." This Union Report will begin to reveal your deeper patterns of relating. As you identify core themes, reflect on the energies you and your partner gave birth to through your union.
- *Within the next seven days, write a love letter, a thank-you letter, or a letter of forgiveness* to all those in your life whom you need to relate to so that you can help create more wholesome encounters. If the person has died or has vanished out of your life, then write a letter and burn it with a little sage to begin to release the vibratory pain or stagnant energies of your past.
- *During your morning meditation and prayers, send love, light, and forgiveness* to those you're sending letters to, or to those who are on your intimate relationship list.
- *Self-worth/self-love must be in place within you* in order to establish any Divine Relationship. It's

not about your relationship with him or her; it's about your relationship with self! Ast, the guardian of Sacred Union, teaches us that loving union with self is the foundation for all other unions in our life. As you do your journal work, ask yourself what it would take to establish a healthy union with Self.

- *Place a family tree on your altar that diagrams the Sacred Unions,* the marriages of body, mind, and spirit, in your immediate and extended family. Meditate on these sacred ancestral unions and ask for guidance and inner light.

- *Daily at sunrise, you and your mate should come together* to perform and to share your journal work to support one another in focusing on the work of strengthening and unfolding Sacred Union.

Thereafter, to maintain the union at a high level, commit to performing this spiritual work weekly. Vow not to get so busy in the world that you forget the importance of creating Sacred Union on a regular basis so you both may be fulfilled.

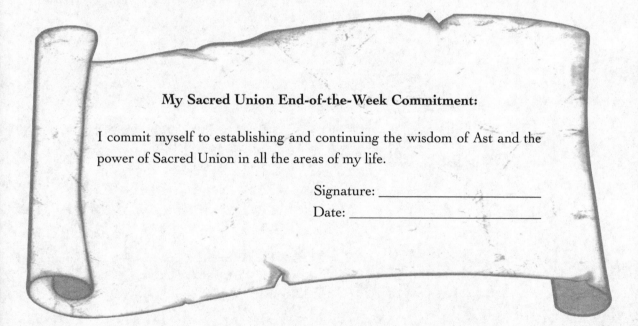

**My Sacred Union End-of-the-Week Commitment:**

I commit myself to establishing and continuing the wisdom of Ast and the power of Sacred Union in all the areas of my life.

Signature: _____

Date: _____

# CHAPTER 14
# GATEWAY 9: NEFER ATUM: THE SACRED LOTUS INITIATION

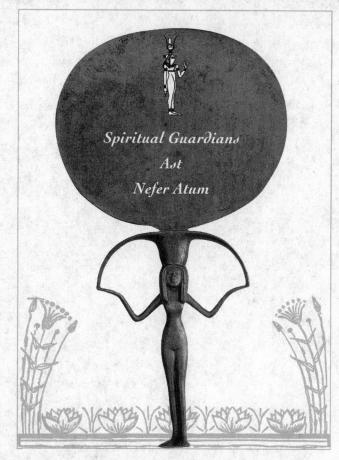

Spiritual Guardians
*Ast*
*Nefer Atum*

**Ancestors**

Queen Hatshepsut

Mary McLeod Bethune

**Elders**

Nana Ansaa Atei

Empress Akwéké

**Contemporary**

Anukua Ast Atum

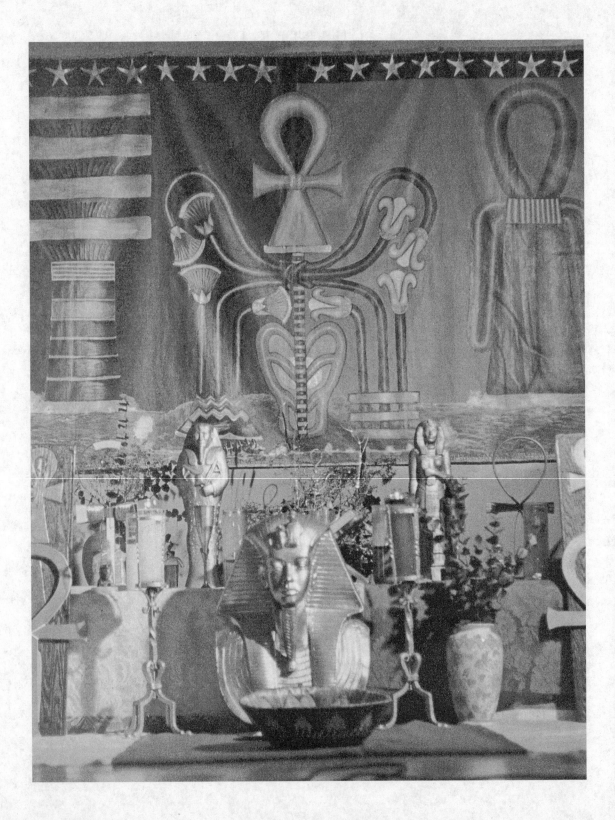

# NEFER ATUM: SACRED LOTUS INITIATION ALTAR WORK
## Face Your Heart to the East—to the Rising Sun
*(Layout from top view)*

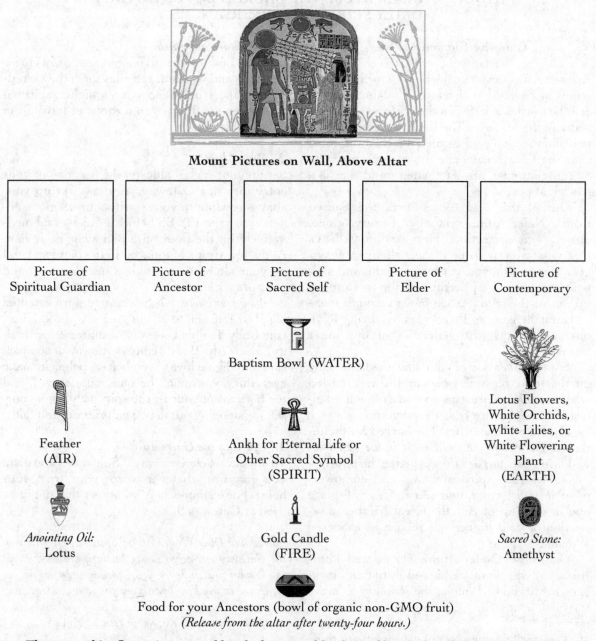

**Mount Pictures on Wall, Above Altar**

Picture of
Spiritual Guardian

Picture of
Ancestor

Picture of
Sacred Self

Picture of
Elder

Picture of
Contemporary

Baptism Bowl (WATER)

Feather
(AIR)

Ankh for Eternal Life or
Other Sacred Symbol
(SPIRIT)

Lotus Flowers,
White Orchids,
White Lilies, or
White Flowering
Plant
(EARTH)

*Anointing Oil:*
Lotus

Gold Candle
(FIRE)

*Sacred Stone:*
Amethyst

Food for your Ancestors (bowl of organic non-GMO fruit)
*(Release from the altar after twenty-four hours.)*

**Float one white flower in a crystal bowl of water, add a drop of lotus oil, and place on your altar.**

Sacred tablecloth (gold) and scarf to wear during prayer.
Sacred color cloth to lay before altar. Sacred instruments to be played as you pray.

# GATEWAY 9: NEFER ATUM: THE SACRED LOTUS INITIATION
## DAILY SPIRITUAL OBSERVANCES

### Gateway Element: Ether

Ancient Afrakan spiritual women adorned themselves by covering with a lotus blossom what we call the third eye, between the eyebrows, but it is actually the first eye. The lotus represents spiritual illumination and beauty. Placing the lotus over the brow means one has a perfected state of consciousness, an illuminated mind that is a garden of peace.

Out of the mud comes forth the Sacred Lotus, Nefer Atum, symbol of beauty, grace, purity, and perfection. Her wisdom tells us that what appear to be life's challenges, struggles, ups and downs, confusion, pain, and sadness are actually opportunities for us to move up out of the mud. As we move through these tests, challenges, and struggles, we bring forth our inner lotus, the reflection of our inner beauty.

For the ascension of your soul, meditate daily on the lotus blossom on your brow. Envision what the lotus represents so that you will manifest Nature's beauty from deep within.

Through Nefer Atum: The Sacred Lotus Initiation Gateway, you will experience Oneness with the Creator/Creatress, divine inspiration, divine wisdom, spiritual unity, and empowerment in body, mind, and spirit. This will place you in the Seat of Ast, the Great Mother, a reflection of your higher self reborn as a Sacred Woman.

Gateway 9: Nefer Atum: The Sacred Lotus Initiation will eliminate Sacred Initiation blockages in the Body Temple: the inability to move forward, or a feeling of being stuck in a rut or trapped.

The spiritual exercises of ascension are to be performed daily for seven days, the number for the spirit. This will awaken your inner Gateways of Divinity so that you may blossom into your full sacred center.

### 1. The Spiritual Bath

Use lotus oil for the divine oneness of NTR inspiration and wisdom. It brings forth the sacredness of the womb and ignites higher spiritual consciousness. Place 4 to 6 drops of lotus oil in your bathwater.

### 2. Your Altar

Set up your sacred altar on the first day of your entry into this Gateway. You may set up your altar according to your spiritual or religious beliefs (see page 18). Sit before it quietly and meditatively on the floor on a pillow, or in a chair. Add a few drops of lotus oil to the baptism bowl on your altar, and sprinkle a few drops around your prayer space.

*Anoint with lotus oil.* Select only pure essential oils. Use lotus oil to anoint your crown, forehead (the Body Temple Gateway of supreme spirituality), heart (the Body Temple Gateway of compassion and divine love), womb area, palms to make everything you touch become more sacred, and the bottoms of your feet to spiritually align yourself for stepping out in power, promise, and faith.

### 3. Opening the Gateway

To invoke each Gateway's Spiritual Guardian, you may use whatever words pour from your heart. For example, here's a prayer that might be used at Gateway 9:

*Sacred and Divine Nefer Atum, Spiritual Guardian of the Gateway of Sacred Lotus Initiation, please accept my deepest gratitude for your healing presence on my altar and in my life. Thank you for your guidance and inspiration, and for your love and blessings, and please accept my love and blessings in return.* Hetepu.

As you offer your prayer, simultaneously shake, ring, beat, or rattle a sacred instrument (sistrum bell, drum, shekere, or bells) to awaken the NTR that is indwelling.

### 4. Libation

Pour a libation for the Nefer Atum: Sacred Lotus Initiation Gateway from a special cup, or sprinkle water from a bowl onto the earth or a plant, as you call out this prayer of praise and adoration.

— *Pour a libation* as you say, *All praise and adoration to the Spiritual Guardians, Ast and Nefer Atum, Protectors of the Sacred Lotus Initiation.*

— *Pour a libation* as you say, *All praise and adoration to the Ancestor of the Sacred Lotus Initiation, Queen Hatshepsut.*

— *Pour a libation* as you say, *All praise and adoration to the Elders of the Sacred Lotus Initiation, Nana Ansaa Atei and Empress Akwéké.*

— *Pour a libation* as you say, *All praise and adoration to my Divine Self and my Contemporary Divine Sister, Anukua Atum, who honors the Sacred Lotus Initiation.*

### 5. Sacred Woman Spirit Prayer

Ring a bell or play another sacred instrument at the beginning and end of this prayer. As you open your palms to the Sacred Spirit or gently place them over your heart, recite:

#### Sacred Woman Spirit Prayer

*Sacred Woman in the making,*
*Sacred Woman reawaken,*
*Sacred Spirit, hold me near.*
*Protect me from all harm and fear*
*beneath the stones of life.*
*Direct my steps in the right way as I journey*
*through this vision.*
*Sacred Spirit,*
*surround me in your most absolute*
*perfect light.*
*Anoint me in your sacred purity, peace,*
*and divine insight.*
*Bless me, truly bless me, as I share*
*this sacred life.*
*Teach me, Sacred Spirit, to be in tune*
*with the universe.*
*Teach me how to heal*
*with the inner and outer elements*
*of air, fire, water, and earth.*

### 6. Sacred Initiation Prayer

Shake bells, beat a sacred drum, or play another instrument at the beginning and ending of this prayer.

*Great and Divine Supreme Mother, thank you for showing me the way to becoming a realized Sacred Woman. I thank you for awakening me to my true nature, for opening the Gateways of Sacred Woman Enlightenment. I thank you for washing my soul at the shore of the Great Ocean of Nu; for charging me with the light of the sun's rays; for delivering me a refreshed breath of life; for helping me to stand on solid ground, as I return to my Sacred Woman seat of stability and strength, poise, ease, and empowerment.*

*I thank you, Great and Divine Supreme Mother, for reawakening and healing my womb; for bringing power back into my words and serenity into my silence. I thank you for giving me the foods that reflect good health and longevity; for cleansing my space and presenting me with a sacred home; for beautifying me and bringing out my creativity in unlimited ways. I thank you for healing my life and giving me the desire to help others to heal themselves; I thank you for restoring all my relations, for giving me the courage to experience Sacred Union, and for filling my spirit with joy and gratitude.*

### 7. Chanting Hesi

Chant this *hesi* four times:

*Nuk Pu Ntrt Hmt* — I am a Sacred Woman.

### 8. Fire Breaths

Prepare for your Fire Breathing by slowly inhaling four times and exhaling four times. Then, when you are totally at ease, begin your one thousand Fire Breaths. Inhale deeply like a pump through your nose (mouth closed) as you expand the breath down into the abdomen, then back up to the chest. Completely exhale out through your nostrils from your abdomen as it contracts and the lungs release your breath completely. Repeat this breath rapidly in and out, in and out.

Allow each deep Fire Breath to represent the opening of the thousand lotus petals of illumination and radiance to reach Nefer Atum—the ultimate Afrakan lotus station of Divinity.

### 9. Gateway 9: Sacred Lotus Initiation Meditation

Increase the length of time you spend in meditation every seven days. The longer you are in meditation, the deeper your inner peace will be, and the more solid your *ba* (spirit) will become. The cleaner your Body Temple, the sooner it will be able to live permanently in the peace and inner balance of the meditative state.

Welcome home, High Queen. Breathe deep. You are finally through. You have risen above many challenges and crossroads, and you may now take your rightful place in your seat of Ast.

Take your amethyst in your right hand, close your eyes, and take a deep breath. You are here now. You have finally arrived.

As you sit in your seat of Divine Power, allow the light within you to emanate from your center as you merge with the dynamic force of unlimited, ever-flowing light and energy from within.

You will never be separated from your seat again—this seat of highest good, where the lotus grows under and around it, where strength is secured, good deeds flow, wisdom soars, excellent health manifests, and compassion and nurturing reside. An enlightened Sacred Woman, you sit upon this seat by your very nature. The light has been awaiting you for thousands of years, for lifetimes gone by. Welcome home to this great seat of our beginnings.

*Color Visualization.* Visualize the color of the Gateway while in meditation: white with light blue, for purification, illumination, and devotion. As you perform your meditation, wear white and/or place a white cloth on your altar.

*Sacred Stone Meditation.* While in meditation, hold an amethyst in your palm over your crown. The amethyst is the sacred healing stone of the Nefer Atum Gateway.

### 10. Herbal Tonics

Drink Solar Water during spiritual prayer work and throughout the week. This is pure water charged by the sun for one to four hours.

### 11. Flower Essences

To deepen your experience of Gateway 9, choose from the following flower essences. Take 4 drops four times per day directly on or under the tongue, or add the same amount to a small glass of purified water and sip. For instructions on how to choose flower essences, see page 23.

- *Star tulip:* Spiritual receptivity, opening the feminine aspect of the self to the higher worlds.
- *Pomegranate:* Creative expression of the feminine aspect of self.
- *Mugwort:* Enhancing and balancing moonlike, receptive qualities of the psyche.
- *Iris:* Creating a chalice or inner vessel for receiving higher inspiration; attunement to feminine forces.
- *Angelica:* Attunement with spiritual beings; protection and guidance from the angelic realms.
- *Alpine lily:* Greater inner space for the feminine self.
- *Lotus:* Spiritual elixir; enhances and harmonizes higher consciousness; open an expansive spirituality; meditative insight and synthesis.

### 12. Diet

Follow the Sacred Woman Transitional Dietary Practices presented for Gateways 7 and 8.

In preparation for Gateway 9: The Sacred Lotus Initiation, choose one of the following dietary observances. Consume 100 percent raw (live/uncooked) food or follow the Sacred Woman Seven-Day Fast (page 175).

### 13. Sacred Initiation Journal Writing

This is best done after internal cleansing (enema) and/or meditation. When you are cleansed and centered, you can receive spiritual messages from the One Most High with grace. When you are in the spirit, messages travel down through your spirit mind, to your heart, into your hand, and onto the paper. (This is how I do all my writing.)

The best time to receive your spiritually inspired written work is after you have completed your altar work, between the hours of 4 A.M. and 6 A.M. Keep your journal and a very special pen by or on your altar to work with the power, force, and stillness at the coming of dawn, the hour of Nebt-Het.

Affirm your daily life. Write in your journal at this time thoughts, activities, experiences, and interactions that present themselves. You can also write down your visions, desires, dreams, and affirmations so that you will be able to draw on these resources when help and support are most needed.

*Consult Sesheta.* If you find that you are unable to contact your inner voice during your journal work, call Sesheta, the keeper and revealer of secrets (who is indwelling), to assist and speak through you.

### 14. Senab Freedom Shawl or Quilt

Choose a new piece of cloth that corresponds to the Gateway color (indicated in exercise 9 of your Daily Spiritual Observances or in Sacred Altar Work) to add to your Senab Freedom Shawl or Quilt. This cloth will serve as a mini-canvas to represent your experience in the Gateway you're working in.

Also, collect meaningful symbols that can be added to your shawl or quilt in appliqué or patchwork style. You can add stones, other natural objects, collectibles, family heirlooms, photographs that have been reprinted on fabric, or any other significant items that embody the essence of your experience. Give your imagination free rein and let your craftswoman spirit tell your story. For more information about the Senab Freedom Shawl or Quilt, see pages 122–125.

### 15. Sacred Tools

Place a sacred feather representing Maat, and shells representing Nu, the ocean, on your altar. Create a scale to weigh the feather against your heart.

### 16. Sacred Reminder

Throughout the week, observe closely the wisdom presented for the Gateway you're in. For maximum results, live freely and harmonize with the various systems of wellness and practice the Seven-Day Transformative Work at the end of the Gateway.

### Closing Sacred Words

*Mother/Father Divine, help me walk through my life as a Sacred Journey of lessons learned and visions realized. Help me to be reborn as a Sacred Woman.*

# OUR ANCIENT
# KHAMITIC HERITAGE AS WOMEN

In ancient times in Khamit (Egypt), women were sacred. They were treated with great respect and reverence. They were lifted up. In the societies of ancient Nubia and Khamit, women were free. These Afrakan women were very successful in their own right. They owned property, stood side by side with their men in business and personal life, and were Priestesses passing on spiritual wisdom. The lineage of the children passed through the mother. You can even see from the shape of the symbolic Ankh how the women of this time were viewed. She was represented as the top loop on the Ankh, supported by her King as the lower part. In this way together they brought forth the future, our children, as a mighty nation. The Ankh was carried religiously by the King and Queen and Priest and Priestess daily to represent our High Order.

### The Ankh—A Symbol of Initiation

Ancient Afrakan Queens, Priestesses, Kings, and Priests thousands of years ago wore and carried the Ankh. The Ankh is the sacred symbol born from the Afrakan Khamitic people that represents the continuity of Life Eternal.

| | | |
|---|---|---|
| Water | Woman | Ast |
| Air | Womb | |
| Fire | Children | Heru |
| Earth | Man (*Djed*) | Asar |

The Ankh is the perennial sign and symbol of unity. It unites all the elements and thus acts as a tool of healing. The Sacred Ankh, Key of Life, calls us to remember the First Afrakan Family (our Adam and Eve)—the Divine Mother Ast, the Divine Father Asar, and the immaculately born child Heru, our cultural hero.

In ancient times we saw the Creator/Creatress represented in both male and female aspects to serve as a model for divine balance throughout society. To put a woman down, suppress her, beat her, not only was considered a societal crime, but was above all a spiritual crime against

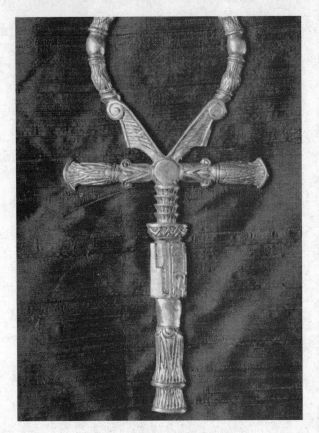

Ankh—The Symbol of Unity

the feminine aspect of the Most High dwelling within all men and women.

The Forty-Two Laws of Maat were named after the female NTRU, Maat, who represented peace, harmony, justice, and righteousness. The laws were designed to establish for us a divine spiritual order for correct living. These laws are found written on the walls of ancient Khamit to this day so that we would never forget the supreme Natural Law.

# A SUPREME INITIATION:
# RETURNING TO THE ANCIENT
# TEMPLES OF MY ANCESTORS

Although it has been a long time coming, through the writing of this book I've been allowed to return home to Khamit. Thousands of years have passed since I lived here, and I have journeyed through numerous incarnations to reach my original destiny. It was so good to go home again, to reacquaint myself with myself in the land that was my beginning.

I revisited ten or more temples in a state of awe and amazement at our ancient way of life. The architectural brilliance left me spellbound. The spiritual adeptness left me in a place of profound gratitude. The cultural vastness, absolute intelligence, and electrifying beauty left me breathless.

The depiction of our way opened me up to the greater possibilities of my life and greater hopes for my people's healing. I kept thinking that maybe we can't all go home again in body, but home is available to us all—if we dare to claim it—in spirit. We can be delivered to our ultimate liberty through the true knowledge of self that this journey brings. As I traveled from temple to temple, I became more and more encouraged and inspired to live out my Afrakan legacy.

Everyone discouraged me from traveling to Khamit during the summer months, yet I soon discovered that the heat of Khamit was part of my initiation. It forced me to go deep inside myself to work through, above, and beyond the extreme transformative healing heat that Sun Ra poured through me. Sun Ra was at its height, which helped me open to all that I received in an unforgettable way. It emblazoned the spiritual, the cultural, and the healing path that our beloved Ancestors walked. The heat seemed a necessary tool to help me experience our potential power and greatness, as the original people of light.

For me, this journey home was like drinking liquid gems—diamonds, rose quartz, and lapis lazuli—poured into a sacred chalice of pure distilled water. I drank my journey down, and it reached into my *aritu* (chakras). With each swallow, clarity and enlightenment emerged. I began to experience, more than at any other time in my life, a clear vision of where I was going, because now I knew where I'd come from.

For years I'd heard many of our historians and spiritual leaders and scholars speaking of Khamit or Egypt. They all spoke of our greatness in the past tense. But for me it is all present; it is all now. Our past greatness is in our present, waiting for us to access it as we begin to clean up our Body Temple where the Most High dwells. As we begin to pray to the Most High in the ancient way, we fly as Hru, the falcon.

Everything in life has been leading me to this journey: the studying, the readings, the workshops, the self-healing, the channeling, the dancing, the sweat lodges, my marriage to my teacher and mentor. It was all leading me back home to my divine ancestral past. All Praise to the Creator/Creatress.

## How Had My Transformation Come About?

The temples of our holy land spoke to my soul, and the interaction was glorious. Everay, my son through marriage, said before my departure that I would never be the same after my journey to Khamit. He was right. I have been touched by the light and the glory of NTR, my Creator/Creatress, because of that pilgrimage.

I wondered to myself in my still moments how and why this journey was having such a profound effect on me. Was it because of the divine souls that I traveled with—Baba Heru, our teacher and Priest, my husband, who also acted as our guide through the sacred temples? Was it due to those I call the Mesu-Heru Sisters (the Mesu-Heru were four female guardian angels who guarded and protected the sacred organs of those traveling from the physical world to the spiritual world)?

These guardian women in my life are Ingani Choice, an Ambassador of Purification; Taen-Ran Anx Cheta, a Khamitic Priestess; and Snt Tehuti, Heal Thyself Ambassador of Purification and my Initiate. We had traveled to Khamit, and now we were homeward bound. These women had vowed to live a pure, culturally and spiritually attuned life. Was it because of them that my journey had been so supremely elevating?

Was it because we had all cleansed, fasted, bathed, prayed, and studied our Nile Valley legacy to prepare for this soul journey? Or was it the constant heat of 105 degrees plus that purged and delivered us to purity? Was it that no matter how challenging the events, we promised to remain in *hotep* (peace)? Was it the white clothing we wore daily with a shawl or head wrap to indicate the cosmic color of the day? Or was it just our time? I believe it was all those things, wrapped into one, that made our trip so utterly *Nefer Atum* (sweet and illuminating).

We were tested to the max as *khepera* (transformation) worked on us daily; through the exercise of patience, tolerance, endurance, we came up *Heru* (victoriously), like falcons flying high above *Set* (challenges). We came through our initiations, each one on a different plane, but all in *NTRT Maat* (divine right order).

All of us, from generation to generation, have been told untruths, or half-truths, or outright lies about our legacy as divine Afrakan beings who once ruled the earth. It was a campaign designed to destroy our relationship with our most powerful sacred self. And yet the entire human family emerged from us, and one day soon we will come to see and know the truth that will set us all free. We, the Afrakan people of the Nile Valley, breastfed everyone, from beloved Moses and the Persians and the Greeks to the Buddha, Mohammed, Jesus, and Mother Mary. The walls of the temples of our Afrakan Ancestors tell the great story of our noble legacy.

For centuries, foreigners have tried to dislocate us from our source of spirituality, but the truth could not be denied to us as our group stood before our massive, powerful, all-encompassing beginnings. We channeled, and we listened and saw. Ast, the Great Mother, and Asar, the Great Father, worked through our

teacher, Baba Heru, as he performed spiritual, psychological, cultural, and surgical work to weave back together all our disconnected parts. For thousands of years our bloodlines have been dismantled. Our self-worth, self-esteem, self-love, pride, and healing were all replenished on our glorious journey to our past and present. We all agreed that the legacy of slavery no longer had a hold on our souls. Our cells had been recharged, our DNA restored. We had become reborn, liberated Nubians.

### The Sacred Woman Speaks: "Go Home, Now!"

As I was coming to the very end of a three-and-a-half-year journey of the writing of *Sacred Woman*, the spirit of the Sacred Woman, the spirit of this book, spoke to me loud and clear: "Go home," she said. "Go home to Khamit. You can no longer procrastinate. The time is now. For I will have one more thing to say to you before I release you. Once you have journeyed home I will speak through you and then you will be done."

The writing of *Sacred Woman* grew out of the process of following a particular life path for twenty-five years. It is a record of my steps as part of an ancient way that I have adopted and accepted and reenacted as a means of healing myself. It has been my way of supporting other women in their healing, particularly the Afrakan woman. As I reached the end of the book, the Sacred Woman demanded in a loving way that I

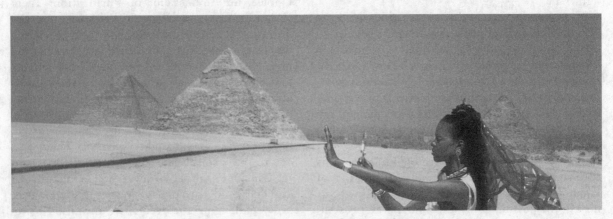

Queen Afua Saluting Ra at the Giza Plateau

undergo an initiation that would end and begin with my journey to and from Khamit, our Mother, Egypt.

"Go home," she said. "Now!"

Seven weeks later, at 105 degrees and on the ninth day of travel, I stood before my royal spiritual family surrounding me on the various temple walls. I wasn't sure which day I had entered which temple, for the nine days had felt like one long, intense coming forth from night to day, of coming out and rising up into myself through my past. It was all leading me to "a great good gettin'-up morning"—a new period of divine bliss. This trip marked the beginning of a new age for me in every sense of the word—a greater opportunity for a richer life on a soul level.

## My Temple Initiations

In Luxor (ancient Thebes), at the vast temple complex of Karnak, built at the beginning of the Twelfth Dynasty (ca. 1785 BCE), I stood inside the Temple of the Holy Family of Ptah, Sekhmet, and Nefer Atum and had an experience that saddened and empowered me all at the same time. I witnessed a living oracle taking place through me.

After much walking through vast columned chambers, we entered Temple Room 1, where the sacred statue of Nefer Atum was supposed to be. But at some point in the past it had disappeared, possibly into some museum. The symbol of the spiritual essence of our people had been removed, and all that was left was an empty room. And because Nefer Atum has been taken, confusion, turmoil, and disease rule the earth. For the planet to ascend, for there to be peace on earth, Nefer Atum must be returned to this holy place. Nefer Atum must stand next to his father Ptah and mother Sekhmet. The Celestial Royal Family must be reborn in us as it is in Nut (Heaven).

In Temple Room 2 we entered into a state of quiet reverence when we saw the NTRU Ptah sitting in a *kes* (a kneeling position of praise). Ptah is the symbol for foundation and building, but his head had been broken off and lost. You cannot, as an Afrakan being, build without your head; without your head there is no direction.

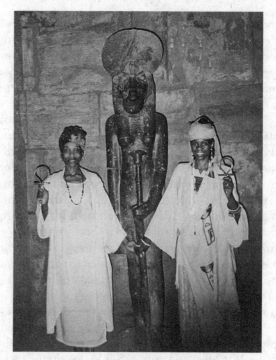

Tehuti and Queen Afua at the
Shrine of Sekhmet

Through study, prayer, fasting, and reclamation of our ancient ways, our missing head shall return to us, making us whole. This is why returning home is a part of the puzzle of our ascension.

In Temple Room 3 we found Sekhmet, the Lion-Headed Female Guardian of all healing. And there she stood totally intact, carrying an Ankh in her left hand. As she rose above us, at least two feet taller than myself and the Mesu-Heru Sisters, we began to weep and to give praise. Through the unspoken power of my Ancestors I was brought to a *kes*, and I began to speak these sacred words in a trancelike state:

"Divine Sekhmet, you are not in a museum in some far-off land, you are home, you are where our Ancestors placed you from the beginning, and it is from this sacred space I speak.

"Sekhmet, healer of all, holy feminine aspect of the Creator/Creatress, we are one and the same. When I see you, I see myself. All that you are I am, for I come forth from your holy limbs. The sun disk of Ra worn on your head, representing divine light, energy, and regeneration—that is me. The lotus scepter that you carry in your hand, representing pure splendor, is mine by nature. And you yourself, a woman lioness, Fearless One who stands here unmoved, you alone, Great Healer, have allowed time to bring me forward with my sisters in spirit so that we may awaken into the remembrance of our true way.

"You, Sekhmet, an aspect of the Divine, still stand here to protect and support righteousness throughout the lands. You, the mother who taught Imhotep, the great architect and healer, through spirit, you opened the way to all healing temples and sanctuaries on our precious land. You were the one who was left behind, knowing that your children's children's children would return to seek out healing and wellness. As a civilization, we may have gone under for a moment, but we've returned in time to heal and to rise up again. Most of our sacred temples have been buried or robbed by ancient and modern thieves, or defaced by various religious sects, or completely destroyed by fire, or inundated by the Nile. But here you stand, Sekhmet, the miracle, Healer of Healers. You have stood strong and undaunted for thousands of years, you who dwell within me. *Tua NTR.*

"I sing praise to sweet NTR, for I acknowledge, live, and teach from the oldest tradition of healing, which you, our divine spiritual reflection, symbolize. We, your daughters, are here to continue in the ancient Afrakan tradition of healing and wellness. We are here to pick up the lotus scepter and continue the legacy of healing and divinity for our people and the people of a world gone astray. The world needs our teachers to return again, for our way is the hope and the light.

"As daughters of Sekhmet, when we depart from this holy ground and return to Amenta [America], we vow to carry your light of healing to everyone we meet. We vow to rebuild the holy land from inside our Living Temples. We vow to carry, share, and spread the remembrance of our way."

At Karnak, at the huge and imposing Temple of Amun, I came face-to-face with the Sacred Lake, which measures eighty by forty meters. For me, this is where purification began—this lake where our Ancestors purified and baptized themselves several times a day. What was most astounding to me was that a large granite scarab, a symbol of transformation, was facing the lake. This told me that our Ancestors believed that in order to bring your life into higher resonance you must first purify yourself in the sacred water for true transformation to take place. The scarab had been dedicated by Pharaoh Amen Hetep II to the Sun NTRU (Ra) Atum Khepera, who was represented by the scarab.

In Aswan, at the temple complex of Kom Ombo, the Temple of Het-Hru had a most profound effect upon my soul. Near the wall of healing was a Birthing House where women experienced natural childbirth. It was there that we acknowledged the spirit of the ancient mothers Ast (Isis) and Het-Hru (Hathor). We felt the anointing from a feminine perspective as we observed wall carvings of Ast sitting upright on the birthing stool.

I had heard New Age mothers speak of birthing stools in the 1970s as though they had invented the concept of allowing the power of gravity to make birthing our babies an easier and more sacred experience. Now I saw that Ast had shown her daughters what to do at the beginning of time so that we might birth our babies in harmony. But out of ignorance and for the convenience of doctors and hospitals, we birth lying on our backs, placing our feet up on stirrups and going against the flow of gravity. As a result, we have long, painful, sometimes dangerous birthing experiences.

Women, follow the ways of our Ancestors in squatting to birth; this is the way to birth our infants, and the way to overall healing.

Next to Mother Ast were surgical instruments that we used thousands of years ago, even though historical records claim that Hippocrates of Greece was the father of modern medicine. In reality, medicine began with the Afrakan race, through Mother Ast and Imhotep.

Across from the Healing Wall was a Wailing Wall, on which was carved a box containing two eyes that see all and two ears that hear all. Brother Mohammed, our guide, told us that this was the wall where we as an ancient people came to cry, to moan, to let go of our pain and so clean and renew our *ba* (soul). As my husband and Mohammed continued to talk about this Wailing

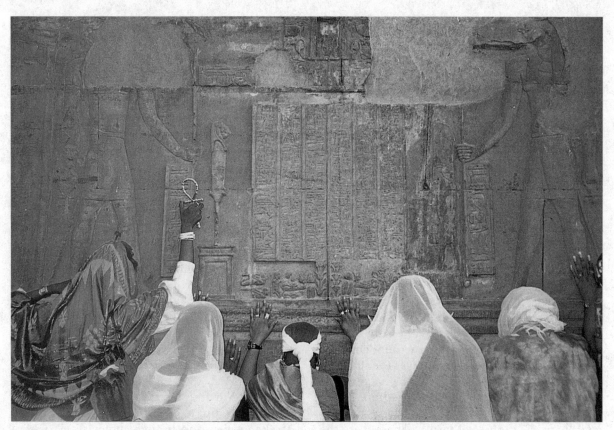

The Wailing Wall at Kom Ombo Healing Temple

Wall, I began to walk toward it with my hands up in a pose of surrender.

Hru Ankh Ra Semahj called out, "What are you doing?"

I replied as I continued to approach and stretch my body across this most sacred wall, "I'm going to wail for myself, for us, our children, and my people, for all that we have gone through as a race—the devastation, the slavery, and the disrespect from the hands of foreigners. I wail for us as a people in captivity. I wail for the rape, anguish, disregard, and lynching and robbery of our culture. I'm gonna wail for the land that is no longer our land in flesh, but always in spirit. I'm just gonna wail."

Priestess Taen-Ra Anx Cheta, Snt Tehuti, and Ingani joined me as we wailed for the past and present condition of our mothers, our aunties, our sisters, our fathers, our men, ourselves, and all our extended family. We women did what we had to do at the Wailing Wall. We let it go with our quiet, soulful tears so that our cups could be refilled with the original way of Maat. We prayed to return to that time when the first people were in tune with the One Most High Creator/Creatress; the time when we were in harmony with Nature and ourselves; the time when peace on earth was supreme and divine; the time when spiritual intelligence was the norm. Back to the sacred time when art and spirit were one, when the world sat at our black feet and in our sacred temples to study the path of light. Back to a time when women were revered, cherished, respected, and held high within society. Back to a time when women shared power and leadership in the governmental and in the spiritual arena.

At Dendera, inside the Temple of Het-Hru (Hathor) on the banks of the Nile, I discovered a wonderful reality. Throughout the life of my healing work, I had always thought about, and meditated on, creating major Healing Centers—

places of wellness that would affect planetary change. But nothing in me thought or perceived of such a vision as the massive institutions and healing temples that our Ancestors manifested thousands of years ago. As I walked around the grounds where healing took place, I stood in the center of one of the small healing rooms, closed my eyes, and entered my spirit as I breathed in and my ancient memories returned. I was in the timeless space and I saw myself at work in this sacred healing temple, living out my past life as a healer. Then, still in a dreamlike reverie, I saw myself bringing others to those same small temple healing rooms in a different land, in my present village and town, Bedford-Stuyvesant in Brooklyn, at *Smai Tawi*, at Heal Thyself / Know Thyself. Suddenly my past and present had become one.

As I grounded myself once more inside Het-Hru's temple, I realized that witnessing this sacred ground was like being surrounded by a huge holistic healing hospital. It was the supreme wellness sanitarium. There was the sacred lake of purification. It had long ago dried up, but in my inner vision I could see our people bathing joyfully in the rapture of purity. There were the ruins of the Birthing House, and the Fasting Rooms where people came from all over to heal under the spiritual guides of Ast and Het-Hru.

Then came the Baptism of Womanhood on the Island of Philae at Aswan, where the Temple of Ast (Isis) "[lay] beneath the water of Lake Nasser, but now due to the technical assistance from, yes, both Italy and West Germany, it was possible for them to save some of the monuments and re-erect them on the higher neighboring island of Agilka."[1]

The Temple of Ast now rests inside a womb-like place, metaphysically speaking. The Great Mother Ast is empowered again as she sits inside of this sacred protected space where she is surrounded by rocks that create the womb shape. The Nile water surrounds her, representing her sacred fluids. At the entrance of the watery womb are felluccas, the small Nile boats that ferry people who come from all over the globe to sit at the feet of the Great Mother and give homage to the Great Afrakan Queen. From every land they come, speaking in their own tongues,

in awe of her magnificence, trying to comprehend the magnitude of it all.

To our regret, the Mother has been physically defaced, her facial image literally chiseled out by the ignorance of people from various spiritual houses. But she still remains and nurtures everyone who looks upon her eyes of light, love, and guidance.

This disrespect for mothers in general that permeates this world, this absolute historical disregard of woman, must come to an end, or we are all doomed. Let the mother in you stand up and demand your just respect, reverence, and proper due. There will be salvation according to the degree that the original Mother returns to sit upon her sacred throne inside of her sacred self and we accept her gifts of spirituality, compassion, peace, and healing. Not a moment before the Black Mother, the Nubian Queen, gets her due in each and every land will there be peace on earth.

This was the message that I received from the Temple of Ast.

All the many temples I traveled to only opened me up to the truth of our spiritual Afrakan selves and brought home to me where the original spiritual concept of our body as a temple of the Living God came from. It was carved into the walls when we, the parents of today's earth people, lived in the belief that everything in life centers around the truth our Ancestors knew and still shared with those of us who come to them to receive these sacred teachings. One very important key was made clear to me. No one needed to come and teach us about spirituality and the power of the One Most High Creator/Creatress, for our entire land, life, government, education, science, and healing were totally centered around the power of the One Creator/Creatress. As reflections and expressions of the Creator/Creatress, the Priestesses and Priests, the Queens and Kings, the teachers and scholars exemplified and reflected the whole spirit of the society of *smai tawi*, of Upper and Lower Khamit (Egypt).

This trip did so much for me personally that I really can't put on paper and into words what's inside my heart, for the mending of my soul and the healing of my Afrakan mind were so very deep. At the great *merkut*, the pyramids at Giza outside Cairo, we went down into the foundations that led into a chamber that our Ancestors used for initiation. There we sang *hesi* (spiritual songs) and gave praise to the Divine for giving us an opportunity to return to this awesome sacred place, our home.

Then there was the empowering experience of standing on the grounds of the magnificent mortuary temple at Deir el Bahrin, where Queen/Pharaoh Hatshepsut had left her vibration. That let me know there was absolutely nothing that we can't achieve, as Afrakan women or as men, because her power, strength, and Maatness is in our bloodline. All of us may share and tap into her eternal spirit at any point to be used to lead and to rebuild, and refortify ourselves and our people into wholeness. It appeared that in nearly every temple we visited, Nut, the Heavenly Mother, ranged across the sky of the ceilings to indicate the holiness of the temples. Nut met us in the same room where Nebt-Het had stood by the head of Asar, Ast at his feet, to create the first recorded resurrection ritual of an Afrakan King Man. It was beyond glorious. The vision of Nut carved into several temple ceilings that we visited expressed to me how highly our ancient society regarded women. It revealed that ancient women were the embodiment of sacredness, and that through our spirit, we womenfolk can "wombnifest" all things.

Our Ancestors left us a legacy of sacredness that I've longed for. Our Ancestors have spoken to us from the walls, telling us to become one with Nature, for air (Shu), water (Nu), earth (Geb), and Fire (Ra) can heal our Body Temple as we drink, bathe in, and consume the Most High in all its glorious manifestation. We will re-create ourselves as we meditate on the heavenly realism of Nut, the house of the One Most High. A positive reawakening of the Afrakan woman's perspective of self was always a part of our healthy Afrakan Nile Valley reality. If we relentlessly seek out the source of our beginnings we can unlock the mystery and tap into our powers as the original Sacred Woman.

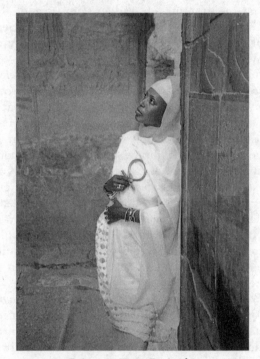

Priestess Taen-Ra in the
Temple of Her Ancestors

## Sacred Initiation: Seven-Day Transformative Work

- *Write your Sacred Woman Initiation speech* in your journal, your testament to what you have learned on this journey into the Eleven Gateways and how it has transformed you. Where are you now, and where are you ultimately going from here? Make your commitment statement sitting on and in your seat of the Great Divine Mother Mut Ast, Sacred Seat of Spiritual Power and High Holy Quality of Wellness.
- *Reflect on each Gateway and identify the greatest challenge you experienced.* Now spread out your freedom shawl and tell the story of each Gateway and its challenge and how you turned its lesson into a blessing. As you take delight in your growth, embrace and appreciate your strides. Remember, with each Gateway you have moved through, you have gained new energy, knowledge, wisdom, and enlightenment. The time has come to cherish and celebrate your experience in each Gateway. Give thanks to the NTRU for a safe journey, and proudly assume your seat as a Sacred Woman about to be unveiled.
- *Begin to contemplate the new name you want to symbolize your rebirth as a Sacred Woman.* Your new name should indicate your goals and aspirations. A name is traditionally given at your first birth, and now again as you are reborn a Sacred Woman. For example, as you take on the quality of the Most High for a balanced, harmonious life, you may take the name of Maat. If you seek divine inner and outer beauty according to your growth and development, you will become Het-Hru and be spiritually empowered by the powerful sacred words that express that aspect of the Creator/Creatress.

  In taking on an Afrakan spiritual name it is advisable to go through a ceremony such as the one presented in Gateway 9. This is because a name will draw a new level of understanding and awareness to you. The name you choose will guide, inspire, enhance, and transform you, so before taking it on, seek counsel from an Elder within your spiritual cultural order. Then you must fast and pray so the appropriate name will come to you through divine guidance.

  Taking such a name is like putting on a crown, so wear it well, represent your name well; represent your family, your community, with dignity and respect as you carry your name. Walk in the spirit of Truth as the Creator/Creatress blesses you through your name. Names are sacred; they tell your history, your past, your present, and your future. So be fully conscious and pure in heart, mind, and body as you receive your sacred name.

  Acquiring a new name is like being awakened, being born again, or coming fully alive. So a welcoming ceremony and rituals are very much in order as you take on this new life, this new responsibility to self and community, and above all to the One Most High.
- *Pour a libation of pure water or rainwater onto the earth outside your home,* or onto a plant indoors, with offerings of prayer and thanksgiving to the Creator/Creatress, then to your Ancestors (your Spiritual Guides), then to your community and the needs of your community.
- *Record your visions.* Each day of your preparation for initiation, particularly at sunrise while in meditation, you will receive visions from on high. Record them in your journal and be prepared to share them on the seventh day at your initiation ceremony.
- *Wear white clothes and accessories.* For seven days wear white from head to toe for purity and spiritual elevation. Cover your crown for spiritual protection.

**My Nefer Atum Sacred Lotus End-of-the-Week Commitment:**

I commit myself to establishing and maintaining the Nefer Atum spirit of my Sacred Lotus Initiation in all areas of my life.

Signature: _____

Date: _____

## PREPARATION FOR THE SACRED LOTUS REBIRTHING CEREMONY

We strengthen and grow with the lessons that come as we pass through each Gateway, each stage of development. We celebrate every new turning of our lives with a ceremony, because it charges us and lights the way. Observe the following:

- Surround yourself with female Elders who can advise you from their life experiences and give you direction and support in your new role. Receive advice about your new path and how to make it blossom.
- Receive a spiritual reading from a Smai Tawi Sacred Woman Priestess or reputable astrologer, numerologist, and/or spiritual reader to gain new insight into your sacred calling— discover the true purpose of your incarnation and what you were born to contribute to life.

During your seven days of preparation for your initiation, you will receive visions that are waiting to be born. Observe your visions, begin to breathe them, stand up and walk them into the world.

### Preparation

- Live-food preparation—supported by two to four other sister Queens.
- White ceremonial cloth for Rebirther(s).
- White ceremonial wrap for Initiate.
- White cloth to cover Birthing Stool.
- Gourd or white bowl for Initiates to drink from and wash in for spiritual bath.
- Wooden Birthing Stool or low stool of some sort.
- Powdered white clay or chalk to circle Birthing Stool.
- Two blue bowls to place inside of the birthing circle.
- Items for the Ceremonial Birthing Altar.
- White garments for everyone participating and attending.

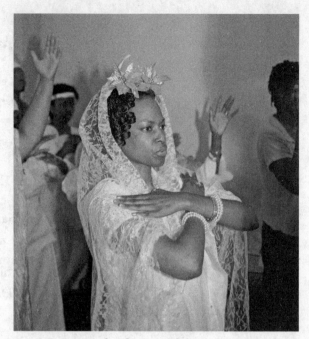

Preparing for the Sacred Lotus Initiation

### And Keep in Mind . . .

- The organizers will need to arrange for one or two rehearsals with everyone involved.
- We recommend making a videotape of the ceremony so the Initiate-to-be can share the experience with her mate and other family members, and for the family archives.
- If you would like to empower your Sacred Relationships, the ceremony may include your extended family members who have supported you and your journey. A ceremony of this sort can be very healing for everyone who is blessed to participate.

*It is very important that you be pure and healthy as you enter the final gate of initiation so that you can appreciate and receive the spirit of khepera, your transformation.*

### NEFER ATUM: THE SACRED LOTUS INITIATION

As we approach the end of the Eleven Gateways of Transformation, it is time to celebrate our birthing ourselves into a new, healthier, and more spiritually centered lifestyle.

The first birthing ceremonies were enacted thousands of years ago in the ancient Nile Valley when a mother-to-be was birthing a child. They were sacred rites that only women attended, and they marked the first recorded appearance of Midwives, Priestesses who were skilled at bringing new life into the world. Traditionally, from two to five Spiritual Midwives were present at the Birthing Ritual. Because these Priestesses lived a spiritual lifestyle, they were able to call forth the Divinity from the celestial realm to assist them in this sacred work. This ensured the safety and protection of both mother and child as they moved through this powerful and dangerous transformation to a new life.

Through rituals, such as breathing, meditating, *hesi* (sacred chant), and prayers, the Divine Child came to the village in the form of the newborn, and everyone's life was by its presence. The continuation of the family was looked upon as divine in ancient Khamit, and was supported from the spiritual realm. The mother was seen as a reflection of Ast, the Great Earthly Mother in the ancient Khamitic holy family. The husband was seen as Asar, the Great Earthly Father, and the child was viewed as Hru, a being of light, a Child of Victory.

Today we perform Birthing Ceremonies to celebrate our passage into Sacred Womanhood. This ceremony is very appropriate for women who have completed their Sacred Woman womb work and transformation. It is for the woman who has worked through her womb journal, danced the Dance of the Womb, consumed the Sacred Womb Nutritional Program, and performed regular meditation and prayer work over the resurrection of her womb. It is for the woman who has experienced healing in each of the Eleven Gateways of Transformation and taken on the Heal Thyself lifestyle, and has experienced a rebirth, becoming the child Heru—the new light reborn on higher and sacred ground.

The Rebirthing Ceremony is a graduation ceremony, for a woman or a circle of women who have completed the Sacred Woman Training. It allows them to feel renewed, reborn, and committed to continue living and sharing Sacred Woman Wisdom. The ceremony is to be presided over by a teacher(s), healer(s), mentor(s), or Elder(s)—women who have experience in guiding others through the Sacred Woman Training.

This ritual is also very much in order for a woman who has independently applied Sacred Woman teachings and techniques and desires to celebrate her rebirth, either by herself or within a circle of women supporters.

This ceremony is equally appropriate for women with intact wombs and for women who have experienced a hysterectomy, for we are all part of the celebration and the resurrection of the spirit of the Sacred Womb—man.

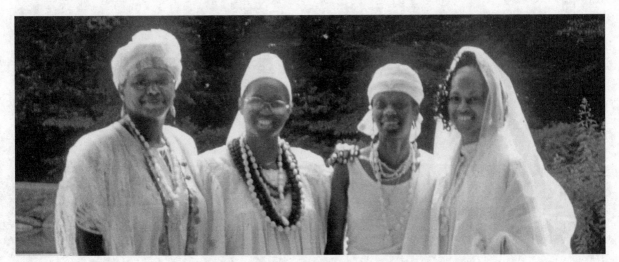

Aspirants prepare for Initiation.

# SACRED WOMAN GATEWAY ALTAR

White Tablecloth

Ast Spiritual Midwife Statue, or any Inspiring Female Symbol that Uplifts the Spirit of the Day

Vase of Lotus-Like White Flowers (lillies, orchids, carnations)

**Place a lotus candle on the altar to symbolize each Gateway and Guardian**

### Gateway Guardians

| Sacred Womb | Sacred Words | Sacred Foods | Sacred Movement | Sacred Beauty | Sacred Space | Sacred Healing | Sacred Realtionships | Sacred Union | Sacred Lotus Initiation | Sacred Time | Sacred Work |
|---|---|---|---|---|---|---|---|---|---|---|---|
| Nut | Tehuti | Ta-Urt | Bes | Het-Hru | Nebt-Het | Sekhmet | Maat | Ast | Nefer Atum into Ast | Seshat | Meskenet |

**Place at center of the altar**

Bowl of Purification Water Representing Nebt-Het, the Guardian of the Body Temple and Spiritual Midwife

**Place at left side of the altar to represent material gestation**

Bowl of Fruit

Bottle of Lotus Oil

Beautiful Box Containing Initiation Ankh

Maat Feather(s)

**Place at right side of the altar to represent Spiritual Works**

Bowl of Fruit

Pot of Incense

Place a bowl of fresh fruit on the altar in a wooden or glass bowl as an energetic offering to Divinity and your Ancestors. Return fruit to the soil, bury into the ground every 7 weeks and place the fruit on the altar for each new gateway you're about to enter into.

# THE SACRED LOTUS INITIATION

## The Rebirthing Ceremony

Sister Midwives, Elders, blood and extended family, and friends who support the Initiates who are Rebirthing are all welcome and requested to participate.

Everyone at the ceremony, both participants and guests, should be dressed in white to represent protection, purification, and spiritual renewal.

### 1. Opening Chant and Entrance of the Conductress

The ceremony is conducted by the presiding Khamitic Priestess and Spiritual Mut (Mother) Queen. She will be assisted by the Priestess of whichever group of sisters is presenting the ceremony. As the Priestess enters, she will signal the beginning of the drumming by a female drummer who accompanies her, along with the "village women" chanting "Ankh" (Eternal Life), their sweet voices making a joyful sound. Friends and extended family may join in the praise song. The Priestess will then give the signal for the entrance of the Initiates.

### 2. Welcoming Prayer

As the Aspirants enter, the village women call out and shout in a festive Afrakan way as the Priestess welcomes the Aspirant into the center of the Circle. As each Aspirant stands in the center, she is greeted by the spontaneous chants, praise songs, and dances of the Divine Midwives.

The presiding Priestess greets the Aspirants, standing before those who represent the Divine Spiritual Midwives. She acknowledges: "Today in Afrakan Khamatic tradition we celebrate your rebirth as a Sacred Woman. May the Creator/Creatress NTR bless you as you are taken through this birthing ceremony on this great day. May you have a safe journey and a beautiful delivery into your new life."

### 3. The Libation

A libation is poured before the Rebirthing Altar (see the Ceremonial Rebirthing Altar chart).

### 4. The Purification and Dressing Ritual of the Aspirants

This Purification Ritual is conducted by the Priestess and the Divine Midwives. This includes:

- Washing each Aspirant's feet
- Smudging her body with sage or frankincense and myrrh
- Placing the white garment of Initiation on her
- Offering her a bowl of purifying herb tea to drink

The village now calls forth the Divine Spiritual Midwives by name to empower the rebirthing ritual:

- Nut, Mother of all Wombs
- Ast, Great Earth Mother
- Nebt-Het, Lady of the Sacred House

- Meshkenet, Keeper of the Womb
  - Ta-Urt, Mother of the Earth
  - Bes, Keeper of Music and Dance, Lover of Children
  - Het-Hru, Keeper of Beauty, Love, the Arts

Each Divine Spiritual Midwife will circle the Aspirants as the purification ritual begins, speaking aloud of the role she performs in this ceremony and the Sacred Gifts that she brings, affirming that she carries the energy and blessings of the Divine.

### 5. Smudging
The Divine Spiritual Midwives then smudge the candidates and the entire village with frankincense and myrrh.

### 6. Blessing
The Priestess now blesses the Aspirants with the Maat feather, touching their crown, their heart center, and their Sacred Womb.

Guests of various other spiritual orders may also bless the Aspirants—for example, with Native American or Tibetan blessing and purification techniques.

### 7. Prayer Request for the Aspirants
Individually or together all of the Aspirants now recite.

Grant that I may reach the heaven of everlastingness and the mountain of thy favored ones, may I be joined with the shining beings, holy and perfect, may I come forth with them to see thy beauties thou shinest at eventide and thou goest to thy Mother Nut.

### 8. Acknowledgment
Now the Aspirant offers her acknowledgment of each of the Divine Midwives and reflects on the lessons learned at each Gateway and how her consciousness has been transformed. She may use her freedom shawl and the lessons embroidered in that cloth to show us the symbols of her story.

The Priestess acknowledges the trials and triumphs in the Initiate's story.

### 9. Formation of the Birth Canal
Divine Spiritual Midwives gather to form a birth canal. They stand in a row facing each other, arms held high, forming an archway for each Aspirant as she approaches the Birthing Stool. The ancient Egyptians sat their mothers-to-be on Birthing Stools, or they squatted on Birthing Bricks to use the power of gravity to help with the birth.

### 10. The Circle of Protection
The Priestess in charge sprinkles a circle of powdered white clay or powdered white chalk around the candidate sitting on the Birthing Stool. She next places two blue bowls with lotuslike flowers inside the sacred circle to help protect the mother.

### 11. Spiritual Offerings
The Priestess places ears of corn before the feet of the candidate for her to give as spiritual offerings to the sisters. This symbolizes that she's prepared to be a reborn child of the Divine.

## 12. Adoration of Inner and Outer Spiritual Guardians

The Divine Midwives representing Ast and Nebt-Het now seat the Mother on the Birthing Stool and sit at her right and left side for her protection.

## 13. Charge to the Aspirants

Each of the Divine Spiritual Midwives comes before the Aspirant, one at a time, to offer the spiritual crown of each Gateway of Divinity.

## Gate 0

*Spiritual Midwife:* "I, Nut, your Heavenly Cosmic Spiritual Mother of the Sacred Womb, ask that, before you sit in your Seat of Ast, you repeat this vow to commit to Nut's Divinity."

*Aspirant:* "I commit and vow from this day forward to establish a sacred relationship with my Sacred Womb in word, action, and deed for now and all eternity."

*Spiritual Midwife:* "So it is. You are now crowned with the Spirit of Nut."

## Gate 1

*Spiritual Midwife:* "I, Tehuti, your Spiritual Guardian of the Sacred Word, ask that, before you sit in your Seat of Ast, you repeat this vow to commit to Tehuti's Divinity."

*Aspirant:* "I commit and vow from this day forward to establish a sacred relationship with my Sacred Word in word, action, and deed for now and all eternity."

*Spiritual Midwife:* "So it is. You are now crowned with the Spirit of Tehuti."

## Gate 2

*Spiritual Midwife:* "I, Ta-Urt, your Spiritual Guardian of Sacred Food, ask that, before you sit in your Seat of Ast, you repeat this vow to commit to Ta-Urt's Divinity."

*Aspirant:* "I commit and vow from this day forward to establish a sacred relationship to divine healthy eating that I may nourish my mind, body, and spirit in word, action, and deed for now and all eternity."

*Spiritual Midwife:* "So it is. You are now crowned with the Spirit of Ta-Urt."

## Gate 3

*Spiritual Midwife:* "I, Bes, your Spiritual Guardian of Sacred Movement and Dance, ask that, before you sit in your Seat of Ast, you repeat this vow to commit to Bes's Divinity."

*Aspirant:* "I commit and vow from this day forward to establish a sacred relationship with my physical body through Sacred Movement and Dance in word, action, and deed for now and all eternity."

*Spiritual Midwife:* "So it is. You are now crowned with the Spirit of Bes."

## Gate 4

*Spiritual Midwife:* "I, Het-Hru, your Heavenly Cosmic Spiritual Mother of Sacred Beauty, ask that, before you sit in your Seat of Ast, you repeat this vow to commit to Het-Hru's Divinity."

*Aspirant:* "I commit and vow from this day forward to establish a sacred relationship with my Sacred Beauty in word, action, and deed for now and all eternity."

*Spiritual Midwife:* "So it is. You are now crowned with the Spirit of Het-Hru."

### Gate 5

*Spiritual Midwife:* "I Nebt-Het, your Spiritual Guardian of Sacred Space, ask that, before you sit in your Seat of Ast, you repeat this vow to commit to Nebt-Het's Divinity."

*Aspirant:* "I commit and vow from this day forward to establish a sacred relationship to create and live within my Sacred Space in word, action, and deed for now and all eternity."

*Spiritual Midwife:* "So it is. You are now crowned with the Spirit of Nebt-Het."

### Gate 6

*Spiritual Midwife:* "I, Sekhmet, your Spiritual Guardian of Sacred Healing, ask that, before you sit in your Seat of Ast, you repeat this vow to commit to Sekhmet's Divinity."

*Aspirant:* "I commit and vow from this day forward to establish a sacred relationship with my Sacred Healing in all areas of my life in word, action, and deed for now and all eternity."

*Spiritual Midwife:* "So it is. You are now crowned with the Spirit of Sekhmet."

### Gate 7

*Spiritual Midwife:* "I, Ast, your Spiritual Guardian of Sacred Relationships, ask that, before you sit in your Seat of Ast, you repeat this vow to commit to Ast's Divinity."

*Aspirant:* "I commit and vow from this day forward to establish and maintain a sacred relationship with all my relationships in word, action, and deed for now and all eternity."

*Spiritual Midwife:* "So it is. You are now crowned with the Spirit of Ast."

### Gate 8

*Spiritual Midwife:* "I, Maat, your Spiritual Guardian of Sacred Union, ask that, before you sit in your Seat of Ast, you repeat this vow to commit to Maat's Divinity."

*Aspirant:* "I commit and vow from this day forward to establish and maintain a sacred relationship with my male reflection in word, action, and deed for now and all eternity."

*Spiritual Midwife:* "So it is. You are now crowned with the Spirit of Maat."

### Gate 9

*Spiritual Midwife:* "I, Nefer Atum, your Spiritual Guardian of Sacred Initiation, Guide to Inner Illumination, Keeper of the Sacred Aromas, Divine Guide of World Healing and Unification (Smai Tawi), ask that, before you sit in your Seat of Ast, you repeat this vow to commit to Nefer Atum's Divinity."

*Aspirant:* "I commit and vow from this day forward to establish my Sacred Divine inner and outer world vision. I vow to continue to rebirth through Sacred Midwife Meshkenet so that I may sit on the Sacred Power Seat of the Divine Mother Ast that is indwelling and so that I may wear the Illuminated Crown of Nefer Atum in word, action, and deed for now and all eternity."

*Spiritual Midwife:* "So it is. You are now crowned with the Spirit of Meshkenet, the Rebirther, Ast, the Great Mother, and Nefer Atum, the Illuminated One."

### 14. Dance of the Womb Representing Labor and Rebirth

The Dance of the Womb representing labor and the rebirthing process is performed to drums and bells by the Spiritual Midwife representing the guardian Mut (Mother) Renenet, who oversees harvest and fertility. This womb dance represents the beginning of labor, and each movement is symbolic of the contractions of birth. The music and the dance flow through Mut Renenet to the Aspirant.

### 15. The Breathing Ritual and Anointing of the Lotus

As the energy of labor is transferred from Mut Renenet to the Aspirant, she is in full labor now, demonstrated through this Breathing Ritual, headed by the Divine Midwife representing Nebt-Het, the Keeper of the Breath. It was Nebt-Het who stood at the head of Asar, helping to breathe life into him along with her sister Ast for his first resurrection after his murder and dismemberment by his brother Seth. She does the same for the Aspirants.

The presiding Priestess now comes forth to lead the village in the Breathing Ritual. The Divine Midwives representing Ast and Nebt-Het go to the mother's side to reenact the birthing with a thousand Fire Breaths of Nefer Atum.

Ast squats before the candidate who represents all the Aspirants, and together all the Aspirants do the Fire Breaths, representing the birthing process. Nebt-Het, with feathers in each hand, stands behind the candidate, and spreads her wings. With each breath, her arms go up for the inhalation and down for the exhalation as the entire village of womenfolk breathe together as one force. This collective breathing ceremony allows the Aspirant and the entire village to experience their own rebirth, sister to sister, for we are each other's reflection. My healing and rebirthing are yours, and I claim yours as mine. *Note:* The village can join the Aspirants on their last one hundred breaths.

### 16. The Rebirth

The Priestess then faces the representative of the Aspirants and asks:

"Sister-Midwives, I ask you now, is there anyone among you who knows a reason why this Sister should not be a candidate for rebirth?"

(If no objections are raised, the Priestess says:)

"Midwives, please take your stations."

(In unison, the Midwives ask their Aspirants:)

"Are you ready to give birth?"

(The Aspirants reply as one in a resounding voice from deep in their wombs:)

*"Yes!"*

"Are you strong enough?"

*"Yes!"*

"Have you truly passed through each Gateway?"

"*Yes!*"

"Are you ready to see who you really are?"

"*Yes!*"

"Are you willing to claim, now and forever, the fullness of your being?"

"*Yes!*"

(The Priestess says:)

"Sister-Midwives, please raise the Sacred Mirror."

(The Midwives hold up the mirror before the faces of the Aspirants and say:)

*"Aspirant, behold the face of your true self!"*

(As the Aspirants gaze at their reflections in the Sacred Mirror, the Priestess says:)

"When you feel ready, speak these *hekau* words of power:

"*'My face is of Nefer Atum. Nuk Pu Ntrt Hmt.'*"

(The drums roll and the shekeres rattle in joyous celebration. Then the Priestess says to the Aspirants:)

"You have now rebirthed yourselves. You have been reborn as Nefer Atum, a divine Sacred Woman."

### 17. *The Naming*

The Spiritual Midwives then offer the Initiate an ancestral charge from the women of the village and ask her:

"By what new name shall we call you?" The Initiate says:

> *I am pure at a place of passage that is*
> *great. I have destroyed my defects. I*
> *have made an end of my wickedness. I*
> *have annihilated the faults that belong to*
> *me. I myself am pure. I am might. Oh*
> *Gatekeepers, I have made the way. I am*
> *like unto you. I have come forth by day.*

"My name is [Sacred Name]. I am a Sacred Woman. *Nuk Pu Ntrt Hmt.*" (The Initiate explains the meaning of her new name.)

The Initiates then say together:

*"I come forth, I shine. I go in and I come to life. My seat is on my throne. I sit in the pupil of my first eye. I have commanded my seat. I rule it by my mouth, speaking and silent. I maintain an exact balance. Season to season, the Creator/Creatress and I are one. I am one coming from one."*

(The Priestess then calls forward each Initiate by her new name and crowns her with the Sacred Lotus Crown.)

### 18. *Honoring and Gifting the New Initiates*

Family members now come forward to acknowledge the new Initiates. The eldest family member drapes the seat of the Sacred Woman with a new cloth. The Initiate then takes her seat to symbolize her return to her throne. Individual family members now offer special gifts at the feet of the Initiate. This is a special time for the family to give praise and acknowledgment for the profound achievement of their Sacred Woman who has dared to reach the heights.

### 19. Address from the Priestess: The Responsibilities

"Our planet is dying because the collective voices of healthy, whole women have not spoken out loudly enough. Newly reborn Sacred

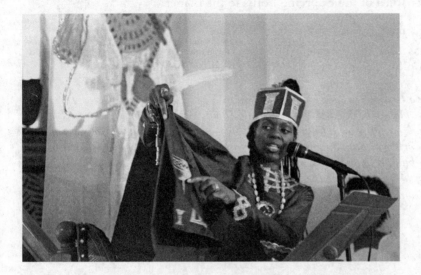

Women can channel a high healing that will cause the planet to vibrate at its highest frequency and bring us all back to life so we may be saved.

"Sacred Women, you have assumed your Sacred Seat of Ast. I now give you a commission for yourself and for planetary wellness:

• Be sure always to take care of yourself first so you will be able to reach out and serve others.
• Create a Sacred Womb Healing Circle or a Sacred Woman Sister-to-Sister Support Group.
• Mothers, draw closer to your daughter(s) and niece(s). Keep the lines of communication open.
• Help a sister! Save a womb, save a breast by sharing information on the Sacred Woman Natural Living lifestyle.
• Help women in need of help. Let the Spirit direct your course.
• Teach brothers, men, sons, and husbands how to cope with a Sacred Woman by helping them to connect to their Sacred Selves.
• Be a mentor or a spiritual friend to other women in need by helping them to connect to their Sacred Selves.
• Devote time at drug and alcohol abuse centers to share holistic wellness teachings.
• Devote time at shelters as you share your Sacred Woman survival knowledge with those in need.
• Raise funds for women in shelters to help them to get a new start, and to aid them in activating their vision.
• Encourage women to start and operate their own businesses.
• Teach the Sacred Woman text by becoming a certified Sacred Woman Priestess/Guide/Advisor/Consultant.
• Be an example of a Sacred Woman all the time to encourage and uplift self and others.

• It's not over. Now that you have gathered your tools of wellness and sacredness, go forth bravely from your Seat of Ast. Place the Lotus of Nefer Atum upon your crown consciousness and spread the good news and the sweet spirit of the Supreme Lotus to the planet."

### 20. Closing Prayers

The Priestess and the Divine Midwives, representing Ast (Isis) the Great Mother, together offer closing prayers, letting Spirit be their guide.

### 21. Sacred Initiate's Prayer

*Divine Holy of Holies, blessed be my arrival to Absolute Divinity so that I may be a vessel for the world to receive through me pure, loving, healing light. May we all be made whole as it was in the beginning, when the world was pure and filled with green land and purified oceans, clean air, rich soil, and magnificent human light beings, melanin-charged, spiritually potent people who inhabited the earth. The world has now come to the end of the road of its destruction. We take our seats as Sacred Women so that we may begin again!*

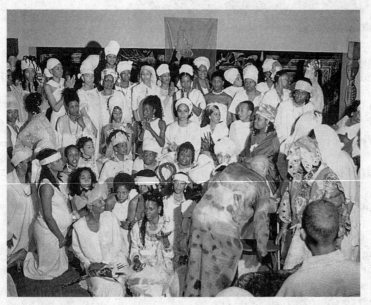

Sacred Women
Initiates

### 22. The Global Sacred Woman Proclamation

Together the Initiates proclaim the truth of their new consciousness through the power of Sacred Words.

# THE GLOBAL SACRED WOMAN
# PROCLAMATION

*We the Sacred Women of the globe declare and proclaim Planetary Healing as we sit on our seats of power and purity. Swiftly gaining control of our lives and thus directing our destiny, we look out over what we have created, and in deep reflection and intense contemplation we see our challenges as numerous sacred opportunities—predestined and necessary as fuel for our present ascension.*

*Through self-healing and self-knowledge—with the tools of divine grace—we gather from the four corners of the globe an illustrious tapestry of Sacred Woman ways envisioned through our inner Gateways. We, the Sacred Women of the world, do not ask for permission, consent, or approval to be who we are.*

*Our hands raised in praise to heavenly Nut, our feet firmly planted as roots in Ta-Urt, the earth, we take our sacred seat as we absorb the earth's power and stability, fortitude, and consistency.*

*Whether we face tidal wave or windstorm, hurricane, monsoon rain, or noncompassionate man-made laws, we shall not be moved from our righteous position. For it is here, in consciousness, that we sit as Sacred Women, upon the seat where planetary resurrection begins.*

## CHAPTER 15

# GATEWAY 10: SACRED TIME

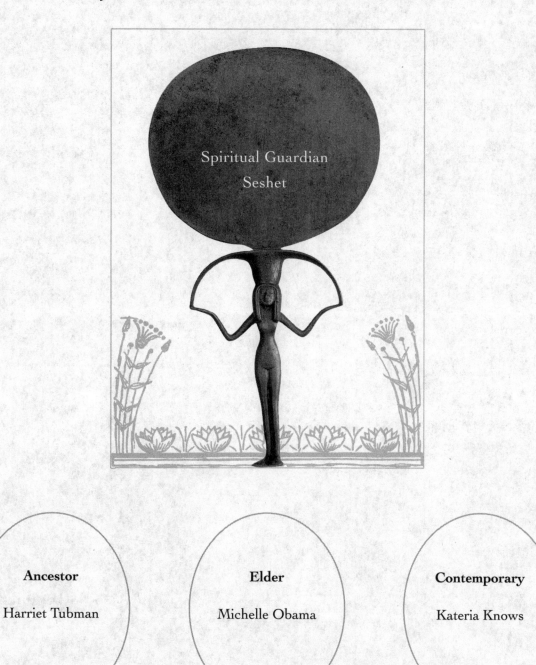

Spiritual Guardian
Seshet

**Ancestor**

Harriet Tubman

**Elder**

Michelle Obama

**Contemporary**

Kateria Knows

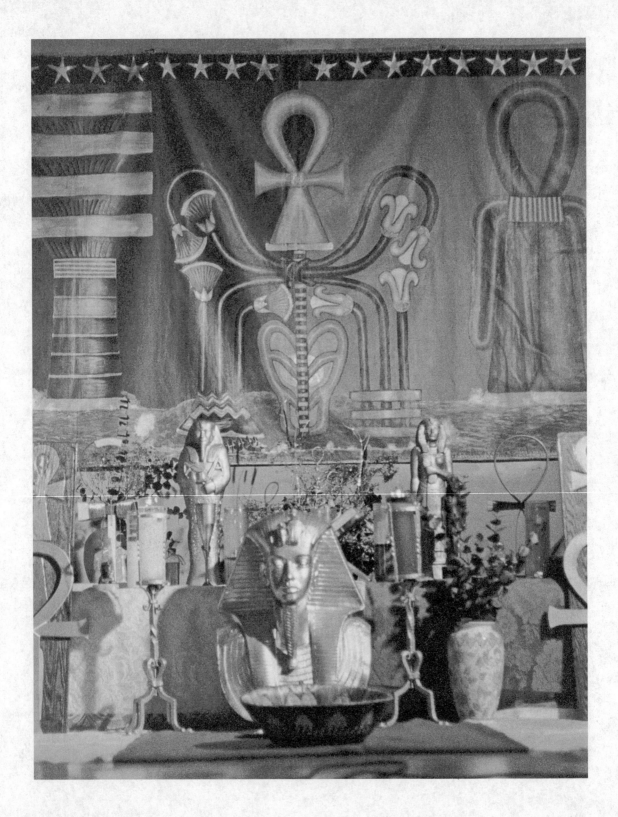

# SACRED TIME ALTAR WORK
## Face Your Heart to the East — to the Rising Sun
*(Layout from top view)*

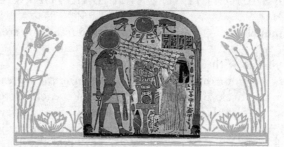

**Mount Pictures on Wall, Above Altar**

Picture of
Spiritual Guardian

Picture of
Ancestor

Picture of
Sacred Self

Picture of
Elder

Picture of
Contemporary

Baptism Bowl (WATER)

Feather
(AIR)

Ankh for Eternal Life or
Other Sacred Symbol
(SPIRIT)

Flowering Plant
(EARTH)

*Anointing Oil:*
Rosemary

Deep Yellow Candle
(FIRE)

*Sacred Stone:*
Topaz

Food for your Ancestors (bowl of organic non-GMO fruit)
*(Release from the altar after twenty-four hours.)*

**Place on your altar a knotted cord to measure an hour.**

Sacred tablecloth (deep yellow) and scarf to wear during prayer.
Sacred color cloth to lay before altar. Sacred instruments to be played as you pray.

# GATEWAY 10: SACRED TIME DAILY SPIRITUAL OBSERVANCES

## Gateway Element: Air

Sacred Time is life. What you do with your time will determine the quality of your life. Time moves within and through the circle of life; it's ongoing, and it never ends. From Life in the body, to Life in the Spirit, time is forever evolving. Time as life is to be cherished and appreciated that your days and nights be filled with peace, joy, and abundance.

Perform spiritual exercises of ascension daily for seven days to awaken the possibility of purpose. Then, for twelve weeks and thereafter, develop and birth your work with the teachings found within this Gateway.

### 1. The Spiritual Bath

Use rosemary oil to attune you to the Divine rhythm of life and to open your crown *arit* (chakra). Add 7 drops of rosemary to your bathwater and to a bowl of purified water on your altar, and sprinkle a few drops around your prayer space.

### 2. Your Altar

Set up your sacred altar on the first day of your entry into this Gateway. You may set up your altar according to your own spiritual or religious beliefs (see page 18). Sit before your altar quietly and meditatively on the floor on a pillow, or in a chair. Add a few drops of rosemary oil to your baptism bowl on your altar, and sprinkle a few drops around your prayer space.

*Anoint with rosemary oil.* Select only pure essential oils. Use essential oil of rosemary to anoint your crown and your third eye (in the center of your forehead between the brows), the Body Temple Gateway of supreme spirituality. Next, anoint the heart (the Body Temple Gateway of compassion and divine love). Also anoint your womb area, the palms of your hands (to make everything you touch become more sacred), and the bottoms of your feet (to spiritually

align yourself for stepping out in power, promise, and faith).

### 3. Opening the Gateway

To invoke each Gateway's Spiritual Guardian, you may use whatever words pour from your heart. For example, here's a prayer that might be used at Gateway 10:

*Sacred and Divine Seshat, Spiritual Guardian of the Gateway of Sacred Time, please accept my deepest gratitude for your healing presence on my altar and in my life. Thank you for your guidance and inspiration and for your love and blessings, and please accept my love and blessings in return.* Hetepu.

### 4. Libation

Pour a libation for the Sacred Time Gateway from a cup, or sprinkle water from a bowl onto the earth or a plant, as you call out this prayer of praise and adoration.

*I pour this libation in praise and adoration of the Sacred Mother Guardian of Gateway 10,* the Great Cosmic Mother of Sacred Time.
*I pour this libation in praise and adoration of the Ancestor of Gateway 10,* Harriet Tubman.
*I pour this libation in praise and adoration of the Elder of Gateway 10,* Michelle Obama.
*I pour this libation in praise and adoration of my Divine Self and my Divine Contemporary,* Kateria Knows.

### 5. Sacred Woman Spirit Prayer

Gently ring your bell, or softly play another sacred instrument at the beginning and end of the prayer.

*Sacred Spirit, NTR, hold me near, close to your bosom. Protect me from all harm and fear, from the blows of life. Direct my steps in the right way as I journey through this vision. Sacred Spirit, surround me in your absolutely perfect light. Anoint me in your sacred pu-*

rity, peace, and divine insight. Bless me, truly bless me as I share this sacred life. Teach me, Sacred Spirit, to be in tune with the Universe. Teach me how to heal with the inner and outer elements of air, fire, water, and earth.

### 6. Sacred Time Prayer

Shake bells, beat a sacred drum, or play another instrument at the beginning and ending of this prayer.

*I am in full gratitude for each moment and beat of time I have spent in my life. Sacred Spirit, may I honor my life by living in harmony and in tune with the moon, sun, and stars, which fill me, my time, my relations, my family, and humanity.*

### 7. Chanting Hesi

Chant this *hesi* four times:

*Nuk Pu Ntrt Hmt* — I am a Sacred Woman.

### 8. Fire Breaths

Prepare your Fire Breaths by slowly inhaling four times and exhaling four times. Then, when you are totally at ease, begin your eleven hundred Fire Breaths. Inhale deeply like a pump through your nose (mouth closed) as you expand the breath down into the abdomen, then back up to the chest. Completely exhale out through your nostrils from your abdomen as it contracts and the lungs release your breath completely. Repeat this breath rapidly in and out, in and out.

Allow each deep Fire Breath to represent the opening of the thousand lotus petals of illumination and radiance, ultimately reaching Nefer Atum — the ultimate Afrakan Lotus station of Divinity.

### 9. Gateway 10: Seshat Meditation

Each day of the twenty-one days you spend working through Gateway 10, increase the length of time you spend in meditation. The longer you are in meditation, the deeper your inner peace will be, and the more vibrant your *ka*

(spirit) will become. The cleaner your Body Temple, the sooner it will be able to live permanently in the peace and inner balance of the meditative state.

Visualize yourself being in harmony in and with time. If you can see from your inner vision, then you can create your reality. Applying and visualizing the Guardians at work in your life will bring forth your excellence.

- Begin by inhaling into the spirit of Nebt Het awakening within you at 4 A.M. as you tap into and receive your inner treasure in the exhalation.
- Inhale Ast at noon as you activate and receive your treasure.
- Inhale the spirit of Het-Hru by 4 P.M. Exhale into self-care and self-love as you receive the results of nurturing your body, mind, and spirit through a vegan dinner, self-massage, healing bath, etc.
- At the closing of your day, inhale into the spirit of Nut as you exhale a night of peace and rest from a powerful day of Divine Wellness.

*Color Visualization.* In Gateway 10, which honors the element of air, visualize deep yellow. Deep yellow is the color for divine wisdom and high intellect. It carries positive, magnetic currents that strengthen your nerves and brain. As you perform your meditation, wear a piece of deep yellow cloth on yourself (scarf or headwrap) and place a deep yellow cloth on your altar.

*Sacred Stone Meditation.* While in meditation, hold a topaz in your palm over your womb. The topaz is the sacred healing stone of Gateway 10.

### 10. Herbal Tonics

Drink herbal tea while you are doing your altar, prayer work, and journal work in Gateway 10. Use the Heal Thyself Woman's Herbal Formula (see the product list in the appendix) for General Womb Wellness.

Alfalfa tea, made from the plant's roots and

leaves, is another useful tonic for Gateway 10 as it strengthens higher vision while purifying the body's anatomy.

Drink your tea for twenty-one days to receive the full benefits of attuning to Gateway 10. Enjoy your herb tea in your favorite mug during or after spiritual writing. Be sure to finish the tea before 1 P.M.

*Preparation.* Use one teabag or 1 teaspoon loose tea to 8 ounces of water boiled in a nonmetallic pot. Boil water, turn off flame, then add tea and steep. Strain herbs from water. Drink before or after your morning bath or sacred shower. Drink with joy and peace as you breathe quietly between sips and settle into easy contemplation.

### 11. Flower Essences

To deepen your experience of Gateway 10, take 4 drops of rosemary essence four times per day directly on or under the tongue, or add the same amount to a small glass of purified water and sip. Rosemary helps you overcome stagnation that blocks forward movement in time. For instructions on how to choose flower essences, see page 23.

### 12. Diet and Movement

Daily, follow the Sacred Woman Natural Living Dietary Laws given in the Womb Wellness Cleansing Food Plan (see page 71) and do the Dance of the Womb movements presented in Gateway 3. Omit soy; limit whole grain and starch. Increase green vegetables to strengthen your purpose.

### 13. Sacred Time Journal Writing

Journal writing is best done after your sacred bath and/or meditation. When you are cleansed and centered, you can receive with grace spiritual messages from the One Most High. When in the spirit, messages travel down through your spirit mind, to your heart, into your hand, and onto the paper. (This is how I do all of my writing.)

The best time to receive your spiritually written work is after you have completed your altar work, between the hours of 4 A.M. and 6 A.M. Keep a very special pen and journal by or on your altar to work with the power, force, and stillness at the coming of the dawn.

At this time, write in your journal the thoughts, activities, experiences, and interactions that occurred previously in your daily life. You might also want to write down your self-inspired hopes, visions, desires, and affirmations so that you can draw on them for help and support when needed. You'll be surprised at how healing and sustaining your journal wisdom can be.

### 14. Senab Freedom Shawl or Quilt

By the time you reach Gateway 10, your Senab Freedom Shawl or Quilt should be completed.

### 15. Sacred Tools

Knotted cord to measure an hour.

### 16. Sacred Reminder

Throughout the next week, you are to observe closely the wisdom presented the Gateway you are in. For maximum results, live freely in tune with the various systems of body, mind, and spirit wellness presented. Honor the Seven-Day Transformative Work at the end of the Gateway.

### Closing Sacred Words

*Divine Creator/Creatress, help me to honor the sacredness of time. Thank you for all the blessings you have granted me.*

## SESHAT AND THE LAWS OF SACRED TIME BY QUEEN ESTHER SARR

*Queen Esther Sarr is the Dean of the Global Village and guide to healing by the light of the moon.*

When we think about the phenomena of life-forms, the planets, the solar system, the Universe, and Cosmic dynamics, we realize it is actually a miracle how all these systems work in harmony and do not collide! Each has its own system and regimen separate from the others, yet at the same time they are connected to one another due to originating in the same source. It is reminiscent of an orchestra where each set of instruments plays their own part, but the conductor has all parts synchronized together in harmony to create beautiful music. When we examine the Orchestra of the Universe on a closer level, we see that it also deals with timing, rhythm, and synchronization. Sixty minutes in an hour, twenty-four hours in a day, seven days in a week, and twenty-eight days in a month (this is what nature provides as a natural month or a lunar month). The moon rotates through eight phases, ascending and descending in a twenty-eight-day span. The ascending phases are the new moon, the crescent moon, the first-quarter moon, the gibbous moon, and the full moon. The descending phases are the disseminating moon, the last-quarter moon, and the balsamic.

Julius Caesar, born in July, gave thirty-one days to the calendar for his birth month. His son Augustus Caesar, born in August, also added more days to his birth month, giving August thirty-one days. With these and other additions, our calendar now has only one accurate month according to the natural lunar cycles. That is February, the only month with twenty-eight days.

Here in the Gateway of Seshat, I lead a class titled "Healing by the Light of the Moon." I educate sacred women on how to identify the different moon phases, what the phases represent, and how to align our lives in order and harmony with natural laws. Working with the moon cycles, we establish consistent regimens for wellness. All women are unified under the moon through our moon cycles and the lunar cycles involved with childbearing. Although the moon is not seen globally by all women at the same time, the ever-present energy radiating from it is a constant and powerful force for unity. The awakening of the Wise Wombman is an integral part of the Sacred Woman Journey that we cherish as we expand toward enlightenment and embrace Sacred Time.

### "Two Thousand Seasons"

*There is no beauty but in relationships. Nothing cut off by itself is ever beautiful . . . All beauty is in the creative purpose of our relationships. The Destroyers will set traps for the body, traps for the heart, traps to destroy the mind. Such a group, a world of creation, of beauty, none of the Destroyers' traps can hold.*

—AYI KWEI ARMAH

Sacred Woman is such a group, and in our awakening, as we become liberated with the Gateways, we get to overcome the traps set. For over two decades, this quote has caused me to ponder our relationships, the Destroyers, beauty, and the traps. In the spirit of Seshat—Sacred Time, *Sacred Woman* is right on time to aid us in healing all our relations. Throughout all seasons, from new moon to full moon, our days flow from Mother Nebt-Het hours (between 4 and 6 A.M., tapping into our intuition) to Mother Ast hour (midday) to manifesting (wombnifesting—what you received from your treasure chest of intuition) to Het-Hru (afternoon—nurturing yourself through acts of love) to Nut (nighttime—when you rest and heal in order to rise up to yet another dawn of Nebt-Het). With each day, following the flow of the Sun rising and setting and integrating the Gateways in one powerful tapestry of inner relationship healing, we get to evolve into optimal beautiful beings. Healing our relationship with ourselves, making ourselves whole, we heal our relationships outside of ourselves as well.

*Sacred Woman* is all about our relationship with ourselves, which reflects in one way or another our relationships with all others, including our mothers, fathers, grandparents (elders), mates, friends, children, coworkers, community, and so forth. I've found that all our relationships are an extension of the past, present, future of our conscious and subconscious mind; also included are our feelings, our emotions, our heart, our states of being. Sacred Woman Gateways hold up the inner and outer mirrors; we can see reflection of ourselves and of our relations. With each Gateway, if we look deeply enough we will learn the lessons that our relationships offer and thereby get an opportunity to heal through those relationships and get out of the traps. We get the chance to overcome, to transform, to undo the traps that we find ourselves in from Gateway to Gateway.

When I think about the word "trap," I think of a bear . . . caught. The animal cannot open the trap to free itself. Locked in, the animal bleeds out and dies. The trap is fatal. Then I think about human beings and how we can be trapped in various ways. In our minds if we lock into toxic, debilitating thoughts from which we can't seem to free ourselves, it can cause us to attract and create toxic patterns such as violence, abuse, lack, and limitation. Toxic thoughts and patterns often are passed down through our bloodlines as if from a DNA stream of life. We must address thoughts and conditions such as lack and limitation, consumption of dietary toxic food, and unconscious living. Each addictive bite of food, each toxic thought is like a bear trap clutching us until we are numb, bleeding out, dying daily.

I have witnessed that as we travel through the Gateways, the traps begin to loosen and melt away. This journey is the passport to deliver us out of the traps and into a beautiful pathway of holistic freedom. As we travel from Gateway to Gateway, our traps magically, mystically begin to melt away. We can free ourselves from the gruesome traps of darkness, downtroddenness, hurt, rage, and revenge. We become more beautiful. Gateway to Gateway, we begin to escape from the mental, physical, spiritual, and financial traps that have been set by the residue of slavery, colonialism, and racism. I am encouraged to report that with each Sacred Woman Gateway we become free of the traps. Liberation is at hand.

Sacred Woman, it is time to take the Harriet Tubman walk. It is time for her daughters to look up at the stars and Mother Nut (the sky mother); to trust their intuition (Mother Nebt-Het, the Lady of the Heavenly Realm); and to walk as herbalists and healers within (Sekhmet). Run off the plantation of disease, pain, and suffering. Like Mother Harriet Tubman, we must run for our freedom, away from the big house, the cotton fields, the whip, and the chain. After our Mother Hero freed herself, she looked back and went back time after time to help others to get out of the trap. Fearlessly, she came back for us despite a ransom on her life. Even with the blood-hungry wolf-dogs sniffing her out for the kill, this woman of courage loved us and led hundreds of us to liberation. Mother Harriet said: "I would have freed more if they knew they were slaves."

The journey of Sacred Woman is a Mother Harriet Tubman Journey, is a King/Queen Hatshepsut Journey, a Queen Mother Moore Journey, a Queen Nzinga Journey. In her own way, each of these freedom-fighting women fought for our wholeness to get us out of the traps.

In Gateway 0: Nut, Sacred Womb Wellness Teachings, we get out of the trap of womb disease and womb pain in order to reach Womb Wellness. The womb pain and dis-ease trap is widespread. Just ask your mother, grandmother, auntie, and/or your sister-friends. Listen and realize you will be sharing womb trap stories. Most women learn not to complain and just suffer in silence. They learn to try to numb the pain with painkillers that ultimately contribute to killing, numbing out the womb. From these sick wombs we attract sick mates and birth sick children. The global cycle of pain continues to birth itself. Nut said, "Come to me and I will help you." It is time to be free from STDs, fibroid tumors, chronic PMS, heavy bleeding, and infertility. It is time to get free from the traps. "I will heal you and get you out of the womb trap, my daughter."

Gateway 1: Tehuti, Sacred Word. Get out of the trap of words of poor communication that destroy, and away from words of abuse to self or others. Reach words that heal, transform, and rejuvenate.

*Gateway 2: Ta-Urt, Sacred Food.* Get out of the trap of craving consumption of toxic debilitating food (flesh, junk, frozen, sugar, fried, microwaved, processed food). Heal with food from the Garden that rejuvenates and detoxifies.

*Gateway 3: Bes, Sacred Movement.* Get out of the trap of stagnation and constipation. Tap into mobility; unblock your life and move forward.

*Gateway 4: Het-Hru, Sacred Beauty.* Get out of the trap of low self-esteem and inner child pain and conflict. Tap into your beauty; love yourself and your inner child and get free.

*Gateway 5: Nebt-Het, Sacred Space.* Get out of the trap of mental confusion causing lack of spiritual confidence and clutter. Learn to trust your intuition as you cleanse and clear your inner and outer space.

*Gateway 6: Sekhmet, Sacred Healing.* Get out of the trap of all forms of disease, such as high blood pressure, hypertension, diabetes, and arthritis. Tap into your inner healer and heal yourself in body, mind, and spirit.

*Gateway 7: Maat, Sacred Relationships.* Get out of the trap of drinking and drugging to suppress your hurt. Get free. Get out of the trap of broken, wounded family relationships; of past mother or father hurts. Tap into attracting and creating vibrant relationships. Tap into the spirit of forgiveness.

*Gateway 8: Ast, Sacred Union.* Get out of the trap of divorce and resentful relationships. Tap into your inner transformation and heal in and through your relationships. Get out of the trap of poverty. Tap into your wealth by unifying left- and right-brain inner power.

*Gateway 9: Nefer Atum, Sacred Lotus.* Get out of the trap of dwelling in the mud of toxicity. Purify yourself and let your light shine.

*Gateway 10: Seshat, Sacred Cosmic Time.* Get out of the trap of procrastination. Spin your *arit* (chakra) wheels of spiritual freedom with each and every day you elevate.

*Gateway 11: Meshkenet, Sacred Work.* Get out of the trap of not living on purpose. Tap into your Sacred Work.

Rather than be trapped in a physical or spiritual prison, as a Sacred Woman continue to live on your Sacred Path. Rather than become homeless through gentrification and other forms of displacement, we will overcome, we will turn to our beautiful holistic selves and rise and shine. Because, Sacred Woman Healer, this is our time!

# IT'S TIME TO GET OUT OF THE TRAPS

## The Mask Maintains the Trap, and the Trap Masks Are Interchangeable

We secure the traps with the mask to hide how lost we are from others. As we purify ourselves through the cleansing of our 7 Aritu, we remove the mask. With each *arit* getting clearer every day, with each *arit* meditation performed, we become whole.

The TRAP is a cover-up of weaknesses, insecurities, hurts, pain. The TRAP represents deception, dishonesty, dis-ease, and division. The TRAP hides the truth as it covers up your true feelings and thoughts. The MASK may be on out of fear of loss . . . lost relationships, lost love, lost finances. The MASK offers a false sense of protection. The MASK can have many appearances: beauty, ugliness, strength, weakness, love, hate, support, control, and so forth. A person may wear the MASK as a means to an end. A person may wear the MASK to gain favor, love, a job, sex, material wealth, opportunities, friendships, marriage, and control.

The MASK cannot be trusted. The MASK may smile at you while cutting your throat. The MASK may offer you the world while stealing you blind. The MASK can operate as your mother, father, mentor, child, friend, lover, husband, wife, confidant, boss, coworker, neighbor, or lover.

To get favor, the MASK will give you whatever you need to give the MASK what it needs from you. The MASK will make you feel that you can't live without it. The MASK from others can capture your heart, get into your business, get into your bed, take over your mind, steal your trust, your identity. The MASK might take over your home, destroy your reputation, take your breath away, and break your heart. The clearer you are, the more purified you are, the less you will attract people who wear the MASK and the more you can discern who they are.

Perpetual disease is a MASK for spiritual and/or emotional damage and pain. The longer we go without healing the spiritual and emotional body, the more calcified and chronic the MASK becomes. This calcification can be called cancer (an eating-away of one's life force), high blood pressure (emotional heart pain), fibroid tumors (deep-seated anger), heart attack (broken heart), or arthritis (stagnation).

To get out of the traps, we must walk diligently through each Gateway and each energy center. Freedom awaits—be diligent with your Gateway and *arit* practice.

## THE MAKING OF THE ARITU SYSTEM FROM ANTIQUITY TO NOW

Now that you have journeyed from Gateway 0: Sacred Woman up and through Gateway 9: Sacred Initiation as a seed of light coming out of the mud, you've reached your full bloom. You are coming into Sacred Time in Gateway 10 to secure, protect, maintain, and magnify your freedom, your liberation.

Through the 7 Aritu Wheels of Power— a Khamitic energy healing system of transformation—you will come out of all traps. Begone, the domestic violence trap, the divorce trap, the zombie music that has locked a generation in a rhythmic trap. Begone, social traps, poverty traps, toxic dietary food traps, depression/anxiety emotional traps, erectile dysfunction trapping the men and fibroid tumor, hysterectomy, and menstrual pain trapping the women. Let us be freed from the broken-family traps, the single-parent traps, the forced-to-live-in-shelters traps. Let us be freed from the incarceration trap and from the inner-child bondage trap. Let us be rid of high blood pressure, diabetes, cancer traps. From Sacred Woman to the 7 Aritu to living out our purpose of Meshkenet, we will overcome all traps and return to being a holistic radiant people. Our brothers, fathers, grandfathers, and sons can join us on a twenty-one-day to eighty-four-day (a season) of Green

Garden Eating shared in Sacred Woman Gateway of Ta-Urt. The family can join in the 7 Aritu daily meditation to support family healing.

The 1960s was a time of profound change in America and the world. We saw the birth of the Civil Rights Movement, the Anti-War Movement, and the African Cultural Movement. The Yoga Meditation and Chakra Healing Movements appeared on the scene as an advanced East Indian spiritual liberation system. As I developed in the teachings of KMT, my study brought me to the understanding that in fact, the chakra system originated with the first people of the black lands in the Nile Valley. These were the mothers and fathers of holistic and allopathic medicine. Their term for the chakra was *"arit"* (for one energy center) or *"aritu"* (for more than one). It was astounding to learn that advanced spiritual practices and purification rites began with my ancestors.

As I was in a quest to find myself and my inner power, I came to the realization that much of what we call New Age is actually Old Age— the lifestyle teachings of antiquity. I recall having a quest moment. I asked Sen Ur Ankh Ra Senahj Su Ptah, an Elder of KMT Teachings, "Did the ancestors have a chakra system?" He told me that indeed they did and advised me about the *Pert M Hru N Gbr,* miscalled *The Egyptian Book of the Dead.* I began to read and read and reflect and then rejoice. To me, a yogini from the 1960s era, this information was one of the greatest discoveries ever! We Afrakans not only birthed aromatherapy, reflexology, hydrotherapy, and color therapy—now known as holistic health—but also birthed the *aritu,* later on in spiritual history known as the chakras.

I began about 1995, twenty-five years ago, to develop or reconstruct the 7 Aritu Afrakan Khamitic Energy Healing System using as my base the Doorkeeper (*ari-aa-s*), or opener of the Way from within; the Watcher (*sati*), the inner observer; and the Herald (*sema*), the inner call-out. Then I connected aromatherapy and the corresponding sacred stones used by our Nile Valley Ancestors and some of the foods of antiquity to construct the 7 Aritu Healing Chart that you are about to encounter. At the inception of writing or channeling *Sacred Woman,* I tried to set this text on the Aritu System, to no avail. Then when I channeled the *Sacred Woman* anniversary edition text, the Sacred Woman Guardians began to talk through me. They placed themselves in the corresponding appropriate energy centers based on their attributes.

For twenty-five years I was on a spiritual excavation to connect, align, discover, channel the original chakra work, the mother/father of the chakra system, the *aritu.* In this research presentation there are 7 Aritu. Mother Guardian Seshat called forth the 7 Aritu System with her seven-star lights. Seshat is "Star Gate" guide, guiding us into her Gateway with much *merr* (love) and care and intelligence. Mut Seshat informed me of the formula, the measurement of practices that would achieve liberation from all the traps. Through this method and these tones, we can be the most beautiful people freed of bondage. Humanity's ascension would take place through the women living the 7 Aritu practice and sharing it with their families. Through these women, humanity can and will come out of the traps that are spoken of in the classic book *Two Thousand Seasons* by Ayi Kwei Armah.

Mother Guardian Seshat is the Keeper of the Moon, of geometry, of mathematics, of measurement, of the House of the Books, the Mother of Architecture who sets the foundation of temples by the stars, Seshat is accompanied by Nefer Atum the Lotus—also an Afrakan Nile Valley spiritual principle of ascension and transformation from out of the mud. Through a process of purification, fasting and prayers, eating, anointing, and sacred wrapping, we come out of the mud and ascend to our most blossomed state of pure illumination. In order to maintain the Blossom, the most spiritual beautiful and liberated state, we are to learn and live daily the 7 Aritu that Mut Guardian Seshat offers from the Ancients. Throughout daily practices we can end all suffering on Planet Earth. We can enjoy a global City of Wellness.

Getting out of the traps was a legacy stolen from the black land of KMT and our earliest ancestors. The original people took the blame for the acts of the Greeks and Romans, who become "Pharaoh" in later dynasties. Remember the quote, "Tell old Pharaoh to let my people go"? The original people were the ones who took Jesuwa (also known as Jesus) into KMT for sixteen years; there he went through his spiritual initiation. The Greeks and Roman burned the library that Mut Guardian Seshat was in charge of. They stole the libraries in order to misrepresent our story and thereby keep the Afrakan Mother and Father lost to spiritual ascension and healing. We were trapped away from our Most High selves. The Journey of the Traps evolved through tribalism. *My tribe against your tribe* evolved into the transatlantic slave trade. For eight generations *millions of the healers of the earth were stolen,* put into slave ships, and sent to the Americas, the Virgin Islands, and Europe.

Free labor, broken backs, broken families, broken lives sunup to sundown, stolen people: my ancestors. Then Willie Lynch entered with his advice on how to keep a people enslaved. This sealed the coffin of slavery. Lynch advised "Gentlemen and Businessmen" to follow his instruction in order to keep slaves for at least three hundred years. From my ancestors' blood, flesh, and tears, American banks were built. America's wealth was built from the plantation to the corporate boardroom. After slavery, we walked off the plantation with a Bible, a knapsack, and the clothes on our backs. From this my people had to build homes, grow crops, create work, build institutions of learning, raise cattle. We were a stolen people. We were considered by the American Constitution to be three-fifths of a person. To this day, more than a hundred years after slavery ended, my people are still fighting for their rights to be whole. Stolen language, stolen culture, stolen families, stolen medicine, stolen mind, body, and spirit. The 1950s and '60s brought in Marcus Garvey, Martin Luther King, and Malcolm X to liberate We, the People. They fought and died for our liberation.

In the 1980s AIDS was injected into our community, as was crack. Crack and AIDS became a part of population control. It hit home. My friends were dying of AIDS all around me, and crack took down my children's father. Single parenting became dominant among many of the mother-friends in my neighborhood. My community. While this was taking place, I was teaching Goddess Circles with Queen Esther and leading women's healing retreats, which led me to ultimately reach the consciousness of Sacred Woman. Hundreds of women took my Sacred Woman Teachings before the book *Sacred Woman* was written. To them, I give thanks for walking with me on the early journey. Before the writing of the text, Sen-Ur Semahj asked me who the women I planned to write about were. How did they live? That question had to have an answer, so I set sail for deep study, fasting, and prayer in order to mend my people starting with the mothers, the Woman. For "As you heal a woman, you heal a nation." Twenty years later, in 2020, *Sacred Woman* is living a twenty-year anniversary with thousands of women around the world awakening the healer within through living the Sacred Woman Gateways rites of passage.

What I witnessed over the years was that many women are able to maintain the teachings and continue to ascend daily, but some women fall off and back into the traps, even after Ascension.

The time has come to fully break the spell. The time has come for the unearthing of the 7 Aritu Transformation System from antiquity to the present day of the Millennials and beyond.

Sacred Guardian Mut Mother Seshat laid the foundation for building the spiritual temples of humanity's beginning. She has now been called to build our inner spiritual temples through the unearthing for *Sacred Woman* of the 7 Aritu, so that we will never again fall asleep on our wholeness and wellness; so that we will never again be a divided people; so that as we spiritually unify from Gateway to Gateway, leading us to our 7 Aritu, we vibrate on the Highest Frequency of protection, of love, of peace, of prosperity, of oneness. Together we women will create Heaven on Earth.

Seshat the Sacred Moon Guardian of writing, mathematics, and astrology is crowned with the seven-pointed star, which represents the source of all creative consciousness.

## THE JOURNEY TO THE GREAT AWAKENING

From the traps of destruction, disease, and suffering to the Great Awakening of wellness, health, and vitality came forth the first energy system names of the *aritu* (predating the chakra system of East India). The Aritu System from the Nile Valley of Khamit of the black land, born of the original Healers of the Planet Earth, comprises the seven energy centers. After thousands of years, the *aritu* have been unearthed in this particular format for all of humanity to come into Maat (balance and harmony).

I give profound appreciation to Sen-Ur Ankh Ra Semahj Se Ptah of the Studio and Shrine of Ptah for his support in making this chart a reality. As a young yogini thirty years ago, I first asked him if there was a chakra system in our Khamitic culture. He replied, "Yes," and advised me to look into *The Book of Coming Forth*. And the rest is—our story.

## IT'S ALL *ME*

The time has come for the most advanced training in order to reclaim our power. Repeat with me four times: "It's All Me!" All relationships are an extension of where you have been and where you are going. Everything we do is in relationship to ourselves and our state of being. From the food we eat to the air we breathe—all is interconnected in the dance of life. All relationships are a creation of our past, present, and future; all are our relationships to ourselves. The relationship that you are having with another person is actually the relationship that you are having with yourself. Get your relationship with yourself in Maat balance and all your relationships will transform to your highest or lowest frequency.

Create your life practice cleansing and rejuvenating with your inner self with the Gateways and the *aritu* daily and overcome the traps. Align with the Freedom Frequency of Wellness.

Tap into your inner self beginnings and chant the ancient tones. Meditate. Eat from the green garden. Harmonize with sacred stones and the healing aroma of our ancient Nile Valley ancestors. Visualize, harmonize, crystallize yourself to your highest frequency and all of your relations will heal one by one or as multitudes. As you shift, so do all of your relationships.

Once you have reached Sacred Time Gateway, for advanced spiritual development you are to perform the 7 Aritu through meditation, visualization, and chanting (*hesi*).

1. Sit comfortably in a chair or on a yoga floor chair. Burn the aromatherapy oil of the Gateway that you are working on for the day or week, or use the aromatherapy oil from one of the 7 Aritu.
2. Center yourself in the breath of the thousand-petaled lotus. Perform 250 Fire Breaths in your morning *arit* meditation. Then perform the breathwork in prayer at midday, afternoon, and sunset, for a total of a thousand breaths a day. After the first round of 250 breaths, visualize the color of the energy center and the gland you are restoring and visualize upon that color the Sacred Woman Gateway Guardian energizing your body, mind, and spirit.
3. Chant or speak out loud the name of the Doorkeeper (the opener of the Way), the Watcher (the inner vision of the self), and the Herald (the spokesperson within).
4. Sit and be still in your heart. Then listen from within to the message, the lesson that *arit* is bringing you.
5. Journal and then give thanks. Release the traps one by one or all at once as you ascend.

## ARI ANKH RA EGYPTIAN KMT YOGA

Perform Ari Ankh Ra—five hundred rapid Fire Breaths—at sunrise, midday, afternoon, and evening daily.

*I am the Lady (Ast) / Lord (Asar) of the double crown (right and left brain). I am in the Utchat (Seat of Ascension). I exist by its strength. I come forth. I shine. I go in (to meditation).*
*I come to life.*

*My seat is on my throne. I sit in the pupil of my eye (sixth arit). I am Heru (the Falcon, the Sun of Asar with keen vision) traversing. I have commanded my seat (my crown consciousness).*

## DAILY PRACTICE TO REMOVE ALL TRAPS

Perform daily the Aritu Meditation Holistic Lifestyle as it appears in the 7 Aritu table on pages 394–395, coupled with five hundred to a thousand Fire Breaths. You will be transformed to optimal well-being.

## GUARDIANS

| | |
|---|---|
| Abtu | The seat of adoration of Asar |
| Anpu | Known as the one who presides over the embalming ceremony |
| Anu | The city known as the City of the Sun |
| Apep | The crystallization of evil and the enemy of Ra (Life) |
| Aritu | Wheels of power (chakras) |
| Asar | Father of humanity, represented by the left hemisphere of the brain |
| Ast | Mother of humanity, represented by the right hemisphere of the brain |
| Ra | Guardian, represented as the Sun |
| Re-Stau | Territory of initiation, a passage that leads from the physical world to the spiritual realm |

# THE 7 ARITU ENERGY HEALING CHART SCROLL FOR BODY, MIND, AND SPIRITUAL AWAKENING

| Color Healing | The Journey to Liberation Through the 7 Aritu Awakening | The Trap The Darkness | The Awakening The Light | Sacred Woman Sacred Man Corresponding Guardians | Energy Centers | Glandular Healing |
|---|---|---|---|---|---|---|
| VIOLET | Crown Healing Liberation The Seat of Supreme Illumination | Alzheimer's, brain fog, depression, attachment issues, disconnected from source, confusion | Surrender to divinity, awakened visionary | Nefer Atum Seshat Ast & Asar Ra | Crown Pituitary | Central nervous system |
| INDIGO | Pineal Healing Liberation The Seat of Ascension | Confusion, headaches | Connected to the Most High, heightened intuition | Nebt-Het | First eye (Utchat) Pineal | Limbic system |
| BLUE | Throat Healing Liberation The Seat of Divine Communication | Poor communication, gossip, verbal abuse, enlarged thyroid, laryngitis | Truth, vibrant communication | Tehuti | Throat | Endocrine system |
| GREEN | Heart Healing Liberation The Seat of Love, Compassion & Forgiveness | Brokenhearted; heart attack, high blood pressure, asthma | Love, trust, compassion, forgiveness | Maat Het-Hru | Heart AB | Cardiovascular system, respiratory system |
| YELLOW | Solar Plexus Liberation The Seat of Protection | Anxiety, constipation, stagnation, fear, colon cancer | Inner sunshine, willpower to process your relations, courageous | Ta-Urt | Solar plexus | Digestive, liver, gallbladder system |
| ORANGE | Sacral Healing Liberation The Seat of Creativity | Shame, womb diseases, PMS, fibroids, prostate cancer | Creativity, pleasure, womb wellness, prostate wellness | Nut Meshkenet Sekhmet Bes Min | Sacral | Reproductive system |
| RED | Coccygeal Healing Liberation The Seat of Stability | Fear, stagnation, isolation, constipation | Fearlessness, grounded, stability | Ta-Urt Ptah | Coccygeal (Root) | Adrenal system |

The Aritu Meditation Holistic Lifestyle for optimal wellness. *Hesi* (chant) and study from the first *arit* (the coccygeal) to the crown *arit* for your daily ascension.

| Door Keeper (Opener of the Way) The Prayer and the *Hesi* from the Doorkeeper, the Watcher, and the Herald | Watcher (Inner Observer) | Herald (Inner Callout) | Food as Medicine Herbs as Medicine | Aromatherapy Anointing | Sacred Healing Stones Meditation |
|---|---|---|---|---|---|
| Sekhem-Matenu-Sen [u] *Arit* Affirmation: "I have come to you, Ast & Asar. I am purified from disease. You revolve around heaven. You see Ra. You see the knowing ones. Only one. Behold, you are in her/his gloried body and it becomes strong. May my ways be prosperous before you." | Aa-Maa Kheru | Khesef-Khemi [u] | Blackberries Gotu-kola herb | Lotus oil | Amethyst |
| Atek-Tau-Kehaq-Kheru *Arit* Affirmation: "I have come daily. I have come daily. I have made the way. I have passed the test of Anpu. I am the lady/lord of the double crown. Without words of power, I—avenger of right—have avenged the eye (Utchat). I have healed the eye of Ast & Asar. I have made the way." | An-Hra | Ates-Hra-Sh | Purple cabbage Ginkgo herb | Frankincense oil | Clear quartz |
| Ankh-F-Em-Fent [u] *Arit* Affirmation: "I have brought your jawbones into Re-Stau. I have brought your backbone into Annu, gathering the pieces there. I have turned back Apep. I have washed the wounds. I have made a way among you. I am the most ancient among the NTRU. Because of me, Ast & Asar is victorious. Her/his bones I have gathered. His/her limbs I have joined together." | Shabu | Teb-Hra Keha | Berries Eucalyptus herb | Eucalyptus oil | Turquoise, aquamarine |
| Khesef-Hra-Ast-Kheru *Arit* Affirmation: "I am a strong one, a child of the ancestors of Ast & Asar. May my Mother Ast and my Father Asar present evidence for my claim. I have brought life to the nostrils forever. I am a child of Ast & Asar. I have made the way. I have passed through the place of divine trials." | Se-Res-Tepu | Khesef At | Green veggies Hawthorne berries herb | Ylang ylang | Emerald, malachite |
| Qeq-Hauatu-Ent-Pehui *Arit* Affirmation: "I have concealed in the great deep, O judge of speech. I have come and I release the defects for Ast & Asar. I bind up his/her standard, which comes forth from the crown. I have opened the way in Re-Stau. I have eased the pain of Ast & Asar. I have made the way, enabling Ast & Asar to shine in Re-Stau." | Se-Res-Hra | Aaa | Okra, melons Cascara sagrada herb | Fennel oil | Yellow topaz, tiger's eye |
| Un-hat *Arit* Affirmation: "I sit to perform the first desire of my heart. I weigh my words as Tehuti. I make offerings along the way. Great that I may pass on to behold Ra like those who make offerings." | Seqet-Hra | Uset | Apricots, mangoes Woman's Herbal, Man's Herbal | Sandalwood oil | Amber, fire opal |
| Sekhet-Hra-Asht-Aru *Arit* Affirmation: "I am great making light. I have come to thee, Ast & Asar. I adore you. Homage to you, Ast & Asar, in your power and dominion in Re-Stau. You rise up and you conquer. O Ast & Asar in Abtu, you go around heaven sailing in the presence of Ra. You see the knowing ones. I am a divine ruler; may I not be turned back at the wall of burning coals. I have opened the way in Re-Stau. I ease the pain of Ast & Asar, causing Ast & Asar to shine." | Metti Heh | Ha-Kheru | Cayenne, ginger Senna & mint herb | Musk oil | Ruby, hematite |

## SHU BREATHING

Perform the following spiritual practice of Shu Breathing throughout the day. For beginner, intermediate, and advanced students—reach an optimal one thousand Nefer Atum Power Breaths.

- *At dawn:* In Nebt Het hour between 4 and 6 A.M., perform 250 Ra/Shu Fire Breaths. Close out in five minutes of open heart meditation.
- *At midday:* In Ast hour, midday/noon, perform 250 Ra/Shu Fire Breaths. Close out in five minutes of open heart meditation.
- *At sunset:* In Het-Hru hour, between 4 and 6 P.M., perform 250 Ra/Shu Fire Breaths. Close out in five minutes of open heart meditation.
- *At evening time:* In Nut's hour between 8 and 10 P.M., perform 250 Ra/Shu Fire Breaths. Close out in five minutes of open heart meditation.

## SACRED TIME: SEVEN-DAY TRANSFORMATIVE WORK

Daily, as you continue to purify your life through sacred words, thoughts, and deeds on the physical, mental, emotional, and spiritual planes, the words coming out of your mouth and back to you will be words of power, light, and healing. You will speak sacred words to sacred souls.

- *Talk fast: Perform a talk fast over the next seven days.* Speak only when necessary; don't talk for hours. Watch as your words become pure and organic. Throughout the week observe a seven- to twelve-hour talk fast, alone or with others who are doing the same practice.
- *Sacred Word affirmations.* Finally, following a daily affirmation, participate in morning and evening prayer. Now begin to reclaim your natural self through your words:

*My life is in harmony through living a life of and in Divine Time.*

*Today, I am transformed in and through Seshat, the Guardian of Sacred Time.*

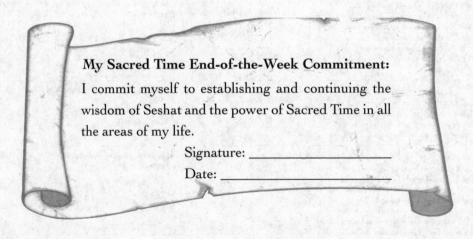

### My Sacred Time End-of-the-Week Commitment:

I commit myself to establishing and continuing the wisdom of Seshat and the power of Sacred Time in all the areas of my life.

Signature: _____

Date: _____

# CHAPTER 16
# GATEWAY 11: SACRED WORK

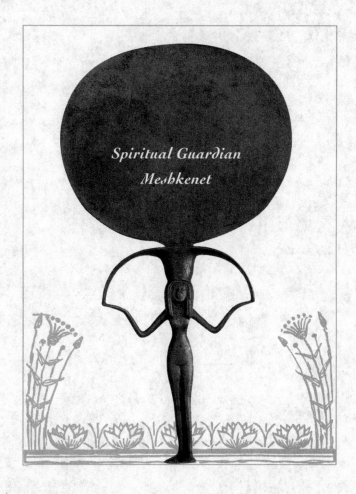

*Spiritual Guardian*
*Meshkenet*

**Ancestor**

Madame C. J. Walker

**Elders**

Maxine Waters

Angela Bassett

**Contemporaries**

Queen Latifah

Jada Pinkett Smith

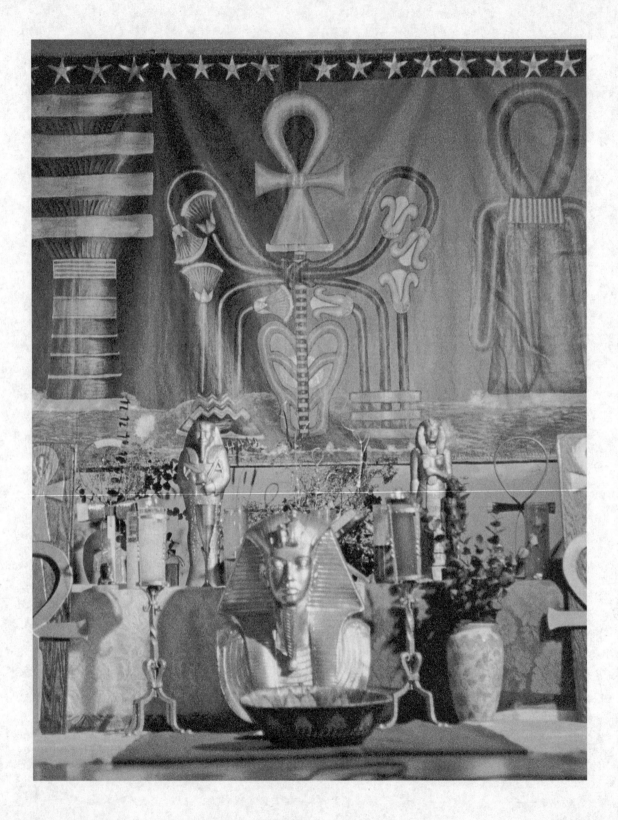

# SACRED WORK ALTAR WORK
## Face Your Heart to the East—to the Rising Sun
### (Layout front top view)

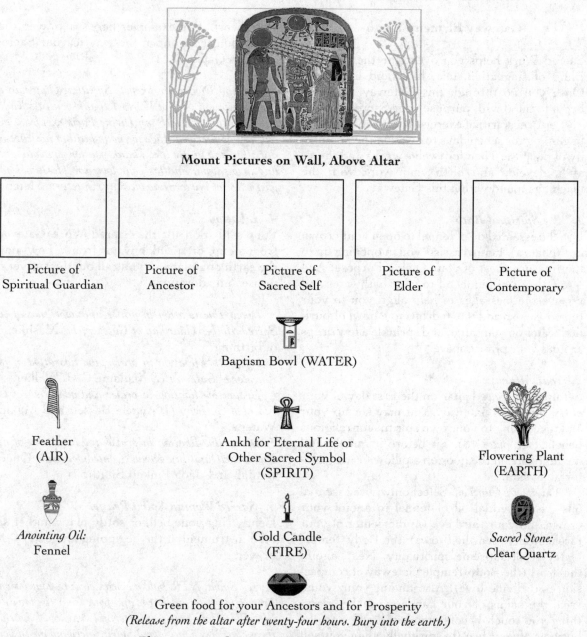

**Mount Pictures on Wall, Above Altar**

Picture of
Spiritual Guardian

Picture of
Ancestor

Picture of
Sacred Self

Picture of
Elder

Picture of
Contemporary

Baptism Bowl (WATER)

Feather
(AIR)

Ankh for Eternal Life or
Other Sacred Symbol
(SPIRIT)

Flowering Plant
(EARTH)

*Anointing Oil:*
Fennel

Gold Candle
(FIRE)

*Sacred Stone:*
Clear Quartz

Green food for your Ancestors and for Prosperity
*(Release from the altar after twenty-four hours. Bury into the earth.)*

**Place on your altar your Vision Quest Business Plan.**

Sacred tablecloth (gold) and scarf to wear during prayer.
Sacred color cloth to lay before altar. Sacred instruments to be played as you pray.

# GATEWAY 11: SACRED WORK DAILY SPIRITUAL OBSERVANCES

## Gateway Element: Earth

Sacred Work helps you overcome the Birthing Blues of stagnation, fear, lack, and limitation. Once you go through this Gateway, you will begin to build with purpose your Sacred Work.

Perform spiritual exercises of ascension daily beginning for seven days to awaken the possibility of purpose. Then for twelve weeks and thereafter, develop and birth your work with the teachings found within this Gateway.

### 1. The Spiritual Bath

Use the essential oil of fennel to open your crown *arit* (chakra). Fennel assists you in opening up to the treasure chest of your Divine Purpose. Add 4 to 6 drops of fennel oil to your bathwater and receive the messages to help align you to your purpose. Also add 4 to 6 drops to a bowl of purified water on your altar, and sprinkle a few drops around your prayer space.

### 2. Your Altar

Set up your sacred altar on the first day of your entry into this Gateway. You may set up your altar according to your own spiritual or religious beliefs (see page 18). Sit before it quietly and meditatively on the floor on a pillow or in a comfortable chair.

*Anoint with fennel oil.* Select only pure essential oils. Use essential oil of fennel to anoint your crown and your third eye (in the center of your forehead between the brows), the Body Temple Gateway of supreme spirituality. Next, anoint the heart (the Body Temple Gateway of compassion and divine love). Also anoint your womb area, the palms of your hands (to make everything you touch become more sacred), and the bottoms of your feet (to spiritually align yourself for stepping out in power, promise, and faith).

### 3. Opening the Gateway

In your prayers to each of the Gateway Guardians, you may use whatever words pour from your heart. For example, here's a prayer that might be used to open the way to your Sacred Work in Gateway 11:

*Sacred and Divine Meshkenet, Spiritual Guardian of the Gateway of Sacred Work, I thank you in advance for presenting me with my Divine Purpose. Please accept my deepest gratitude for your healing presence on my altar and in my life. Thank you for your guidance and inspiration, and for your love and blessings, and please accept my love and blessings in return. Hetepu.*

### 4. Libation

Pour a libation for the Sacred Work Gateway from a cup, or sprinkle water from a bowl onto the earth or a plant, as you call out this prayer of praise and adoration.

*I pour this libation in praise and adoration of the Sacred Mother Guardian of Gateway 11,* Meshkenet of birthing.

*I pour this libation in praise and adoration of the Ancestor of Gateway 11,* Madame C. J. Walker.

*I pour this libation in praise and adoration of the Elders of Gateway 11,* Angela Bassett and Maxine Waters.

*I pour this libation in praise and adoration of my Divine Self and my Divine Contemporaries,* Queen Latifah and Jada Pinkett Smith.

### 5. Sacred Woman Spirit Prayer

Gently ring your bell, or softly play another sacred instrument at the beginning and end of the prayer.

*Sacred Spirit, NTR, hold me near, close to your bosom. Protect me from all harm and fear, from the blows of life. Direct my steps in the right way as I journey through this vision. Sacred Spirit, surround me in your absolutely perfect light. Anoint me in your sacred purity, peace, and divine insight. Bless me, truly bless me as I share this sacred life. Teach me, Sacred Spirit, to be in tune with the Universe. Teach me how to heal with the inner and outer elements of air, fire, water, and earth.*

## 6. Sacred Work Prayer

*Nuk Pu Nuk Meshkenet*
(I am that I am Meshkenet)

*Blessings reign from birth. I have been given a Sacred Work that was designed specifically for me. A work that was passed down by my ancestors who have gone before me. A work that reflects who I am, my mission on earth, my gratitude of living, my passion, and my purpose. O Creator/Creatress, if by chance I am unconscious of my Sacred Work, I commit to fast and pray until it is revealed to me in a dream or a vision, by night or day. I will purify until You show me the way to my Sacred Work. For when my Sacred Work makes itself known to me, I vow to have courage to live it, to be about my Mother's/Father's work. I vow to cherish the gifts that are bestowed upon me through my Sacred Work. May the works that come through me not only be a blessing to me, but also received, used, and shared—a blessing—by all others. This I pray.*

## 7. Chanting Hesi

Chant this *hesi* four times:

*Nuk Pu Ntrt Hmt*—I am a Sacred Woman.

## 8. Fire Breaths

Prepare your Fire Breaths by slowly inhaling four times and exhaling four times. Then, when you are totally at ease, begin your twelve hundred Fire Breaths. Inhale deeply like a pump through your nose (mouth closed) as you expand the breath down into the abdomen, then back up to the chest. Completely exhale out through your nostrils from your abdomen as it contracts and the lungs release your breath completely. Repeat this breath rapidly in and out, in and out.

Allow each deep Fire Breath to represent the opening of the thousand lotus petals of illumination and radiance, ultimately reaching Nefer Atum—the ultimate Afrakan Lotus station of Divinity.

## 9. Gateway 11: Meshkenet Meditation

Each day of the twenty-one days you spend working through Gateway 11, increase the length of time you spend in meditation. The longer you are in meditation, the deeper your inner peace will be, and the more vibrant your *ka* (spirit) will become. The cleaner your Body Temple, the sooner it will be able to live permanently in the peace and inner balance of the meditative state.

**The Sacred Womb Meditation**
Squat while pressing down on birthing bricks, one on each side, right and left. Bear down as you inhale and exhale. With each breath, visualize your vision through your womb as you continue to breathe deep in and out. See yourself crowning a golden bright light of your vision—your purpose, your work, emerging from your womb. Then take a final deep breath in and out as the fullness of your baby, your purpose, is born. With your hands by your womb catch your vision and then bring her to your breast, your heart, and hold her close. Lovingly commit to nurse your vision as she grows day by day. Give thanks to the Divinity Within for birthing your Divine Purpose.

*Color Visualization.* In Gateway 11, which honors the element of earth, visualize gold for prosperity and wealth. As you perform your meditation, wear a piece of gold cloth on yourself (scarf or headwrap) and place a gold cloth on your altar.

*Sacred Stone Meditation.* While in meditation, hold a clear quartz in your palm over your womb. The clear quartz is the sacred healing stone of Gateway 11. It amplifies the clarity of your inner vision, giving you the ability to see your purpose clearly.

## 10. Herbal Tonics

Drink herbal tea while you're doing your altar, prayer work, and journal work in Gateway 11. Use the Heal Thyself Woman's Herbal Formula (see the product list in the appendix) for General Womb Wellness.

Alfalfa tea, made from the plant's roots and leaves, is another useful tonic for Gateway 11 as it strengthens higher vision while purifying the body's anatomy.

Drink your tea for twenty-one days to receive the full benefits of attuning to Gateway 11. Enjoy your herb tea in your favorite mug during or after spiritual writing. Be sure to finish the tea before 1 P.M.

*Preparation.* Use one teabag or 1 teaspoon loose tea to 8 ounces of water boiled in a nonmetallic pot. Boil water, turn off flame, then add tea and steep. Strain herbs from water. Drink before or after your morning bath or sacred shower. Drink with joy and peace as you breathe quietly between sips and settle into easy contemplation.

### 11. Flower Essences
To deepen your experience of Gateway 11, take 4 drops of chlorophyll essence four times per day directly on or under the tongue, or add the same amount to a small glass of purified water and sip. For instructions on how to choose flower essences, see page 23.

### 12. Diet and Movement
Daily, follow the Sacred Woman Natural Living Dietary Laws given in the Womb Wellness Cleansing Food Plan (see page 71) and do the Dance of the Womb movements presented in Gateway 3. Omit soy; limit whole grain and starch. Increase green vegetables to strengthen your purpose.

### 13. Sacred Work Journal Writing
Journal writing is best done after your sacred bath, and/or meditation. When you are cleansed and centered, you can receive spiritual messages from the One Most High with grace. When in the spirit, messages travel down through your spirit mind, to your heart, into your hand, and onto the paper. (This is how I do all of my writing.)

The best time to receive your spiritually written work is after you have completed your altar work, between the hours of 4 A.M. and 6 A.M.

Keep a very special pen and journal by or on your altar to work with the power, force, and stillness at the coming of the dawn.

At this time, write in your journal the thoughts, activities, experiences, and interactions that occurred previously in your daily life. You might also want to write down your self-inspired hopes, visions, desires, and affirmations so that you can draw on them for help and support when needed. You'll be surprised at how healing and sustaining your journal wisdom can be.

### 14. Senab Freedom Shawl or Quilt
By the time you reach Gateway 11, your Senab Freedom Shawl or Quilt should be completed.

### 15. Sacred Tools
Your support team and your Business Plan Birthing Wheel of your vision are your most Sacred Tools. Embrace them as they embrace you and together grow your purpose.

### 16. Sacred Reminder
Throughout the next twenty-one days to a season, you are to observe closely the wisdom presented in Gateway 11. For maximum results, live freely in tune with the various systems of body, mind, and spirit wellness presented.

### Closing Sacred Words

*Divine Creator/Creatress, help me to honor and treat my purpose in a most sacred way. Thank you for all the blessings you have granted me on this sacred journey as I bring my purpose to full term.*

## BIRTHING OUR LIVES

*Did you hear?!*
*We're about to birth a new world!*
*Become one with yourself, your work, and birth*
*your vision.*

*Get in line with the Divine —*
*The creative force within you, through the help of*
*the Great Spirit Meshkenet —*
*the Spiritual Guardian and Caretaker of Sacred*
    *Wombs*
*that houses the life of woman and man.*
*The Great Spirit will guide you to your Sacred*
    *Vision*
*if you dare to step to your natural rhythm.*

## Family: The Root of Your Sacred Work

In ancient tradition, work was considered family business. In this regard, as people developed in work, particularly entrepreneurship, it was expected that they pass on their skills to blood relatives or extended family. As you grow into your own Sacred Work, teach your children so that they will get firsthand direction and inspiration about working in a divine family. Be an example to your children as well as to your community in creating your life's work. Don't procrastinate. Liberate yourself. Let Spirit guide you. Be brave and begin now, conceiving and birthing your purpose, your Sacred Work.

Create inner works that support you and your family. Create works that support your health, bring forth financial abundance, and restore your harmony.

*Smai tawi* (unity) is essential for healthy living. You must become emancipated. You must no longer allow your work (your job) to enslave you. When you live your Sacred Work, you will ensure a dis-ease-free existence. As you establish your freedom and live out your destiny, encourage others to do the same. Live your Sacred Work and witness your body grow in health and transform. Gratitude and joy will take over because you will be living out your true destiny.

If you've spent several years working to receive a degree in a particular area and discover that you really have a distaste for your present job, then call on the ancient spirit of *khepera* (transformation). Go forth and make *khepera*, the change in your work that will give both you and your community fulfillment. Behold! You do not have to remain trapped in that job. Be led by Spirit. Move forth and re-create your world as you would mold and reshape clay. Your life's work, your vision, is your clay. Change each step of the way as needed to become your Divine Self. Think pure thoughts, eat pure non-GMO, organic foods, and perform pure actions to result in pure work. Grow your Sacred Work inside of you.

Do not fear the vastness of your vision. The Creator/Creatress has a divine place for you. Step through and beyond your fear and embrace your divine plan. Step out in faith. Be creative. It's all there! Everything you need to create your own business is in your circumference. Start small and grow or start large and expand. Reach out for help; help will come. Be bold in spirit. Leap to your success in the work force that you created, and your life's work will grow immeasurably.

Your vision: Become the Boss Lady. Take higher those who are at one with your purpose, those who share your vision. Activate.

Your Sacred Work must be an ongoing development process of acknowledgment, acceptance, empowerment, projection, and sharing. Live your Sacred Work. Your natural talent, your gift, is your divine right. Through activation of your Sacred Work, you will experience hard work and you also will experience wholeness, serenity, success, harmony, and prosperity. Activating your Sacred Work is living your truth. To give up on your Sacred Work, or to put it under a rock or aside, is to deny yourself from being born. Denial of the birthing is what makes us unfulfilled, frustrated, and impotent. Come alive; be encouraged and enlightened as you go within to discover the power and joy of living on purpose.

## Birth a Divine Vision

The birthing of your Divine Vision is the Most High's goal for you. Through appropriate use of the Meshkenet birthing principle, we may unleash and birth the gift of our Sacred Work upon the earth: work that uplifts, empowers, strengthens, restores, charges, and transforms humanity into true goodness. However, if you misuse the Birthing Wheel and birth visions to manipulate, enslave, dominate, and devalue humanity in any way, you will ultimately receive the *shai* (karma) for your actions. Wrong deeds will turn back onto the maker. Such destruction and misuse poison your bloodline for generations to come. What you create and pass on to others must be of highest order to create health, light, and bliss on your pathway homeward to your Sacred Self.

*The Realization*
*Your Life's Work is a Sacred Mission*
*Free Yourself*
*You Must Live Your Sacred Work*
*Warning! There is no rest for those who do not live*
*    their Sacred Work.*
*You must live your Sacred Work to be fully alive!*
*If you ignore, avoid, suppress or hold back on what*
*    the Creator/Creatress has blessed you with*
*(your work, your gifts), you will experience dis-*
*    ease in body, mind and spirit.*
*You will be internally blocked or constipated.*

## SACRED WORK

*Work is love made visible. If you cannot work with love but only with disdain, it is better that you should leave your work and sit at the gate of the temple and take alms of those who work with joy.*

— KHALIL GIBRAN, *THE PROPHET*

Since 1977, I've carried this powerful sacred quote with me on my many journeys. It has assisted and inspired me with the unfolding of my Sacred Work, which is teaching people how to heal themselves. When I found that many of my clients, devotees, and students on the Heal Thyself Path of Purification continued to have physical, emotional, and spiritual blockages although living a lifestyle of Natural Living and fasting, I reviewed the state of their relationship to their occupations. In many cases, the lack of living their Sacred Work was the culprit.

It is *not* just diet alone—be it vegetarian, vegan, or flexitarian, live food or cooked food— that makes you sick. You may be eating and drinking correctly, and you may release negative relationships from your life, but if you are putting in 40 hours, weekly, 160 hours monthly, 1,920 hours yearly on a job that feeds your depression, unfulfillment, rage, suppression, disap-

pointment, racism, and/or resentment, you will still have blockages. You can end up carrying twenty-five to a hundred excess pounds caused by emotions and toxins that poison your thoughts, your feelings, and your spirit. You are also susceptible to high blood pressure, premature aging, strokes, heart conditions, brain tumors, skin eruptions, stress, and depression, to name a few dis-eases.

Being a conscious woman and man, you must perform the work that the Most High Creator/ Creatress has given you. If you march to the beat of another's drum, you will be out of rhythm. As you purify your Body Temple, your work will be revealed to you. If you are already aware of your gift but don't know how to actualize it fully, that, too, shall be revealed. The how, what, and where will be answered as your inner light comes forth through your Sacred Work Birthing Wheel. Your thoughts and your visions will become pure as you live a high-frequency life, a life of Maat in all ways.

## MY PERSONAL
## SACRED WORK JOURNEY

From artist to healer to spiritualist to businesswoman to Sacred Woman. I am air, fire, water, and earth; I transform through all seasons; I am the sun and the moon. I am unlimited dimensions of every possibility. I birth that which is inside of me. The 1960s was a time for freedom fighters, revolutionaries, spiritualists, and health activists to emerge, to bring balance to a troubled Western world. I was caught up in the glorious time of truth, freedom, and self-knowledge. I could not help but birth that which was inside of me. It was my time to awaken.

As a teenager, I became an artist. It was art in the form of dance that ignited my inner fires, which led me to become one with the rhythm of the drum. On these shores of "America the free," four hundred years ago during the period of chattel slavery, drums had become taboo for Afrakans to make and/or play. In the 1960s, I became part of an African Cultural Spiritual Revolution; we were breaking free. We began to love ourselves, our hair, our color, our drums and dance, our heritage, ourselves. Afrakan Dance and Drum sprang forth from my culture and inspired my rebirth; it was the beginning of reclaiming myself. The denial of Afraka within me was over. I was Black and Proud.

*Ise Oluwa Kolabajo.*
*The work of the Creator cannot be destroyed.*
*—traditional Yoruba spiritual*

I danced self-doubt, self-hate, and rage out of me. Then one day while dancing "Yanvalou" (traditional Haitian rhythm and dance), a beautiful harmonic melody of peace began to dance inside of me. I recalled my Afrakan Mind and I became *we;* I danced to *our* liberation. Therefore, I wanted *us,* my people who had been beaten down, to experience a state of wholeness. I formed a dance company and created choreography for my company members, and we danced a spirit love, we danced a liberation dance to the sound of the drums.

I was Black and Proud.

I was drafted as a member into a senior company, which led me to perform in *Aida* at the Metropolitan Opera House in New York City. In my early twenties, I became a member of the Syvilla Fort Dance Company and performed with my Ast/Nebt-Het, Queen Esther. As I matured, I became a dancer with the Olatunji Dance & Drumming Company. My art did not stop with dance. Before getting married and having my babies, I became the lead singer of an all-male singing group and live band, which led me to travel and perform throughout New York City. Over time, all my works intertwined. Our leader was Joseph Walker—a Broadway actor and screenwriter. I auditioned for and become a member of a professional theater company named the Demi Gods. Within the company we studied all forms of art—voice, dance, acting, playwriting—in order to master our crafts as total artists. My experience with this theater company exposed me to the discipline associated with the arts. All I wanted was to be an artist, to be living in my purpose. Well, so how in the world did I become a healer?

I was chronically sick throughout my youth. During my involvement with the arts, I learned about holistic health as a way to heal myself. I cleansed, I fasted, I detoxed; I healed and re-healed. I changed my lifestyle from toxic living to Natural Living while I continued to develop within the arts. I began to study yoga for self-healing and eventually became a Hatha Yoga teacher. I performed house calls for couples to help them establish harmony in the home. I began to study holistic health formally and over some years, I became a holistic health consultant, fasting instructor, colon therapist, polarity practitioner, and lay midwife.

All this prepared me to open up Heal Thyself Natural Living Center, a holistic center. During this early period of natural healing, I was able to eliminate dis-ease of body, mind, and spirit for myself and for members of my community. I was gaining the knowledge that as human beings we have unlimited potential.

I kept growing and exploring new possibilities of healing naturally. The healing took a lead role and the artist became the supporting cast of my growing wellness. In my thirties, I became a holistic lab worker, and within one year I created nine Heal Thyself natural formulas. As I matured on my path of living, I met my third husband, a Khamitic Priest. I felt he had knowledge that could guide me toward being more spiritually in tune with my Afrakan culture. I studied with him and, after some time had passed, he ordained me as an Afrakan Khamitic Priestess. Finding my spiritual path completely charged my soul.

In 1990, I authored *Heal Thyself for Health and Longevity* and began traveling internationally, offering motivating lectures in holistic health. Just when I thought I had completely arrived at my destination within my Sacred Work, I was encouraged to write the *Sacred Woman* text. After seven years of hard labor, I birthed *Sacred Woman: A Guide to Healing the Feminine Body, Mind, and Spirit.*

In spring 2000, this body of work led me to found and direct the Global Sacred Woman Village. Through retreats, seminars, and workshops, thousands of women worldwide have been initiated (as Sacred Women) onto the Path of Holistic Liberation.

Throughout the years, I have continued cleansing and healing my life, reaching deeper and deeper inside myself for my Truth, my Purpose. My Work.

In 2002, Art resurfaced through me and I dared to become a songwriter for healing. I produced the *Sacred Woman Medicine Song* CD. I now reclaim my beginnings as a Sacred Artist who intertwines with who I am, a Natural Healer, a Spiritual Teacher, all directed by the Businesswoman. The Artist and Healer and Spiritualist and Businesswoman became one. There was born Healing Arts.

This is the tapestry of my Sacred Work, which is all interwoven into what makes me, "ME!" On my journey to discovering my Sacred Work, I learned to allow Spirit to guide my steps.

When I reflect on the magnificence of it all, I can see clearly how every part of my life was a necessary journey that led me to manifest my many Sacred Works. In my career expansions within holistic health, I've discovered that life is constantly in transition and transformation. Due to our personal inner growth, our Sacred Work expands and changes; likewise, it takes on new direction and various forms. When we are not afraid of ourselves and stand strong in our greatness and uniqueness, a new and exciting life is bound to come through. With each breath, like nature, we are in transformation; we expand, we grow and take on new forms that are revealed through our Sacred Works. As sure as the seasons within nature change, so do we.

If you block the change and growth that's stirring up in you, you will be stunted, and you will "die" while living. Each time the light of change returns, I gather all the courage within me. I ask to be guided about how to move on and expand into my inner rooms. As light turns on in my unused, previously unlit rooms, I ask for courage to tap into yet another Sacred Work. I feel so close to the Divine when I completely trust the Divine's guidance. I open the door and enter into the unknown of myself: a once dark space inside my house that is now illuminated. By the lantern of purification of my body, mind, and spirit, I get ready to live more of my Sacred Work. It is truly exciting as each conception and birth brings me closer to my Divine Self. I use all previous works and lessons as the unending bridge that will carry me to my next Sacred Work, the love of my life.

The purpose of this chapter is not so much to give you the mundane practice of beginning, holding on to, and growing your work. Many great thinkers and successful entrepreneurs have presented the knowledge you need for that. My purpose is to encourage and inspire you to pick up your lantern, to encourage, inspire, and motivate you, the seeker of self-knowledge, to reach for your highest self, your truth, your work, your Sacredness. I encourage you to let yourself experience the light of your birth and rebirth in such a way that your spirit will guide you to a life's work reflecting you and your purpose for being. This work will encourage you to be yourself freely, to birth yourself despite your fears and beyond your apprehensions.

Once you realize your purpose and go forth with your work that was given to you at birth, you will really begin to live. May the ancestors continue to travel with you as you crack open your Sacred Work, within your heaven on earth. May you meet the spirit of Meshkenet, the Divine Midwife within you, as I have. May she bless you to join with your Sacred Work that awaits you, as you tap into the All-Amazing You!

## BLESSINGS OF LIVING YOUR SACRED WORK

In the Afrakan Khamitic tradition, the Healer, the Sacred Artist, and the Spiritual Priestess were one. As such, the Healer's work was manifested through dance, song, and drama. Prayers were spoken, songs were sung, herbs were used, and spiritual baths were performed.

It took me thirty years to discover the absolute truth and vastness of my work. I have embraced *smai tawi* (unity) within my work. I have accepted that there is no need to choose one work over another, for my work is a fusion of my Vision. I am a Spiritualist, an Artist, and a Healer. In relationship to my Afrakan ancestry, I heal through Art. All of my expressions are working in Maat. I know bliss while I work. Pray that it does not take you a lifetime to realize what your Divine Work is. Pray that you may recognize your Sacred Work and begin to birth it, so you can know your bliss.

*Do not settle.* Search until your true work reveals itself to you, for then your life's mission will be fulfilled, and your joy will be realized. If everyone were about their Sacred Mission, as they really should be, this world would be a place not of fear, pain, frustration, and disease, but of light, joy, wellness, and plenty.

*Bond.* Become one with what you love. When you find what you love to do, you will want to do it all the time. You will do it even if you don't get paid for it. Then you will have found your "life's work." Your life's work feeds and nourishes your soul with wholeness, with peace, power, and, yes, even prosperity. Stay loyal to your calling even if it takes a lifetime. Through you the Most High has spoken into you your Sacred Work. Accept it and the abundance; the prosperity will shine through. Accept your calling with a resolved state of courage.

In Afrakan tradition, you are born into your work. In contemporary times, we often need guidance to see our work. You may live for several years not knowing your mission, who you are, or what you should be doing. The family into which you were born established your destiny. Your elders taught you and revealed to you your grand purpose at birth. The purpose of your work from the beginning was to strengthen the clan, tribe, community, and nation. Names were chosen to keep you mindful of your purpose for being. The Elders showed you the way. Your work was ordained; it was necessary.

The ways in which you can tell if you have found your life's work are:

- You are in love with it. Your great love of your work will draw all abundances to support you and your mission, which are one and the same.
- It feels like a gift; special. Your work appears as the gift from the Most High that it is.
- You devote time to your work. You feel like you can do it all the time.

Your Sacred Work must be an ongoing developmental process of acknowledgment, acceptance, empowerment, projection, expounding, exposing, and sharing. Living your Sacred Work, your natural talent, your gift by Divine Right, is a necessity for you to experience wholeness, serenity, success, harmony, and prosperity. Activating your Sacred Work is living your truth.

### How to Identify a Person Living Their Sacred Work Vision

- They are excited about living.
- They have tapped into their creativity.
- They are healthy and vibrant.
- They are joyous.
- They are fulfilled.
- They have unlimited vision.
- They are free.
- They are radiant.
- They are loving.
- They are at their appropriate weight. (Generally, when you are spiritually, mentally, and emotionally fed by living your Sacred Work Vision, your body weight is appropriate for your age and height.)

### FINDING YOUR SACRED WORK

If you are unaware of your life's work, then begin to fast and rise up between 4 A.M. and 6 A.M., Nebt-Het's Hours of Intuition, and listen deeply for your work to reveal itself to you. As you become cleaner and cleaner, the answers that you seek about your purpose will be revealed to you in as much detail as you are ready to receive. If you are still unclear about your work, then have someone you trust refer you to a minister, priest, priestess, spiritualist, astrologer, numerologist, or your local "bush doctor" for direction.

Once you receive your message, your calling, don't hesitate to listen and obey, for you have been spiritually instructed. Be confident to act on faith and know that all you need to do to bring forth your Divine Work will be given to you as you grow into your true self.

### THE BIRTHING BLUES: PART 2 OF YOUR SACRED WORK

The Birthing Blues are not physical; they are metaphysical. Throughout this section, I am not talking about a physical hysterectomy or a physical abortion. The Birthing Blues speaks of what we do that does not allow our purpose to come spiritually or emotionally to full term.

There is no blame. Birthing Blues is about taking responsibility for our condition. Within each Birthing Blues state, from morning sickness to abortion, take quiet meditation time to reflect on what that state means to you. As you listen from within, use your Nebt-Het intuition to discover your inner Birthing Blues conditions and focus on how you can arrest and release each of them.

Gateway 11 is all about helping you to transform out of the Birthing Blues into Meshkenet, where you get a chance to live your purpose. In other words, to fulfill Gateway 11 is to get unstuck, to break through, to reach your Divine Destiny. After identifying your Birthing Blues blockage, this Gateway will empower you to take your life into your own hands and heart.

The power to transform your Birthing Blues into your Meshkenet Birthing Wheel is the power to live your purpose within you.

### Beware

Beware the Birthing Blues. Your own fears will bite you in the butt and attract to you your "impossible" state of consciousness.

Beware the Naysayers in your DNA, telling you why you can't make it happen. They say you couldn't, so you can't. Look, study, reflect on the Birthing Blues so you can uproot and overcome with total awareness.

### Affirmation

*I accept that I am overcoming all birthing traumas*
*I accept that I am learning the lessons of all my*
*    creations*
*I accept that I will open myself up to healing beyond*
*    the*
*Birthing Blues.*

The Birthing Blues crisis indicates the lack of preparation and readiness to conceive, carry, and deliver your Sacred Work. What are you doing to block your Sacred Work? What are

your Birthing Blues and how are you going to recover and heal from them? Inside of you are all the answers.

By way of Sacred Work Birthing Exploration, the Sacred Work Journal is going to help you reveal to yourself the root of your Birthing Blues. You will discover from within all that you need to overcome your Sacred Work challenges. You will become in tune with how to make your dream a reality and successfully birth and nurture your Sacred Work into its adulthood.

Allow this process to take seven days for clearance.

### Prayer

*Oh, Divine that dwells in me, assist me in*
*    overcoming the Birthing Blues,*
*that I may unblock my blessings and live out my*
*    Sacred Destiny.*
*Oh, Divine that dwells in me, I pray for freedom*
*    from what's ailing me.*
*Help me to trust that my Vision can, in fact, be.*

### SACRED WORK / MESHKENET QUESTIONNAIRE

For self-inventory, fill out this questionnaire. Observe your level of blockage. Reflect on how much releasing you will need in order to reach your Meshkenet and birth yourself to your purpose.

Check all those entries that are true for you. Record the time and date of your responses. You can change them when appropriate.

☐ My work makes me feel ill, depressed, and angry.
☐ When at work, I wish I were elsewhere.
☐ I'm not living out my life's work/mission.
☐ I keep making excuses for why I can't succeed in my mission.
☐ I feel that I'm unable to feed, clothe, and house (support) myself.
☐ I am working in a dead-end job.
☐ I am dissatisfied with my work.
☐ I dislike the people I work with.

☐ I feel consistently overwhelmed with my work.

☐ My current work suppresses my creativity.

☐ I feel stifled.

☐ I feel depressed beginning on Sunday night because I have to prepare to go to work on Monday.

☐ I feel resentful that other people seem to live out their dreams while I live a status quo life.

☐ I am experiencing jealousy of other people's work rather than focusing on my own mission.

☐ By suppressing my life's work from coming through, I feel like I am a self-abuser.

☐ Accepting other people's limited opinions of me causes me mental and spiritual pain.

☐ I'm experiencing so many mixed messages about my life's work, I am confused.

If you checked two or more of these items, then you are in danger of not being in Meshkenet, your Sacred Work. Keep going; you will overcome the Birthing Blues.

## Physical Work Blockages

As a result of not living your purpose—not being in your Sacred Work—the following diseases and dis-eases could manifest within:

- Drug or alcohol use
- Ulcers
- Impotency
- Infertility
- Migraines
- Unhappiness about work environment
- Working in a dead-end job
- Work that is not economically prosperous
- Being overworked and underpaid
- Feeling overwhelmed
- Obesity
- Job-hopping
- Constipation
- Forms of cancer

Keep going on your journey to heal yourself and manifest your Meshkenet (Sacred Work).

## Understanding the Birthing Blues

Sacred Work Journal questions will help you reflect on and overcome your Sacred Work challenges. Answering the following questions will help you form a clear picture of what blocks you have, along with what you must unblock and overcome to manifest your dreams, your visions, and your Sacred Work, thereby overcoming the Birthing Blues.

## Sacred Work Blockages

If you are experiencing Sacred Work blockages, take a look at the following rationales that we often use to prevent ourselves from living out our Sacred Work. They can catch us up in the web of the Birthing Blues.

What has prevented you from doing your ideal work? Write about it in your journal.

- I don't have enough money.
- I don't have energy after work.
- I don't have support from my family.
- I am afraid to act, because I will probably fall away.
- I have a secure job with benefits; why rock the boat?
- I don't believe that I can do what I really want to do.
- I don't think I deserve to do what I really want to do.
- I don't have a degree in the area of work that I want to pursue.

## Childhood Approval Syndrome

Beware of limitations created during your childhood. Others may say, "Be safe, don't stretch"; "You can't . . ."; "We haven't . . ." Our parents/elders taught us what their vision was for us. Perhaps we did not necessarily believe their vision of who or what we were to become. They might have been right; they may have been wrong. Yet it was that vision that formed us. Study the Birthing Blues, plus the Birthing Wheel, and your truth will be revealed. Grow through this Gateway; uproot and clean up the cancer that has stopped you from living your divine most powerful Destiny.

# PEOPLE THAT STUNT YOUR GROWTH

Be careful with whom you share your vision. People may discourage your vision. They may not be able to see what you see. If they don't reflect your ideals, they may block the fulfillment of your purpose.

Answer the following questions:

1. In my youth, did anyone encourage or discourage me from living my life's work? Who and how?
2. In my adulthood, did anyone encourage or discourage me from living my Sacred Work? Who and how?
3. What are some of the hurdles that I must overcome to live my Sacred Work?
4. What are my fears about living my Sacred Work?
5. How long have I been in fear about living my Sacred Work?

Believe in yourself. Answering these questions is the beginning of birthing your Sacred Work!

## BIRTHING BLUES CHART

The Birthing Blues chart is arranged according to danger depending on where you are in your development. Keep in mind that we may be misguided from within (ourselves) and/or without (others). It is by lack of faith in our Divine purpose that we birth our blues.

### Hysterectomy

A hysterectomy indicates that your Sacred Work is in danger of never birthing itself. Your Sacred Work Vision has been completely rooted out and you are now convinced that you will never manifest it. You have completely given up hope of conceiving, carrying, or birthing your Sacred Work. Someone may have said to you as you were establishing your vision, "You'll never be successful," "Why bother, you'll never make a living from that," "You're living a pipe dream," and other non-supportive phrases. You may say, "Vision work is bigger than me, I can't..." These are inner and outer reflections that create or destroy your potential to manifest and birth your work.

**Sacred Work Affirmation (Antidote)**

My Sacred Work Vision is rooted firmly within me. Nothing, no one, not even I, will hinder the conception and the birth of my Divine Sacred Work.

You can have your uterus but have closed down the door of possibilities of bringing purpose to your life.

**Journal Work**

Identify the Vision Work that experienced a hysterectomy.

- When did I create this Sacred Work blockage?
- How and why did I create this Sacred Work blockage?
- What am I willing to do to overcome this Sacred Work blockage?

### Infertility

Infertility indicates that you are not acting on your vision; your vision is stagnated. An infertile state is also one in which you're mentally, physically, and emotionally blocked, therefore unable to conceive ideas. You might say, for example, "I don't know what my Sacred Work is." And no matter how often you ask the question, you come up empty.

The Infertility Birthing Blues is a condition of lack. Infertility is not being enough, having enough, or knowing enough.

**Sacred Work Affirmation (Antidote)**

Divine light that dwells in me, I affirm today that I am enough, I have enough, and I know enough. I'm open enough to unblock myself and birth my Sacred Work Vision.

You can be fertile and conceive a child, but not able to conceive a vision, your purpose.

**Journal Work**

Identify the Vision Work that was infertile.

- When did I create this Sacred Work blockage?
- How and why did I create this Sacred Work blockage?
- What am I willing to do to overcome this Sacred Work blockage?

## Abortion

Abortion indicates that the seed and egg of your Sacred Work Vision germinated; you conceived, but after conception, out of hopelessness and fear, lack of consciousness or lack of preparedness, you feel you don't have what it takes to support your vision. You terminated your Sacred Work Vision midstream; you eradicated the Sacred Work Vision from the womb of your mind, the womb of your heart, and therefore the womb of your Sacred Seat, even though it was oh, so painful to do.

### Sacred Work Affirmation (Antidote)

I am no longer running scared of my birth. I embrace myself completely; therefore, I will absolutely prepare myself to take my Sacred Work Vision full term.

The question here is: Will I or will I not carry my vision through? A mother once said in the midst of a Sacred Woman healing circle, "I am a seamstress, a designer of sorts, and I have a lot of cloth sitting around at home unfinished. I start a project, then midway through finishing my work, I put it on the shelf and start up sewing on another project. Starting and stopping is my internal conflict." This repeated pattern represented her "unfinished work that didn't go full term." She realized she'd been aborting her vision, her gift, over and over again.

How many of us have conceived our Sacred Works with enthusiasm, then begun to second-guess our conception and terminate our Sacred Work pregnancy out of fear and insecurity? How many of us have shared our vision with company who did not believe in us? So we, too,

begin to doubt ourselves. We begin feeling the vision is too awesome a responsibility to bring to full term. Aborting it seems to be the only answer.

You can be abortion-free but, upon conceiving your purpose, decide to terminate that purpose midterm.

**Journal Work**

Sit still, breathe, relax, let go—tap into your Sacred Center and bring forth your truth. Identify the Vision Work that was aborted.

- When did I create this Sacred Work blockage?
- How and why did I create this Sacred Work blockage?
- What am I willing to do to overcome this Sacred Work blockage?

## Miscarriage (Spontaneous Abortion)

Miscarriage indicates that the weight of your vision was too heavy to carry. Develop the muscle, the consciousness, and the skills to carry your Sacred Work through. To go full term, you must spend a great deal more time in Cycle 1—Purification Preparation (the cycles are described later in this chapter).

### Sacred Work Affirmation (Antidote)

*Because I nurtured myself appropriately in Cycle 1—Purification Preparation, I have the power to carry the weight and force of my Sacred Vision Work.*

You can conceive a baby and lose it during the third or fourth month; you can also conceive your purpose and then lose it along the way.

**Journal Work**

Identify the Vision Work that miscarried.

- When did I create this Sacred Work blockage?
- How and why did I create this Sacred Work blockage?
- What am I willing to do to overcome this Sacred Work blockage?

## Morning Sickness

Morning sickness indicates a lack of preparation of your Sacred Work. The vision is overwhelming, so you feel incapable of carrying it, and you enter a state of disease due to lack of mental, physical, and spiritual cleansing before conception.

To overcome morning sickness, continue to activate Cycle 1—Purification Preparation through your pregnancy.

### Sacred Work Affirmation (Antidote)

*My Temple is pure, healthy, and united in body, mind, and spirit, capable of preventing morning sickness.*

You can go through pregnancy to full term without experiencing morning sickness, but many get pregnant with vision and purpose and then grow weak while carrying the heaviness of their burden.

### Journal Work
Identify the Vision Work that experienced morning sickness.

- When did I create this Sacred Work blockage?
- How and why did I create this Sacred Work blockage?
- What am I willing to do to overcome this Sacred Work blockage?

## Edema/Preeclampsia

Edema/preeclampsia indicates that you are extremely overwhelmed by your Sacred Work Vision. You conceived your Sacred Work in fear and doubt and carried it throughout your pregnancy, resulting in a terminal dis-ease, a shutting down of your creative capacity.

### Sacred Work Affirmation (Antidote)

*My Sacred Work and I are in NTR Maat (Divine Order). I have uprooted the fears and doubts of carrying and birthing my Sacred Work.*

### Journal Work
Identify the Vision Work that experienced edema/preeclampsia.

- When did I create this Sacred Work blockage?
- How and why did I create this Sacred Work blockage?
- What am I willing to do to overcome this Sacred Work blockage?

## Premature Birth

Premature birth indicates that your Sacred Work came out too soon and was underdeveloped, but it lives by grace. For your Sacred Work to survive, you must give it extreme care as it matures.

### Sacred Work Affirmation (Antidote)

*My Sacred Work Vision is developed, strong, and powerful. This is accomplished through absolute love, devotion, dedication, and care for the coming forth of my Sacred Work Vision.*

### Journal Work
Identify the Vision Work that experienced a premature birth.

- When did I create this Sacred Work blockage?
- How and why did I create this Sacred Work blockage?
- What am I willing to do to overcome this Sacred Work blockage?

## Stillbirth

Stillbirth indicates lack of nourishment, faith, knowledge (training), and enthusiasm. You fear you're not enough to carry your vision to its zenith. You carried your Sacred Work full term, but on its birth it died due to Lack Syndrome (see Infertility, above).

### Sacred Work Affirmation (Antidote)

*My Sacred Work Vision is alive and well. I have faith, knowledge, enthusiasm, and support to maintain and grow my vision.*

A newborn can live a vibrant life, but you can see your purpose pass away after its birth.

## Journal Work

Identify the Vision Work that experienced a still-birth.

- When did I create this Sacred Work blockage?
- How and why did I create this Sacred Work blockage?
- What am I willing to do to overcome this Sacred Work blockage?

## Crib Death

Crib death indicates that the death of your vision came after birth. Now that the vision is born, you are still lacking the appropriate knowledge of your Sacred Work to carry it through its many levels of growth, so it dies unexpectedly. Throughout, there were signs that the vision was challenged. You weren't tuned into the signs. Due to lack of appropriate support—promotion, marketing, advertisements, economics, love, nurturing—your Sacred Work lost its momentum while in its infancy, resulting in its burial.

### Sacred Work Affirmation (Antidote)

*I affirm that my Sacred Work Vision lives through me, fully alive. Daily I strengthen my vision as I grow, expand, and breathe appreciation, joy, and vitality into my Sacred Work.*

### Journal Work

Identify the Vision Work that experienced a crib death.

- When did I create this Sacred Work blockage?
- How and why did I create this Sacred Work blockage?
- What am I willing to do to overcome this Sacred Work blockage?

## BIRTH YOUR SACRED WORK

*Your gift is your life.*
*Your work is your life mission waiting to be born.*
*We all have been given a Divine Work to do.*

*If you do the work that Spirit has given you,*
*Then your work will heal, lift, and inspire*
*You and all others to live their Sacredness.*

Your Sacred Divine Work has the capacity to mold and remake you. Take care of your health so you may enjoy your true destiny. Living your Sacred Work is an act of worship and prayer and a Sacred Union with the soul, waiting to be born.

### The Sexuality, the Conception, and the Fulfillment of My Sacred Work

I'm fulfilled! Today I had intercourse with the light and together we conceived my dream. I cleaned, I prayed, I trusted, and I opened myself up to my Divinity; for I am not afraid. If fear sets in at any point in my conception, I will breathe the breath of the anointed, I will relax and let go, that I may conceive the fullness of my purpose.

I'm ready. I close my eyes to feel the seed of my dream enter in NTR (the light of the One Most High within). I cry, I release, I open my petals of new beginning. Thank you, Divine within me. As I open my eye (*Udjat*) to the light, the vision is being planted. I begin to swell up inside due to the light of my vision. As it is getting clearer, I breathe deeper. The light of my vision is getting stronger. I'm excited, I cannot hold back. I'm on fire as the vision builds up inside the womb of my mind. It's expansive, this womb of my heart; explosive, this womb of my Sacred Seat. It's impregnating. I place my hand over my abdomen, and I grab my womb from the outside in, as I contract and release my soul to meet the orgasm (the light) with bliss. It's there! The vision has been planted. I see it and it's lovely. I feel it; I can taste and smell the aroma of my Sacred Work. I am submerged in bliss, listening to the cosmic sounds, connected to the Divine's Creation. I am with child; I'm devoted to carrying my vision through all the cycles; as I grow this vision inside myself, it is protected within my Body Temple. I nurture my vision daily, I'll birth a radiant, beautiful, profound, crystal-clear Sacred Vision, and everyone will come from far and near to share in it. Now that I have conceived, the Deeper Work begins to birth.

It is now time to take my full journey from Cycle 1 to Cycle 9.

## ENTER INTO SACRED WOMAN RITES OF PASSAGE

### Level 2

#### 12 Weeks to Self-Purpose Activation

### 12 WEEKS TO BIRTHING

### BIRTHING YOUR SACRED WORK

**Enter Into Sacred Woman Rites of Passage**

#### Level II

**Self-Purpose Activation to 12 Weeks of Birthing**

**My Sacred Work—My Life's Purpose**

### MESHKENET'S BIRTHING WHEEL OF ENLIGHTENMENT: ACTION CYCLE TO BIRTHING MY SACRED WORK

You have finally arrived. You were able to travel through and learn from the pain and pitfalls of the Birthing Blues. You are now ready to come into alignment with birthing your Meshkenet, your Sacred Work, your purpose. From Cycle 1 through Cycle 9, you will be guided on how to birth your Self.

Allow this process to unfold a full season during Gateway 11, Sacred Work.

The quality of the birthing of your Sacred Woman and how well you experienced the birthing cycle determine the quality of your Sacred Work. You can get stuck in any one cycle of birth and experience the Birthing Blues if you are not ready to ascend to the freedom of your Sacred Self. Traveling the Birthing Wheel, your

Sacred Work will be anything but easy. Regardless of the challenges, however, you must believe in the blessing of living your Sacred Work in order to overcome. In the end, it will be worth every bit of the effort it took to conceive, birth, and grow your Sacred Work. I've been privileged to birth many works over the years. At times I've experienced great disappointment; pain came in the form of financial challenges, lack of confidence, fear of the unknown, procrastination, and stagnation. By the grace of the Divine, I could not, would not, let the visions die inside of me. It is through my visions that I am fully beautiful—that I am able to be all of myself.

Reading through the following birthing cycles will assist you in actualizing your Sacred Work. Cycle 9 represents completion, coming of age, going full circle, indicating that your vision has fully ripened according to the state you're in. Each birthing stage (cycle) must be completed and charged before you proceed to the next. Set your schedule. Keep your Divine discipline happening whatever occurs. Keep moving forward and upward. Take nine days, more or less, to move through each cycle. It will take a minimum of nine weeks and as much as nine months to open up the gates and birth your Sacred Work. Put yourself on a Sacred Clock—a practical spiritual timetable to accomplish your goal.

### Meshkenet Journal and Sacred Work Exploration

Before you enter into Birthing Wheel Cycles 1 through 9, Meshkenet Journal Reflection is a work of exploration and self-evaluation that will assist you in birthing your Sacred Work. As you move through this body of work, you will come to hear your inner voice, the All-Knowing Sacred Self that has the answers to the birthing of your Sacred Work. As you work through this text through meditation practice, cleaning rituals, visualization activities, and journal writing, you will birth your Divine Purpose in the form of your Sacred Work. Let us bear down on the ancient birthing bricks of our first ancestors of the Nile Valley, as we release from our loins the answer that unblocks the secret to our birthing our Sacred Work Vision.

As you answer the following questions, you will receive a clear and concise picture of the Sacred Work Birthing process, therefore birth a healthy work. Journal outside in an open space of nature or journal in a room that is clean, clear, and uncluttered so that your mind and heart have the space to flow. Breathe deeply several times, then open up your heart and speak your truth as you answer these questions.

- How long have I been longing to live my ideal work?
- How can I improve and strengthen my Sacred Work?
- What benefits are there in my performing my Sacred Work?
- How am I going to overcome my fears and apprehensions?
- Am I willing to live without manifesting my life's work?
- Do I have a guide that reflects my Sacred Work?
- Do I have contracts to help me live my Sacred Work?
- How do I see my Sacred Work manifesting in:

  — A week?
  — One month?
  — Six months?
  — One year?
  — Two years?
  — Five years and beyond?

- Do I have the education (information) to birth my Sacred Work?
- Do I have enough training to commit to and strengthen my Sacred Work?
- What will I do to master my Sacred Work?
- Do I have enough money (finances) to live in my Sacred Work?
- What do I need financially to make it happen? (Write out the details.)

### How to Use the Birthing Wheel

Take one wheel and one vision at a time. Place the name of your vision in the wheel and place an approximate date of birth expectancy under your Sacred Work Vision. You may conceive and birth two to four births simultaneously. If this is so, be aware that it will be more challenging, but if you're really focused, the birthing of your Sacred Works can be done effectively. Fill in the circles according to your inner vision. (You may use these as a sample of seeing your vision on paper.)

Carry only what you can handle. The fewer wheels you spin at one time, the better you can birth meaningful work in a strong and timely way. Because I had so many visions at once, it took longer for them to birth. I had to develop profound patience and focus so as not to lose sight of any one of my visions.

### Become a Midwife for Self and Others

Independently or collectively, create a Sacred Work Support Circle. You can meet once a week, or every new moon, or every full moon. Interact via meditation, visualization, brainstorming, networking, clarifying, reviewing, and growing. Discuss your daily Meshkenet Sacred Work checklist as you go forward to rebirth your Sacred Work Visions. Be sure to spend quality time developing and rebirthing your Sacred Work. As you work independently or collectively as a Sacred Work Collective of midwives, you may be at different points of birth. Some may have to spend more time in conception than others; some may be in the second trimester of gestation of their Sacred Work. Others may require a longer or a shorter labor. Wherever you find yourself in the spectrum of your birthing process, know that in Divine time your work will birth and flourish according to your devotion, dedication, enthusiasm, and tenacity. As Lady Prema, my sister-friend on the Purification Journey, says: "Hold on to your inner vision and over time it will come to light. Just don't give up on yourself, for in you is the truth, the light."

# CYCLE 1: THE WOMBNIFEST OF PURIFICATION PREPARATION

The only way to birth your Sacred Work is to be prepared to focus, to center, to open yourself as you birth yourself through all nine cycles. Give yourself twenty-one days to prepare for the conception of your purpose in order not to conceive a distortion of it.

During this time, you will detox and purify in order to conceive, maintain, and birth a Divine Thought Seed for a Sacred Work Vision. In this way, you can create an inner environment for your Sacred Work Vision to flourish.

Clear your energy field of negative thoughts, emotions, reactions, and relations so that you don't birth your fear or rejection, or pour hurts into the conception of your Sacred Work. Remember, these negativities cause involuntary abortion, miscarriage, morning sickness, or any of the other possible Birthing Blues.

## Eat to Feed Your Purpose

Green foods feed your purpose. For breakfast, have fresh fruits and Juiced Greens Live Formula.

For lunch and dinner, eat salad, steamed greens, avocados, lentils, peas, and sprouts. Serve with 8 to 16 oz. of green juice.

*Avoid* meats, junk food, fast food, GMO food, processed food, starch, and sugar.

## Spiritual Surgery Through Daily Affirmations

The following process of breathing, relaxation, and affirmations helps undo the psychological and emotional damage that hinders our Meshkenet development.

Begin with the appropriate Sacred Work Affirmation.

### Sacred Work Affirmations

- My work is my Sacred Vision.
- Realization of my Sacred Work is my life's quest.
- I take on my Sacred Work with courage.
- I and my Sacred Work are one.
- My Sacred Work acts as my devotional service to the Divine no matter how humble or grand.
- My Sacred Work is my service to the enhancement of humanity.
- My Sacred Work is my passion.
- I have unwavering faith that I will go full term and birth my Sacred Work.
- I am entitled to and deserve to live my Sacred Work.

Then continue: *"My energy field inside the womb of my mind is filled with light."* In the middle of each affirmation, breathe in, then out. Release the vibrations you're feeling in and around the work that you are releasing from your womb center.

Proceed to the Release Phase.

### Spiritual Detoxification Release Affirmations

- I release hostility (breathe) from the womb of my mind, heart, and seat of Creation.
- I release rage (breathe) from the womb of my mind.
- I release insecurity (breathe) from the womb of my mind.
- I release hurt (breathe) from the womb of my mind.
- I release resentment (breathe) from the womb of my mind.
- I release fear (breathe) from the womb of my mind.
- I release doubt (breathe) from the womb of my mind.

Follow with the Recharge Phase. Repeat these two phases—Release and Recharge—as you create spiritual energy in the womb of your heart, mind, and Sacred Seat.

### Spiritual Detoxification Recharge Affirmations

- I bring the breath of light into the womb of my mind.
- I bring the breath of life into the womb of my heart.
- I bring the breath of life into the womb of my Sacred Seat.
- I bring the breath of light into the womb of my mind, heart, and Seat of Creation.
- I bring the breath of love into the womb of my mind, heart, and Seat of Creation.

- I bring the breath of serenity into the womb of my mind, heart, and Seat of Creation.
- I bring the breath of peace into the womb of my mind, heart, and Seat of Creation.
- I bring the breath of strength into the womb of my mind, heart, and Seat of Creation.
- I bring the breath of joy into the womb of my mind, heart, and Seat of Creation.
- I bring the breath of pure energy into the womb of my mind, heart, and Seat of Creation.

## CYCLE 2: THE WOMBNIFEST OF THE CONCEPTION

Through the Seeker of Light, open your heart center, the location of your Sacred Work. Through channeling meditation, see and receive your purpose. Breathe deeply into your heart center seven or more times, then breathe one hundred Fire Breaths. Return to slow deep breathing. Rest in your heart.

See a door. Open it up. Go inside. Before you is an altar where the Divine dwells. Breathe. Ask the question, "What is my Sacred Work?" Listen closely. Keep breathing. "Seek and you shall find." If you don't see or hear your Sacred Work, continue to perform Cycle 1 — Purification Preparation to ready yourself for seeing and conceiving your Sacred Work.

The Seeker and the Conceiver are two sides of the same coin. Now that you see the vision, will you accept it? The acceptance of your Sacred Work Vision allows you to conceive the life of your Sacred Work. Locate your Sacred Work through the Sacred Woman Gateways of Enlightenment. If you asked and you've witnessed your Sacred Work Vision, then you've experienced enlightenment.

Impregnate the womb of your mind, the womb of your heart, and the womb of your Sacred Seat with your vision according to the Gateways.

- *Gateway 0 Nut, Sacred Womb:* obgyn, nurse-midwife, astrologer, astronomer, rebirther, doula, Womb Yoga Dancer, Womb Yoga Dance instructor
- *Gateway 1 Tehuti, Sacred Word:* scholar, motivational speaker, writer, publicist, editor, computer specialist, teacher
- *Gateway 2 Ta-Urt, Sacred Food:* food preparation, chef, agriculturist, dietitian, farmer, chef
- *Gateway 3 Bes, Sacred Movement:* dancer, sacred performer, physical therapist, exercise specialist, Womb Yoga Dance teacher, practitioner, artist, fitness coach
- *Gateway 4 Het-Hru, Sacred Beauty and Inner Child:* clothing designer, makeup artist, musician, beauty care specialist, child care specialist, beautification worker, seamstress
- *Gateway 5 Nebt-Het, Sacred Space:* interior decorator, architect
- *Gateway 6 Sekhmet, Sacred Healing:* healer herbalist, nurse, doctor, reflexologist, energy worker
- *Gateway 7 Maat, Sacred Relationships:* psychotherapist, judge, court system worker
- *Gateway 8 Ast, Sacred Union:* marriage therapist/consultant, tantric sexual guide, Spiritual Healer, meditation practitioner
- *Gateway 9 Nefer Atum:* media person, public relations, advertising marketing specialist, meditation teacher (guide), spiritualist, rebirther
- *Gateway 10 Seshat, Sacred Time:* practitioner of Sacred Time, astrologer, numerologist
- *Gateway 11 Meshkenet, Sacred Work:* career coach, a Queen Afua Meshkenet Coach

If you are versed in pendulum readings, then you may use a pendulum to help divinely select your work. (See pages 273–276 for suggestions on using a pendulum.)

## CYCLE 3: THE WOMBNIFEST OF THE DIVINE PLAN OF YOUR PURPOSE

Conception is acceptance of your divine connection. This cycle is about strengthening the Conception by writing out your business plan. To receive enlightenment, it takes time to open up the womb of your mind, the womb of your heart, and the womb of your Sacred Seat. To conceive your vision, you must open your womb to receive the light of your Sacred Work Vision.

Once you see or hear the enlightenment of your Sacred Work Vision, then connect your heart and your womb as one stream of light. As above, so below. Begin to breathe deeply from your heart down to your womb several times for the Divine Plan to take hold. As you breathe more and more, allow your heart center to become larger and allow your womb to be more subtle and receptive. Breathe deeply that your Sacred Work may now begin to take form. Follow your intuition when you sense that the Divine Plan is manifesting. Gently place your hand over your heart center and your womb center for a few minutes as you breathe through your palms into your conception centers to seal in the Conception of the Divine Plan. The Divine Plan Conception is completed.

Once you receive your message and conceive your Sacred Work Plan, your calling, don't hesitate to listen and obey. Further spiritual instruction on how to bring forth your Sacred Work on a material plane will come to you as you travel through Meshkenet's Birthing Wheel.

Freely and creatively fill in your Sacred Work Commitment statement to assist the birth of your Sacred Work. Read your statement to focus and remind you to go forward when the challenges of growth occur. The review of your commitment will also inspire you to go full term, regardless of the hurdles you must climb to reach your ultimate goal.

### My Sacred Work Commitment

Right now, I commit myself to establish the Wisdom of Meshkenet and thereby awaken the midwife within me, that I may bring forth and birth my Sacred Work.

Signature _____

Date of Commitment _____

### Transformative Sacred Work Journal Writing

Part of the Divine Plan of Conception is the development of your Sacred Work Mission Statement. Begin doing this now through your Sacred Work Journal.

- Write down, for seven days, how you feel about your present work and what it would take for you to be totally in line with your Vision.

- In the next seven days, write your Life's Work Mission Statement in as much detail as possible. As you strive to do this, limit or eliminate the intake of starch and flesh protein for seven days so that you will be able to receive clear unblocked visions. Always perform your sacred writing after your morning meditation.
- Once your mission statement is written, place it on your altar to stay consistently, spiritually connected to your vision.
- If need be, receive spiritual guidance during the next seven days. Seek consultation or career advice from an astrologer, numerologist, priest or priestess, minister or imam for further clarification, or read with a pendulum if you have the skill. (See pages 273–276 for suggestions on using a pendulum.)

### Daily Spiritual Development of Your Work

Every morning upon rising, perform this spiritual ritual to assist in bringing forth your Sacred Work. Perform this during Meshkenet Birthing Cycles 3 through 7.

#### 1. The Spiritual Bath
Perform a spiritual bath with frankincense and myrrh or with lotus oil to promote physical and mental clarity. It's uplifting and motivational. Place a few drops of the oil in your bathwater. Add a few drops to a bowl of water as well, and sprinkle a few drops around your prayer space. (Use only essential oils.)

#### 2. Your Altar
Set up your sacred altar according to your own spiritual or religious beliefs (see page 18). Sit before it quietly and meditatively on the floor on a pillow or in a comfortable chair.

*Anoint with lotus oil.* Anoint your crown, forehead (the Body Temple Gateway of supreme spirituality), heart (the Body Temple Gateway of compassion and divine love), womb area, palms, and the bottoms of your feet to make everything your touch become more sacred.

Shake, ring, beat, or rattle your sacred instrument (i.e., drum, sistrum, shekere) to awaken the angelic host that is indwelling.

### 3. Libation

Pour a libation for the Sacred Work Gateway from a cup or sprinkle water from a bowl into the earth or into a plant as you call out by giving adoration.

— *Pour a libation* as you say, Adoration to the Sacred Guardian, Meshkenet, who assisted humanity in our birth and rebirth, and in the rebirthing of our Sacred Work, and Heru, for protecting us on our spiritual journey of life.

— *Pour a libation* as you say, Adoration to the Ancestors. (Name the ancestors who inspire you to develop your Sacred Work.)

— *Pour a libation* as you say, Adoration to the Elders. (Call out those who are your living examples.)

— *Pour a libation* as you say, Adoration to my Divine Self and my Contemporaries who express their Sacred Work. (Name those you wish to emulate.)

### 4. Sacred Woman Spirit Prayer

Gently ring your bell, or softly play another sacred instrument at the beginning and end of the prayer.

*Sacred Spirit, NTR, hold me near, close to your bosom. Protect me from all harm and fear, from the blows of life. Direct my steps in the right way as I journey through this vision. Sacred Spirit, surround me in your absolutely perfect light. Anoint me in your sacred purity, peace, and divine insight. Bless me, truly bless me, as I share this sacred life. Teach me, Sacred Spirit, to be in tune with the Universe. Teach me how to heal with the inner and outer elements of air, fire, water, and earth.*

### 5. Fire Breaths

Prepare your Fire Breaths by slowly inhaling four times and exhaling four times. Then, when you are totally at ease, begin one to one thousand Fire Breaths. Inhale deeply like a pump through your nose (mouth closed) as you expand the breath down into the abdomen, then back up to the chest. Completely exhale out through your nostrils from your abdomen as it contracts and the lungs release your breath completely. Repeat this breath rapidly in and out, in and out.

Allow each deep Fire Breath to represent the opening of the thousand lotus petals of illumination and radiance, ultimately reaching Nefer Atum—the ultimate Afrakan Lotus station of Divinity.

### 6. Meshkenet Sacred Work Birthing Meditation

Close your eyes and sit still as you hold a pink tourmaline stone over your holy womb. Visualize the color pink and your spiritual midwife Meshkenet as you visualize your life's work inside your womb waiting to be born. Perform this meditation daily before your journal work.

The longer you are in meditation, the deeper will be your inner peace and the more solid your spirit (*ka*). The cleaner your Body Temple, the easier it is to go into and live in a state of meditation.

Each time you perform this meditation, more self-knowledge is revealed to you. Record new information that is born out of your meditation; it will be useful as you develop your Sacred Work.

---

### Sacred Vision Birthing

If you are not aware of your life's work at this point, it's time for a Sacred Vision birthing. With your eyes closed, breathe into your heart center, the Gateway of your passion for your Sacred Work. Relax and enter into the Gate of your heart; if you are ready in spirit, your work will be revealed to you. Breathe deeply into your heart center seven or more times, then breathe one hundred Fire Breaths. Now that you know and you have heard the breath inside your womb, it's time for your Sacred Vision to be born.

Begin to breathe into your womb and out for four counts. Breathe deeply and slowly. Make it fuller and stronger with each breath, to represent your contractions and the coming (birthing) of your work (your Vision).

Mother, separate your legs (she's coming). See the crown of your Sacred Work Vision coming through your vagina. The contractions are getting stronger. You may be nervous and apprehensive—what if your work isn't received? Keep your mind centered; worry not. Meshkenet is there for you with open hands and heart, able to help you in a safe, satisfying, and supportive delivery. Open your mouth and raise your voice and breathe, "Ankh . . . Ankh!" Keep breathing stronger and fuller with each contraction.

Now bear down and make the final push. Ah . . . there she is—a beautiful Vision, a wondrous Work. Such genius. Pick up your Sacred Work from your lap and embrace her to your heart. Know that the world will embrace her, and that your good works will be received. Meshkenet will oversee your work in prayer and spirit as your Sacred Work grows. You are not alone.

*Color Visualization.* Visualize soft pink for Divine Love. As you perform your meditation, wear pink and/or place a pink cloth on the altar to birth your true love as Sacred Work. Then visualize white light to clear inner muddy waters, or purple for high spiritual vision.

*Sacred Stone Meditation.* While in meditation, hold a ruby or pink tourmaline in your palm over your heart. At birth (when ideas are born from your womb), this stone directs you on how to be guided from your heart, allowing your heart to open up your true mission. You may also use clear white quartz for inner clarity, or amethyst for enlightenment and clear vision.

### Birthing Meditation for Men

Men, go through the entire meditation, but visualize your seed becoming potent, pure, and enriching. Now release your seed (your Vision, your Divine Works) from your loins, through your careful cultivation of healthy awareness of Meshkenet's Birthing Wheel.

### 7. Herbal Tonics

Drink a cup of herbal tea in your favorite mug daily during or after spiritual writing. Choose one per day among red clover, chaparral, and burdock to help you detox your negative state and rejuvenate and build your Body Temple to house and carry through your powerful vision.

*Preparation.* Use one teabag to 1 cup of water. Boil water, turn off flame, and steep before or after your morning bath or sacred shower. Strain herbs from water then drink with joy and peace as you breathe between sips and unfold in your Sacred Work Journal Workbook.

### 8. Sacred Work Journal Writing

Record new information that you gathered from your meditations to enhance your Sacred Work.

Journal work can best be done after internal cleansing: taking an enema or herbal laxative. Enemas are always recommended before a mother gives birth, which will make delivery easier. Another choice is to take 3 tablets of cascara sagrada with 8 to 12 oz. distilled water two or three times a week until the birth of your work. Do this to keep yourself open and clear. Also plan to take an enema one to three times until the birth of your work.

When you are cleansed and centered, you receive spiritual messages from the One Most High with grace on the issue of your Sacred Work. When in the Spirit, messages travel down through your Spirit Mind to your heart, into your hand, and onto the paper. (This is how I do all my writing).

The best time to receive your spiritually written work is after you have completed your altar work, between the hours of 4 A.M. and 6 A.M. Keep a special pen and journal on your altar to work with the power, force, and stillness at the coming dawn.

Affirm your life daily. Write down your thoughts, activities, experiences, and interactions; or write down your hopes, visions, desires, and affirmations so that you will draw from them for help and support when in need.

# DAILY MESHKENET SACRED WORK CHECKLIST

Follow this structure for a season and observe the miracles.

| | S | M | T | W | Th | F | S |
|---|---|---|---|---|---|---|---|
| 1. Shower in alternating hot and cold water, or take a tub bath in 4 to 8 lbs. Epsom salt or 1 to 2 lbs. Dead Sea salt. | | | | | | | |
| 2. Anoint with lemon or fennel oil. | | | | | | | |
| 3. Libation to the Sacred Guardian, Ancestors, Elders, and Contemporaries. | | | | | | | |
| 4. Recite Sacred Work Prayers and Affirmations. | | | | | | | |
| 5. Fire Breaths, 1,000 to 1,200 over the course of the day: 300 Fire Breaths each at dawn, sunrise, midday, and sunset. | | | | | | | |
| 6. Perform the Meshkenet Breathing Meditation. | | | | | | | |
| 7. Herbal tonics of dandelion and gotu kola. | | | | | | | |
| 8. Sacred Work Journal Writing (work on business plan and/ or website). | | | | | | | |
| 9. Closing Sacred Work (share with Sacred Work Team daily/weekly). | | | | | | | |
| 10. Follow Meshkenet Natural Living Dietary Laws to support the birth and radiant health of your Sacred Work. Live primarily on live, organic greens to nourish properly. | | | | | | | |
| 11. Study/research Sacred Work. | | | | | | | |
| 12. Network/outreach Sacred Work. | | | | | | | |
| 13. Promote/develop marketing for Sacred Work. | | | | | | | |
| 14. Sacred Work environment development (Sacred Space for Sacred Work). | | | | | | | |
| 15. Consumption of Asar Prosperity Green Vegetable Juice (1 pint). | | | | | | | |
| 16. Consumption of 1 quart of distilled water and 2 limes for clarity of vision. | | | | | | | |
| 17. Building Sacred Work economic fund via proposals, savings, investments, fundraising. | | | | | | | |
| 18. Reach out to Meshkenet Birthing Circle Support. | | | | | | | |

Make twelve copies of this Sacred Work checklist to cover one season. On a daily basis, strive to complete your checklist throughout and after Sacred Work conception and afterbirth, to keep you focused on the growth of your vision.

## Sacred Work Daily Checklist

It's time to prepare for leaving your present career or position.

- Build your savings account.
- Start your own business in evenings and weekends.
- Before resigning, do your homework; become well versed and knowledgeable in your Sacred Work. Go to the library. Read books on business for inspiration and knowledge. Surround yourself with people who are successful in their careers. Take trainings or get a certification or degree in your prospective field.
- Gain experience: Volunteer in your field for on-the-job experience and training.
- Affirm that prosperity and abundance shall come from you, aligning yourself and your true calling.

Remember that your life's work is what you love best. Why not develop it and get paid for it? If it's truly your destiny—your *shai*—just as you love performing it, someone (or many) will love receiving it.

## CYCLE 4: THE WOMBNIFEST OF GESTATION

### Develop Your Meshkenet Business Plan

You're growing. Be confident; your vision's getting stronger. Continue to act on your faith and know that all you need to bring forth your Divine Work will be given to you as you grow into your true self, through pure, natural living and being.

Continue to work on performing your morning spiritual observances. Continue also to rewrite, embellish, and perfect your Sacred Work Mission Statement. You may need to create several drafts before you reach your final document. The clearer and more precise your mission statement, the more precise the manifestation of your Sacred Work.

### *Growing into Your Divine Destiny*

- Be in association with those you aspire to emulate.

- Network with skilled professionals who can support your vision.
- Read, explore, and study up on your prospective career.
- Affirm daily your birthright to live your Sacred Work.
- Acquire the necessary skill to support your work.
- Speak your Sacred Vision with like minds for encouragement, inspiration, and knowledge.
- Watch out who you share your vision with.
- Invest time, energy, and resources into your vision.
- Visit the library to study and enhance your vision.
- Develop a business plan as a road map in order to know where you are going and how to reach your destination.
- Always beware of the Birthing Blues (described earlier in this chapter), which can enter in through doubt or fear and contaminate your vision, causing your birth to be unsuccessful and incomplete.
- Study the works, pitfalls, and successes of other businesspeople as a guideline for success.

## One of My Personal Economic Triumphs

My desire to start my own business and carry out my Sacred Work was met with various forms of financial advice from many different people. My mother said, "Keep your credit clean." My father said, "Pay your taxes and purchase the building that houses your work." A business owner said, "Get a loan." A wise one said, "Become a not-for-profit organization and get funded by your community and by large corporations." I did it the old-school way. I relied on myself for funding, meaning I sold my products and services and reinvested the profits to build my business my Sacred Work. I was forced to move my business eleven times, from one location to the next, whether it was as a result of a fire on the premises, a flood washing my business out, or a padlock placed on my door by the city due to lack of funds. Yet I stayed focused on my vision. Through the years, because of poor credit or lack of funds, I rented after each move. Finally in 1993, my mother purchased the building I am now in and put it in my name. Between the support of my husbands' building of the infrastructure and my mother's purchase of the building, my work stabilized immeasurably. Despite the countless challenges I went through to get where I am today, it has been a wonderful, exciting, frightening, loving, transforming, "make you want to holla" Sacred Work Journey.

In the early days of my work, I had a staff of eight that included four colon therapists, two masseuses, and a secretary/manager. The location was in an affluent neighborhood, and I had plenty of business and more clients than I could handle. This was the heyday of my work. Unfortunately, due to poor business management, I had to close down my business abruptly. The city came with padlocks in hand and gave me only thirty minutes to pack my children and my business and move. I went to my mother's home. One week later I returned to move my things out. After moving expenses, I was left with $30, three children, and no business. I was not deterred! I may have been short on money, but I was not short on creativity and faith. In those areas, I've always been abundantly wealthy. Creativity and faith are what ultimately brought me financial stability.

With the $30 I had left to my name, I invested in a bag of clay and herbal extracts that went into producing twelve jars of clay. I sold the clay at a seminar I gave one month after being escorted out of my house by the city. I had no money to rent out space to present the seminar, so I sat down with the rental office at Bed-Stuy Restoration Company and explained to them my story and my desire to continue to serve the community. They supported my vision, and I was able to pay them from my proceeds after my presentation. The presentation was a success. The people came out hungry for healing. And I earned enough profit from the clay sales and the seminar to pay for my space, purchase food for my children, and triple my clay inventory. After a year of working consistently, I built my business back up again.

When I think back now to the city locking me out of my living and working space, having to say goodbye to my devoted staff, being temporarily out of work, and having to carry my children with me to my mother's home, all I can say is "I give thanks," for that was the beginning of a new level of my work altogether. It was in that apparently dark moment that I had the time and space to write my first book and create my line of products. The writing of *Heal Thyself for Health and Longevity* changed my life forever. It became the catalyst by which I reached out and inspired thousands worldwide to journey on the path of Holistic Wellness. It has allowed me to leave a healing legacy for my children's children and for Planet Earth when I am gone.

I have lived through many stories. I have experienced my portion of hard times and good times. Nevertheless, I was and am committed to live my vision. For my vision and I are in a Sacred Union of love and devotion, and together we reach for the heights. This gives us wings and lets us fly.

## CREATE YOUR OWN PERSONAL ECONOMIC TRIUMPH

### Seek Economic Support

- Is your cash flow coming from OPM (other people's money), investors, or YOM (your own money)? Create a budget as part of your business plan.
- Create an environment to support your Sacred Work.
- Create a Sacred Work Team (circle), a Birthing Team to help you progressively build your work, such as the following:

  — *A Meshkenet Guide* is the key or master guide who has knowledge, know-how, and experience on how to develop and birth your vision.
  — *A Het-Hru Guide* loves your vision as you do and will protect it through supportive words and actions.
  — *A Ptah Guide* protects your growing vision in the form of people such as lawyers, accountants, bookkeepers, and business investors.

- Establish your business type so that your Sacred Work team can best support your vision:

  — For profit
  — Not-for-profit

— Single proprietorship
— Joint proprietorship

## CYCLE 5: THE WOMBNIFEST OF THE TRIMESTERS

### Daily Physical Development of Your Sacred Work

- Continue to strengthen your business plan.
- Experience is the best teacher: Continue volunteering in the field of your calling for on-the-job experience and training. This is the best way to get the hands-on experience needed for the cultivation of your vision.
- Continue to connect with those who can help your business grow.
- Take intensive training to support your Sacred Work Vision. The more knowledge and skills you acquire in your field, the more confident and secure your birth will be. Receive the most appropriate, effective training, certification, diplomas, and guide development in your field.
- Update your skills and become computer-educated.
- Take business workshops in management, bookkeeping, office procedures, marketing, and promotion.
- Become a part of an association that focuses on your career.
- Keep your body well nourished and cleaned. Saturate your blood, tissues, bones, brain, and heart with liquid sunlight (green live foods and green live juices) throughout the day.
- Beware: To avoid Sacred Work damage, keep your vision in *sesheta* (secret); conceal it from nonbelievers in order to prevent Birthing Blues from coming into the picture. The world will be made aware of your vision at its birth.
- Be patient with your growth. Know that although you can't see your Sacred Work Vision with the mundane physical eye, it does exist. Life begins in the Spirit; if it's properly and consistently nourished, it will manifest on the material plane.

### Final Release Work for a Successful Birthing

You deserve to live your vision!

Affirm: *I release and let go of all of my fears and apprehension and all other emotions that block the birth of my Sacred Work. I release, I let go, and I let Spirit run my life.*

- Keep yourself encircled with people you want to emulate, people who encourage and inspire you to grow.
- Write an advance letter of your appreciation for bringing forth your Sacred Work.
- Smudge. Use frankincense and myrrh to smudge your crown and heart clean of all fear and doubt as and when they come up.
- Sweat it out in a sauna or steam bath for one hour off and on between showers as you wash your doubts away. Do this once or twice a week or as often as necessary to keep yourself receptive to birthing your vision.
- Walk it off. When in doubt, work it out. Let negativity and fear of being your true self flow as you fight them out of your mind and heart with each step.
- Recite your Sacred Womb Prayer and allow yourself to weep. After the tears, you will clear your heart and thereby see clearly.
- When in doubt, fast your way through on nutrients, herbs, and green vegetable drinks.
- Watch your thoughts and words. Keep your inner house clean and your mind on high.
- Hydrate your vision:

  — Drink 8 to 16 oz. of freshly pressed green juice followed by 8 to 16 oz. of distilled water or alkaline water.
  — Drink 8 to 12 oz. of freshly pressed fruit juices with 8 to 12 oz. of distilled water or alkaline water.
  — Drink 1 quart of warm water with the juice of 2 limes.

Be confident. Remember, you can create anything you desire out of your vision.

## CYCLE 6: THE WOMBNIFEST OF LABOR PAIN

### Riding the Waves of Your Birth

Affirm: *I am not afraid; I have complete trust in the birth of my Sacred Work.*

Ready your soul for the birth; relax and let go. You have come to the place of the deadline or, better said, the "lifeline." It's time to move beyond all excuses about why your Sacred Work cannot happen and how unready you are, for nature is taking its course and you are birthing your work. Fear not: It's time to bring your Sacred Work to the world.

In labor, your fears may heighten. Call on the Divine. Trust yourself. Breathe deeply. Push yourself through. Let go. You've done the necessary work to have a beautiful birth, so just stay in prayer. As you keep on letting go, circle yourself with only the strongest, most positive reflections to help you open up to your greatness. Trust that you and your Sacred Work are going to be fine. Stay within your breath as you follow the legacy of Nut by giving birth to the light of the sunlight that swells in the womb of your consciousness. No matter how intense the birthing contractions, ride them. When you look back, you will reflect that it was worth everything you went through to reach the illumination of your vision.

Oh, your vision has crowned itself. Bear down, commit completely. Push down and out real strong, for you are about to become a *mut*—a mother.

## CYCLE 7: THE WOMBNIFEST OF THE BIRTH

### Ready Your Soul for the Birth

Congratulations! The most challenging labor is over. Your vision is here; you've done it. You are the victor. Check to see if your work is intact. Count its toes, its fingers, and its spirit. Your Sacred Work has survived your inner journey. Now you must ready yourself for the next journey as your vision begins to grow.

## CYCLE 8: THE AFTERBIRTH OF AST AND HERU

All is well now.

According to the legacy of the Nile Valley of Khamit, Ast, the Great Mother of power from within, and Asar, the Great Father of power from within, are the parents of Heru. Heru is the light, the falcon that soars to great heights. Heru

is the true vision that is born out of an evolved soul. At birth, the light of Heru suckles on Mother Ast's breast for strengthening and nourishment. Heru and Ast are reflected in us as we mother and nurture our work, our vision, our "baby" into maturity, strength, and power. Check for your support team. Are they still active in your life after the birth of Heru, your Sacred Work? Your village and the midwives must continue to assist in the ongoing development of raising Heru, your newborn Sacred Work of light and truth.

### The Embrace: Nursing Heru

Watch out for postpartum blues. Heru, the light of your vision, is born out of your being. Therefore, as you care for Ast (the Nurturer within you), then you will care for Heru. You've delivered the life (your Sacred Work); now rest and reflect and regain your balance (i.e., take hot baths, light a candle and meditate as you soak in and appreciate birth). To avoid postpartum blues, embrace the birth soulfully as you give thanks for it.

### The Celebration

Have a community welcome, presentation, or open house. Have a release party. Have a press party. Have a viewing.

Send out announcements for all to witness your newly arrived Sacred Work, via promotion, via internet, radio, cable TV, newspaper, magazine, email, mailing, distribution, informational postcards, and so on. All of these communication approaches will assist in the growth of your Sacred Vision.

## CYCLE 9: MATURING YOUR SACRED WORK

Now that your Vision is born and the world has received it, the greatest task is to continue supporting your Sacred Work to maturity—a level where your work is well established and supports you spiritually, physically, and financially.

If you get worn out, if you run out of funding or faith and become tired of growing your vision, just rest and recharge. Then get back on the road to success with everything you have in you. Build your Sacred Work to the fullest and it will be worth all of your efforts. Fight the odds, for you really are a winner and you can do it. It is a known fact in business that, if you can maintain your work for at least two years, then you are home free. Your Sacred Work has passed the test of time and has the potential to reach maturity.

### Growing Up Heru

According to the Afrakan teachings from antiquity, Heru is the inner victor, the inner light; the falcon who soars to great heights; the one with keen, clear vision.

In order for your Sacred Work to mature, you must water and nurse it daily. Do this through constant promotion, advertisement, re-evaluation, and shaping your work to meet the needs of the people. Stay connected to the voice of the people, and their quest will help you shape your Sacred Work into what is relevant to the times. To maintain, keep your works in the eye of your community, and in the eye of the world. Continue to study and expand in your field and witness your Sacred Work growing as you develop yourself from the inside out.

Be one with Heru, the Victor, and don't turn back. "Forward ever, backward never."

## LIVE YOUR SACRED WORK

I am listed as a healer, an author, a spiritualist, a midwife. Unlimited is what I am, and we all are. Stretch yourself as I've stretched myself over a forty-five-year span, doing what I love best, performing sacred dance. January 23, 2003, at Howard University in Washington DC, I was center stage as the curtains came up and lights were shining down on my dance company, Abut Em Anksamble. What a wonderful experience! My work opened the National Dance Conference, and we danced, and we danced, and we danced our Sacred Work, out of our souls. Before an anticipating audience we performed the Nile Valley River Dance, a contemporary, yet ancient healing art form inspired by our Afrakan Ancestors. Some naysayers tried to limit me; *this* one with her fears and *that* one with her doubts. Some said, "You can't do that, it's too much." "Stay in the box," my subconscious whispered.

But the Spirit within me encouraged, "I am the Victor, your purpose, your Sacred Work." My Sacred Work insisted, "Let me go free to create and re-create a life of physical, mental, and spiritual prosperity." I did exactly that, I kept birthing and re-creating and discovering more levels of my purpose, my sacred world, for freedom.

So I am here to encourage you to stand strong in your Vision. Wherever you reside in the realm of your Sacred Work Vision, it is there your Birthing Wheel lives. Know that we are all, each one of us, entitled to live out every bit of our Sacred Work. Birthing our Divine true purpose is our prayer, our destiny. Know that you will hit rocks and bumps along the way, and you will climb steep hills. Regardless of the apparent obstacles, rise anyway. Move courageously forward; for what appears as obstacles are the lessons needed to help you cultivate your Sacred Work. Open up soulfully and allow the Divine in you to walk you through your glorious and most fulfilling Sacred Work. You can make it happen. Just trust and listen from within as you allow yourself to be guided spiritually to your Sacred Work, your dearest and closest friend. Radiate and know. Live your Sacred Work!

## SACRED WORK: SEVEN-DAY TRANSFORMATIVE WORK

As you continue to purify your life daily through sacred words, thoughts, and deeds on a physical, mental, emotional, and spiritual plane, the words coming out of your mouth and back to you will be words of power, light, and healing. You will speak Sacred Words to sacred souls.

• *Talk fast: Perform a talk fast over the next seven days.* Speak only when necessary; don't talk for hours. Watch as your words become pure and organic. Throughout the week observe a seven- to twelve-hour talk fast, alone or with others who are doing the same practice.

• *Choose the appropriate flower essences* to support your transformative work.
• *Sacred Word affirmations:* Finally, following a daily affirmation, participate in morning and evening prayer. Now begin to reclaim your natural self through your words:

*My life reflects the levels of the words.*

*Today I am transforming my life to a higher good*

*Through energizing, healing words.*

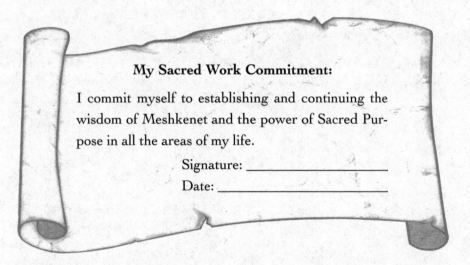

### My Sacred Work Commitment:

I commit myself to establishing and continuing the wisdom of Meshkenet and the power of Sacred Purpose in all the areas of my life.

Signature: _____

Date: _____

# UNTIL WE MEET AGAIN

To the One Most High, to our NTRU, our Ancestors, our Elders and mentors, *tua* (thank you) for walking with us, your daughters. *Tua Het-Hru* (love) for pouring blessings upon our journey through the pages of this book. All hail to our ancient Afrakan way, the Path of Nefer Atum (the lotus of Divinity that comes forth from the mud). Hail to Imhotep and his mother, the Healer within you and the light of the Most High that continued to guide you. I am grateful for all the many spiritual visitations I've received in the channeling of *Sacred Woman*.

We have journeyed deep within our Sacred Wombs and listened to her voice and her wisdom. She ushered us through the Gateways of Initiation to become Sacred Afrakan Women. All women can learn from us as a foundation for growth. We have prayerfully moved into the

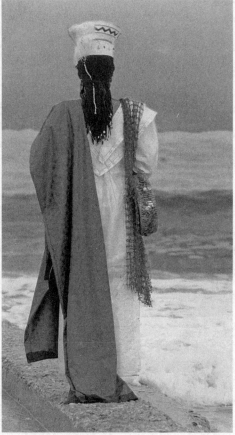

upper room of our lives. We have reclaimed our traditions, our heritage, our culture, our sacredness, and our healing with absolute joy and delight. We have saved ourselves and protected ourselves from every adversity, and finally come full circle to empower ourselves through the guidance of Maat. May the living rituals, concepts, affirmations, techniques, recipes, formulas, and tools offered in this work become a part of your journey back to self.

Whatever your religious affiliation, spiritual direction, or cultural connections, may you be reborn and renewed. Allow your Sacred Lotus Initiation to work through you, so that you will ultimately come into the greatness of who you were destined to be. In the words of our great and beloved Ancestors, until we meet again, *hetepu*, Nefer Atum Lotus Flower Blossom.

## THERE IS A SACRED PART OF ME
### Queen Afua

There is a Sacred part of me
It's a gift from our ancestors from the Hapi Nile
    Valley

There is a Sacred part of me that nothing can discour-
    age
No one can disturb my peace.
That sacred part of me
She is Nut, the sky mother who is indwelling.
She is Tehuti, who guides my divinely inspired words.

There is a perfect part of me that nothing can discour-
    age
No one can disturb my peace.
That perfect part of me
She is Ta-Urt, the earth mother who nourishes my
    Body Temple.
She is Nebt-Het, the guardian who purifies my space.

Where is she?
Where is she?
Go within.
Go within.
She's there.
She's there.

There is a Sacred part of me that is deep within my
    heart
So deep that nothing can disturb my peace.
That sacred part of me
She is Het-Hru, most beautiful.
She is Sekhmet, the healer.
She is Ast, the Great Mother who heals my
    relationships.

There is a Sacred part of me that no one can mislead
No one can destroy my peace.
That sacred part of me
She is Meshkenet, guardian of birthing.
She is Maat, who keeps my heart serene.

Where is she?
Where is she?
Go within.
Go within.
She's there.
She's there.

There is a Sacred part of me that no one can
    discourage
No one can disturb my peace.
That sacred part of me

She is Sesheta, who heals and reveals all.
She is Nefer Atum, Indwelling Lotus of Divinity.

There is a Sacred part of me that resides within my
    crown that
No wickedness, or venom or anger or mistrust,
No evil doings or wickedness can touch.
There is a sacred part of me that is graced with
    harmony.
There is a Sacred part of me filled with serenity.

Where is she?
Where is she?
Go within.
Go within.
She's there.
She's there.

Close your eyes
She's here.

Thank you, Divine Mother/Father.
Thank you, Ancestor.
Thank you, all my guides and Sacred Sisters.

Tua-Ntr
Tua Ancestors, Tua.

# APPENDIX A:
# SACRED WOMAN PRODUCTS AND TOOLS

## HEAL THYSELF NATURE PRODUCTS

- [ ] Green Life Super Nutritional Formula I
- [ ] Master Herbal Formula II
- [ ] Inner Ease Colon Deblocker Formula III
- [ ] Cascara Sagrada Herbal Laxative Tablets IV
- [ ] Queen Afua's Rejuvenation Clay 8 oz. V
- [ ] Queen Afua's Rejuvenation Clay 4 oz. V
- [ ] Breath of Spring Mucus Decongestor VI
- [ ] Woman's Life Herbal Formula VIII
- [ ] Heal Thyself 3-Day Pre-measured Supply of Formulas: Formula I; Formula II; Formula III; Formula IV; Instructional Natural Living and Nutritional Fasting Card
- [ ] Heal Thyself 21-Day Cleansing Kit Includes 21-Day Supply of Formulas: (3) Formula I; (3) Formula II; (3) Formula III; (1) Formula IV; (1) Breath of Spring; (1) 4 oz. Clay; (1) *Heal Thyself* Book; (1) Manual
- [ ] Heal Thyself 7-Day Cleansing Kit Supply of Formulas: (1) Formula I; (1) Formula II; (1) Formula III; (1) Formula IV; (1) Manual
- [ ] Womb Works 3-Step Wellness Pack Includes Womb Works Audiotape, Womb Works Newsletter, and Womb Progress Chart

## HEAL THYSELF HOLISTIC EDUCATION LITERATURE

- [ ] *Heal Thyself for Health and Longevity,* by Queen Afua
- [ ] *Heal Thyself Cookbook,* by Diane Ciccone
- [ ] Dance of the Womb Exercise Chart
- [ ] Heal Thyself Home Study Manual

## HEAL THYSELF AUDIOTAPES

- [ ] Womb Works Audiotape
- [ ] Indwelling Healer Audiotape

## HEAL THYSELF VIDEOTAPES

- [ ] Kitchen Power Cooking Class Video
- [ ] 21-Day Fasting Video Course—8 hours
- [ ] Liberation Through Purification Video

## HEAL THYSELF APPAREL

- [ ] Heal Thyself T-Shirts
- [ ] Heal Thyself Tote Bags

## NEBT-HET TEMPLE AROMATHERAPY

- [ ] Sandalwood
- [ ] Jasmine
- [ ] Rosemary
- [ ] Cinnamon
- [ ] Eucalyptus
- [ ] Lavender
- [ ] White Rose
- [ ] Frankincense
- [ ] Myrrh Oil
- [ ] Lotus Oil

## SACRED WOMAN BOUTIQUE PRODUCTS

- [ ] Candles for each Gateway
- [ ] Essential oils for each Gateway
- [ ] Maat Feather
- [ ] Nebt-Het/Ast Sister-to-Sister Sacred Shawls—raw silk in purple or white with gold glyphs
- [ ] Sacred Woman 10-Week Curriculum Binder
- [ ] Incense Burners
- [ ] Libation Bowls
- [ ] Sacred Music Instruments
- [ ] Stones for each Gateway
- [ ] Sacred Woman's Womb Scroll Chart
- [ ] Womb Works Kit

- [ ] Meditation and Healing Audiotapes
- [ ] Queen Afua's Rejuvenation Clay: 4 oz.; 8 oz.
- [ ] *Heal Thyself for Health and Longevity*, by Queen Afua
- [ ] *Heal Thyself Cookbook*, by Dianne Ciccone
- [ ] Kitchen Power video
- [ ] Global Sacred Woman Fast
- [ ] Sacred Work / Meshkenet Manual
- [ ] Sacred Woman Video Series of the Gates
- [ ] Dance of the Womb Chart
- [ ] Sacred Woman Fashion Show Video
- [ ] Sacred Woman Graduation Video
- [ ] Sacred Woman Living Drama Video
- [ ] Sacred Woman Music Audiotape
- [ ] Sacred Woman Music CD

*For the prices and orders of the following tools, please contact the Studio of Ptah: (212) 226-8487; (212) 343-9706; (718) 604-0027. All Designs by Hru Ankh Ra Semahj Se Ptah.*

- [ ] Sacred Woman's Initiation Silver Rings and Gold Rings
- [ ] Ast and Nebt-Het Pendant (for those men who support their Sacred Woman)—Gold/Silver/Platinum
- [ ] Toe-Rings (14K gold)
- [ ] Sacred Woman's Coin—Bronze/Silver/Gold
- [ ] Engagement Rings and Wedding Bands—Bronze/Silver/Gold (14K or 18K) or Platinum
- [ ] Ankh Pendants—Silver/Gold/Platinum
- [ ] Meditation Ankhs (sterling silver)
- [ ] Sacred Woman's Earrings—Gold/Silver
- [ ] Divine Sacred King Man's Rites of Passage

## WOMB WELLNESS REVOLUTION

### The Womb Care Classified Love Kit for Womb Wellness

- [ ] Womb Care Love Nutritional Formula
- [ ] Womb Care Love Herbal Detox Formula
- [ ] Womb Care Love Colon Cleanse Formula
- [ ] Womb Care Love Rejuvenation Clay Formula

Radiate, luminate, and awaken with your Sacred Woman Ceremony Kit for all your feminine body, mind, and spiritual needs. Light your aromatherapy candle, spray your magical essential mist, and drink your detox herb. Relax as you bask in your spiritual bath, behold your sacred stone, and recite your sacred prayers. Overcome, become one with your inner natural divinity.

For prices or information about Heal Thyself or Sacred Woman Boutique Products, log on to www.queenafua.com.

## ELEVATE HUMANITY: BECOME AN ARITU (CHAKRA) HEALING PRACTITIONER

You can become a certified Aritu Healing Practitioner and restore yourself and your community. For more information, contact (929) 351-2140 or visit www.queenafua.com.

As a prerequisite, you should complete Sacred Women Practitioner or Man Heal Thyself Wellness Warrior Rites of Passage training.

# APPENDIX B:
## BIOGRAPHIES OF SACRED WOMAN ANCESTORS, ELDERS, AND CONTEMPORARIES

## GATEWAY 0: THE SACRED WOMB

### Sacred Womb Ancestors

**BIDDY MASON.** Nurse-midwife. Biddy Mason learned her legendary midwifery and nursing skills on different southern plantations from older slave practitioners knowledgeable in the use of medicinal herbs, exercise, and healing diet. In 1848, Mason's owner moved his household from Mississippi to Utah, then, in 1851, to California. Mason gained her freedom in California, settling in Los Angeles. In her new home, Mason's consistently high standards in her successful practice of midwifery were quickly established among all social classes. Her homestead became a dispensary and base for her generous charitable work, often providing a refuge for needy people of all races.

**QUEEN MOTHER MOORE.** Volunteer nurse, political organizer, and pan-Afrakanist crusader. Queen Mother Moore was a highly intelligent and courageous woman whose long career of political activism merged Black Nationalism and Pan-Afrakanism. Born in New Iberia, Louisiana, in 1898, she worked as a volunteer nurse in the 1918 influenza epidemic. Becoming an active member of Marcus Garvey's Universal Negro Improvement Association (UNIA) while living in New Orleans, she was a founding member of the UNIA's Black Cross Nurses corps. Queen Mother moved to Harlem in the 1920s and remained a committed Pan-Afrakanist right up to her death in Brooklyn in 1997, championing struggles for self-determination, housing, unjust imprisonment, nutrition, and women's issues throughout the diaspora.

### Sacred Womb Elders

**AUNT IRIS O'NEAL.** Midwife extraordinaire, registered nurse, healer, and keeper of the womb. The tenth child in a very large family, Aunt Iris O'Neal was born in 1920 in Tortola, Virgin Islands. Her midwifery practice was centered on Virgin Gorda and Annie Gorda, Virgin Islands, but after 1939 when she completed her studies, she started work in Peebles Hospital in Tortola. O'Neal delivered more than seven hundred babies during her long career. "I think that God wants us to work with each other," Aunt Iris O'Neal has said, "but we must do it with a heart of love."

**JOSEPHINE ENGLISH.** MD specializing in obstetrics and gynecology, a humanitarian and institution builder. Born in 1920, Dr. English spent her early childhood in Englewood, New Jersey, graduating from high school in 1937. She attended Meharry Medical College in Nashville. Dr. English established her practice in Brooklyn, New York, and has successfully delivered thousands of children (including all of Malcolm X's daughters), and provided care for just as many mothers over the past forty years. She founded a comprehensive Health Care Center in 1975 and throughout the years has developed and continues to nurture the following community organizations: The Adelphi Medical Center, The Bushwick Medical Office, and the Health Is Right for Everyone Program.

### Sacred Womb Contemporaries

**JEWEL POOKRUM.** MD and natural health leader. Dr. Pookrum's stated purpose is to "see the perfection of every person's present state of health." When she began practicing Western medicine in 1981, she observed that surgery did not always cure acute pain. She also discovered that examining certain parts of the body—the iris of the eyes, or the feet, for example—gave her a barometer of the body's current condition. She quickly understood that we are whole entities and that the body, mind, and spirit are interdependent and reciprocal. In other words, people get well when they initiate and create their own healing. Dr. Pookrum founded the Perfect Health Institute of Nutritional Medicine in 1986.

**NONKULULEKO TYEHEMBA.** Certified nurse-midwife. One of the Keepers of the Shrine of Meshkenet, who lives and works in Harlem and is the director of the Harlem Birth Action Committee (HBAC). Nonkululeko has been a midwife for the past eighteen years. She has also worked with women giving birth in Senegal, Navajo-Hopi Homeland in Arizona, St. Croix, upstate New York, and the southern part of the United States. She is dedicated to the revolutionizing of women's reproductive rights. HBAC sponsors births and is a woman's resource center for woman's empowerment.

## GATEWAY 1: SACRED WORDS

### Sacred Word Ancestors

**ZORA NEALE HURSTON.** Foremother, anthropologist, folklorist, novelist, and autobiographer. Born in the all-black town of Eatonville, Florida, in 1891, Zora Neale Hurston was one of the most colorful and complex figures of the Harlem Renaissance. After studying at Morgan Academy in Baltimore, Howard University in Washington, DC, and Barnard College in New York City, she developed as an adept folklore fieldworker and gifted writer. Her remarkable body of writings—such as her masterpiece *Their Eyes Were Watching God* (1937) and the two volumes of folklore, *Mules and Men* (1935) and *Tell My Horse* (1938)—has earned her a place of honor in the pantheon of exceptional writers. She died in Florida in 1960.

**MARGARET WALKER.** Poet, novelist, essayist, and educator. Margaret Walker, born in Birmingham, Alabama, in 1915, grew up in a family that emphasized education and the intellectual life. She submitted a collection of poetry *For My People*, for her master's thesis at the University of Iowa. With its publication in 1942, Walker made history. Her dissertation at Iowa State was a novel about the Civil War Reconstruction era, *Jubilee*, which was published in 1965. *Jubilee* had been a work-in-progress for more than thirty years. Walker also had a long and distinguished career as an educator. She retired from Jackson State in 1990. She died in 1998.

### Sacred Word Elders

**MAYA ANGELOU.** Autobiographer, poet, playwright, theatrical and film director, producer, performance and recording artist, public speaker, and educator. Born in St. Louis in 1928, Maya Angelou is a prolific author who became one of America's most famous poets when, at the request of President Bill Clinton, she wrote and delivered the poem *On the Pulse of the Morning*, at the 1993 presidential inauguration. Her literary reputation stems from the first volume of her serial autobiography, *I Know Why the Caged Bird Sings* (1970). Other autobiographical fictions include *Gather Together in My Name* (1974), *Singin' and Swingin' and Gettin' Merry Like Christmas* (1976), *The Heart of a Woman* (1981), and *All God's Children Need Traveling Shoes* (1986).

**TONI MORRISON.** Novelist, essayist, editor, lecturer, educator, and Nobel Prize laureate. Toni Morrison, born Chloe Anthony Wofford in Loraine, Ohio, in 1931, established herself in American and African American literature with the publication of her first novel, *The Bluest Eye*. Morrison has also published *Sula* (1975), which won the National Book Award; *Song of Solomon* (1977), winner of the National Book Critics Circle Award; *Tar Baby* (1981); and *Beloved* (Pulitzer Prizer winner in 1988, made into a movie a decade later by Oprah Winfrey, directed by Jonathan Demme); and *Paradise*. Morrison won the Nobel Prize in literature in 1993 after the publication of *Jazz* in 1992.

**CAMILLE YARBROUGH.** Community activist, writer, composer, and radio talk show host. Camille Yarbrough is best known for the books she has written for children, such as *Cornrows* (1979) and *The Shimmershine Queens* (1988). Knowing how children tease and taunt one another whenever they gather, sometimes humorously, sometimes leading to hurt, anger, and confusion, Yarbrough uses the power of the Sacred Word to explore these taunts and the circumstances and feelings that arise from them. In all of her works, Afrakan American children are encouraged by adults to acquire knowledge about their histories so that they can protect both their psyche and their spirit. Yarbrough is a multifaceted griot elder who has worked with children in various programs, performing in plays, and writing lyrics and composing music for young audiences.

**NIKKI GIOVANNI.** Poet, essayist, lecturer, and educator. Born Yolande Cornelia Giovanni in Knoxville, Tennessee, in 1943, Nikki Giovanni's early reputation grew from her black militant revolutionary poems included in her first volumes, *Black Feeling, Black Talk* (1968), *Black Judgement* (1969), *Re-Creation* (1970), and the award-winning poetry-and-gospel album *Truth Is on Its Way* (1971). Giovanni books of poetry include *Love Poems* (1997), for which she received a NAACP Image Award, and *The Selected Poems of Nikki Goivanni.* Her early success led to two important conversations with her Sacred Word elders: *A Dialogue: James Baldwin and Nikki Giovanni* (1972) an *A Poetic Equation: Conversations Between Nikki Giovanni and Margaret Walker* (1974).

### Sacred Word Contemporaries

**EDWIDGE DANTICAT.** Award-winning novelist. Since the publication of her debut work, *Breath, Eyes, Memory,* in 1994, Edwidge Danticat has been praised as one of America's brightest, most graceful, and vibrant writers. Born in Haiti in 1969, at the age of twelve she left her birthplace for New York to reunite with her parents. She earned a degree in French literature from Barnard College, where she won a 1995 Woman of Achievement Award, and later an MFA from Brown University. Danticat's collection of stories from 1995, *Krik? Krak?* was nominated for a National Book Award. *Breath, Eyes, Memory* was selected by Oprah Winfrey for her book club. Her second novel, *The Farming of Bones* (1997), based on the 1937 massacre of Haitians at the border of the Domician Republic, was published to great acclaim.

**JESSICA CARE MOORE.** Spoken-word performance artist and publisher. Jessica Care Moore, born in Detroit in 1972, began her poetic journey hitting the open-mike scene in her hometown, then struck out for New York City in 1995 to immerse herself in its growing spoken-word circuit. Career fireworks began for Moore after she won first place five consecutive weeks during the amateur contest component of *Showtime at the Apollo.* Since then she has participated in a number of poetry events, such as the National Black Arts Festival in Atlanta and the Yari Yari Women Writers Conference in New York City. Moore and her poetry were also featured in the gospel musical *Born to Sing Mama 3* at Madison Square Garden with Shirley Ceasar and CeCe Winans. In 1997 she established her own publishing company, Moore Black Press, with the release of *The Words Don't Fit My Mouth.*

## GATEWAY 2: SACRED FOOD

### Sacred Food Ancestor

**AST (ISIS).** Her name means "seat" or "throne," which means that she is the embodiment of the throne. Ast (Isis) is the sister-wife of Asar (Osiris) and the mother of Heru (Horus). She is the personification of the female creative power that conceived and brought forth every living creature and thing. She is also the noblest example of a faithful and loving wife and mother, and it was in that role that she was most highly honored by the Khamites. As the mighty earth NTRU her name was Usert; as the NTRU of cultivated land and fields she was Kekhet; as the NTRU of the harvest she was Renenet; and as the NTRU of the food that was offered to the gods she was Tcheft. Ast is usually shown with her breast exposed to signify that she is the Divine Nurturer. She is of special significance, for kings regarded her as their symbolic mother.

### Sacred Food Elder

**AMON d RE A.** Culinary artist and living food caterer. Founder of Hapi Sun Food Caterers in Chicago, Amon d Re A is a specialist in the preparation of "living foods." Her delectable creations, coupled with her innovative and imaginative approach to food preparation, have made her a popular lecturer and workshop leader. The sacred food she serves up includes the highest-quality ingredients: fresh fruits and vegetables (organic when possible), and nuts and spices from the world over.

### Sacred Food Contemporaries

**ATURAH BAHTIYAH** has for years applied the power of natural medicine and living food. She earned a Bachelor's in data management. She is a transformational coach; contributing author in Planet Heal; vegan for 22 years and a certified raw foodist; wife of Prince Rahm; loving mother, grandmother; a Crowned Sister in the African Hebrew Israelite of Jerusalem nation. She traveled across the Mediterranean Sea and Atlantic Ocean over 60 times, visiting and researching wellness centers extensively in more than 19 countries in her search for the best holistic healing practices and modalities. She founded Tikeyah Regenerative Health & Wellness Center (Sacred Woman satellite) (tikeyah.com).

**CHER CARDEN.** Wellness consultant and living food instructor. Through education and wellness therapies, Cher Carden, based in New York City, encourages her students to discover, heal, and develop their unique expression of God-Essence. She is committed to helping people all over the world enhance the quality of their lives and make healthy lifestyle choices.

**DIANE CICCONE.** Mother, healer, lawyer, and gourmet cook. An excellent example of the Natural Living lifestyle in action, Diane Ciccone has been on a path of purification for more than twenty years, having studied with Dr. John E. Moore, the Reverend Philip Valentine, and Queen Afua. A graduate of Colgate University and Hofstra School of Law, Ciccone is in private practice in New York City. When not working or studying, she can be found in her kitchen, cooking new and healthy recipes for her husband and daughter.

**CHEF LAUREN VON DER POOL**'s hunger for healthy living began in Washington, D.C., where she grew up in a food desert—an environment totally lacking fresh, healthy options. When Von Der Pool realized that what was going on in her life and community was happening globally, she began to educate herself, her community, and the world about healthy living. A passionate humanitarian, artist, and author of *Eat Yourself Sexy* and *Fresh City Kids*, Von Der Pool dedicates her life to raising awareness about living a conscious, creative, green life. Chef Lauren Von Der Pool has been on the path of healing through plant medicine for decades, working with the likes of Serena Williams, Stevie Wonder, Common, and many more! In addition to being a world-renowned celebrity chef who has catered the Oscars, American Music Awards, and countless award shows and movie premieres, Von Der Pool is now a Reiki Master, Health and Wellness influencer/public speaker, Holistic Healer, and Herbal Medicine woman.

Lauren offers an array of services centered around raising the consciousness awareness of humanity starting with what we typically do daily, like eating, breathing, talking, thinking, and visualizing! Von Der Pool believes that everything we need we have, we just have to be aware of it! With a clean plant-based diet, proper breathing, positive affirmations, meditation, visualization, and a happy and willing heart, the sky is the limit! Lauren guides people on their wellness journey by offering food as medicine.

## GATEWAY 3: SACRED MOVEMENT

### Sacred Movement Ancestors

**JOSEPHINE BAKER.** Dancer, singer, and actress. Josephine Baker was a multitalented and supremely charismatic performer who was a forerunner of today's contemporary superstars. Born Josephine Carson in St. Louis, Missouri, in 1906, she was raised primarily in the city's slums. By age fifteen she had relocated to New York City and joined the chorus of Sissle and Blake's all-black cast musical *Shuffle Along*. After appearing in another Sissle and Blake production, *Chocolate Dandies*, Baker went to Paris in 1925 with *La Revue Negre* and became an overnight sensation — typically clad only in a skirt of feathers, representing the exotic spirit of the Jazz Age. After gradually evolving into a sleek, sophisticated jazz chanteuse, Baker returned to the United States in 1936 to star in the Ziegfield Follies. She was a war hero during World War II and a tireless humanitarian who emerged as a central figure in the Civil Rights Movement. While touring the Far East in 1953, Baker adopted a pair of Asian war orphans; over the years that followed she adopted more children of various racial and cultural backgrounds, nicknaming them her "Rainbow Tribes."

**PEARL PRIMUS.** Dancer, choreographer, and anthropologist. Born in Trinidad in 1919, Pearl Primus grew up in the United States. While at the New School for Social Research, she began to study what were then called "primitive dances." Beginning in 1948, she studied dance in Africa for eighteen months, and went on to travel the South observing the lifestyles of the common people, living with sharecroppers, and visiting black churches. Inspired by these experiences, her choreography chronicled black experience in the United States and the traditional dances of Africa and the Caribbean. In 1959, on her second major trip to Africa, Primus was named director of Liberia's Performing Arts Center, a position she held for two years. While in Liberia, Primus married Percival Borde, a dancer and choreographer. They returned to the United States and later formed the Earth Dance Company in the 1970s. Pearl Primus died in 1994.

### Sacred Movement Elders

**KATHERINE DUNHAM.** Anthropologist, dancer, choreographer, and teacher. Katherine Dunham is an influential leader in black theatrical dance. Born in Chicago in 1909, she studied anthropology at the University of Chicago and did extensive dance fieldwork in Haiti, Jamaica, Martinique, and Trinidad. She moved to New York City in the late 1930s. Forming a highly acclaimed all-black dance troupe in the 1940s, she and her troupe worked in motion pictures and Broadway musicals and performed African and Caribbean dances for diverse audiences around the world through the 1950s. From 1965 to 1967, she was in Senegal, representing the United States at the Festival of Black Arts and training the national Ballet of Senegal. In the 1970s she became artist in residence and then professor at Southern Illinois University. After serving as executive director of an arts training center named in her honor, she died in 2006.

**CARMEN DeLAVALLADE.** "Total" dancer, actress, and singer. Carmen DeLavallade was born in Los Angeles in 1931. She was a protégée of the late modern dance pioneer Lester Horton, and came to be known as a "total" dancer, equally at home in ballet, modern, and theatrical dance. Because she could also sing and act, DeLavallade had a reputation as a well-rounded performer. She has been featured with the Metropolitan Opera Ballet, the Boston Ballet, the Alvin Ailey Dance Theater, and her own company. She has danced in four films, including *Carmen Jones* (1955). DeLavallade is married to the widely acclaimed dancer, choreographer, and artist Geoffrey Holder.

### Sacred Movement Contemporaries

**JUDITH JAMISON.** Dancer, choreographer, and artistic director of the Alvin Ailey Dance Theater. Born in Philadelphia in 1944, Judith Jamison began dance classes at age six, with black ballet pioneer Marion Cuyjet. After graduating from high school, she briefly attended Fisk University, but soon returned home to dance full-time at the Philadelphia Dance Academy. While auditioning for a Harry Belafonte television special in New York, she was spotted by Alvin Ailey, who asked her to join his company. In 1971 Ailey choreographed a signature solo work for Jamison, *Cry*. After a distinguished career as a dancer, Jamison left Ailey to establish her own company, the Jamison Project, in 1987. She returned to become artistic director of the Alvin Ailey Dance Theater in 1988, right before the ailing Ailey died, becoming the first Afrakan American woman to direct a major modern dance company.

**DEBBIE ALLEN.** Award-winning choreographer, actress, director, and producer. Debbie Allen started taking dance lessons at age three in her hometown of Houston, Texas. After studying privately with a former dancer with the Ballet Russes, and attending the Ballet Nacional de Mexico in Mexico City, at age fourteen she became the first black student admitted to the Houston Ballet Foundation. She studied speech and theater at Howard University, while a member of choreographer Mike Malone's dance troupe. Graduating cum laude from Howard in 1971, she immediately left for New York. Over the decades she has proven herself to be a Renaissance woman, dancing with George Faison's Universal Dance Experience; appearing numerous times on Broadway; winning two Emmy Awards for the series *Fame;* directing and producing NBC's *A Different World;* and co–executive producing the film *Amistad,* directed by Stephen Spielberg.

**QUEEN ESTHER.** Dancer and "The Beauty Doctor." Queen Esther is an extraordinary movement artist with a background in dance spanning decades. Along with several years of study and training under the tutelage of Queen Afua of Heal Thyself, Queen Esther has used her knowledge as a Sacred Woman of diet and nutrition, healing herbs, cleansing, and purifying to develop her title as "The Beauty Doctor." Queen Esther has the ability to see the hidden beauty in others. She inspires both men and women to allow their inner magnificence to shine as it reflects self-love and self-confidence.

## GATEWAY 4: SACRED BEAUTY

### *Sacred Beauty Ancestor*

**QUEEN TIYE** (ancient Egypt, 1415–1340 BCE). A princess of Nubian birth, she married the Khamitic King Amenhotep III, who ruled during the New Kingdom Dynasties around 1391 BCE. Described by contemporaries as black and gorgeously beautiful, she was one of the most influential queens ever to rule Khamit. Queen Tiye held the title of "Great Royal Wife" and, following the end of her husband's reign, held sway over Khamit during the reign of her three sons, Amenhotep IV, Smenkhare, and the famous child-king, Tut-ankh-amen. For nearly half a century, Tiye governed Khamit, regulated her trade, and protected her borders. During this time, she was believed to be the standard of beauty in the ancient world.

### *Sacred Beauty Elders*

**KAITHA HET-HERU.** Holistic beauty expert Kaitha Het-Heru is founder, director, and chief priestess of Pa Nefer Het Em Het Heru, the Temple Beautiful of Het Heru ministries. She is keeper of the Shrines of Het Heru, Sekhmet, Ta-Urt, and Ast. She is a carrier of the sacred symbol of the Royal House of Khamit (Smai Tawi), the "Ankh," which she received from Kera Ptah (Shrine of Ptah). Het-Heru is also an ordained minister of the Ancient Hapi (Nile) Valley Order, Het Ptah Ka. Her ministry is dedicated to the remembrance of the Sacred Divine Feminine NTRT: Het-Hru. She is author of *I Love My Beautiful Body Temple,* written to inspire respect for the indwelling Divine self and the Sacred Body Temple. As a holistic beauty consultant, she motivates, educates, and empowers women through the "Beauty from the Inside Out" program, which is based on Wat Nefer / The Beauty Path, a contemporary interpretation of ancient Afrakan beauty traditions.

**LENA HORNE.** Actress, recording artist, and concert performer. Lena Horne was born in Brooklyn, New York, in 1917. Forced to quit school at age sixteen to bring money into the household, she got a job at the Cotton Club, solely on the basis of her beauty. She danced in the chorus line and took singing lessons. At eighteen, Horne joined Noble Sissle's Society Orchestra as a singer. In 1940 she started her recording career singing with Charlie Barnett's band. Accepting an offer to appear in a club in Los Angeles, she found work in Hollywood. She starred in the all-black cast classics *Cabin in the Sky* and *Stormy Weather,* both in 1943. By the late 1940s and throughout the '50s, Horne was at the top of her form, artistically and financially. In 1981, at the age of sixty-four, she opened on Broadway with *Lena Horne: The Lady and Her Music,* which became the longest-running one-woman show in the history of Broadway.

**NEKHENA EVANS.** Beauty consultant, lecturer, author, and entrepreneur. Nekhena Evans has long been considered one of the great pioneers of the locked-hair-care industry, opening doors to rare hairlocking knowledge, education, and quality hair-care services. Evans uses her wealth of experience to help young and old recognize their true greatness through the natural beauty of locked hair. Her book, *Everything You Need to Know About Hairlocking,* is a rare treasury of information on locked hair care, its history, and its impact on building self-awareness and pride.

### Sacred Beauty Contemporaries

**ERYKAH BADU.** Award-winning recording artist, actress, and contemporary stylemaker. Born Erica Wright in Dallas, Texas, Erykah Badu captured the world's attention in 1997 with the release of her album *Baduizm,* which quickly rose to the top of the charts, achieving platinum status in under a month. With hit singles, the much programmed music videos "On and On" and "Next Lifetime," and numerous magazine cover features, she became one of the most recognizable figures in popular music, with her Afrakan headwraps and ornate jewelry. She walked away with four awards at the Soul Train Lady of Soul Awards ceremony that same year. In November 1997 she released her second album, *Live,* which is composed of live tracks from *Baduizm* in addition to a couple of new songs, "I'll Be The Moon" and "Tyrone." She gave birth to her first child, Seven, in 1997.

**LAURYN HILL.** Award-winning recording artist, songwriter, producer, and contemporary

stylemaker. Born in South Orange, New Jersey, Lauryn Hill appeared at the Apollo Theater when she was thirteen, performing Smokey Robinson's "Who's Loving You" during an amateur competition. While she was in her midteens, she and her childhood friends Wyclef Jean and Pras Michael formed the group the Fugees. Their first album, *Blunted on Reality,* didn't top the charts, but the group created quite a buzz on the underground club scene, largely on the strength of Hill's onstage charisma. The Fugees' second release, in 1996, *The Score,* sold more than seventeen million copies and gave Hill a chance to stretch as a singer. Following the birth of her first son, Zion, Hill concentrated on motherhood while maintaining a low profile in the music world. Then she released a solo album in 1998, *The Miseducation of Lauryn Hill,* which was instantly hailed as a masterpiece. Lauryn's debut album swept all of the music award shows in 1998 and 1999, landing the Grammy awards for Album of the Year and Best New Artist.

## GATEWAY 5: SACRED SPACE

### Sacred Space Ancestor

**QUEEN NEFERTARI AAH-MES.** Her marriage to the great Rameses II of lower Ancient Egypt is known as one of the greatest royal love affairs ever. This marriage also brought an end to the hundred-year war between Upper and Lower Ancient Kemet (Egypt), which unified both kingdoms into one great nation. Monuments of this love affair still remain today in temples that Rameses built for his wife at Abu Simbel. The immense structures, known as the temples of Abu Simbel, are among the most magnificent monuments in the world, hewn from the mountain that contains them as an everlasting dedication to King Rameses and his wife Nefertari. These structures remain the largest, most majestic architecture ever built to honor a wife.

### Sacred Space Elder

**BARBARA ANN TEER.** Actress, director, writer, and founder / executive director of the National Black Theater. Barbara Ann Teer's credits include Broadway and television appearances. She has appeared in the motion pictures *The Pawnbroker* and Ossie Davis's *Gone Are the Days*, but she is best known for her work with the National Black Theater (NBT), also known as the Sun People's Theater, in Harlem. Through the NBT, Teer created her ritualistic theater, known as "The Teer Technology of Soul," as a technique for teaching "God Conscious Art." She has also worked to use the arts as a source of community economic development in Harlem, with the expansion of the NBT and affiliate retail and commercial spaces.

### Sacred Space Contemporary

**QUEEN AFUA MUT NEBT-HET.** Queen Afua's Sacred Space is the Body Temple. On the Path of Purification for decades, she is a practitioner of the art of Natural Healing and is founder and director of the Heal Thyself Natural Living Center in Brooklyn, New York. Believing in our ability to heal ourselves from all disease through proper education, guidance, support, and application of natural healing tools, such as herbs, water, fasting, proper nutrition, divine prayer, and meditation, Queen Afua is well versed in Natural Living and fasting techniques as a way of total body, mind, and spirit wellness.

## GATEWAY 6: SACRED HEALING

### Sacred Healing Ancestors

**ANKH HESEN PA ATEN RA.** Royal princess. The third daughter of Pharaoh Akhenaten, who believed in one God, and Queen Nefertiti. Her father founded a new capital for Egypt, new beliefs, and a new culture in what came to be known as the Amarna Heresy.

**DR. ALVENIA FULTON.** Naturopath and nutritionist. Dr. Fulton was among the first of the Afrakan American naturopaths in the United States. She was a trailblazer in all aspects of the quality-of-life movement and has served as nutritionist to such stars as Josephine Baker, Ossie

Davis, and Ruby Dee, among others. Dr. Fulton was one of the first recipients of the Roots Award presented by the city of Berkeley, California, in recognition of contributions of African-derived cultures to the well-being and quality of life in the Bay Area.

### Sacred Healing Elder

**BERLINA BAKER.** Colon therapist, reflexologist, and educator. Berlina Baker manages and owns the Stream of Life Colonic Center along with her partner Alva Saafir. The director of group-healing programs and retreats, she trains colon therapists, and offers "Heal Thyself" adult education classes at the Chicago City colleges, where she teaches the use of herbs as a path to healing.

### Sacred Healing Contemporaries

**DR. SHARON OLIVER.** Holistic medical doctor. Dr. Oliver gave up a thriving emergency medicine practice because she couldn't spend enough quality time with her young daughter. Her emergency room experience made her aware of her calling to move to a higher level of healing. Dr. Oliver believes that all healing occurs through the application of universal truths and wishes to guide and support others with the use of herbs, nutrition, and a holistic approach. She is the mother and director of the Whole Life and Health Center, an institution devoted to combining the best principles of holistic care to optimize the health of her clients.

**EARTHLYN MARSELEAN MANUEL.** Healer, educator, writer, and creator of The Black Angel Cards: A Healing Tool for African American Women. Born and raised in Los Angeles and nurtured in a Creole/Haitian tradition, along with a strong belief in Spirit, Earthlyn has been honored for her passionate belief and work on behalf of African American women and girls.

She was gifted with The Black Angel Cards by Ancient Black Women Spirits in a dream. They are based on a new indigenous base of wisdom called Shoke. She created the extraordinary artwork that appears in this oracle deck as well. As Earthlyn says of this gift, "The Black Angel Cards are here to help us nurture our intuitive selves and to assist us in trusting what we know. Let's begin the healing."

## GATEWAY 7: SACRED RELATIONSHIPS

### *Sacred Relationship Ancestors*

**SOJOURNER TRUTH.** Foremother and abolitionist. She was born Isabella Baumfree around the year 1797 in Ulster County, New York. Her exact date of birth is unknown, because she was born into slavery. She had many owners, her last being Isaac Van Wagener. About the time she was freed, one of her sons was sold illegally in Alabama. With much determination, she instituted a lawsuit against the man who sold her son, and gained his freedom. In 1843 she changed her name to Sojourner Truth, and, answering what she considered to be a calling from God, she joined the Methodist Church and became a traveling evangelist. From then on, she "traveled up and down the land," speaking in many towns in the Northeast and Midwest on women's rights and against slavery. She supported her travels by selling copies of her book, *The Narrative of Sojourner Truth.*

**SARAH AND ELIZABETH DELANY.** Siblings extraordinaire, a doctor and a teacher. Sarah Delany and her "little" sister Dr. Elizabeth (Bessie) Delany grew up with eight other siblings in turn-of-the-century North Carolina; their father was born in slavery, yet became the nation's first black Episcopal bishop. As young women, they moved to New York City, rising to professional prominence in Harlem during its heyday in the 1920s and '30s, "Queen Bess" as a doctor and Sarah as a teacher. Choosing careers over marriage, the sisters remained single throughout their long and amazing lives. When the book *Having Our Say: The Delany Sisters' First 100 Years* was published, the world was introduced to these irrepressible sisters, who, although fragile at the time of publication, were still fiercely independent and devoted to each

other. The Delany sisters embody the Ast-Neb-Het sister-to-sister relationship.

### *Sacred Relationship Elder*

**QUEEN NZINGA RATABISHA HERU.** Egyptologist and conference organizer. Nzinga Ratabisha was instrumental in organizing the First Annual Ancient Egyptian Studies Conference. Queen Nzinga Ratabisha Heru believes in bringing people together to raise their consciousness. She served as the international president of the Association for the Study of Classical African Civilization (ASCAC). Ms. Heru was also cofounder of Rivers Run Deep Institute, which provides professional development for teachers and staff of schools in urban settings, focusing on the effective and academic needs of Afrakan American students. She took the name of Nzinga (a warrior-queen who unified her people and fought for forty years to keep the Portuguese out of Angola), combined with Ratabisha, which means "she who corrects things and makes things right." She believed, "It is better to live one brief moment in truth than to live an entire lifetime in lies." This is the perfect recipe for lasting relationships.

### *Sacred Relationship Contemporaries*

**OPRAH WINFREY.** Television host, actress, and producer. Oprah Winfrey's Emmy-winning television show established her as one of the most important figures in popular culture. Her contributions are felt beyond the world of television, in such areas as publishing, music, film, philanthropy, education, health and fitness, and social awareness. She used *The Oprah Winfrey Show* to enlighten, entertain, and empower her viewers. Oprah began her broadcasting career at the age of nineteen, when she became the youngest and first Afrakan American woman to anchor the news at Nashville's WTVF-TV. In 1984, she moved to Chicago to host WLS-TV's morning talk show, *AM Chicago*, which became the number one talk show one month after Oprah began hosting. In 1985 she was nominated for an Oscar for her performance in *The*

*Color Purple* and in 1999 she starred in *Beloved*. In 1998 she launched the Oprah Book Club.

**IYANLA VANZANT.** Writer and nationally honored inspirational speaker. As founder and executive director of Inner Visions Spiritual Life Maintenance Network, Iyanla Vanzant inspires others to transform their lives through workshops, lectures, and her books, *One Day My Soul Just Opened Up, The Value in the Valley,* and *In the Meantime.* Vanzant's personal experiences have given her profound insight into life. After she left her abusive husband, she went to Medgar Evers College and the City University of New York Law School. She moved to Philadelphia with her children and practiced as a public defender for three years. She later became an ordained minister, committed to a message based on the principles of divine power and self-determination.

**LADY PREMA.** Producer, singer, songwriter, actress, and transformational workshop leader. The author of *Jewel from Within* and *My Soul Speaks,* Lady Prema has been a Heal Thyself supporter for years. A crystal and gemstone therapist, and a practitioner of yoga and tai chi, she practices aromatherapy, does macrobiotic cooking, and is a skilled musician on various African instruments.

## GATEWAY 8: SACRED UNION

### Sacred Union Ancestor

**BETTY SHABAZZ.** PhD, wife, mother, and college professor. Betty Shabazz was not a black nationalist when she first met Malcolm X in 1956 at a Harlem mosque, nor was she involved in the struggle for civil rights. She was a dedicated Muslim studying to be a nurse. She gave up her studies in 1958 to marry Malcolm X and raise a family. Betty Shabazz put Sacred Union above all else, and made the sacrifice of caring for their four daughters as Malcolm X traveled all over the country and to Afraka spreading the word of the right of black people to defend themselves against racist oppression. After Malcolm X's death, she worked to keep her husband's legacy

alive, defending his teachings from those who sought to misinterpret and misrepresent his words. Dr. Betty Shabazz was deeply respected for her efforts to heal the black community after the loss of her husband and Dr. Martin Luther King, Jr.

### Sacred Union Elders

**RUBY DEE.** Actress, poet and writer, television host, mother, and wife. Ruby Dee brought a mark of dignity, determination, and intelligence to the roles she played on the stage and screen. Born Ruby Ann Wallace in Cleveland, Ohio, in 1924, she and her family moved to Harlem when she was an infant. By the time she was a teenager, Ruby Dee—the name she adopted when she went onstage—was submitting poetry to the *Amsterdam News* and became involved in political activities. After high school, she attended Hunter College in New York City, majoring in French and Spanish, and began studying acting. Joining the American Negro Theater (ANT), she appeared in many ANT productions from 1941 to 1943, and made her Broadway debut in *South Pacific* in 1943. She married fellow actor Ossie Davis in 1949, and often worked with her husband onstage and in movies. Ruby Dee and Ossie Davis's spirited memoir, *With Ossie & Rubie* (1997), depicts how their thriving careers and family life were blended into a marriage of many years. It offers invaluable insights into how to make a Sacred Union work.

**CORETTA SCOTT KING.** Civil rights activist, wife, and mother. As the wife of civil rights leader Martin Luther King, Jr., Coretta Scott King was ready to continue his work and perpetuate his ideals after his 1968 assassination. In the early years of their marriage, her primary role was to raise their four children. However, over the years, her devotion to Sacred Union involved her more and more in her husband's work, and she performed his lectures in song as he did in speech. When demands became too much for him, she began to fill the speaking engagements when he could not. After his death, she became a dynamic activist and peace crusader, founding the Martin Luther King Center for Social Justice. Mrs. King is often honored for keeping her husband's dream alive.

### Sacred Union Contemporary

**SUSAN TAYLOR.** Editor, writer, and public speaker. Susan L. Taylor served as the editor in chief of *Essence* magazine from 1981 to 2000, helping to make it into the most influential magazine for black women, especially in the areas of achievement, style, beauty, and personal relationships. Through her column "In the Spirit," her extensive travels, and numerous public appearances, she offers inspiration and guidance to millions of readers and other women. She is the author of *In the Spirit: The Inspirational Writings of Susan L. Taylor, Lessons in Living,* and *Confirmation: The Spiritual Wisdom That Has Shaped Our Lives,* the book she co-authored with her husband, Khephra Burn. This book offers a collection of the wisdom of diverse cultures that has been at the core of this inspiring couple's spiritual growth.

Ms. Taylor's ability to balance her professional responsibilities with her loving spiritual union with Khephra is an inspiration to us all.

## GATEWAY 9: NEFER ATUM: THE SACRED LOTUS INITIATION

### Sacred Lotus Initiation Ancestors

**QUEEN HATSHEPSUT.** One of the most fully realized Sacred Women of her time, Queen Hatshepsut became an extraordinary Pharaoh and enlightened peace-bringing ruler. Daughter of Thothmes I, she proclaimed herself king, not queen, of Khamit after the death of her husband and during the minority of her stepson Tuthmosis III. She is often depicted wearing the false beard associated with kingship. In order to establish her position as a ruler, she built the magnificent temple complex at Deir-el-Bahri, and had inscribed on the walls the tale that she was a daughter not of Thothmes I but of the god Amon and Queen Aah-Mes.

**MARY McLEOD BETHUNE.** Foremother, educator, organizer of women's groups, and philanthropist. This Sacred Lotus Woman picked cotton for eight to ten hours a day from the age of ten. Her life took a miraculous turn when Miss Emma Wilson, a schoolteacher at the local Presbyterian Church in Mayesville, South Carolina, offered Mary's mother an education for one of her children. In three years, after teaching her brothers and sisters to read, Mary went to the Scotia school in Concord, North Carolina, graduating in July 1894. She set her heart on establishing a school for black girls. She opened the doors to her Daytona Beach, Florida, Literary and Industrial School for Training Negro Girls in 1904. Her husband, Albertus Bethune, shared her vision and later helped to establish what became Bethune-Cookman College. Bethune's work moved to the national stage when in 1936 she was appointed director of the Division of Negro Affairs by President Franklin Roosevelt. Her life philosophy of ennobling labor and economic independence was rooted in her firm belief in the doctrine of universal love.

### Sacred Lotus Initiation Elders

**NANA ANSAA ATEI.** Akan Priestess and Registered Nurse. In 1954, Nana Ansaa Atei received her practical nursing license from Montefiore Hospital. In 1959, she went to Fordham Nursing School to further her education and become a registered nurse. Between 1970 and 1972, Nana Ansaa Atei experienced her long and difficult training under Nana Okomfopayin Akua Oparebeah, Akan Priestess of the Akonedi Shrine, to become a full-fledged Akan Priestess. She was the first African American woman to learn psychic and traditional healing to graduate from the Nana Akonedi Shrine. Nana Ansaa has since continued her spiritual development through other systems, such as the Khamitic system. She performs naming ceremonies, healing circles, and spiritual consultation, gives herbal remedies and supplements, and uplifts people wherever she can.

**EMPRESS AKWÉKÉ.** Cultural healer. Empress Akwéké has devoted most of her life to helping people heal and transform. She uses holistic healing modalities in the areas of education, health, family, food, housing, and cultural/creative arts, and spiritual support, to help sustain the lives of people and families with whom she has worked over the years. Her community service work includes teaching at the Bedford Hills Women's Correctional Institute, Lincoln Correctional Facility, and numerous community-based organizations, churches, and community health centers.

### Sacred Lotus Initiation Contemporary

**ANUKUA AST ATUM.** Natural Living expert and priestess. Inliss Weh AnukUa Kyte, presently called Anukua, has spent years of her life unveiling the mysteries of self and the earth. She has assisted countless seekers on the path of natural living. Developing transformational skills through art, the study and practice of spirituality, an intense study of the body, and healing modalities of natural living (decades of being a vegetarian) all contribute to her success. Tepi-Arit Priestess and keeper of the Kra Nt Htp in Los Angeles, California, she was presented an Ankh in 1989 by the Shrine of Ptah. Founder of "Heal Your Hair" and braiding and hair-locking practice since 1979, she stands among those who gave birth to the popularity of braids. Her Life Lover Healing Company offers assistance to those who are on a natural path with food preparation workshops, new life counseling, and cultural and healing transformational workshops.

## GATEWAY 10: SACRED TIME

### Sacred Time Guardian

**SESHAT,** the Scribe. The Lady of Mathematics who presided over the House of Life. Seshat's most prominent task was to assist the king in stretching the cord for the layout of all temples and other royal buildings. She is a Magician carrying a wand with its seven-pointed star, a symbol that presents the course of all creative ideas and consciousness. Her powers of cause and effect were legendary before the founding of Egypt. She was the feminine aspect of Thoth and the essence of cosmic intuition, creating the geometry of the heavens alongside Thoth. She became a goddess of writing, astronomy, astrol-ogy, architecture, and mathematics. Her title of "Mistress of the House of Books" indicates that she also took care of Thoth's library of scrolls. She is the patron of libraries and all forms of writing, including census, accounting work, and record keeping.

### Sacred Time Ancestor

**HARRIET TUBMAN.** Born between 1820 and 1825, the Great Mighty Mother of Freedom Harriet Tubman was born to enslaved parents in Dorchester, Maryland, during the Civil War. She became a dedicated soldier in the liberation of Afrakans. Harriet's life was nothing but a calling from the most high! By way of the Underground Railroad, she freed more than seven hundred slaves in South Carolina alone. Despite a life of pain and struggle, she overcame. Hers are among the shoulders that we stand upon today.

### Sacred Time Elder

**MICHELLE LaVAUGHN ROBINSON OBAMA.** The world knows Michelle Obama as the First Lady married to the forty-fourth president, the first black president of the United States, Barack Obama. Mrs. Obama graduated from Princeton University and later served as the dean of student affairs at the University of Chicago. She has worked diligently to empower women, children, and families to achieve greater wellness.

### Sacred Time Contemporary

**KATERIA KNOWS.** Royal greetings, my name is Kateria Knows, I'm an Astrologer, Spirit Interpreter, Intuitive Counselor, and Reiki Healer. I have over twenty years of Astrology study under my belt. When we align with the Stars, we live a life of a Heavenly existence. It is time.

## GATEWAY 11: SACRED WORK

### Sacred Work Guardian

**MESHKENET** was a goddess of childbirth and destiny, a divine midwife, and the protector of the birthing house. She was also a goddess of fate who could determine a person's destiny. She had the power to protect newborn babies and their mothers. Her name means "birthing place," and she was generally depicted as a birthing brick with a human head, or as a woman wearing the headdress of a cow's uterus. She is the one who breaths *ka* (spirit) into a child as it enters the world.

### Sacred Work Ancestor

**MADAME C. J. WALKER.** The first black woman millionaire in the United States, Ms. Walker was an extraordinary inventor. Born in 1867, she invented her own line of cosmetics and hair products for brown and black women all over the globe, including women who suffered from scalp ailments. By traveling around the country, she established successful laboratories and manufactories during the years of the Harlem Renaissance.

### Sacred Work Elders

**MAXINE WATERS.** Born in St. Louis, Missouri, on August 15, 1938. The fifth out of thirteen children, she was raised by a single mother. Maxine graduated from high school in Missouri, in 1961, before her family moved to Los Angeles, California. Ten years later, in 1971, she received a bachelor's degree in sociology from Los Angeles State College (now California State University). She has held various jobs in the service and educational fields. An elected official, Waters has served in the US House of Representatives (California) since 1991. She is cofounder of the Black Women's Forum, and Community Build. Ms. Waters received the Bruce F. Vento Award from the National Law Center on Homelessness & Poverty for her work to decrease the homeless population.

**ANGELA EVELYN BASSETT.** Renowned producer, writer, actress, and activist. Ms. Bassett began her career in 1980 after she earned her BA from Yale University and an MFA from the Yale School of Drama.

### Sacred Work Contemporaries

**QUEEN LATIFAH.** A multitalented queen, a famous musician, songwriter, actress, singer, rapper, and activist. She has always been at the forefront of liberation for black women.

**JADA PINKETT SMITH.** Actress. Born in Baltimore, Maryland, the talented Mrs. Pinkett Smith is known around the world for her work in projects including *In A Different World* and *Set It Off*. She attended the School of the Arts in Baltimore, which led to big roles on the screen where she keeps evolving in her craft.

# NOTES

## PREFACE

1. K. J. Carlson, D. H. Nichols, and I. Schiff, "Indications for Hysterectomy," *New England Journal of Medicine* 328, no. 12 (1993): 856–60.
2. K. Kjeruklff, G. Guzinski, P. Langenberg, et al., "Hysterectomy and Race," *Journal of Obstetrics and Gynecology* 82, no. 5 (1993): 757–64.

## CHAPTER 1.
## KHAMITIC NUBIAN PHILOSOPHY

1. A. E. Wallace Budge, *The Egyptian Book of the Dead* (New York: Dover Publications, 1967 [1895]), 215–18.
2. A. E. Wallis Budge, *Books on Egypt and Chaldea: The Book of the Dead*, vol. 3 (London: Keagan, Paul, Trench, Trubner and Co., 1909), 594.
3. Budge, *Books on Egypt and Chaldea*, 612.

## CHAPTER 2.
## GATEWAY 0: THE SACRED WOMB

1. A. E. Wallace Budge, *The Egyptian Book of the Dead* (New York: Dover Publications, 1967 [1895]), 134–35.
2. Budge, *Egyptian Book of the Dead*, 21.
3. Budge, *Egyptian Book of the Dead*, 242.

## CHAPTER 3.
## THE SPIRIT OF THE WOMB

1. Langston Hughes, "Harlem," *Book of Langston Hughes* (New York: George Braziller, 1958), 123.
2. Dr. Frances Cress Welsing, *The Isis Papers: The Key to the Colors* (Chicago: Third World Press, 1991), 231–41.

## CHAPTER 4.
## THE CARE OF THE WOMB

1. Both these illustrations come from a Colon Health Chart created by my late colon therapy teacher, Dr. Robert Wood.
2. From "Breast Cancer Basics," African American Women's Speakers Bureau, on the internet at http://trfn.clpgh.org/aawsb/breast.html.

## CHAPTER 5.
## THE COMMITMENT

1. Elizabeth Wayland Barber, *Women's Work, the First 20,000 Years* (New York: W.W. Norton, 1994), 180.

## CHAPTER 6.
## GATEWAY 1: SACRED WORDS

1. This and all flower essences are from Patricia Kaminski and Richard Katz, *Flower Essence Repertory: A Comprehensive Guide to North American and English Flower Essences for Emotional and Spiritual Well Being* (Nevada City, CA: Flower Essence Society Earth-Spirit, 1994).
2. English translation appears in A. E. Wallace Budge, *The Egyptian Book of the Dead* (New York: Dover Publications, 1967 [1895]), 157.

## CHAPTER 7.
## GATEWAY 2: SACRED FOOD

1. Sally Price, *Co-wives and Calabashes* (Ann Arbor: University of Michigan Press, 1984), 52.
2. Price, *Co-wives and Calabashes*, 20, 52, 87.

## CHAPTER 8.
## GATEWAY 3: SACRED MOVEMENT

1. A. E. Wallace Budge, *The Egyptian Book of the Dead* (New York: Dover Publications, 1967 [1895]), 215.

## CHAPTER 9.
### GATEWAY 4: SACRED BEAUTY

1. R. B. Amber, *Color Therapy: Healing with Color* (Santa Fe, NM: Aurora Press, 1983), 42.
2. Ann K. Copeland and Glenn E. Markoe, eds., *Mistress of the House, Mistress of the Heaven: Women in Ancient Egypt* (New York: Hudson Hills Press, in association with Cincinnati Art Museum, 1996), 85, 87.
3. Maulana Karenga, *Selections from the Husia: Sacred Wisdom of Ancient Egypt*, selected and retranslated (Los Angeles: University of Sankor, 1984), 67–71.

## CHAPTER 11.
### GATEWAY 6: SACRED HEALING

1. Barbara S. Lasko, *Remarkable Women of Ancient Egypt* (Berkeley, CA: B. C. Scribe, 1996).
2. A. E. Wallace Budge, *The Egyptian Book of the Dead* (New York: Dover Publications, 1967 [1895]), 151.

## CHAPTER 12.
### GATEWAY 7: SACRED RELATIONSHIPS

1. A Metu-NTR Khamitic phrase.

## CHAPTER 13.
### GATEWAY 8: SACRED UNION

1. Maulana Karenga, *Selections from the Husia: Sacred Wisdom of Ancient Egypt*, selected and retranslated (Los Angeles: University of Sankor, 1984), 44.
2. Alvin F. Poussaint, MD, "Prostate Cancer: Male Killer Hits Famous and Not So Famous," *Ebony*, April 1997. Dr. Poussaint is a clinical professor of psychiatry at the Harvard Medical School.
3. Nik Douglas and Penny Slinger, *Sexual Secrets: The Alchemy of Ecstasy* (Rochester, VT: Inner Traditions, 1985).

## CHAPTER 14.
### GATEWAY 9: NEFER ATUM: THE SACRED LOTUS INITIATION

1. *Baedeker's Egypt* (Englewood, NJ: Prentice-Hall, 1998), 94.

# ACKNOWLEDGMENTS

For those who directly supported me in the coming of *Sacred Woman*.

Tua NTR, whose body contains the light of the Sacred Guardians and Ancestors. Thank you for so lovingly guiding my heart, hands, and feet on this Sacred Journey.

To the Elders and Contemporary Divine Sisters who are living examples of Divinity. Profound gratitude to you, Brother Gift, for your vision and your insistence that I turn my Sacred Woman Training Manual into a book.

Sen-Ur Ankh Ra Semahj Se Ptah. To my beloved, brilliant husband, kingman, and divine mentor, Semahj, for your tireless, loving, and patient assistance in supporting me in every term and breath of *Sacred Woman*'s birth, I say, *Tua NTR. Tua NTR,* I married my hero.

Ida and Ephraim Robinson. Eternal blessings to my mother, Ida Robinson, for being a professional, perfected, and loving mother toward every aspect of my development. To my father, Ephraim Robinson, who is now an Ancestor, thank you for your loving guidance from the spiritual world.

Children. To my cubs—SupaNova, Sherease, and Ali, my beloved children, your love helped me to keep going when I got tired, and when I thought there was nothing left, you gave me the spark to keep on keepin' on. Mama loves you.

Cheryl Woodruff. Associate Publisher, One World / Ballantine, and my editor, who embodies Sekhemet and walks in the world as a Healing Warrior / Queen. Thank you for being my literary midwife and choreographer. And blessings for your masterful work, pure devotion, and commitment in making this book a reality. Much love for helping me grow.

Marie Brown. Agent. A Nefer Atum/Lotus Queen and my precious agent, thank you for knowing what I needed at every step of the way and for believing in the *Sacred Woman* project.

Kristine Mills-Noble. Art Director. Much gratitude for your brilliant cover and text design and for believing and seeing the vision of *Sacred Woman*. You went far beyond the call of duty in such a powerful and Sacred way.

Barbara Shor. Line Editor. My eternal gratitude for your sweet, humble, and loving hand and heart in the line-editing of the final text.

Michael Brown, artist extraordinaire. For your artistic genius in creating the cover painting for *Sacred Woman*.

Eileen Gaffney. Managing Editor. Much gratitude to you for your impeccable work and attention to detail. And most especially blessings to you for your generosity of spirit. We could have never crossed the finish line without you.

Greg Tobin. Editor in Chief, Ballantine Publishing Group. Sincere appreciation for your ongoing support.

Beverly Robinson. Director of Publicity, One World Books. For getting the word out and taking *Sacred Woman* to the world. Thank you for keeping me in divine order as I travel with the *Sacred Woman* movement.

Allison Glismann. Editorial Assistant, Ballantine Books. Thank you for so closely supporting Cheryl Woodruff and getting us to the finish line.

Lady Prema. My true and devoted sister-friend who had my back on every step of the *Sacred Woman* journey.

Empress Akwéké. Appreciation for boldly and beautifully living a Sacred Life that first inspired my Afrakan Sacredness to live and breathe.

Bob and Muntu Law. Community Leaders. For their magnificent support of the Heal Thyself healing crusade.

Baba Ishangi. Reverend Elder and Inspiration. For being such an inspiration to us all in the restoration of our Afrakan culture.

My extraordinary and humble Heal Thyself staff: Ntreshah Elsa Bernal, Heru Pa-Ur Tehuti Se Ptah, TaMera Het-Heru; Ast Nebt-Het Maat my right hand and *Sacred Woman* assistant; and my videographer, Khadiatou (Terry Wisdom).

David Jackson. For all his literary skill and dedication in the coming of the *Sacred Woman* biographical text at the eleventh hour.

Dr. Sharon Oliver and Dr. Cheryl Scott. For your medical expertise and support.

Gerianne Frances Scott. For being my first literary midwife in helping me to birth the rough draft for the *Sacred Woman* text.

Maxine Tehuti Campbell. For your years of commitment to excellence and your editorial typesetting work.

Yolanda M. Tribble (Tribal). For your relentless devotion in typesetting and researching this text. I am in gratitude.

Portia Davis (BaSheBa Earth). For typesetting when you'd rather be baking in the sun.

Chester Higgins and Anthony Mills. My brilliant photographers. For being so tuned in and for knowing exactly what was needed to speak visually in this text.

Dianne Pharr. For your spiritual guidance and for insisting that I reach out to Marie Brown for her expertise.

Hazelle Goodman. My spiritual sister. For your support and for keeping my heart light with laughter through the most trying times of the creating of this book.

Litina Egun-Gun, designer of the Sacred Woman's Medicine Bag pictured on page 279.

To the Sacred Woman Study Group who shared their Womb Stories and Womb Journal Work so generously: Marie Brown, Lillian Cortez, Kristine Mills-Noble, Cheryl Woodruff, Astede Elegba, Dr. Ellis, Tonya Reid, and Janine Smalls.

Also, my deep gratitude to those who supported my life and my work over the years. My blood brothers, James and Albert Robinson; my spiritual brothers, Tunde-Ra and TaharQa Aleem (the twins); the Sacred Woman Smai Tawi Priestesses; Elder Mother of Purification Etta Dixon; the Sacred Musicians, Laraaji, Nadi, and Entrfied; my spiritual daughters, Erykah Badu and Dawn Coleman; Keisha and Karla Williams; Natalie from Park Slope Copy; my masseuse, Najami; the twin angels Princess and Don; my husband's blood children, Everay, El-Aton, Ptah, Ka-Mena, Sesheta; and his grandbabies; and finally to all my Divine Sacred Sisters and Sacred Brothers, Elders, and Contemporaries who contributed to the *Sacred Woman* text.

# IMAGE CREDITS

The author gratefully acknowledges permission to use illustrations
(listed by page number) by the following individuals and institutions.

228: Nekhena Evans waist beads, © Anthony Mills. All rights reserved
229: Woman in green headwrap, © Gerianne Scott
229: Woman in white headwrap, © Chester Higgins Jr. All rights reserved
231: Mud clan woman, © Anthony Mills. All rights reserved
234: Beautiful African locks, © Anthony Mills. All rights reserved
236: Eye care/radiant eyes, © Anthony Mills. All rights reserved
238: Facial adornments and clothing Kaitha Ket-Heru, © Anthony Mills. All rights reserved
238: Erykah Badu, © Kevin Westenberg
242: Sacred Altar, © Chester Higgins Jr. All rights reserved
254: Sacred Altar, © Chester Higgins Jr. All rights reserved
265: Laying on of hands, © Anthony Mills. All rights reserved
269: Gathering of healers, © Hru Ankh Ra Semahj
279: Healing medicine bag, © Anthony Mills. All rights reserved
288: Sacred Altar, © Chester Higgins Jr. All rights reserved
298: A village of mothers and daughters, © Anthony Mills. All rights reserved
300: Queen Afua and her sons, © Chester Higgins Jr. All rights reserved
301: Queen Afua and her daughter, © Anthony Mills. All rights reserved
304: Sacred Voices, © Anthony Mills. All rights reserved
306: The Bitch is a woman in need of healing, © Chester Higgins Jr. All rights reserved
311: Transformation of the Bitch, © Chester Higgins Jr. All rights reserved
316: Sacred Altar, © Chester Higgins Jr. All rights reserved
327: A sacred union, Queen Afua and Hru Ankh Ra Semahj, © Anthony Mills. All rights reserved
335: The wedding bands of sacred union, © Aaron White
347: Talking it out ritual, © Chester Higgins Jr. All rights reserved
352: Sacred Altar, © Chester Higgins Jr. All rights reserved
358: Ankh, © Chester Higgins Jr. All rights reserved
360: Queen Afua saluting Ra at the Giza Plateau, © Esu Amn-Ra Hru Ma'at
361: Queen Afua and Tehuti at the Shrine of Sekhemet, © Ingani (Virginia) Maat Choice
363: Wailing Wall at Kom Ombo Healing Temple, © Ingani (Virginia) Maat Choice
365: Priestess Taen-Ra in the Temple of her ancestors, © Ingani (Virginia) Maat Choice
368: Preparation for Sacred Lotus Initiation, © Chester Higgins Jr. All rights reserved
369: Aspirants prepare for initiation, courtesy of Merra Khusa
377: Queen Afua's address, © Chester Higgins Jr. All rights reserved
378: Sacred Woman Initiates, © Robert L. Bowden, Jr.
382: Sacred Altar, © Chester Higgins Jr. All rights reserved
398: Sacred Altar, © Chester Higgins Jr. All rights reserved
429: Queen Afua: Until We Meet Again, © Anthony Mills. All rights reserved

# INDEX

## ABOUT THE AUTHOR

QUEEN AFUA is a Master Holistic Healer and Herbalist, Polarity Practitioner, and lay midwife. She is the author of seven bestselling wellness books, *Sacred Woman* being the most well-read text. Queen Afua is also the Mother of Womb Wellness Movement and is founder of Womb Yoga Dance, and thousands of women worldwide have joined Queen Afua in The Sacred Woman Rites of Passage, from America, Africa, London, and The Virgin Islands. Queen Afua is the Chief Priestess of The Nile Valley of Khemet, who teaches her healing works of the in-dwelling healer. Among her many celebrity clients are Erykah Badu, Vanessa Williams, Stevie Wonder, Lauren London, India Arie, and Common. Queen Afua has also been invited to appear on Essence Wellness Expo to share her holistic gifts, and was given the opportunity by renowned DJ Beverly Bond to host a weekly show on the Black Girls Rock platform, offering The Sacred Circle with Queen Afua, including celebrity guests and other wellness warriors with the intentions of elevating the greater community.

## ABOUT THE TYPE

This book was set in Cochin, a typeface named for Charles Nicolas Cochin the younger, an eighteenth-century French engraver. Henry Johnson first arranged for the cutting of the Cochin type in the United States to be used in *Harper's Bazaar*.

Cochin type is a commendable effort to reproduce the work of the French copperplate engravers of the eighteenth century. Cochin is a versatile and attractive face.

# ALSO BY QUEEN AFUA

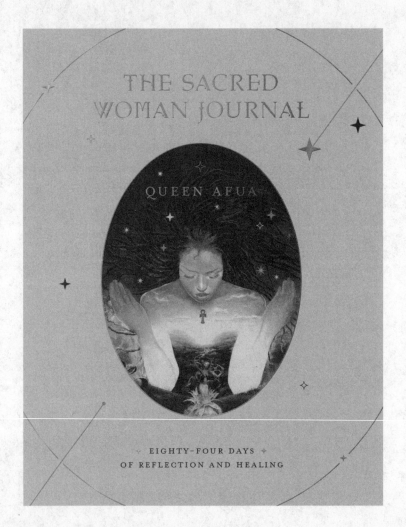

A beautifully formatted, interactive companion
to Queen Afua's *Sacred Woman*, offering readers
a journaling space and a blueprint for healing with daily
mantras, checklists, meditations, and prayers